Current Progress in Gastroenterology Research

Current Progress in Gastroenterology Research

Editor: Phillip Lawson

AMERICAN
MEDICAL PUBLISHERS
www.americanmedicalpublishers.com

AMERICAN
MEDICAL PUBLISHERS
www.americanmedicalpublishers.com

Cataloging-in-Publication Data

Current progress in gastroenterology research / edited by Phillip Lawson.
p. cm.
Includes bibliographical references and index.
ISBN 979-8-88740-035-8
1. Gastroenterology. 2. Gastroenterology--Research. 3. Digestive organs--Diseases.
4. Gastrointestinal system. 5. Gastrointestinal system--Diseases. 6. Internal medicine.
I. Lawson, Phillip.
RC801 .C87 2023
616.33--dc23

American Medical Publishers,
41 Flatbush Avenue,
1st Floor, New York,
NY 11217, USA

ISBN 979-8-88740-035-8 (Hardback)

Contents

Preface

Gastroenterology is the branch of medicine which deals with the digestive system and its disorders. The focus of this speciality is the diseases that affect the gastrointestinal tract, which includes the organs from mouth to anus as well as alimentary canal. The common diseases that are handled under this medical speciality include colorectal cancer, gastroesophageal reflux disease (GERD), malignant tumours, gastric and duodenal ulcers, inflammatory bowel diseases, and rectal disorders. There are several diagnostic and therapeutic procedures performed under this field, such as endoscopic retrograde cholangiopancreatography (ERCP), liver biopsy, colonoscopy, esophagogastroduodenoscopy (EGD) and endoscopic ultrasound (EUS). Advanced endoscopy which is a sub-specialty of gastroenterology, focuses on advanced endoscopic techniques for treating gastrointestinal, pancreatic and hepatobiliary diseases. This book explores all the important aspects of gastroenterology in the modern day. The topics included herein are of utmost significance and bound to provide incredible insights to readers. The extensive content of this book provides the readers with a thorough understanding of the progress in research within this discipline.

This book has been the outcome of endless efforts put in by authors and researchers on various issues and topics within the field. The book is a comprehensive collection of significant researches that are addressed in a variety of chapters. It will surely enhance the knowledge of the field among readers across the globe.

It gives us an immense pleasure to thank our researchers and authors for their efforts to submit their piece of writing before the deadlines. Finally in the end, I would like to thank my family and colleagues who have been a great source of inspiration and support.

Editor

1

Model Based Targeting of IL-6-Induced Inflammatory Responses in Cultured Primary Hepatocytes to Improve Application of the JAK Inhibitor Ruxolitinib

Svantje Sobotta [1†], Andreas Raue [2†], Xiaoyun Huang [1†], Joep Vanlier [3,4], Anja Jünger [1], Sebastian Bohl [1], Ute Albrecht [5], Maximilian J. Hahnel [5], Stephanie Wolf [5], Nikola S. Mueller [6], Lorenza A. D'Alessandro [1], Stephanie Mueller-Bohl [1], Martin E. Boehm [1], Philippe Lucarelli [1], Sandra Bonefas [1], Georg Damm [7], Daniel Seehofer [7], Wolf D. Lehmann [1], Stefan Rose-John [8], Frank van der Hoeven [9], Norbert Gretz [10], Fabian J. Theis [6,11], Christian Ehlting [5], Johannes G. Bode [5], Jens Timmer [3,4†], Marcel Schilling [1*†] and Ursula Klingmüller [1*†]*

[1] Division Systems Biology of Signal Transduction, German Cancer Research Center, Heidelberg, Germany, [2] Discovery Division, Merrimack Pharmaceuticals, Cambridge, MA, United States, [3] Institute of Physics, Albert Ludwigs University of Freiburg, Freiburg, Germany, [4] BIOSS Centre for Biological Signalling Studies, Albert Ludwigs University of Freiburg, Freiburg, Germany, [5] Clinic of Gastroenterology, Hepatology and Infectious Diseases, University Hospital, Heinrich Heine University of Düsseldorf, Düsseldorf, Germany, [6] Institute of Computational Biology, Helmholtz Zentrum München, Neuherberg, Germany, [7] Department of Hepatobiliary Surgery and Visceral Transplantation, Leipzig University, Leipzig, Germany, [8] Institute of Biochemistry, University of Kiel, Kiel, Germany, [9] Transgenic Service, Center for Preclinical Research, German Cancer Research Center, Heidelberg, Germany, [10] Medical Research Center, Medical Faculty Mannheim, University of Heidelberg, Mannheim, Germany, [11] Department of Mathematics, Technical University of Munich, Garching, Germany

***Correspondence:**
Jens Timmer
jeti@fdm.uni-freiburg.de
Marcel Schilling
m.schilling@dkfz.de
Ursula Klingmüller
u.klingmueller@dkfz.de

† These authors have contributed equally to this work.

IL-6 is a central mediator of the immediate induction of hepatic acute phase proteins (APP) in the liver during infection and after injury, but increased IL-6 activity has been associated with multiple pathological conditions. In hepatocytes, IL-6 activates JAK1-STAT3 signaling that induces the negative feedback regulator SOCS3 and expression of APPs. While different inhibitors of IL-6-induced JAK1-STAT3-signaling have been developed, understanding their precise impact on signaling dynamics requires a systems biology approach. Here we present a mathematical model of IL-6-induced JAK1-STAT3 signaling that quantitatively links physiological IL-6 concentrations to the dynamics of IL-6-induced signal transduction and expression of target genes in hepatocytes. The mathematical model consists of coupled ordinary differential equations (ODE) and the model parameters were estimated by a maximum likelihood approach, whereas identifiability of the dynamic model parameters was ensured by the Profile Likelihood. Using model simulations coupled with experimental validation we could optimize the long-term impact of the JAK-inhibitor Ruxolitinib, a therapeutic compound that is quickly metabolized. Model-predicted doses and timing of treatments helps to improve the reduction of inflammatory APP gene expression in primary mouse hepatocytes close to levels observed during regenerative conditions. The concept of improved efficacy of the inhibitor through multiple treatments at optimized time intervals was confirmed in primary human hepatocytes. Thus, combining quantitative data generation with mathematical modeling suggests that repetitive treatment with Ruxolitinib is required to effectively target excessive inflammatory responses without exceeding doses recommended by the clinical guidelines.

Keywords: IL-6, mathematical modeling, acute phase response, ruxolitinib, primary hepatocytes

INTRODUCTION

Increased activity of interleukin (IL)-6 has been associated with chronic inflammatory diseases including rheumatoid arthritis (Hirano et al., 1988), multiple sclerosis (Frei et al., 1991; Navikas et al., 1996), and Crohn's disease (Ito, 2003). High IL-6 levels are also frequently found and correlate with poor outcome in patients with sepsis, an acute systemic inflammatory response (Waage et al., 1989; Calandra et al., 1991; Damas et al., 1992; Norrby-Teglund et al., 1995). Accordingly, abrogation of glycoprotein 130 (gp130)-dependent signaling in hepatocytes was shown to prolong survival and to reduce liver damage in an *in vivo* sepsis model (Klein et al., 2007). Persistent inflammation can initiate or promote (Grivennikov and Karin, 2011) malignant progression and a pro-tumorigenic role of IL-6, which is elevated in many types of cancer, has been suggested (Heikkila et al., 2008). Thus, increased IL-6 levels can have detrimental effects. On the other hand, a certain amount of IL-6 is required for efficient immune defense (Kopf et al., 1994) and liver regeneration (Cressman et al., 1996; Sakamoto et al., 1999; Zimmers et al., 2003). Central target cells of IL-6 are hepatocytes, where IL-6 regulates the production of acute phase proteins (APPs) by first activating the IL-6 receptor complex with the signal-transducing subunit gp130. Signals are further transduced via janus kinase 1 (JAK1) and signal transducer and activator of transcription 3 (STAT3; Bode and Heinrich, 2001).

However, other cytokines such as Oncostatin-M (OSM), IL-11, IL-10, and IL-22, also induce STAT3 phosphorylation (see Nakamura et al., 2004; Sabat et al., 2010; Nishina et al., 2012; Rao et al., 2014) and therefore could contribute to the complex regenerative and inflammatory signaling in the liver. OSM is also able to induce IL-6 expression and therefore additionally feeds into JAK1/STAT3 signaling. However, OSM is primarily involved in developmental processes (Nakamura et al., 2004) and presumably only contributes to a lesser extent to the immediate activation of the acute phase response upon liver damage. IL-11 was shown to be mainly involved in hepatocellular responses upon oxidative stress and hepatotoxic drugs (Nishina et al., 2012). The anti-inflammatory cytokine IL-10 is an essential factor controlling inflammation (Murray, 2006). After partial hepatectomy Yin et al. observed after 1 h an increase in *Il10* mRNA expression, but the concentration of IL-10 protein was not examined (Yin et al., 2011). Distinct from IL-6, IL-10 apparently does not induce the expression of suppressor of cytokine signaling 3 (SOCS3), (Ichikawa et al., 2002) and in mice lacking a functional *Socs3* gene in macrophages or neutrophils no obvious alteration in IL-10 signal transduction is observed (Yasukawa et al., 2003). For IL-22 Rao et al. observed in hepatectomized mice in comparison to sham operated mice an increase of *Il22* mRNA after 1 h and a further increase after 3 h, whereas *Il6* mRNA was already maximally induced after 1 h (Rao et al., 2014). On the other hand Ren et al. did not detect a statistically significant increase of *Il22* mRNA in mice in response to hepatectomy, but rather reported a statistically significant increase of IL-22 protein in the serum starting at 6 h post hepatectomy with a peak at 12 h (Ren et al., 2010). Further, in response to LPS injection a very low level of induction of *Il22* mRNA was observed in the liver with a peak at 4 h post injection, whereas a much stronger activation of *Il22* mRNA with comparable kinetics was observed in the spleen (Wegenka et al., 2007). Likewise, Dumoutier et al. reported that IL-22 is primarily produced by innate spleen cells in mice. These studies showed a peak of *Il22* mRNA in the serum after 2–3 h post LPS injection and elevated serum levels of IL-22 at 4 h post treatment (Dumoutier et al., 2011). Analysis of IL-22 knockout mice revealed that in the absence of IL-22 hepatocellular proliferation at 48 h post hepatectomy is reduced (Kudira et al., 2016). Further, 6 h post LPS injection a very heterogeneous decrease in STAT3 phosphorylation is observed in IL-22 knockout mice compared to wild type mice (Wallace and Subramaniam, 2015) and the authors concluded that the IL-22 knockout mice display appropriate inflammatory responses to LPS in the liver. Together these studies suggest that IL-22 is a mediator of the cross-talk between immune cells and hepatocytes and contributes to efficient liver regeneration but potentially distinct from IL-6 primarily contributes to long-term recovery.

IL-6/STAT3-dependent target genes encode the APPs fibrinogen-γ (*Fgg*), serum amyloid P (*Apcs*), haptoglobin (*Hp*), hemopexin (*Hpx*; Alonzi et al., 2001), hepcidin (*Hamp*; Wrighting and Andrews, 2006; Pietrangelo et al., 2007), as well as *Socs3*, the negative feedback regulator of IL-6 signaling (Starr et al., 1997; Croker et al., 2003). Although, APPs fulfill beneficial roles in host defense and tissue repair (Bode et al., 2012), several adverse effects have been reported for different APPs. Hepcidin, for instance, a crucial regulator of iron homeostasis (Sakamori et al., 2010; Ganz and Nemeth, 2012), contributes to the development of anemia under inflammatory conditions (Weinstein et al., 2002; Kemna et al., 2005). Elevated expression of fibrinogen was related to formation and progression of atherosclerotic plaques (Levenson et al., 1995) and serum amyloid P, the major APP in mice, was suggested to contribute to the persistence of amyloid deposits (Tennent et al., 1995). Dysregulated APP production may thus foster pathologic changes during uncontrolled inflammatory responses.

Triggered by its involvement in several pathologies, therapeutic targeting of IL-6 signaling is a focus of ongoing

RESULTS

Physiological IL-6 Concentrations during Liver Regeneration and Inflammation

A broad range of circulating IL-6 concentrations has been reported during liver regeneration (Slotwinski et al., 2002; Nechemia-Arbely et al., 2011; Yin et al., 2011) and inflammation (Waage et al., 1989; Damas et al., 1992; Piao et al., 2013), but a direct comparison of regenerative and inflammatory conditions has not been performed yet. To provide a basis for our *ex vivo* experiments and to enable model predictions of physiological relevance, we determined physiological IL-6 concentrations in mice following partial hepatectomy (PHx; Mitchell and Willenbring, 2008) and lipopolysaccharide (LPS) injection (Fattori et al., 1994; Copeland et al., 2005), which trigger liver regeneration and acute inflammation, respectively. Serum IL-6 levels were measured using a bead-based immunoassay. We observed rapid but transient induction of serum IL-6 in response to PHx and LPS treatment (**Figure 1A**). Peak IL-6 levels were detected 2 h post PHx with 1.4 ng/mL (±0.3 ng/mL *SD*; $n = 3$). Similarly, IL-6 amounts in response to LPS injection peaked at 2 h, but reached considerably higher concentrations of 201.8 ng/mL (±77.8 ng/mL *SD*; $n = 5$). Following the peak, IL-6 levels dropped quickly and returned to baseline levels at 8–24 h. For comparison, sham surgery and NaCl injection as control treatments for PHx and LPS, respectively, caused serum IL-6 levels to increase only slightly. Less than 0.4 ng/mL IL-6 after sham surgery and <0.1 ng/mL IL-6 after NaCl injection were measured. The background IL-6 concentration in untreated mice was <10 pg/mL, which corresponds to previously reported values (Huang et al., 2003). To conclude, IL-6 levels in response to PHx and LPS treatment increased in a fast but transient manner. Similar dynamics were observed for PHx and LPS treatment. However, LPS caused 100-fold higher peak IL-6 levels, compared to PHx.

In addition to serum IL-6 levels, we developed a strategy to determine the IL-6 concentrations present in the hepatocytes' microenvironment. We analyzed STAT3 activation (Tyr-705 phosphorylation) as read-out in livers from PHx and LPS-treated mice. Phospho-STAT3 levels were measured using multiplexed bead-based arrays (**Figure 1B**), revealing rapid and transient induction of STAT3 activation after PHx and LPS treatment. Peak levels were reached at 2 h following PHx and even earlier, after 1 h following LPS injection. Thus, the conversion of IL-6 signal to STAT3 activation is very efficient. The amplitude of STAT3 activation after LPS treatment was more than twice as high as in the case of PHx. After peaking, the phospho-STAT3 signal decreased likewise in PHx and LPS treated livers, and returned to levels close to baseline at 24 h. STAT3 activation was also detectable in animals treated with sham surgery, which has been reported previously (Cressman et al., 1996; Heim et al., 1997), and which is likely due to stress caused by the surgical procedure.

To compare the contribution of IL-6 and of the other STAT3 activating cytokines IL-22, OSM, or IL-11, on STAT3 phosphorylation in the liver, we performed additional time-resolved qRT-PCR measurements of liver lysates from LPS or PHx treated mice. In comparison to the induction of IL-6 protein expression (**Figure 1A**) and *Il6* gene expression (Appendix Figure S14) no major induction of OSM, IL-22, or IL-11 was elicited by partial hepatectomy or by LPS (Appendix Figure S14).

In parallel, phospho-STAT3 levels were determined in primary mouse hepatocytes stimulated with 0.1–500 ng/mL recombinant human IL-6 (hIL-6) for 20 min to capture the maximal phospho-STAT3 signal (**Figure 1C**). When the work of the presented study was initiated, recombinant murine IL-6 was not yet commercially available. Therefore, human IL-6, produced as described in Vandam et al. (1993), was utilized and was kept for the entire study to ensure consistency.

Samples from mouse livers (**Figure 1B**) and from primary mouse hepatocytes (**Figure 1C**) were analyzed simultaneously in a 96-well plate format using equal lysis conditions for direct comparability of the measured phospho-STAT3 signal. Dose-dependent STAT3 activation in primary mouse hepatocytes followed a sigmoidal behavior in response to IL-6. It was detectable from 2.5 ng/mL hIL-6 on, then steeply increased and quickly reached saturation at 25–50 ng/mL (**Figure 1C**). Approximation of the IL-6/phospho-STAT3 dose-response curve from primary mouse hepatocytes by a 4-parameter Hill regression function enabled to correlate phospho-STAT3 signal intensities in livers from PHx or LPS-treated mice to IL-6 concentrations that elicited the observed STAT3 response. The peak phospho-STAT3 signal (average ± SEM of 2 and 3 h time points) after PHx approximately corresponded to an IL-6 concentration equivalent to 6.8–7.9 ng/mL hIL-6. In the case of LPS, the peak phospho-STAT3 signal (average ± SEM of 1 and 2 h time points) approximately corresponded to a signal obtained with 28.1–500 ng/mL hIL-6. The STAT3 signal detected after NaCl injection was out of range of our reference curve and corresponded to <0.1 ng/mL hIL-6 (**Figure 1C**).

To convert the responses elicited by hIL-6 to the concentrations relevant in the mouse, we performed dose response experiments comparing the potency of increasing doses of human and murine IL-6 in stimulating STAT3 phosphorylation in primary mouse hepatocytes. As shown in **Figure 1D**, this revealed that murine IL-6 is more potent to elicit STAT3 phosphorylation in murine hepatocytes compared to hIL-6 with an overall shift of the dose-response curve to lower IL-6 concentrations. Collectively, STAT3 was activated rapidly, efficiently and transiently in mouse livers after PHx and LPS treatment. In line with IL-6 serum concentrations (**Figure 1A**), peak phospho-STAT3 signals corresponded to human IL-6 concentration ranges for PHx (6.8–7.9 ng/mL; average: 7.4 ng/mL) and LPS (28.1–500 ng/mL; average: 264.1 ng/mL). This corresponds to a mouse IL-6 concentration of 1.8 and 50 ng/mL, respectively (**Figure 1D**).

Time-Resolved Characterization of Key IL-6 Target Genes

To investigate the APP gene signature induced by hIL-6 in primary mouse hepatocytes, and to establish the time-dependent

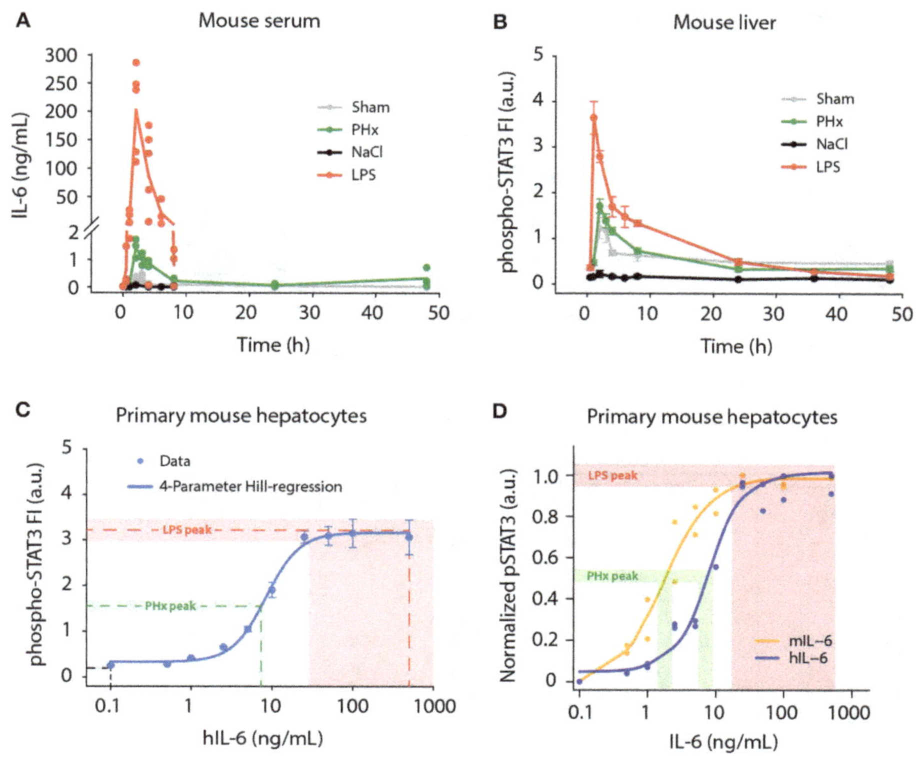

FIGURE 1 | Physiological IL-6 concentrations during liver regeneration and inflammation. Mice were subjected to control (Sham) surgery or partial hepatectomy (PHx), and control (NaCl) or lipopolysaccharide (LPS, 1 μg/g body weight) treatment. Serum and livers were collected at indicated time points. **(A)** Absolute serum IL-6 levels were measured by a bead-based immunoassay. Filled circles represent data from individual mice, solid lines connect average values of biological replicates. Sham, PHx, and LPS-treatment: $n = 3$–6 per time point; NaCl: $n = 1$ per time point. **(B)** STAT3 phosphorylation at Tyr-705 was quantified by multiplexed bead-based arrays in lysates of frozen mouse liver samples. Per time point or IL-6 dose, 3–6 biological replicates were measured and scaled by normalizing to their average signal. Filled circles represent average ±standard error of the mean (SEM) of biological replicates; solid lines are shown for visual guidance in the mouse liver data set. **(C)** Primary mouse hepatocytes were stimulated with 0.1–500 ng/mL of recombinant human IL-6, and lysed after 20 min. The 4-parameter Hill regression function **(C)** was generated using SigmaPlot software, and served to convert phospho-STAT3 signals to IL-6 concentrations. Dashed lines represent average phospho-STAT3 signals of the 1 and 2 h time points (NaCl, LPS), or 2 and 3 h time points (PHx), and corresponding derived IL-6 concentrations. Shaded areas represent standard error of the mean. **(D)** Primary mouse hepatocytes were stimulated with mouse IL-6 or human IL-6 to derive the doses of human IL-6 mimicking regenerative and inflammatory conditions, indicating that 1.8 ng of mouse IL-6 is equally potent to 7.5 ng of human IL-6 on mouse hepatocytes. FI, fluorescence intensity; a.u., arbitrary units.

regulation of respective genes, we performed microarray analysis of primary mouse hepatocytes stimulated with hIL-6 (40 ng/mL) for up to 32 h. Global analysis of the genome-wide transcriptome profiling was performed using principal component (PC) analysis (PCA). In the two most relevant PCs the samples were separated by time and by condition (control vs. hIL-6) and biological duplicates were clustered (**Figure 2A**) indicating high reproducibility. The individual contributions of genes to the two PCs are shown in the respective rotation space for PC1/2 (**Figure 2B**). We found well-established IL-6 targets, such as *Socs3* and the APP genes *Apcs*, *Fgg*, and *Hamp* to be major contributors to both, stimulus-specific and time-dependent, regulation (**Figure 2B**).

Differential gene expression analysis of the microarray data set was performed using a linear regression model with gene-wise Bayesian variance estimation (Ritchie et al., 2015). We classified the IL-6-regulated genes as early (0.5–2 h), intermediate (4–16 h), and late (24–32 h) response genes to establish optimized time frames for the measurements (**Figure 2C**). In total 1,728 genes were significantly regulated upon hIL-6 stimulation (Appendix Figure S1A), while 723, 779, and 694 genes were IL-6-regulated at early, intermediate, and late time points, respectively. Intermediate and late IL-6-response genes showed more than 40% overlap. Enrichment analysis of respective gene lists showed that the late IL-6 response was enriched for genes relevant in the acute phase response (Appendix Figure S1B). Significantly regulated genes included *Socs3*, which was induced at early, intermediate, and late time points. Another early-induced gene was *Cxcl10*. We found the APP genes *Fgg*, *Hamp*, and *Il33* to be induced at intermediate and late time points, whereas compared with control *Apcs* was increased only at late time points. Interestingly, the gene encoding the C reactive protein (CRP), displayed a similar expression pattern as *Apcs*. Hierarchical clustering of significantly regulated genes and further APP genes of interest (Heinrich et al., 1990) revealed that especially late APP

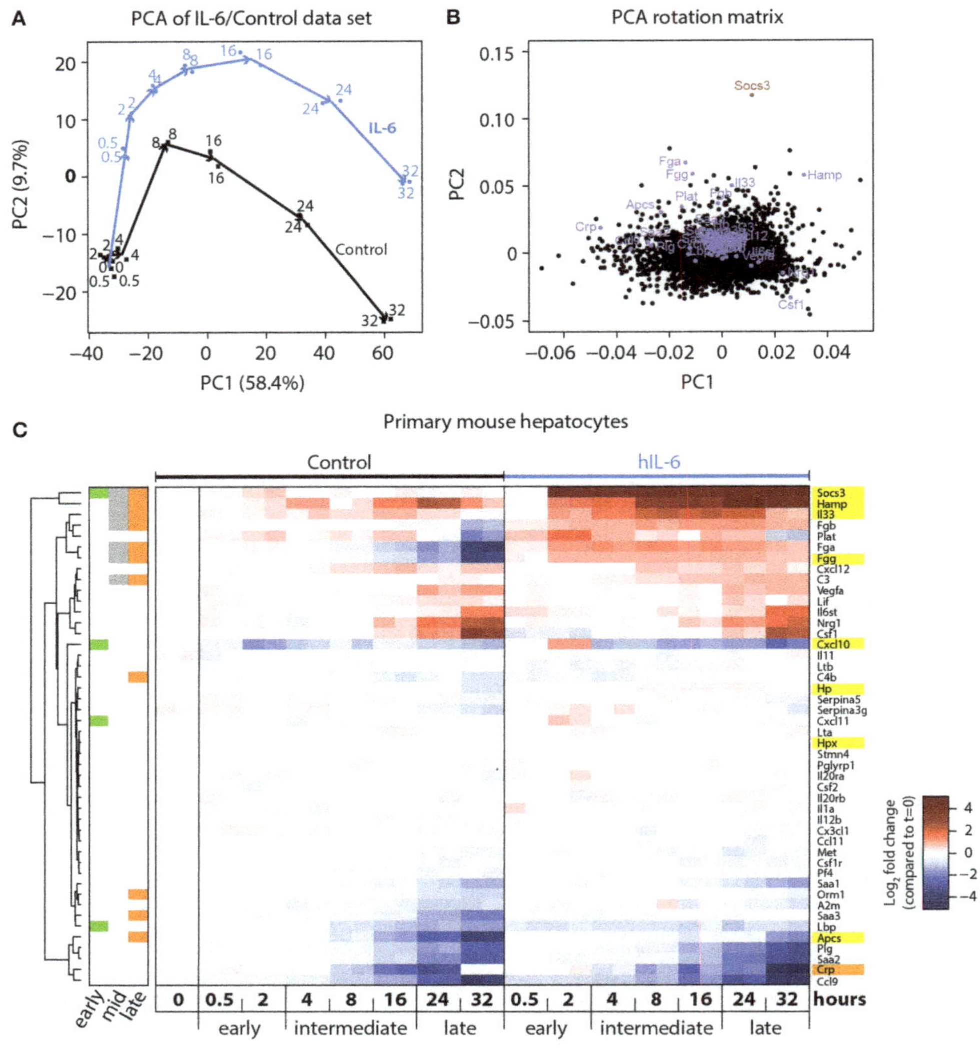

FIGURE 2 | Genome-wide analysis of IL-6-induced transcriptional responses. **(A)** Primary mouse hepatocytes were stimulated with 40 ng/mL hIL-6 or left untreated (Control), and RNA was isolated at indicated time points. Transcriptome profiling was performed using GeneChip Mouse Genome 430 2.0 Arrays (Affymetrix). Samples were projected onto the first two principal components (PC) of the data set, and values in PC1/2 are plotted. Arrows connect subsequent time points for Control and IL-6 condition, and are shown for visual guidance. **(B)** Contributions of individual genes to the respective PCs are shown. Genes of interest are labeled and highlighted in blue (APP), or dark red (*Socs3*). **(C)** Hierarchical clustering of expression patterns of APP genes of interest. Expression values are centered to mean expression of $t = 0$ Control samples. Sidebar color-codes whether genes were significantly regulated at early, intermediate, or late time points. APPs that are most relevant in the murine context are highlighted in yellow. CRP, an important APP in the human context, is highlighted in orange.

genes clustered and were mostly induced upon hIL-6 treatment (**Figure 2C**).

Taken together, we present a comprehensive list of IL-6 target genes that are expressed in response to hIL-6 stimulation in primary mouse hepatocytes. Of these we obtained detailed time-resolved expression profiles of previously known (*Apcs, Fgg, Hamp, Hp, Hpx, Socs3*) and less well-established (*Cxcl10, Il33*) IL-6 target genes. These selected genes served as read-out for the IL-6-induced hepatic acute phase response in the following experiments, and the recorded temporal dynamics enabled the choice of optimal time points for dose-dependent analysis.

Dynamic Mathematical Model of IL-6 Signaling Capturing Inhibitor Effects

To link the observed physiological IL-6 concentrations to activation of signal transduction and induction of target genes and to quantitatively predict the impact of the pathway inhibitors Ruxolitinib and Stattic, we generated a mathematical model of IL-6-induced JAK1-STAT3 signaling in primary mouse hepatocytes (**Figure 3A**). Assuming the law of mass-action kinetics, we translated the previously established molecular interactions (Heinrich et al., 2003) in response to IL-6 into a set of ODEs. Two compartments were modeled to describe the shuttling of STAT3

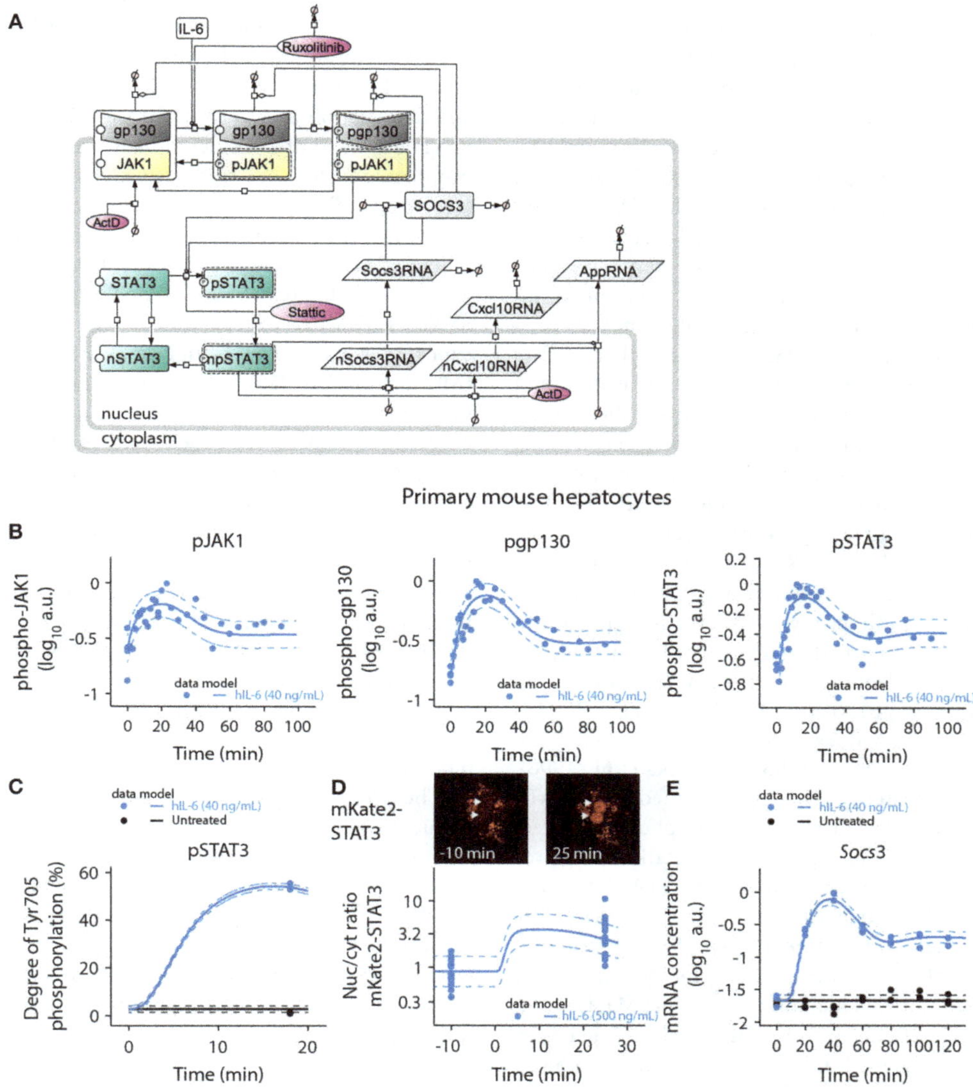

FIGURE 3 | Mathematical model of IL-6-induced JAK1-STAT3 signaling and model calibration with time-resolved signaling data. **(A)** The ODE-based model is represented as process diagram (Kitano et al., 2005). Individual reactions of species (arrows) can be induced (circle-headed lines) or inhibited (bar-headed lines). Dashed line borders highlight active species. AppRNA is representative for the different intermediate/late APP mRNAs *Fgg*, *Hamp*, *Il33*, *Apcs*, *Hp*, and *Hpx*. The production of cytoplasmic *Socs3* and *APP* mRNAs was modeled using a delay (τ), corresponding to five additional processing steps of intermediate nuclear RNA species. Inhibitors are shown in red color. ActD, actinomycin D; Prefix p, phosphorylated species; Prefix n, nuclear species. **(B)** Primary mouse hepatocytes were treated with 40 ng/mL of hIL-6 and lysed for protein or RNA isolation at indicated time points. Phosphorylated JAK1, gp130, and STAT3 were measured using quantitative immunoblotting preceded by immunoprecipitation to enrich for the target proteins. Recombinant calibrator proteins were used for normalization. **(C)** Primary mouse hepatocytes were treated with 40 ng/mL of hIL-6 for 18 min, lysed and subject to immunoprecipitation. Enriched proteins were separated by SDS-PAGE, in-gel digested, and analyzed by mass spectrometry to determine the degree of Tyr-705 phosphorylation of STAT3. **(D)** Example widefield fluorescent microscopic images of primary hepatocytes from mKate2-STAT3 mice unstimulated (left panel) or stimulated with 500 ng/mL hIL-6 for 25 min (right panel). White arrows indicate positions of nuclei. The ratio of nuclear to cytoplasmic mKate2-STAT3 was determined by live-cell imaging in 20 hepatocytes isolated from mKate2-STAT3 heterozygous mice 10 min prior to and 25 min after stimulation with hIL-6 (500 ng/mL). **(E)** Primary mouse hepatocytes were treated with 40 ng/mL of hIL-6 and lysed for RNA isolation at indicated time points. *Socs3* mRNA was quantified by qRT-PCR ($n = 3$). Filled circles: experimental data; solid lines: model trajectories. Dashed lines indicate the measurement noise as estimated by the error model. a.u., arbitrary units. For additional experimental data used for model calibration see Appendix Figures S26–S81. In total, the model was calibrated with 3090 data points.

between cytoplasm and nucleus, as well as the nuclear export of newly synthesized mRNAs. The model contained four input variables: IL-6, Ruxolitinib, Stattic, and actinomycin D (ActD). Based on immunoassays of human IL-6 in mouse hepatocyte supernatants (Appendix Figure S2), constant IL-6 concentrations and complete removal of ligand after stimulation pulses were assumed. Because Ruxolitinib was reported to have a plasma half-life of ~3 h in humans (Shi et al., 2011), Ruxolitinib degradation was included in the model. Considering that inhibition by Stattic is irreversible, its concentrations were modeled as constant. The temporal evolution of the dynamic variables was described by 25 ODEs, the detailed steps were as follows (**Figure 3A**): gp130 and JAK1 were described to be pre-associated (Behrmann et al., 2004) and were modeled as one complex JAK1_gp130 with different activation states, as described previously for the interaction of JAK2 with the erythropoietin receptor (Bachmann et al., 2011). The alpha receptor subunit IL-6R was not considered in the model, because it is not directly involved in the dynamic phosphorylation events that initiate IL-6 signaling (Taga et al., 1989). IL-6 promotes activation and phosphorylation of JAK1, causing generation of the species pJAK1_gp130. Additionally, there is also a low level of basal activation. Subsequently, also gp130 is phosphorylated by JAK1 to create the fully activated receptor complex pJAK1_pgp130. Stimulus-independent negative regulatory mechanisms at the receptor level, as reported for JAK1 (Simoncic et al., 2002; Lehmann et al., 2003), were taken into account by including two deactivating steps. Both partly active pJAK1_gp130 and fully active pJAK1_pgp130 are directly converted to inactive JAK1_gp130. This simplification is based on the assumption that dephosphorylation of gp130 and JAK1 is coupled. STAT3 is activated by JAK1 only after docking to phosphorylated gp130 (Lutticken et al., 1994; Stahl et al., 1995; Yamanaka et al., 1996). Thus, double-phosphorylated pJAK1_pgp130 mediates STAT3 activation. The species pSTAT3 represents phosphorylated, active, and dimeric STAT3. A separate dimerization step was neglected, because the oligomerization state of STAT3 was not assessed by experiments. Active, dimeric pSTAT3 subsequently translocates to the nuclear compartment, and npSTAT3 promotes transcription of *Socs3* and APP genes. The generation of cytoplasmic RNA was modeled including a delay (τ; MacDonald, 1976; Bachmann et al., 2011) for both *Socs3* and APP genes to account for processing and nuclear export of these early-induced transcripts. Based on repeated profile likelihood analysis, we concluded that *Socs3*, *Cxcl10*, *Fgg*, *Il33*, *Hp*, and *Hpx* required an explicit delay in the model to describe the available data, while *Apcs* and *Hamp* did not. *Socs3* was expressed earlier than any of the APP genes. For the APP genes, *Cxcl10* had the shortest delay, followed by *Fgg*. The other APP genes exhibited slower dynamics (see Appendix Figure S24). Cytoplasmic Socs3RNA promotes synthesis of SOCS3. SOCS3 inhibits the signaling pathway by increasing degradation of the receptor complex as well as inhibiting phosphorylation of STAT3 by the fully activated receptor complex (Starr et al., 1997; Babon et al., 2012; Kershaw et al., 2013). Therefore, SOCS3 enhances degradation of all receptor states and inhibits the STAT3-activating reaction converting STAT3 to pSTAT3. Production of APP proteins was not assessed experimentally and was thus not considered in the model. The target RNA and protein species Socs3RNA, SOCS3, and Cxcl10/AppRNA are furthermore subject to degradation.

Deactivation of nuclear STAT3 was suggested to be mediated by phosphatases (Yamamoto et al., 2002). A combined dephosphorylation and dissociation step was therefore modeled in the nuclear compartment, converting dimeric, active npSTAT3 to monomeric, inactive nSTAT3. Based on model identifiability analysis, it was concluded that dephosphorylation and dissociation of STAT3 in the nucleus is very fast. Therefore, npSTAT3 was not considered as a state variable, but modeled proportional to the cytoplasmic concentration of pSTAT3 (see Appendix for more information). STAT3 was shown to continuously shuttle between cytoplasm and nucleus independent of its activation state (Liu et al., 2005; Reich and Liu, 2006). Accordingly, we allowed nuclear import for both, inactive STAT3 and active pSTAT3, while only inactive nSTAT3 can be exported back to the cytoplasm. The previously determined (Mueller et al., 2015) ratio of cytoplasmic to nuclear volume of primary mouse hepatocytes (12.67/0.5 pL, for frequently binucleated hepatocytes) facilitated modeling of concentration changes due to inter-compartmental transport processes.

The pathway inhibitors Ruxolitinib and Stattic were incorporated into the model according to their published molecular modes of action. The JAK inhibitor Ruxolitinib (Lin et al., 2009; Quintas-Cardama et al., 2010) negatively influences JAK1-dependent reactions in the model, specifically the generation of pJAK1_gp130 and pJAK1_pgp130. Stattic blocks activation and dimerization of STAT3 (Schust et al., 2006) and therefore in our model inhibits the respective conversion of STAT3 to pSTAT3. All transcriptional processes are furthermore blocked by ActD.

The protein abundances of the pathway components gp130, JAK1, STAT3, and SOCS3 were determined by quantitative immunoblotting (Schilling et al., 2005a) according to standard curves of recombinant calibrator proteins. The determined number of molecules per cell (Appendix Figure S3) provided the absolute scale for model predictions of those specific states. Remaining unknown model parameters were estimated based on time- and dose-dependent experimental data, as described in the following sections.

Model Calibration with Time-Resolved Signaling and Gene Expression Data

The mathematical model depicted in **Figure 3A** was calibrated with quantitative experimental data describing the time-resolved dynamics of IL-6-induced JAK1-STAT3 signaling in primary mouse hepatocytes. Cells were treated with hIL-6 for up to 120 min in a continuous or pulsed manner. The levels of phosphorylated and total protein species were measured by quantitative immunoblotting (Schilling et al., 2005a), including randomized sample loading and normalization to suitable housekeeping proteins or, in case proteins were enriched by immunoprecipitation, to recombinant calibrator proteins. hIL-6-induced phosphorylation of gp130, JAK1, and STAT3 was transient displaying a peak at around 20 min. Phospho-gp130, -JAK1, and -STAT3 subsequently declined, but did not reach basal levels within the observed time frame (**Figure 3B**). Further, SOCS3 protein expression was determined upon treatment with different concentrations of IL-6 (Appendix Figures S43–S45) and we observed a transient protein expression dynamic that resembles the mRNA expression profiles. Using quantitative mass spectrometry (Hahn et al., 2011), we determined the site-specific degree of Tyr-705 phosphorylation of STAT3 at the time point of maximal activation (54.4% at 18 min, 40 ng/mL hIL-6; **Figure 3C**). We also quantified the nuclear translocation of STAT3 by live-cell imaging of hepatocytes isolated from heterozygous mKate2-STAT3 knock-in mice (**Figure 3D** and Appendix Figure S11). In mKate2-STAT3 mice, the wild type STAT3 locus is replaced by an mKate2-STAT3 knock-in reporter gene. The expression and phosphorylation of the fusion protein was validated by immunoblotting in primary mouse hepatocytes that were isolated from the knock-in reporter mice and wild-type animals (Appendix Figure S13). Cells were treated with hIL-6 and the phosphorylation of endogenous and tagged-STAT3 was compared. These studies showed that mKate2-STAT3 is expressed at a slightly lower level than the endogenous protein but the phosphorylation dynamics correlated with the phosphorylation dynamics of the endogenous STAT3. The mKate2-STAT3 reporter mice so far have only been obtained as heterozygous mice. For the generation of the mKate2-STAT3 reporter mice we identified seven positive ES clones and out of these two generated germline transmission. The crossing of the heterozygous animals resulted in 66.8% WT and 33.2% heterozygous animals ($n = 232$) and these heterozygous mice showed no phenotype, also concerning viability in comparison to WT animals. Due to the strong autofluorescence in the cytoplasmic compartment of primary mouse hepatocytes (see dot-like structures in Appendix Figure S13C), we focused on the quantification of the IL-6-induced translocation of mKate2-STAT3 to the nucleus. In unstimulated cells, mKate2-STAT3 was equally distributed between cytoplasm and nucleus (STAT3 nuc/cyt ratio of 1), in accordance with the previously reported continuous shuttling of STAT3 independent of its activation state (Liu et al., 2005; Reich and Liu, 2006). We tested continuous shuttling of STAT3 between nucleus and cytoplasm, independent of its activation state in our initial mathematical model. However, based on identifiability analysis (see Appendix Figure S15), we found that export of phosphorylated STAT3 could be made arbitrarily small and was therefore omitted from the final model. Following hIL-6 stimulation, mKate2-STAT3 quickly accumulated in the nucleus. At 25 min (500 ng/mL hIL-6), the nuclear mKate2-STAT3 concentration exceeded cytoplasmic mKate2-STAT3 by a factor of 3 (STAT3 nuc/cyt ratio of ≈ 3; **Figure 3D**). *Socs3* mRNA was measured by qRT-PCR, revealing rapid induction after IL-6 stimulation with a peak time of 40 min. Afterwards, *Socs3* mRNA levels declined, but stayed elevated throughout the observed time frame. Background *Socs3* mRNA expression in unstimulated hepatocytes did not change over time, indicating a specific response (**Figure 3E**). The trajectories of the calibrated model accurately represented the experimental data describing multiple levels of IL-6-induced signaling (solid lines in **Figures 3B–E** and Appendix Figure S9).

To validate the microarray analysis and to obtain detailed time-resolved expression profiles, we analyzed selected significantly regulated genes by quantitative real-time quantitative PCR (qRT-PCR) in a time-resolved manner. In agreement with the microarray analysis, we found *Cxcl10* and *Socs3* to be early-response genes. *Cxcl10* was transiently induced by hIL-6. After an initial peak at 1 h *Cxcl10* expression levels decreased below those observed in untreated cells. *Socs3* expression showed a sharp peak with high amplitude at 1 h of hIL-6 treatment. Subsequently, its levels declined but stayed elevated up to 24 h. This is consistent with our microarray analysis, which identified *Socs3* to critically contribute to overall regulation (**Figure 2B**) and to be significantly IL-6-induced at all time points (**Figure 2C**). The genes *Fgg*, *Hamp*, and *Il33* were induced by IL-6 and were clearly detectable from 3 to 6 h on, as shown by qRT-PCR analysis. All three genes showed sustained activation with high expression levels up to 24 h of IL-6 treatment, thus validating our microarray analysis which identified *Fgg*, *Hamp*, and *Il33* to be significantly regulated at intermediate and late time points. *Apcs* was found to be a late-regulated gene. qPCR-based validation revealed a steady decrease of *Apcs* expression in untreated cells. IL-6 treatment rescued this decrease and caused elevated *Apcs* expression at 24 h relative to untreated cells (**Figure 4** and Appendix Figure S10). The APP genes *Hp* and *Hpx* were not significantly regulated in our microarray analysis (**Figure 2C**), but have previously been reported to be IL-6 responsive and STAT3-dependent (Alonzi et al., 2001). qPCR analysis identified *Hp* and *Hpx* to be late-response genes with increased expression at 24 and 48 h of IL-6 treatment (**Figure 4** and Appendix Figure S10).

Model Calibration with Dose-Dependent Target Gene Expression Data from Normal and Perturbed Conditions

In addition to time-resolved data, we calibrated the mathematical model with dose-dependent expression data for the IL-6 target genes shown in **Figure 5** and Appendix Figures S4, S5. Primary mouse hepatocytes were treated with a wide range of hIL-6 concentrations covering basal, regenerative, and inflammatory physiological levels (**Figure 1**) for 1, 6, or 24 h to capture strong expression of early, intermediate, and late responsive genes, respectively. Based on the experimental data, we identified the nuclear dephosphorylation rate to be high. Since nuclear STAT3 dephosphorylation is so rapid that the level of nuclear phosphorylated STAT3 exactly follows the cytoplasmic concentration of phospho-STAT3, the model was reduced by one equation.

We further identified *Socs3* mRNA to respond to IL-6 treatment in a highly sensitive manner (**Figure 5A**). The other early-induced gene *Cxcl10* responded at 25–50 ng/mL hIL-6, and did not reach saturation within the observed hIL-6 range. Compared with *Socs3*, it thus showed lower sensitivity toward hIL-6 (**Figure 5A**). In contrast, the sensitivities of intermediate and late APP genes were similar to that of *Socs3*—*Fgg*, *Hamp*, *Il33*, *Apcs*, *Hp*, and *Hpx* mRNAs were induced from 1 to 10 ng/mL hIL-6. All showed sigmoidal dose response curves and saturation at high IL-6 concentrations (100–500 ng/mL). The dose-dependent behavior of all target genes was accurately described by the model (**Figures 5A–C** and Appendix Figure S4).

We also calibrated our model with experimental data describing the impact of the two pathway inhibitors Ruxolitinib

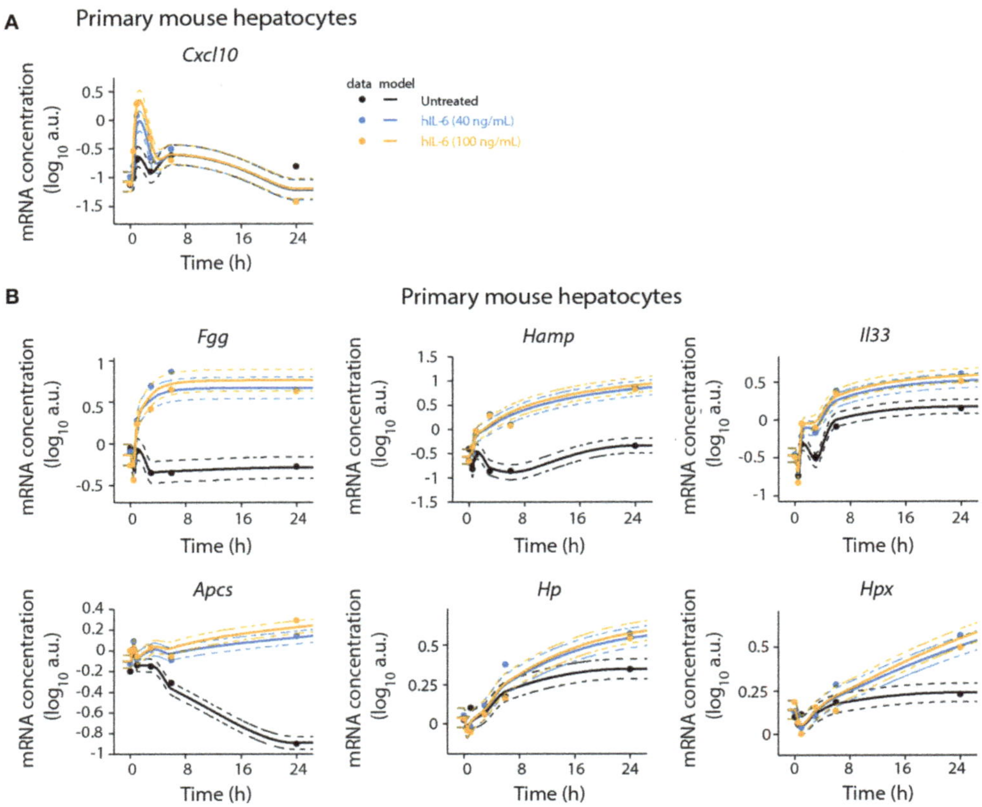

FIGURE 4 | Detailed time-resolved analysis of selected IL-6 target genes. Primary mouse hepatocytes were stimulated with hIL-6 or left untreated and RNA was isolated at indicated time points. Target mRNA expression was analyzed by qRT-PCR (qPCR) (**A** *Cxcl10*; **B** *Fgg*, *Hamp*, *Il33*, *Apcs*, *Hp*, and *Hpx*). Data were normalized to the geometric mean (Vandesompele et al., 2002) of *Hprt* and *Tbp* expression. Filled circles represent individual replicates ($n = 2$); solid lines are model fits; dashed lines indicate errors estimated from the model. The expression level in the control is modeled using a monotonic spline. Additional replicate is displayed in Appendix Figure S10.

and Stattic on dose/time-dependent *Socs3* mRNA induction and STAT3 phosphorylation dynamics in primary mouse hepatocytes (**Figure 5D**). The inhibitor Stattic shows toxic effects and is not used in the clinic. In our experiments we applied Stattic for a maximum of 2 h to primary mouse hepatocytes to avoid general toxicity. Though Stattic was used to calibrate the model, experimental results with this inhibitor are only shown in the Appendix (Appendix Figures S9, S46, S52–S53, S62–S69, S83–S84, S89).

Inhibitor pre-treatment for 1 h caused a reduced basal level of *Socs3* mRNA and a reduced sensitivity and peak magnitude of the dose-dependent *Socs3* response upon IL-6 stimulation (**Figure 5**). *Socs3* expression at 1, 6, and 24 h was detectable from 1 ng/mL hIL-6, steadily increased, and reached saturation at 50 ng/mL hIL-6. In line with the previous observation in a clinical trial (Shi et al., 2011), the efficacy of Ruxolitinib decreased with increasing incubation time. The experimental data of *Socs3* expression in response to hIL-6 alone or hIL-6 and Ruxolitinib was described by the model trajectories (**Figure 5D**).

To summarize, the model was calibrated in two stages. First the upstream model of IL-6 signaling was developed and calibrated. The upstream model also termed "core model" consists of the receptor level, the STAT3 pools and SOCS3 and is calibrated on both wild type as well as inhibitor data. The downstream model, which consists of the APP genes, was included in a second step. Since none of the APP genes feed back into the system, these were parameterized separately to keep the analyses computationally tractable. The downstream model was parameterized while keeping the upstream model parameters fixed. Parameter profile likelihood curves for all APP genes are presented in the supplement (Appendix Figures S15–S22).

Designing Improved Ruxolitinib Treatment Schedules

Following calibration with quantitative experimental data, our mathematical model was able to describe IL-6-induced signaling responses at multiple levels, including the impact of pathway inhibitors on STAT3 (Appendix Figure S9A) and *Socs3* activation (**Figure 5**). We next employed the model to predict the inhibitor impact on hIL-6 dose-dependent APP gene expression in murine hepatocytes. In analogy to the inhibition of *Socs3* mRNA induction (**Figure 5D**), the model predicted that Ruxolitinb treatment reduces sensitivity of the response for most APP genes (**Figure 6**). Importantly, subsequent experimental analysis

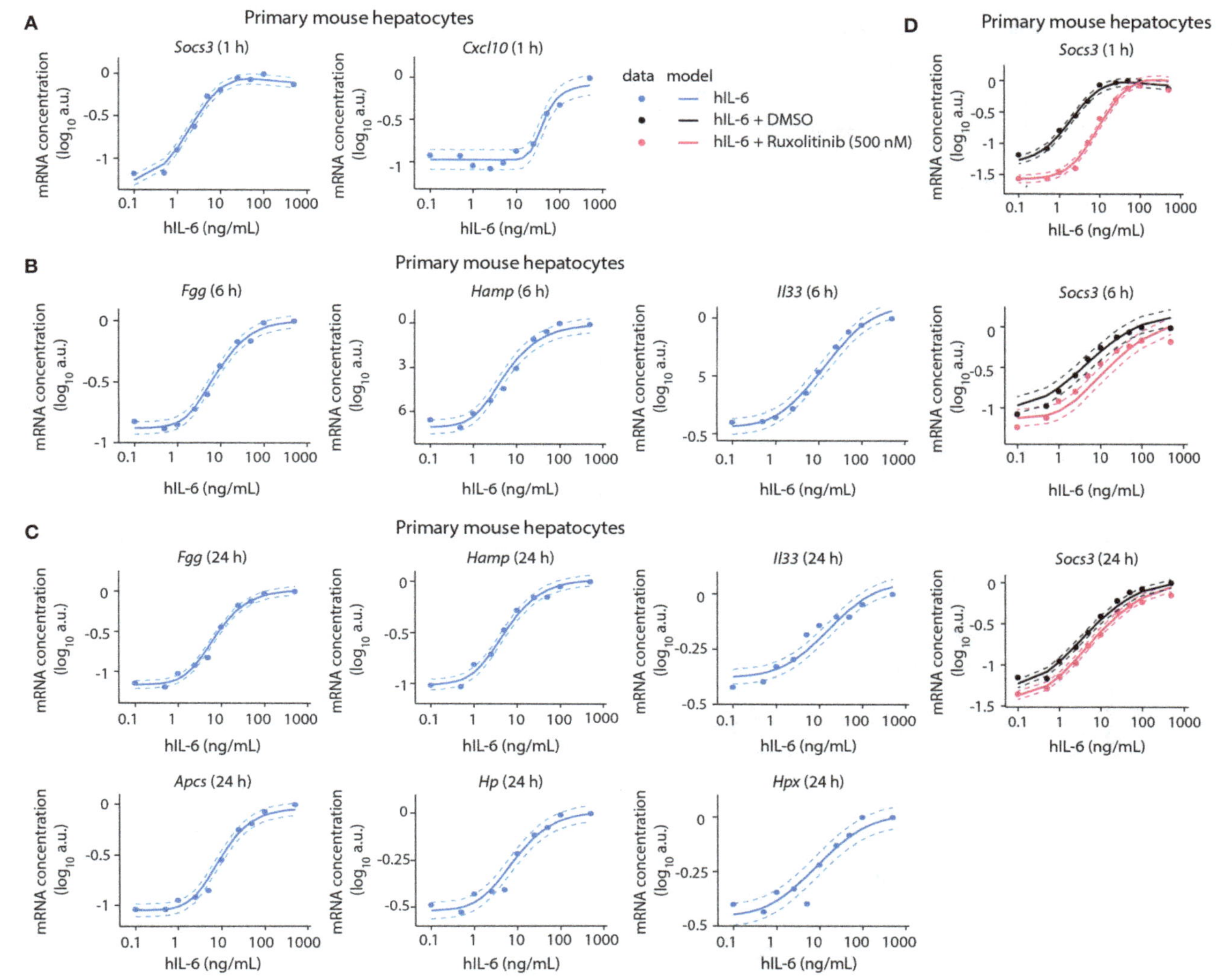

FIGURE 5 | Model calibration with dose-dependent target gene expression data from normal and perturbed conditions. Primary mouse hepatocytes were pre-treated with Ruxolitinib or DMSO control for 1 h prior to hIL-6 stimulation, or left untreated. Dose-dependent analysis of target gene expression was performed by applying 0.1–500 ng/mL hIL-6. At indicated time points (1, 6, and 24 h), target mRNAs were quantified by qPCR (**A** *Socs3* and *Cxcl10*; **B** *Fgg*, *Hamp*, and *Il33*; **C** *Fgg*, *Hamp*, *Il33*, *Apcs*, *Hp*, and *Hpx*; **D** *Socs3*). Filled circles: log-transformed experimental data; solid lines: model trajectories. Dashed lines indicate the measurement noise as estimated by the error model. a.u., arbitrary units. For additional replicates used for model calibration see Appendix Figure S4.

validated the model-predicted effects of Ruxolitinib treatment on all analyzed APP genes (**Figure 6** and Appendix Figure S5). As observed previously in the case of *Socs3* mRNA expression at 1, 6, and 24 h (**Figure 5D**), the long-term efficacy of Ruxolitinb in primary mouse hepatocytes was reduced in the case of intermediate/late APP genes (**Figures 6B,C** and Appendix Figures S5B,C).

To assess the suitability of different targets in reducing the APP response, we performed a sensitivity analysis. If one considers the APPs to be very stable, then the protein levels will approximately be proportional to the integral of the expression of the APP genes. We performed a Local Parameter Sensitivity Analysis with respect to the model parameters, which is shown in **Figure 7A**. Here we can observe that inhibiting production and activation of the receptor, inhibiting the activation of STAT3 and reducing the degradation of *Socs3* (mRNA) are all predicted to lead to additional attenuation of the APP response. To further inhibit STAT3 activation, we decided to apply additional doses of Ruxolitinib.

Continuous suppression of elevated IL-6-induced APP gene expression would be required to counteract inappropriate inflammatory responses, but Ruxolitinib-mediated reduction of hIL-6 target gene expression in murine hepatocytes was less effective at advanced time points (**Figures 5, 6**). The model predicted that higher single doses of Ruxolitinib would lead to larger suppression of the APP genes. However, since higher doses

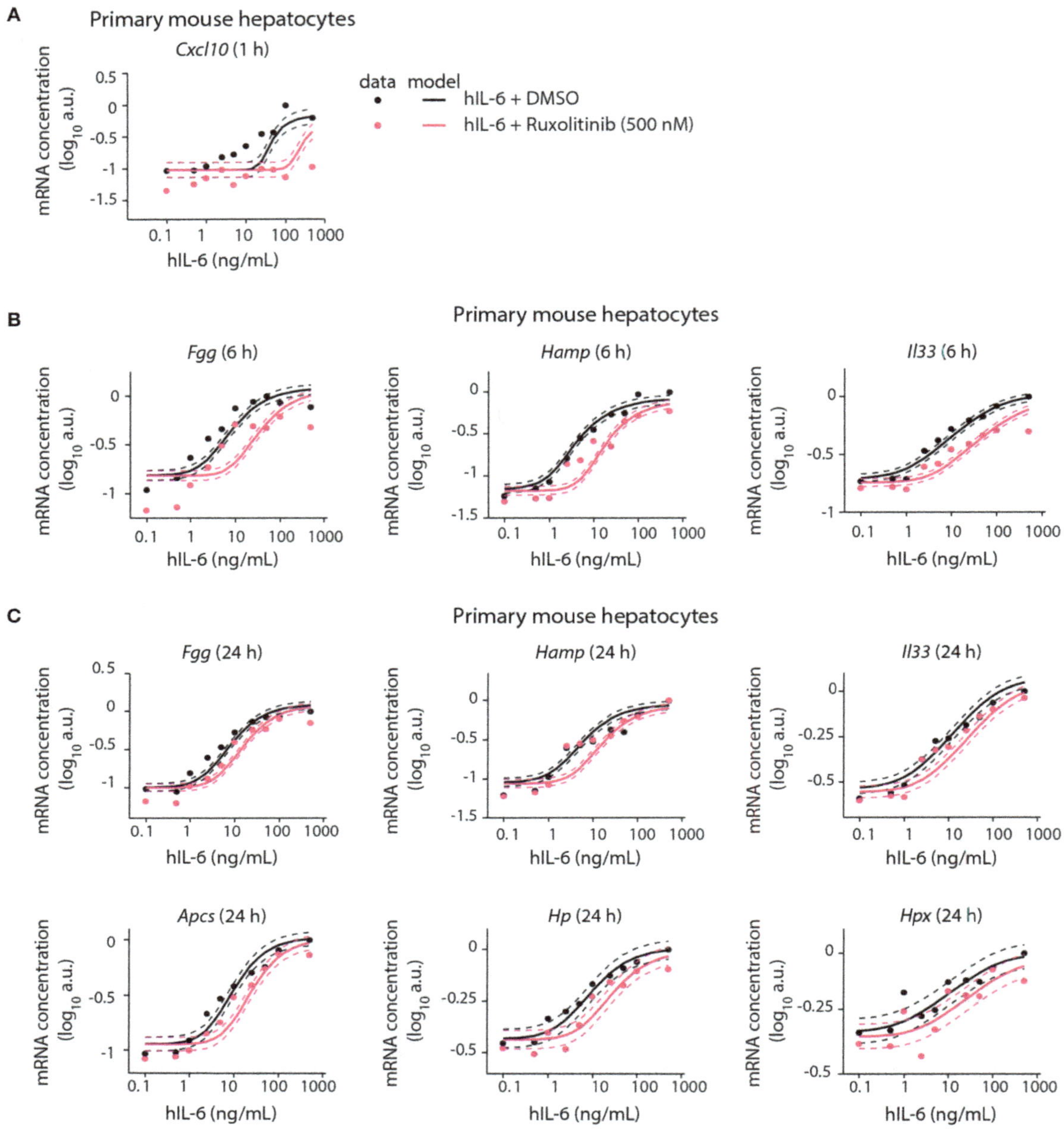

FIGURE 6 | Model prediction and experimental validation of the inhibitor impact on dose-dependent APP gene expression. Solid lines represent model predictions for dose-dependent APP gene expression with or without Ruxolitinib pre-treatment. For experimental validation (filled circles), primary mouse hepatocytes were pre-treated with Ruxolitinib or DMSO control for 1 h prior to hIL-6 (0.1–500 ng/mL) stimulation. APP mRNA expression was quantified at indicated time points by qPCR (**A** *Cxcl10*; **B** *Fgg*, *Hamp*, and *Il33*; **C** *Fgg*, *Hamp*, *Il33*, *Apcs*, *Hp*, and *Hpx*). Dashed lines indicate the measurement noise as estimated by the error model. a.u, arbitrary units. For additional replicates see Appendix Figure S5. For additional experimental data used for model validation see Appendix Figures S82–S88.

of the inhibitor could have detrimental side-effects, we employed our mathematical model to design treatment schedules for Ruxolitinib where the concentration of Ruxolitinib in the system does not exceed a maximal dose. The aim was to continuously suppress elevated IL-6-induced APP gene expression, while not exceeding a maximal level of 500 ng/mL Ruxolitinib. As objective, the integral up to 24 h of the APP mRNA levels in response to 100 ng/mL hIL-6 was used as a proxy for APP expression during inflammation. In this way, inappropriate inflammatory responses could be counteracted without completely abrogating APP gene expression. Ideally, continuous administration of Ruxolitinib would be preferred. However, due to practical considerations, we restricted the search to a maximum of three injections. The model predicted which three Ruxolitinib doses in even time

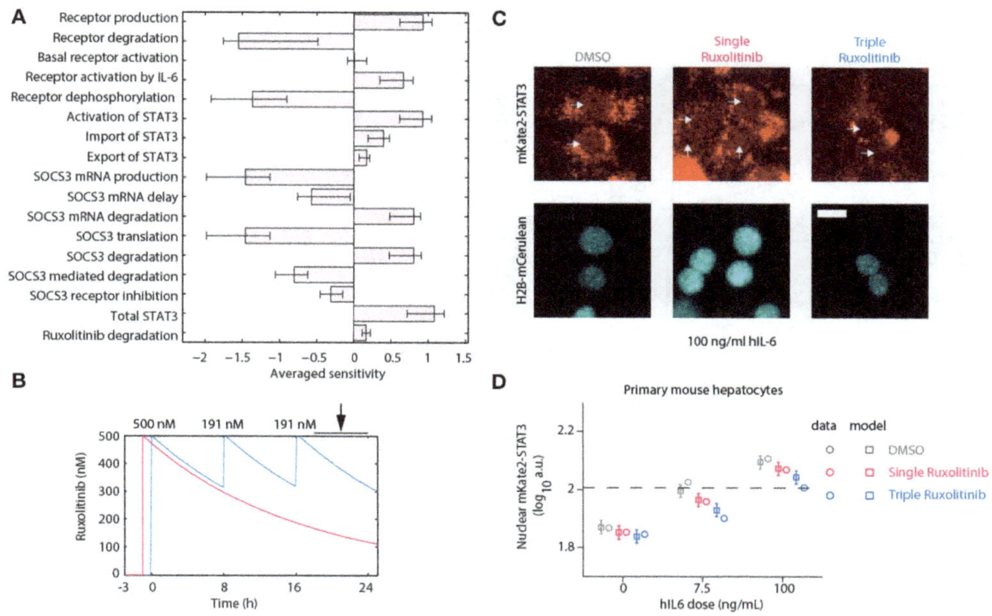

FIGURE 7 | Optimized inhibition of STAT3 nuclear translocation. **(A)** Averaged Local Parameter Sensitivity Analysis for the integrated APP response. Bars indicate model sensitivities to a 50% perturbation in model parameter. Error bars indicate maximum and minimum sensitivity along parameter likelihood profiles. Large perturbations were performed since we are interested in parameters that would have a substantial impact on dynamics. **(B)** Model predictions for Ruxolitinib concentrations over time after single treatment with 500 nM at $t = -1$ h (Single), or using the optimized triple treatment scenario, including Ruxolitinib treatments at $t =$ 0 h (500 nM), 8 h (191 nM), and 16 h (191 nM) (Triple). Arrow indicates the time window of nuclear STAT3 profiling. **(C)** Example widefield fluorescent microscopic images of primary hepatocytes from mKate2-STAT3 mice during the long-term quantification of IL-6-induced mKate2-STAT3 translocation in presence or absence of Ruxolitinib. Cells were stimulated with 100 ng/ml hIL-6 for 24 h, either treated with solvent control (DMSO), pre-treated for 1 h with 500 nM Ruxolitinib (Single Ruxolitinib) or co-treated with 500 nM Ruxolitinib and re-treated with 191 nM at 8 and 16 h (Triple Ruxolitinib). Inhibitor treatment was performed as suggested by the model **(B)**. Image quantification of nuclear mKate2-STAT3 was conducted from 20 to 24 h after hIL-6 stimulation. White arrows indicate positions of nuclei. H2B-mCerulean was used to indicate the positions of nuclei. Scale bar: 20 μm. **(D)** Squares represent model predictions for nuclear STAT3 after treatment with the indicated hIL-6 concentrations in combination with DMSO control, single or triple Ruxolitinib treatment. For experimental validation, primary mouse hepatocytes from mKate2-STAT3 mice were treated accordingly with DMSO or Ruxolitinib and hIL-6. Circles represent average nuclear STAT3 measured with time-lapse microscopy 20–24 h after hIL-6 stimulation. Error bars indicate the measurement noise as estimated by the error model. a.u., arbitrary units. Data presented corresponds to the average of at least 45 imaging fields per condition. For additional replicates see Appendix Figure S6. For additional experimental data used for model validation see Appendix Figures S93–S98.

intervals would effectively counteract loss of the inhibitor due to degradation (**Figures 7B, 8A**).

Therefore, in the presented study, the objective was to minimize the integral of APP mRNA levels. However, we did not use an optimization procedure as a means of determining the treatment schedule, because it is not clear how to prioritize the different APP genes. Instead we made response curves for each of the APP genes and determined the ideal point via visual inspection. Depending on which APP gene is considered therapeutically most important, deviations from this design may be more optimal (see section 3.7 of the Appendix). Predictions for the integrated target gene expression at time point 24 h furthermore revealed that applying the first treatment at $t =$ 0 h, simultaneously with the start of IL-6 treatment, would be superior to the previously applied pre-treatment with Ruxolitinib at 1 h before IL-6 stimulation (Appendix Figure S8). Thus, an optimized Ruxolitinib treatment would include three subsequent treatments at $t = 0$, 8, and 16 h. Given that 500 nM Ruxolitinib would be applied as first bolus at $t = 0$ h, the model predicted that 191 nM Ruxolitinib would be required to replenish the full inhibitor potential at each, 8 h, and 16 h. The initial dose of 500 nM Ruxolitinib was selected based on dose response experiments (Appendix Figures S70, S71) in primary mouse hepatocytes and closely relates to the determined IC_{50}.

Using two experimental readouts, namely nuclear translocation of STAT3 as an indicator of activated STAT3, and IL-6 target gene expression, we validated the predicted advantage of Ruxolitinib triple treatment over the previously applied single pre-treatment (**Figures 7**, **8**). Compared to the single treatment (q24h), the triple treatment (q8h) induced a more sustained inhibitory effect, utilizing considerably lower doses for the repetitive treatment after the initial bolus. Primary mouse hepatocytes were either treated with a single dose (500 nM) of Ruxolitinib at $t = -1$ h (Single), or with three doses at time points $t = 0$ h (500 nM), 8 h (191 nM), and 16 h (191 nM; Triple). Cells were stimulated with hIL-6 concentrations resembling basal (0 ng/mL), regenerative (7.5 ng/mL) or inflammatory (100 ng/mL) physiological levels

The maximal tolerable dose of Ruxolitinib in healthy volunteers was described to be 100 mg once daily, already inducing severe side effects as neutropenia (Shi et al., 2011). This amount corresponds to a concentration of 65 nM assuming an average blood volume of 5 L per human body. The dose-dependent effect of Ruxolitinib on STAT3 phosphorylation in primary human hepatocytes revealed that 50 nM of the inhibitor is in the range of the IC_{50} determined in cells co-treated with hIL-6 (1 or 10 ng/mL) and increasing doses of Ruxolitinib (up to 5,000 nM; Appendix Figure 12). Hence, primary human hepatocytes show an increased sensitivity toward the treatment with Ruxolitinib in comparison to primary mouse hepatocytes. Therefore, we reduced the initial dose of Ruxolitinib from 500 nM as applied in primary mouse hepatocytes to 50 nM for primary human hepatocytes (**Figure 9A**) and the subsequent second and third dosing of 191 nM Ruxolitinib was reduced to 19 nM accordingly.

We measured the expression of the four previously analyzed genes *SOCS3* (**Figure 9B**), *HAMP*, *HP*, and *FGG* (**Figure 9C**), which are established as IL-6 responsive genes both in mouse and human. Additionally the IL-6 induced expression of *CRP* (**Figure 9C**) was examined in primary human hepatocytes due to its routine clinical determination as an indicator of inflammatory responses. For several of the genes of interest almost maximal expression was already achieved with the lower hIL-6 concentration applied suggesting that their expression saturated at lower IL-6 doses in human hepatocytes compared to murine hepatocytes. In line with the model-based insights, the triple Ruxolitinib treatment at equivalent time intervals was again more effective compared to the single treatment to suppress IL-6 induced *SOCS3* and APP gene expression in primary human hepatocytes, confirming our concept.

DISCUSSION

While IL-6 has repeatedly been suggested to contribute to inflammatory or malignant diseases, targeting this central mediator needs to be carefully evaluated to maintain its beneficial regenerative functions (Hunter and Jones, 2015). Here we developed a mathematical model of IL-6-induced JAK1-STAT3 signaling in primary mouse hepatocytes, which adequately predicted how inflammatory gene expression could be reduced to regenerative levels by optimized Ruxolitinib treatment.

Determination of *in vivo* circulating and the IL-6 concentrations during liver regeneration and inflammation enabled to study IL-6 signaling pathway activation within relevant IL-6 concentration ranges. Determined serum levels agree with previously reported values after PHx (1–2 ng/mL; Nechemia-Arbely et al., 2011; Yin et al., 2011) and LPS treatment (175 ng/mL; Piao et al., 2013) of mice. Importantly, simultaneous analysis of samples from PHx- and LPS-treated mice, as performed here, enabled direct comparison of the regenerative and inflammatory scenarios. Thus, we established distinct IL-6 concentration ranges during liver regeneration and inflammation. By quantifying the hepatic IL-6 concentrations, we provide evidence that IL-6 accumulates in the hepatocyte microenvironment after PHx (serum: 1.4 ng/mL, local: 6.8–7.9 ng/mL). This is likely a result of an increased IL-6 secretion by Kupffer cells (Aldeguer et al., 2002) to promote an efficient regenerative response. In contrast, IL-6 levels were similar in serum and hepatocyte microenvironment after LPS injection (serum: 201.8 ng/mL, local: 28.1–500 ng/mL). Local hepatic IL-6 levels following PHx in liver tissues at mRNA and protein level were reported previously (Yin et al., 2011). However, the published IL-6 levels represent both, extra- and intracellular IL-6, and are thus not directly equivalent to IL-6 levels that actively stimulate hepatocytes. Here we inferred the IL-6 concentrations from STAT3 phosphorylation levels in whole liver lysates. Because IL-6 appears to be the main inducer of STAT3 activation in hepatocytes (Cressman et al., 1996), the major hepatic cell type, this approach provides a good estimate of IL-6 concentrations in the hepatocytes' microenvironment.

To exclude the contribution of other cytokines to the activation of STAT3, we performed a qPCR analysis of *Il11*, *Osm*, and *Il22* mRNA expression in liver lysates from LPS or PHx mice (Appendix Figure S14). In these experiments we did not observe an elevation of the mRNAs encoding these cytokines within the time frame of maximal STAT3 phosphorylation detected in the liver lysates from the corresponding mice, at 1 h in LPS treated mice and at 2 h in hepatectomized mice, respectively (**Figure 1B**). On the contrary a very rapid induction of *Il6* mRNA was detected particularly in response to LPS injection that was already maximal after 1 h of LPS injection (Appendix Figure S14) and coincided with maximal STAT3 phosphorylation observed at 1 h post treatment (**Figure 1B**). These results are in line with the studies of Ren et al. reporting that there is no statistically significant increase of *Il22* mRNA in response to hepatectomy, but rather an increase of IL-22 protein is observed in the serum at late time points post hepatectomy starting at 6 h post treatment with a peak at 12 h (Ren et al., 2010). Others observed a peak of *Il22* mRNA induction in the liver at ~3 h post hepatectomy (Rao et al., 2014) or 4 h after LPS injection (Wegenka et al., 2007) and thus much later than the rapid maximal phosphorylation of STAT3 we observed in our study in the liver of hepatectomized or LPS treated mice. Furthermore, 4 h post LPS injection peak levels of IL-22 were detected by ELISA measurements corresponding to ~600 pg/mL (Dumoutier et al., 2011) whereas, in agreement with the study by Wegenka et al., we observed already at 2 h post LPS injection a peak concentration of IL-6 in the serum of 201.8 ng/mL suggesting that the induction of IL-6 in response to LPS is more rapid and more than two orders of magnitude higher compared to IL-22. Further, a major contribution of IL-10 to the early activation of STAT3 and the induction of the acute phase response in hepatocytes appears unlikely. Although it has been observed that the expression of *Il10* mRNA can be induced by PHx (Yin et al., 2011), the ability of IL-10 to induce signaling via JAK1/STAT3 appears primarily restricted to cells of the immune system, such as macrophages and dendritic cells, due to the expression of the IL-10 receptor that is most prominent in these cell types (Murray, 2006; Sabat et al., 2010). In light of these observations we propose that IL-6 is the mediator of immediate early responses in hepatocytes involving STAT3 phosphorylation during liver regeneration whereas other cytokines such as IL-22

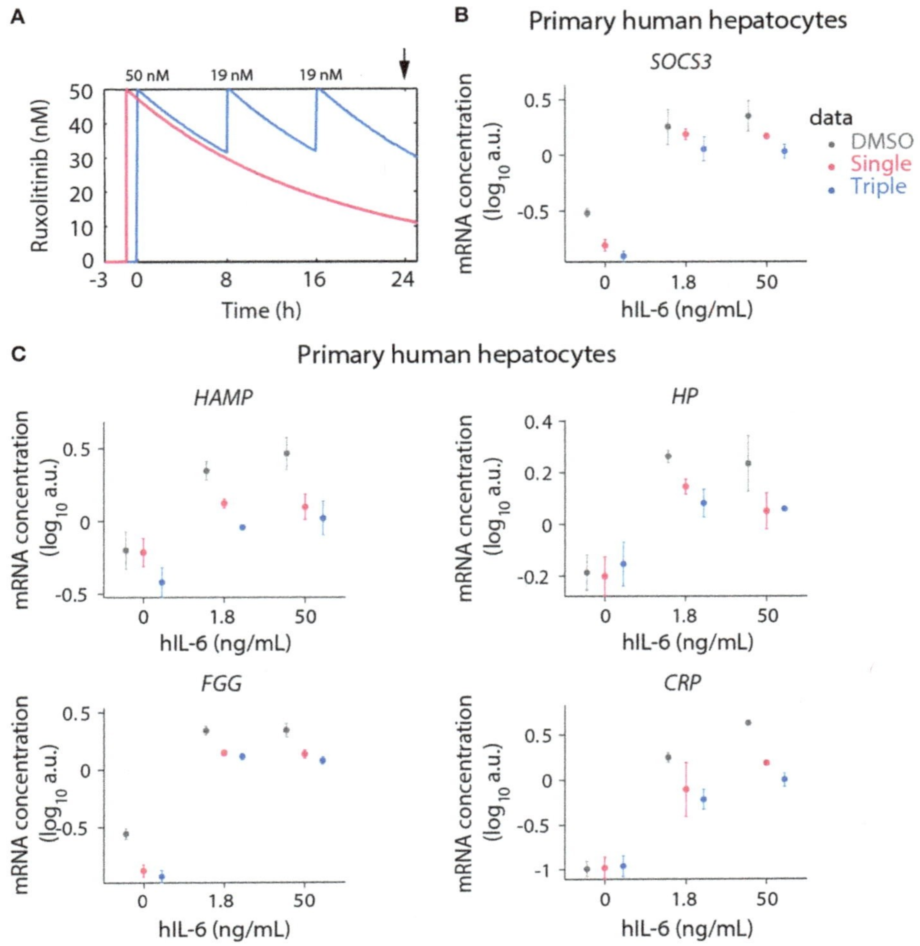

FIGURE 9 | Optimized inhibition of APP gene expression in primary human hepatocytes. **(A)** Model predictions for Ruxolitinib concentrations over time after single treatment with 50 nM at $t = -1$ h (Single), or using the optimized triple treatment scenario, including Ruxolitinib treatments at $t = 0$ h (50 nM), 8 h (19 nM), and 16 h (19 nM) (Triple). Arrow indicates the time point of gene expression analysis. **(B,C)** Expression of *SOCS3* **(B)** and APP genes **(C)** at 24 h after inhibitor treatments as described in **(A)**. Data from primary human hepatocytes of three different donors are shown as mean ± SEM.

or IL-10 may contribute to STAT3 phosphorylation at later time points or in other cell types than hepatocytes.

Because the hepatic acute phase response is largely regulated at the transcriptional level (Andus et al., 1988; Heinrich et al., 1990), we studied IL-6-induced mRNA expression changes in primary mouse hepatocytes. We established the time-dependent regulation of previously known IL-6 targets including *Socs3* (Starr et al., 1997), *Hamp* (Wrighting and Andrews, 2006; Pietrangelo et al., 2007), *Fgg*, *Apcs*, *Hp*, *Hpx* (Alonzi et al., 2001) as well as of two less well-established targets, *Cxcl10* and *Il33*. IL-6-induced genes were grouped into early, intermediate, and late responsive genes, according to their expression levels at 1, 6, and 24 h after IL-6 stimulation. CXCL10 was described previously to be secreted by macrophages in an IL-6/STAT3-dependent manner (Xu et al., 2012, 2015). In the context of hepatitis C virus infection, CXCL10 was suggested to contribute to persistent liver inflammation and fibrosis (Zeremski et al., 2008, 2009; Brownell and Polyak, 2013). Here, we provide evidence that IL-6 stimulated hepatocytes might be a crucial source for CXCL10. In line with the reports by Zeremski et al. (2008, 2009) and Brownell and Polyak (2013), linking CXCL10 and inflammation, *Cxcl10* mRNA was selectively induced by inflammatory IL-6 concentrations, while all other analyzed target genes responded to both, regenerative and inflammatory IL-6 stimuli (**Figure 5**). In addition to *Cxcl10*, we identified *Il33* to be expressed in response to IL-6 in primary mouse hepatocytes. This IL-1-like cytokine (Schmitz et al., 2005) was described to be induced in fibrotic livers, and hepatic stellate cells were suggested as major IL-33 producer in this context (Marvie et al., 2010). Our results indicate that also hepatocytes might produce IL-33. We observed strong and sustained induction of *Il33* mRNA (**Figure 4**), which together with its suggested role of IL-33 as a general alarm signal (Miller, 2011), highlight this gene as an interesting IL-6 target and APP gene in hepatocytes. Both, CXCL10 and

IL-33 secretion by hepatocytes should be investigated in the future to better understand the potential link between IL-6 and chronic inflammation. By acting on T-cells and innate immune cells (Miller, 2011; Brownell and Polyak, 2013), CXCL10 and IL-33 might contribute to the amplification of inflammatory responses.

Signal processing in hepatocytes translates extracellular IL-6 levels to JAK1-STAT3 signaling dynamics and to changes in gene expression. We could quantitatively link these different levels by implementing a mathematical model, which not only described experimentally observed signaling dynamics, but also the impact of the pathway inhibitors Ruxolitinib and Stattic on STAT3 and its target gene activation. While previous mathematical models of IL-6 signaling incorporated IL-6-induced JAK-STAT as well as mitogen-activated protein kinase (MAPK) cascades (Singh et al., 2006; Moya et al., 2011; Xu et al., 2015), we focused our model scope on the JAK-STAT pathway, which according to Dierssen et al. is relevant for IL-6-induced APP expression whereas MAPK activation is dispensable (Dierssen et al., 2008). To obtain a predictive mathematical model, the relation of considered species and experimentally measured components as well as the amount of experimental data needs to be appropriate (Aldridge et al., 2006; Bachmann et al., 2012). Compared to the earlier approaches (Singh et al., 2006; Moya et al., 2011; Xu et al., 2015) that partly relied on literature derived parameter values obtained from different cell types and stimulating agents, the amount of experimental data used for calibration and validation of the model presented here is more extensive. As an example, we assessed the protein concentration of key players of the signal transduction pathway in primary mouse hepatocytes. The obtained value for STAT3 is in good agreement with recently published data from a mass spectrometry approach to determine molecules per cell in primary human hepatocytes (Wisniewski et al., 2016). For the presented study an extensive amount of experimental data was generated using different technologies ranging from quantitative immunoblotting, multiplexed bead-based arrays and quantitative mass spectrometry to qRT- PCR and microarray analysis in order to assess the dynamics of signal transduction and target gene expression. Whereas quantitative immunoblotting, multiplexed bead-based arrays, and qRT-PCR permit very detailed time-resolved analysis, omics technologies will be increasingly employed for quantitative analysis and to facilitate the link to primary patient material (Iwamoto et al., 2016; Adlung et al., 2017).

The nuclear translocation of STAT3 is a crucial aspect of signal transduction in response to IL-6 stimulation. Therefore the determination of the spatial dynamics of STAT3 and inclusion in the mathematical model are of importance. To quantitatively assess this behavior in the context of primary hepatocytes expressing endogenous amounts of fluorescently labeled STAT3, we generated the mKate2-STAT3 reporter mouse line. Since the fluorescently labeled STAT3 was created as knock-in into the endogenous STAT3 locus, its expression should mirror the expression of STAT3 in different organs. Therefore, the reporter mouse model offers a wide range of possible applications to study STAT3 in multiple organs and could especially be useful to track the dynamics of STAT3 at the single cell level.

We established a mathematical representation of the signaling network and could confirm its high predictive power by experimentally validating previously untested scenarios. Specifically, a model-predicted treatment with a high initial bolus and two following lower doses is necessary for a long-term effect of the clinically applied inhibitor Ruxolitinib, thus counteracting its rapid metabolism (Shilling et al., 2010) resulting in its short half-life (Shi et al., 2011).

Multiple-dose Ruxolitinib treatment with equal doses was shown earlier to have a more sustained effect on STAT3 signaling, compared with single treatment (Shi et al., 2011). Importantly, Shi et al. found negligible accumulation of Ruxolitinib after multiple doses, thus minimizing the risk of potential side effects. A twice-daily dosing regimen was furthermore successfully applied in the treatment of myelofibrosis patients (Verstovsek et al., 2012). Notably, previous treatment planning was based on preclinical data and empirical results from clinical trials (Quintas-Cardama et al., 2010; Shi et al., 2011).

While the single treatment with Ruxolitinib did reduce the APP response after treatment with IL-6, more sustained inhibition may still be of importance, but an increase in dose is not desirable due to harmful side-effects such as neutropenia (Shi et al., 2011). If we consider the parameter sensitivity analysis (see **Figure 7A**), we can observe that additional alternatives exist to further suppress the APP response. One option would be to selectively reduce the *Socs3* mRNA degradation rate to benefit from synergistic effects between the pathway's natural inhibitor SOCS3 and the drug Ruxolitinib. However, since selective inhibition of mRNA degradation for one specific mRNA species may not be feasible, a more practical option could be to reduce receptor accessibility. This may be achieved by additional application of a therapeutic antibody against the IL-6 receptor.

In silico analyses, based on mathematical models represent promising approaches to optimally exploit an inhibitor's potential and pre-assess drug safety, prior to testing the drug in patients or healthy individuals. Our established mathematical model represents a starting point for further adaptation to the human system, and could facilitate *in silico* drug treatment planning in the future.

MATERIALS AND METHODS

Chemicals

Chemicals were purchased from Sigma-Aldrich, if not specified otherwise.

Partial Hepatectomy (PHx) and LPS Treatments of Mice

C57BL/6J mice (Janvier) were housed in the animal facility of the Heinrich-Heine-University of Düsseldorf under a constant light/dark cycle, maintained on a standard mouse diet, and allowed *ad libitum* access to food and water. Male, 8–12 week old mice were used for PHx and LPS experiments. Procedures were approved by the North Rhine-Westphalia State Agency for Nature, Environment and Consumer Protection (reference number 87-51.04.2010.A279 for PHx experiments; reference number 84-02.04.2011.A096 for LPS injections). PHx was performed based on the standardized procedure described by Mitchell and Willenbring (2008). Mice were anesthetized using isoflurane (Abott) and received 5 mg/kg body weight carprofen (Pfizer) subcutaneously for analgesia during surgery and the three following days. During the operation, mice were placed on a warming pad. The abdominal cavity was opened applying a 3 cm incision. The left lateral liver lobe was removed by applying a ligature (time point 0 h) close to the base of the lobe followed by cutting the tied lobe just above the suture. A second ligature was placed around the median lobe above the gall bladder but with at least 2 mm distance to the suprahepatic vena cava. The tied median lobe including gall bladder was then resected by cutting just above the suture. Ringer's lactate solution (B.Braun) was applied to detect possible abdominal bleeding which, if present, was stopped before closing peritoneum and skin by over-and-over sutures. The weight of the resected left lateral and median liver lobes was determined. Mice were monitored during awakening and the following days including daily determination of body weight. Sham surgeries were performed analogous to PHx, but without placing ligatures and liver lobe removal. Liver lobes were moved as during PHx operations (time point 0 h).

For LPS-injections, LPS (*Escherichia coli* 0111:B4) was dissolved in 0.9% NaCl (Baxter) and injected intraperitoneally at a concentration of 1 μg/g body weight. At indicated time points after Sham/PHx surgery or LPS-injection mice were anesthetized as outlined above and blood was collected from the vena cava. After clotting, blood serum was obtained by two centrifugation steps at 10,000 × g for 10 min. Livers were perfused in an antegrade direction with cold PBS (Biochrom) supplemented with 0.1 mM Na_3VO_4 until perfusate was clear. Livers were extracted from mice, flash frozen in liquid nitrogen, and stored at −80°C.

Isolation of Primary Mouse Hepatocytes

Primary mouse hepatocyte isolation was performed in a standardized way according to Klingmuller et al. (2006) or according to the refined protocol described by Huard et al. (2012). C57BL/6N mice (Charles River) were housed at the DKFZ animal facility under a constant light/dark cycle, maintained on a standard mouse diet, and allowed *ad libitum* access to food and water. Hepatocyte isolation from mice was approved by the governmental review committee on animal care of the state Baden-Württemberg, Germany (reference number A24/10). For standard time course and dose response experiments, 2×10^6 cells were seeded in 6 cm collagen I-coated tissue culture plates (BD Biosciences) in 2 mL of adhesion medium [phenol red-free Williams E medium (Biochrom) containing 10% (v/v) fetal bovine serum (Life Technologies), 0.1 μM dexamethasone, 10 μg/mL insulin, 2 mM L-glutamine and 1% (v/v) penicillin/streptomycin 100 × (both Life Technologies)]. Cells were maintained at 37°C, 5% CO_2, and 95% relative humidity. After 4 h of adhesion, unattached hepatocytes were removed by washing 3 × with DPBS (PAN Biotech) followed by over-night cultivation (14–16 h) in pre-starvation medium [phenol red-free Williams E medium containing 0.1 μM dexamethasone, 2 mM L-glutamine, and 1% (v/v) penicillin/streptomycin 100 ×]. The next day cells were washed 3 × with DPBS and cultured for 5 h in starvation medium [phenol red-free Williams E medium supplemented with 2 mM L-glutamine, 1% (v/v) penicillin/streptomycin 100 × and 25 mM HEPES] prior to inhibitor/IL-6 treatment. Hepatocytes were always isolated as described and cultivated on collagen I-coated tissue culture plates (BD Biosciences). Differing cell numbers and plate formats or extended pre-starvation periods are indicated in respective methods sections.

Isolation of Primary Human Hepatocytes

The isolation of primary human hepatocytes was performed as described in Iwamoto et al. (2016). For the isolation of the primary human hepatocytes macroscopically healthy tissue was used that originated from resected tumor-free tissue from human livers of three patients (Donor 1: age 65, gender male, disease hepatocellular carcinoma with cirrhosis and diabetes; Donor 2: age 68, gender male, disease hepatocellular carcinoma with nutritive-toxic liver cirrhosis, diabetes, arterial hypertonia; Donor 3: age 78, gender female, disease Klatskin tumor with Steatosis hepatis grade 2, diabetes, arterial hypertonia). Informed consent of the patients was obtained according to the ethical guidelines of the Medical Faculty of the University of Leipzig. Primary human hepatocytes were shipped as cell suspension in ChillProtec Plus (Biochrom) on ice overnight to DKFZ Heidelberg. Primary human hepatocytes were serum- and dexamethasone-depleted and cultivated using the protocol described above for primary mouse hepatocytes, with an adhesion time of 6 h.

Inhibitor and IL-6 Treatments

The STAT3 inhibitor Stattic (Merck Millipore) and the JAK inhibitor Ruxolitinib (Cayman Chemical) were reconstituted in DMSO and primary mouse hepatocytes were pre-treated with the indicated concentrations of inhibitors or DMSO control for 1 h prior to IL-6 stimulation. Actinomycin D was dissolved in DMSO and cells were pre-treated with 1 μg/mL actinomycin D or DMSO control for 10 min prior to addition of IL-6. Human recombinant hIL-6 was manufactured as described in Vandam et al. (1993). Mouse IL-6 was purchased from R & D (406-ML-005). IL-6 stock solutions were diluted in starvation medium and cells were stimulated with the indicated IL-6 concentrations and time spans. Pulsed stimulation was achieved by carefully washing the cells 3 × with starvation medium to remove unbound IL-6 ligand at indicated time points. For treatment durations of up to 2 h, cells were kept at 37°C in a bench-top incubator after inhibitor and/or IL-6 stimulation. During long-term experiments cells were incubated at 37°C, 5% CO_2, and 95% relative humidity.

Immunoassays for the Quantification of IL-6 Levels in Serum and Hepatocyte Supernatants

IL-6 concentrations in mouse serum were quantified using the MILLIPLEX mouse cytokine/chemokine magnetic bead panel (EMD Millipore) according to the manufacturer's instructions. Samples were incubated with antibody-coupled beads overnight. Washing procedures were performed using the ELx405 wash station (BioTek) and fluorescence intensity was detected by a

Luminex 200 System in combination with xPONENT Software version 3.1 (Millipore). IL-6 concentrations in hepatocyte supernatants were measured using the Bio-Plex Pro human IL-6 assay in combination with the Bio-Plex Pro reagent kit (both Bio-Rad) according to the manufacturer's instructions. A dilution series of the recombinant human IL-6 used for stimulation was used as standard curve. Washing was performed using the Bio-Plex Pro II wash station (Bio-Rad) and fluorescence intensity was acquired using the Bio-Plex 200 system and Bio-Plex Manager software version 6.1 (both Bio-Rad). Alternatively, IL-6 concentrations in hepatocyte supernatants were determined using the Quantikine Human IL-6 Immunoassay (R&D Systems). Stabilization of ligand in medium samples was achieved by supplementing 450 μL conditioned medium with 50 μL of 40 mM HCl and 10 mg/mL BSA.

Quantitative Immunoblotting

At precise time points cells were lysed in 1% Nonidet P-40 lysis buffer [1% (v/v) Nonidet P-40 (Roche Applied Sciences), 150 mM NaCl, 20 mM Tris pH 7.4, 10 mM NaF, 1 mM EDTA (Applichem) pH 8.0, 1 mM $ZnCl_2$ pH 4.0, 1 mM $MgCl_2$, 1 mM Na_3VO_4, 10% glycerol; freshly supplemented with 2 μg/mL aprotinin and 200 μg/mL 4-(2-aminoethyl)benzenesulfonylfluorid] and cleared lysates were either directly subjected to SDS-PAGE or used for immunoprecipitations. For cellular fractionation, cytosolic extracts were prepared as described above using Nonidet P-40 lysis buffer. Pelleted nuclei were washed once with Nonidet P-40 lysis buffer and then resuspended in nuclear lysis buffer [420 mM NaCl, 20 mM HEPES pH 7.9, 10 mM KCl, 1 mM EDTA pH 8.0, 1 mM Na_3VO_4, 10% (v/v) glycerol) supplemented with 2 μg/mL aprotinin, 200 μg/mL 4-(2-aminoethyl)benzenesulfonylfluorid and 1 mM DTT]. Nuclei were lysed by pulsed sonication and cleared nuclear lysates were subjected to SDS-PAGE or used for immunoprecipitations. Quality of fractionation was checked by correct subcellular localization of marker proteins Sp1 (nuclear; Santa Cruz Biotechnology, #sc-59) and Eps15 (cytosolic; Santa Cruz Biotechnology, #sc-534).

Protein concentrations of lysates were quantified by BCA assay (Pierce, Thermo Scientific). To immunoprecipitate target proteins, lysates were incubated with anti-gp130 (C20, Santa Cruz Biotechnology, #sc-655), anti-JAK1 serum (Upstate/Merck Millipore, #06-272), anti-STAT3 (Cell Signaling Technology, #9132) or anti-SOCS3 (clone 1B2, Invitrogen, #37-7200) antibodies, protein-A sepharose (GE Healthcare), and recombinant calibrator proteins. For immunoprecipitation experiments the following recombinant proteins were added as calibrator proteins directly to the cell lysates to enable normalization of immunoblot data: Glutathione S-transferase (GST)-tagged gp130ΔN (cytoplasmic domain); GST-STAT3 (full length protein) and Streptavidin binding protein (SBP)-tagged SOCS3 (full length protein). Precipitated proteins and cytoplasmic or nuclear lysates (40–50 μg) were resolved by 10% SDS-polyacrylamide gel electrophoresis and transferred to nitrocellulose membranes according to previously described recommendations for quantitative immunoblotting (Schilling et al., 2005a). Membranes were incubated with anti-phosphotyrosine antibody (4G10, Upstate/Merck Millipore, #05 321) to detect the phosphorylated forms of gp130 and JAK1, anti-gp130 (C20, Santa Cruz Biotechnology, #sc-655), anti-JAK1 (Cell Signaling Technologies, #3332), anti-phospho-STAT3, anti-STAT3 (both Cell Signaling Technologies, 3E2 #9138, #9132) and anti-SOCS3 (Abcam, #ab16030) antibodies. For normalization in cell lysate samples, anti-calnexin and anti-Hsc70 (both Stressgen, #ADI-SPA-860, #SPA-816) antibodies were applied. Nuclear marker proteins were detected by anti-Sp1 and anti-Eps15 antibodies (both Santa Cruz, #sc-59, #sc-534). Horseradish peroxidase coupled secondary antibodies (anti-mouse, anti-rabbit, protein A) were derived from GE Healthcare. Antibodies were removed by β-mercaptoethanol/SDS-treatment prior to re-probing for a different protein. Phosphorylated species were detected first, followed by total proteins and normalizers. Proteins were visualized using enhanced chemiluminescence substrate (GE Healthcare) and signals were detected using a CCD camera (LumiImager F1, Roche; or ImagequantLAS4000, GE Healthcare). For band quantification, LumiAnalyst 3.1 (Roche) or ImagequantTL (GE Healthcare) software was used. Quantitative immunoblotting data were either processed using GELINSPECTOR software (Schilling et al., 2005b) or directly used for mathematical modeling.

Bead-Based Immunoassays for the Analysis of STAT3 Activation

IL-6 concentrations in the liver were determined by measuring STAT3 activation as read-out. Livers from Sham/PHx or NaCl/LPS-treated mice as well as primary mouse hepatocytes were lysed in total cell lysis buffer [136 mM NaCl, 20 mM Tris-HCl, 10% glycerol, 2 mM EDTA, 50 mM β-glycerophosphate, 20 mM sodium pyrophosphate, 1 mM Na_3VO_4, 1% Triton X-100, 0.2% SDS, 1 tablet/10 mL complete Mini EDTA-free protease inhibitors (Roche), pH 7.4]. For other experiments, hepatocytes were lysed using Nonidet P-40 lysis buffer as described above. Livers were homogenized using a microcentrifuge tube-pestle followed by passing through QIAshredder (Qiagen) columns. Cleared liver and hepatocyte lysates were subjected to BCA assay (Pierce, Thermo Scientific) to determine protein concentrations. Relative phospho-STAT3 levels were quantified using the bead-based Bio-Plex phospho-STAT3 (Tyr-705) assay in combination with the Bio-Plex phosphoprotein detection reagent kit, or using the magnetic bead-based Bio-Plex Pro phospho-STAT3 (Tyr-705) set (all Bio-Rad) according to the manufacturer's instructions. Equal amounts of protein (16.67 μg/well or 10 μg/well in a 96-well plate format) were incubated with antibody-coupled beads overnight. For washing steps, the Bio-Plex Pro II wash station (Bio-Rad) was used. The fluorescence intensity corresponding to relative phospho-STAT3 levels was acquired using the Bio-Plex 200 system and Bio-Plex Manager software version 6.1 (both Bio-Rad).

Quantification of Target Gene Expression by Quantitative Real-Time PCR (qRT-PCR)

Cells were collected in RLT Plus lysis buffer and lysates were homogenized using QIAshredder spin columns (both Qiagen). Homogenized lysates were immediately placed on dry-ice and stored at −80°C until RNA isolation. RNA was extracted using the RNeasy Plus Mini Kit (Qiagen) according to the manufacturer's instructions. Reverse transcription was performed using either the High Capacity cDNA Reverse Transcription Kit (Applied Biosystems) or the QuantiTect Reverse Transcription Kit (Qiagen). Diluted cDNA was analyzed applying the Universal ProbeLibrary System on a LightCycler 480 (both Roche), cycling conditions can be found in Appendix Table S2. Relative mRNA concentrations were calculated according to a cDNA dilution series with the Absolute Quantification Second Derivative Maximum method of the LightCycler 480 Basic Software (Roche). Target mRNA concentrations were normalized to the geometric mean of *Hprt*/*Tbp* concentrations or to *Hprt* concentrations. Primer/probe combinations were designed using the Universal ProbeLibrary Assay Design Center (Roche) and are listed in Appendix Table S3.

Microarray Experiment

Primary mouse hepatocytes (2×10^6 cells per 10 cm dish) were cultivated in pre-starvation medium for 24 h before ligand treatment. hIL-6 was added directly to cells in pre-starvation medium at 40 ng/mL and untreated or IL-6-treated samples were collected at time points 0 (4 replicates), 0.5, 2, 4, 8, 16, 24, 32 h (2 replicates each). Results are shown in duplicates, for time point 0 the first two replicates were utilized. RNA was isolated as described above (RNeasy, Qiagen) and gene expression was analyzed on GeneChip® Mouse Genome 430 2.0 Arrays (Affymetrix). The microarray data is accessible via the following URL: https://www.ncbi.nlm.nih.gov/geo/query/acc.cgi?acc=GSE69939.

Microarray Analysis

Principal component analysis was performed on the global transcriptional profiles. The first two principal components explained most of the variance in the data set (PC1: 58.4%, PC2: 9.7%, 68.1% in total).

To analyze significant gene regulation, we applied a linear regression model with the Limma package (Ritchie et al., 2015). Gene expression values y_i were modeled to be explained by time frames t (early, intermediate and late) and condition c (IL-6 and control). The significance threshold of Benjamini–Hochberg adjusted $p < 0.01$ was implemented. For example "early IL-6 response" was extracted from the global linear model by performing contrast analysis of early IL-6 vs. respective (unpaired) early control samples.

All analyses were performed in R Statistical software (www.r-project.org).

Ontology analysis of the three response lists was performed using a model-based ontology analysis (*http://nar.oxfordjournals.org/content/early/2010/02/19/nar.gkq045.full*) using Wiki Pathways and implementing an enrichment threshold using pathways with a probability of being regulated > 0.5.

Mass Spectrometric Analysis

Primary mouse hepatocytes (5×10^6 cells per 10 cm dish) were cultivated for 40 h in serum-depleted medium. Cells were then serum- and dexamethasone-depleted for 5 h in starvation medium, stimulated with 40 ng/mL hIL-6 for 18 min, and lysed in Nonidet P-40 lysis buffer. STAT3 immunoprecipitations were subjected to 10% SDS-PAGE and proteins were stained with SimplyBlue SafeStain (Life Technologies). STAT3-α bands were excised, cut into small pieces (~1 mm^3) and destained with 0.07 M NH_4HCO_3 buffer/30% acetonitrile. Gel pieces were dehydrated in 0.1% trifluoroacetic acid/50% acetonitrile, followed by protein in-gel reduction with 10 mM dithiothreitol (45 min at 56°C) and alkylation with 55 mM iodoacetamide for 30 min in the dark. Digestions were performed with AspN + LysC in 0.05 M NH_4HCO_3 buffer at 37°C overnight. Following incubation, internal peptide-/phospho-peptide one-source ratio standards for quantification of STAT3 Tyr-705 phosphorylation were added. The standard consists of the isotope labeled [$^{13}C_5$,^{15}N] peptides DPGSAAP-**pY**-[L+6Da]-K and DPGSAAP-**Y**-[L+6Da]-K at an exact molar ratio of 1:1. Following standard addition to the gel pieces and 15 min of shaking the supernatant of each sample was collected. Peptide extraction was finished by sequentially adding appropriate volumes of eluents to the gel pieces, shaking them and combining all the supernatants for each sample. The eluents were (i) acetonitrile, (ii) 5% formic acid, and (iii) acetonitrile. The collected sample volumes were reduced by speedvac and purified by applying the ZipTip method (Millipore) according to the manufacturer's recommendations. Final sample volumes of 5 µl were injected into an ultra-performance liquid chromatography (nanoUPLC, nanoAcquity, Waters) online coupled to a Q Exactive Plus-Orbitrap mass spectrometer (Thermo). For details about preparation and application of peptide-/phosphopeptide one-source ratio standards see Hahn et al. (2011) and Boehm et al. (2014).

Generation of mKate2-STAT3 Knock-In Mouse

To generate the mKate2-STAT3 reporter gene, we based the fusion construct on earlier studies (see Herrmann et al., 2007; Samsonov et al., 2013) and inserted the mKate2-coding sequence in front of the first exon of STAT3 by BAC recombineering. An insert harboring mKate2 and part of STAT3 as well as the Neomycin selection cassette flanked by homologous arms was retrieved into PL253 vector (NCI Frederick; Liu et al., 2003) to obtain the gene targeting construct. Gene targeting was performed in the mouse embryonic stem (ES) cell line JM8A3 (Pettitt et al., 2009) by electroporation of the linearized gene targeting construct followed by selection with G418 (Life Technologies) and Ganciclovir. Correctly targeted ES cell clones were identified by long-range PCR and confirmed with southern blot. Chimera were generated by blastocyst injection of correctly targeted ES clones. Male chimera were bred with female wild type C57BL/6N mice to promote germline transmission of the reporter gene. Germline transmission was identified by genotyping PCR. The selection cassette was removed by subsequently crossing heterozygous mice with Cre expressing mice (Schwenk et al., 1995). Only heterozygous mice were used for the experiments, because it was so far not possible to obtain homozygous mKate2-STAT3 reporter mouse offsprings.

See Appendix for more information about gene targeting and genotyping.

Live-Cell Imaging

Primary hepatocytes (15,000 cells per well, 96-well plate format) derived from mKate2-STAT3 heterozygous knock-in mice (Appendix Supplementary Experimental Procedures and Table S1) were infected with adeno-associated viruses encoding mCerulean-labeled histone-2B during adhesion. Cells were cultivated as described above, stimulated with inhibitor/ligand, and imaged using a Nikon Eclipse Ti Fluorescence microscope in combination with NIS-Elements software. Temperature (37°C), CO_2 (5%), and humidity were held constant through an incubation chamber enclosing the microscope. Three channels were acquired for each position: bright-field channel, STAT3 channel (mKate2), and nuclear channel (CFP). Image analysis was performed using Fiji software (Schindelin et al., 2012), and data were processed using R software (The R Foundation). The ratio of nuclear to cytoplasmic (nuc/cyt) mKate2-STAT3 was determined in 20 cells, facilitated by manual segmentation of nuclei (histone-2B-mCerulean signal) and whole cells (bright-field channel). The mean concentration of cytoplasmic STAT3 was derived assuming constant overall mKate2-STAT3. mKate2 background was determined in wild-type nuclei and cytoplasm and subtracted accordingly.

Mathematical Modeling

A mathematical multi-compartment model describing IL-6 signaling in primary mouse hepatocytes was developed. The model is described by a set of coupled non-linear differential equations implemented using the Data2Dynamics software package (Raue et al., 2015) In each simulated experiment, the model is equilibrated to steady state prior to treatment with inhibitors or stimulation. Considering the size and complexity of the model and experimental data, model calibration was performed in two separate stages. The core model describes receptor production, degradation and phosphorylation as well as activation and translocation of STAT3, negative feedback by SOCS3 and the effect of inhibitors, while the downstream model describes the transcription of the various APP genes. Parameters for the upstream and downstream model were estimated separately. All model parameters were estimated directly from the experimental data using Maximum Likelihood Estimation. Several experiments required the use of scaling, offset and error model parameters that were estimated simultaneously with the dynamic parameters. For the core model, 270 parameters (of which 22 dynamic parameters) were estimated on a total of 2220 data points. For the downstream components, we estimated 471 additional parameters (of which 29 dynamic parameters) on a total of 2,288 data points.

To evaluate that parameters are identifiable (Maiwald et al., 2016), profile likelihood calculation followed by either model reduction or additional data acquisition were iteratively applied. For a full mathematical description of the model, including a detailed description of the iterative model building and reduction steps see Appendix section 3.5.

Local Parameter Sensitivity Analysis (LPSA) was performed with respect to model parameters. The local parameter sensitivity for a single APP gene / parameter pair is defined as:

$$S_{app} = \frac{\left(y - y_{ref}\right)/y_{ref}}{\left(p - p_{ref}\right)/p_{ref}} \qquad (1)$$

Here y refers to the model output at the perturbed parameter, while y_{ref} indicates the reference output. As model output, we selected the integral of the mRNA levels. Analogously, p and p_{ref} refer to the parameter value in the perturbed and reference state. These sensitivities are then computed for each of the APP genes and averaged. To assess how much uncertainty there is in these sensitivities, we computed an LPSA for each parameter set in our parameter profile likelihoods and reported the maximum and minimum value encountered within the confidence intervals of all parameters.

The mathematical model is available to the community at the biomodels database as well as on www.data2dynamics.org.

AUTHOR CONTRIBUTIONS

SS, AR, XH, JV, SeB, JT, MS, UK were responsible for study conception and design. SS, AR, XH, AJ, SeB, UA, MH, SW, LAD, SM, MB, PL, SaB, WL, JB acquired the data. GD, DS provided primary human hepatocytes. SR provided recombinant human IL-6. NG conducted the microarray experiments. XH and FvdH generated the recombinant mouse line. SS, AR, XH, JV, SaB, UA, MH, SW, NM, LAD, SM, MB, PL, WL, FT, JT, MS, UK performed the analysis and interpretation of data. SS, AR, XH, JV, AJ, JT, MS, UK drafted the manuscript and all authors critically revised the manuscript.

FUNDING

This study was supported by the following grants from the German Federal Ministry of Education and Research (BMBF): the Virtual Liver Network (0315731, 0315745, 0315766), the Liver Systems Medicine network (LiSyM, 031L0042, 031L0047, 031L0048), the e:Bio collaborative research projects "Multi-Scale Modeling of Drug Induced Liver Injury" (MS_DILI, 031L0074A, 031L0074B) and ImmunoQuant (0316170B), the EraSysAPP consortium IMOMESIC (031A604A, 031A604B, 031A604C). Further, the study was funded by the "Mechanism-based Integrated Systems for the Prediction of Drug-Induced Liver Injury" (MIP-DILI) project, a European Community grant under the Innovative Medicines Initiative (IMI) Programme (Grant Agreement Number 115336) and by the SFB/Transregio grant TRR179 of the Deutsche Forschungsgemeinschaft (DFG).

ACKNOWLEDGMENTS

We thank Susen Lattermann, Marvin Wäsch, and Maria Muciek for excellent technical assistance as well as

Dirk Grimm, Kathleen Börner, and Johanna Meichsner for providing histone-2B mCerulean encoding adeno-associated viral particles. We thank the Nikon Imaging Center (Heidelberg University) for providing access to their facility.

REFERENCES

Adlung, L., Kar, S., Wagner, M. C., She, B., Chakraborty, S., Bao, J., et al. (2017). Protein abundance of AKT and ERK pathway components governs cell type-specific regulation of proliferation. *Mol. Syst. Biol.* 13:904. doi: 10.15252/msb.20167258

Aldeguer, X., Debonera, F., Shaked, A., Krasinkas, A. M., Gelman, A. E., Que, X., et al. (2002). Interleukin-6 from intrahepatic cells of bone marrow origin is required for normal murine liver regeneration. *Hepatology* 35, 40–48. doi: 10.1053/jhep.2002.30081

Aldridge, B. B., Burke, J. M., Lauffenburger, D. A., and Sorger, P. K. (2006). Physicochemical modelling of cell signalling pathways. *Nat. Cell Biol.* 8, 1195–1203. doi: 10.1038/ncb1497

Alon, U., Surette, M. G., Barkai, N., and Leibler, S. (1999). Robustness in bacterial chemotaxis. *Nature* 397, 168–171. doi: 10.1038/16483

Alonzi, T., Maritano, D., Gorgoni, B., Rizzuto, G., Libert, C., and Poli, V. (2001). Essential role of STAT3 in the control of the acute-phase response as revealed by inducible gene inactivation [correction of activation] in the liver. *Mol. Cell. Biol.* 21, 1621–1632. doi: 10.1128/MCB.21.5.1621-1632.2001

Andus, T., Geiger, T., Hirano, T., Kishimoto, T., Tran-Thi, T. A., Decker, K., et al. (1988). Regulation of synthesis and secretion of major rat acute-phase proteins by recombinant human interleukin-6 (BSF-2/IL-6) in hepatocyte primary cultures. *Eur. J. Biochem.* 173, 287–293. doi: 10.1111/j.1432-1033.1988.tb13997.x

Babon, J. J., Kershaw, N. J., Murphy, J. M., Varghese, L. N., Laktyushin, A., Young, S. N., et al. (2012). Suppression of cytokine signaling by SOCS3: characterization of the mode of inhibition and the basis of its specificity. *Immunity* 36, 239–250. doi: 10.1016/j.immuni.2011.12.015

Bachmann, J., Raue, A., Schilling, M., Becker, V., Timmer, J., and Klingmuller, U. (2012). Predictive mathematical models of cancer signalling pathways. *J. Intern. Med.* 271, 155–165. doi: 10.1111/j.1365-2796.2011.02492.x

Bachmann, J., Raue, A., Schilling, M., Bohm, M. E., Kreutz, C., Kaschek, D., et al. (2011). Division of labor by dual feedback regulators controls JAK2/STAT5 signaling over broad ligand range. *Mol. Syst. Biol.* 7:516. doi: 10.1038/msb.2011.50

Becker, V., Schilling, M., Bachmann, J., Baumann, U., Raue, A., Maiwald, T., et al. (2010). Covering a broad dynamic range: information processing at the erythropoietin receptor. *Science* 328, 1404–1408. doi: 10.1126/science.1184913

Behrmann, I., Smyczek, T., Heinrich, P. C., Schmitz-Van De Leur, H., Komyod, W., Giese, B., et al. (2004). Janus kinase (Jak) subcellular localization revisited: the exclusive membrane localization of endogenous Janus kinase 1 by cytokine receptor interaction uncovers the Jak.receptor complex to be equivalent to a receptor tyrosine kinase. *J. Biol. Chem.* 279, 35486–35493. doi: 10.1074/jbc.M404202200

Bode, J. G., Albrecht, U., Haussinger, D., Heinrich, P. C., and Schaper, F. (2012). Hepatic acute phase proteins–regulation by IL-6- and IL-1-type cytokines involving STAT3 and its crosstalk with NF-kappaB-dependent signaling. *Eur. J. Cell Biol.* 91, 496–505. doi: 10.1016/j.ejcb.2011.09.008

Bode, J. G., and Heinrich, P. C. (2001). "Interleukin-6 signalling during the acute phase response of the liver," in *The Liver: Biology and Pathobiology*, eds I. M. Arias, J. L. Boyer, F. V. Chisari, N. Fausto, D. Schachter, and D. A. Shafritz (Philadelphia, PA: Lippincott Williams Wilkins), 565–580.

Boehm, M. E., Hahn, B., and Lehmann, W. D. (2014). One-source peptide/phosphopeptide ratio standards for accurate and site-specific determination of the degree of phosphorylation. *Methods Mol. Biol.* 1156, 367–378. doi: 10.1007/978-1-4939-0685-7_24

Borisov, N., Aksamitiene, E., Kiyatkin, A., Legewie, S., Berkhout, J., Maiwald, T., et al. (2009). Systems-level interactions between insulin-EGF networks amplify mitogenic signaling. *Mol. Syst. Biol.* 5:256. doi: 10.1038/msb.2009.19

Brownell, J., and Polyak, S. J. (2013). Molecular pathways: hepatitis C virus, CXCL10, and the inflammatory road to liver cancer. *Clin. Cancer Res.* 19, 1347–1352. doi: 10.1158/1078-0432.CCR-12-0928

Calandra, T., Gerain, J., Heumann, D., Baumgartner, J. D., and Glauser, M. P. (1991). High circulating levels of interleukin-6 in patients with septic shock: evolution during sepsis, prognostic value, and interplay with other cytokines. The Swiss-Dutch J5 immunoglobulin study group. *Am. J. Med.* 91, 23–29. doi: 10.1016/0002-9343(91)90069-A

Chen, W. W., Niepel, M., and Sorger, P. K. (2010). Classic and contemporary approaches to modeling biochemical reactions. *Genes Dev.* 24, 1861–1875. doi: 10.1101/gad.1945410

Copeland, S., Warren, H. S., Lowry, S. F., Calvano, S. E., Remick, D., Inflammation and The Host Response to Injury (2005). Acute inflammatory response to endotoxin in mice and humans. *Clin. Diagn. Lab. Immunol.* 12, 60–67. doi: 10.1128/CDLI.12.1.60-67.2005

Cressman, D. E., Greenbaum, L. E., Deangelis, R. A., Ciliberto, G., Furth, E. E., Poli, V., et al. (1996). Liver failure and defective hepatocyte regeneration in interleukin-6-deficient mice. *Science* 274, 1379–1383. doi: 10.1126/science.274.5291.1379

Croker, B. A., Krebs, D. L., Zhang, J. G., Wormald, S., Willson, T. A., Stanley, E. G., et al. (2003). SOCS3 negatively regulates IL-6 signaling *in vivo*. *Nat. Immunol.* 4, 540–545. doi: 10.1038/ni931

Damas, P., Ledoux, D., Nys, M., Vrindts, Y., De Groote, D., Franchimont, P., et al. (1992). Cytokine serum level during severe sepsis in human IL-6 as a marker of severity. *Ann. Surg.* 215, 356–362. doi: 10.1097/00000658-199204000-00009

Dierssen, U., Beraza, N., Lutz, H. H., Liedtke, C., Ernst, M., Wasmuth, H. E., et al. (2008). Molecular dissection of gp130-dependent pathways in hepatocytes during liver regeneration. *J. Biol. Chem.* 283, 9886–9895. doi: 10.1074/jbc.M705483200

Dittrich, A., Quaiser, T., Khouri, C., Gortz, D., Monnigmann, M., and Schaper, F. (2012). Model-driven experimental analysis of the function of SHP-2 in IL-6-induced Jak/STAT signaling. *Mol. Biosyst.* 8, 2119–2134. doi: 10.1039/c2mb05488d

Dumoutier, L., De Heusch, M., Orabona, C., Satoh-Takayama, N., Eberl, G., Sirard, J. C., et al. (2011). IL-22 is produced by gamma C-independent CD25(+) CCR6(+) innate murine spleen cells upon inflammatory stimuli and contributes to LPS-induced lethality. *Eur. J. Immunol.* 41, 1075–1085. doi: 10.1002/eji.201040878

Fattori, E., Cappelletti, M., Costa, P., Sellitto, C., Cantoni, L., Carelli, M., et al. (1994). Defective inflammatory response in interleukin 6-deficient mice. *J. Exp. Med.* 180, 1243–1250. doi: 10.1084/jem.180.4.1243

Frei, K., Fredrikson, S., Fontana, A., and Link, H. (1991). Interleukin-6 is elevated in plasma in multiple sclerosis. *J. Neuroimmunol.* 31, 147–153. doi: 10.1016/0165-5728(91)90020-8

Ganz, T., and Nemeth, E. (2012). Hepcidin and iron homeostasis. *Biochim. Biophys. Acta* 1823, 1434–1443. doi: 10.1016/j.bbamcr.2012.01.014

Grivennikov, S. I., and Karin, M. (2011). Inflammatory cytokines in cancer: tumour necrosis factor and interleukin 6 take the stage. *Ann. Rheum. Dis.* 70 (Suppl. 1), i104–i108. doi: 10.1136/ard.2010.140145

Hahn, B., Bohm, M., Raia, V., Zinn, N., Moller, P., Klingmuller, U., et al. (2011). One-source peptide/phosphopeptide standards for accurate phosphorylation degree determination. *Proteomics* 11, 490–494. doi: 10.1002/pmic.201000569

Heikkila, K., Ebrahim, S., and Lawlor, D. A. (2008). Systematic review of the association between circulating interleukin-6 (IL-6) and cancer. *Eur. J. Cancer* 44, 937–945. doi: 10.1016/j.ejca.2008.02.047

Heim, M. H., Gamboni, G., Beglinger, C., and Gyr, K. (1997). Specific activation of AP-1 but not Stat3 in regenerating liver in mice. *Eur. J. Clin. Invest.* 27, 948–955. doi: 10.1046/j.1365-2362.1997.2100770.x

Heinrich, P. C., Behrmann, I., Haan, S., Hermanns, H. M., Muller-Newen, G., and Schaper, F. (2003). Principles of interleukin (IL)-6-type cytokine signalling and its regulation. *Biochem. J.* 374, 1–20. doi: 10.1042/bj20030407

Heinrich, P. C., Castell, J. V., and Andus, T. (1990). Interleukin-6 and the acute phase response. *Biochem. J.* 265, 621–636. doi: 10.1042/bj2650621

Herrmann, A., Vogt, M., Monnigmann, M., Clahsen, T., Sommer, U., Haan, S., et al. (2007). Nucleocytoplasmic shuttling of persistently activated STAT3. *J. Cell Sci.* 120, 3249–3261. doi: 10.1242/jcs.03482

Hirano, T., Matsuda, T., Turner, M., Miyasaka, N., Buchan, G., Tang, B., et al. (1988). Excessive production of interleukin 6/B cell stimulatory factor-2 in rheumatoid arthritis. *Eur. J. Immunol.* 18, 1797–1801. doi: 10.1002/eji.1830181122

Huang, M., Pang, X., Karalis, K., and Theoharides, T. C. (2003). Stress-induced interleukin-6 release in mice is mast cell-dependent and more pronounced in Apolipoprotein E knockout mice. *Cardiovasc. Res.* 59, 241–249. doi: 10.1016/S0008-6363(03)00340-7

Huard, J., Mueller, S., Gilles, E. D., Klingmuller, U., and Klamt, S. (2012). An integrative model links multiple inputs and signaling pathways to the onset of DNA synthesis in hepatocytes. *FEBS J.* 279, 3290–3313. doi: 10.1111/j.1742-4658.2012.08572.x

Hunter, C. A., and Jones, S. A. (2015). IL-6 as a keystone cytokine in health and disease. *Nat. Immunol.* 16, 448–457. doi: 10.1038/ni.3153

Ichikawa, T., Nakao, K., Nakata, K., Yamashita, M., Hamasaki, K., Shigeno, M., et al. (2002). Involvement of IL-1beta and IL-10 in IFN-alpha-mediated antiviral gene induction in human hepatoma cells. *Biochem. Biophys. Res. Commun.* 294, 414–422. doi: 10.1016/S0006-291X(02)00502-8

Ito, H. (2003). IL-6 and Crohn's disease. *Curr. Drug Targets Inflamm. Allergy* 2, 125–130. doi: 10.2174/1568010033484296

Iwamoto, N., D'alessandro, L. A., Depner, S., Hahn, B., Kramer, B. A., Lucarelli, P., et al. (2016). Context-specific flow through the MEK/ERK module produces cell- and ligand-specific patterns of ERK single and double phosphorylation. *Sci. Signal.* 9:ra13. doi: 10.1126/scisignal.aab1967

Kemna, E., Pickkers, P., Nemeth, E., Van Der Hoeven, H., and Swinkels, D. (2005). Time-course analysis of hepcidin, serum iron, and plasma cytokine levels in humans injected with LPS. *Blood* 106, 1864–1866. doi: 10.1182/blood-2005-03-1159

Kershaw, N. J., Murphy, J. M., Liau, N. P., Varghese, L. N., Laktyushin, A., Whitlock, E. L., et al. (2013). SOCS3 binds specific receptor-JAK complexes to control cytokine signaling by direct kinase inhibition. *Nat. Struct. Mol. Biol.* 20, 469–476. doi: 10.1038/nsmb.2519

Kitano, H., Funahashi, A., Matsuoka, Y., and Oda, K. (2005). Using process diagrams for the graphical representation of biological networks. *Nat. Biotechnol.* 23, 961–966. doi: 10.1038/nbt1111

Klein, C., Medina, E., Sander, L., Dierssen, U., Roskams, T., Mueller, W., et al. (2007). Contribution of interleukin-6/gp 130 signaling in hepatocytes to the inflammatory response in mice infected with *Streptococcus* pyogenes. *J. Infect. Dis.* 196, 755–762. doi: 10.1086/520090

Klingmuller, U., Bauer, A., Bohl, S., Nickel, P. J., Breitkopf, K., Dooley, S., et al. (2006). Primary mouse hepatocytes for systems biology approaches: a standardized *in vitro* system for modelling of signal transduction pathways. *Syst. Biol.* 153, 433–447. doi: 10.1049/ip-syb:20050067

Kopf, M., Baumann, H., Freer, G., Freudenberg, M., Lamers, M., Kishimoto, T., et al. (1994). Impaired immune and acute-phase responses in interleukin-6-deficient mice. *Nature* 368, 339–342. doi: 10.1038/368339a0

Kralovics, R., Passamonti, F., Buser, A. S., Teo, S. S., Tiedt, R., Passweg, J. R., et al. (2005). A gain-of-function mutation of JAK2 in myeloproliferative disorders. *N. Engl. J. Med.* 352, 1779–1790. doi: 10.1056/NEJMoa051113

Kreutz, C., Raue, A., and Timmer, J. (2012). Likelihood based observability analysis and confidence intervals for predictions of dynamic models. *BMC Syst. Biol.* 6:120. doi: 10.1186/1752-0509-6-120

Kudira, R., Malinka, T., Kohler, A., Dosch, M., De Aguero, M. G., Melin, N., et al. (2016). P2X1-regulated IL-22 secretion by innate lymphoid cells is required for efficient liver regeneration. *Hepatology* 63, 2004–2017. doi: 10.1002/hep.28492

Lehmann, U., Schmitz, J., Weissenbach, M., Sobota, R. M., Hortner, M., Friederichs, K., et al. (2003). SHP2 and SOCS3 contribute to Tyr-759-dependent attenuation of interleukin-6 signaling through gp130. *J. Biol. Chem.* 278, 661–671. doi: 10.1074/jbc.M210552200

Levenson, J., Giral, P., Razavian, M., Gariepy, J., and Simon, A. (1995). Fibrinogen and silent atherosclerosis in subjects with cardiovascular risk factors. *Arterioscler. Thromb. Vasc. Biol.* 15, 1263–1268. doi: 10.1161/01.ATV.15.9.1263

Lin, Q., Meloni, D., Pan, Y., Xia, M., Rodgers, J., Shepard, S., et al. (2009). Enantioselective synthesis of Janus kinase inhibitor INCB018424 via an organocatalytic aza-Michael reaction. *Organ. Lett.* 11, 1999–2002. doi: 10.1021/ol900350k

Liu, L., McBride, K. M., and Reich, N. C. (2005). STAT3 nuclear import is independent of tyrosine phosphorylation and mediated by importin-alpha3. *Proc. Natl. Acad. Sci. U.S.A.* 102, 8150–8155. doi: 10.1073/pnas.0501643102

Liu, P., Jenkins, N. A., and Copeland, N. G. (2003). A highly efficient recombineering-based method for generating conditional knockout mutations. *Genome Res.* 13, 476–484. doi: 10.1101/gr.749203

Lutticken, C., Wegenka, U. M., Yuan, J., Buschmann, J., Schindler, C., Ziemiecki, A., et al. (1994). Association of transcription factor APRF and protein kinase Jak1 with the interleukin-6 signal transducer gp130. *Science* 263, 89–92. doi: 10.1126/science.8272872

MacDonald, N. (1976). Time delay in simple chemostat models. *Biotechnol. Bioeng.* 18, 805–812. doi: 10.1002/bit.260180604

Maiwald, T., Hass, H., Steiert, B., Vanlier, J., Engesser, R., Raue, A., et al. (2016). Driving the model to its limit: profile likelihood based model reduction. *PLoS ONE* 11:e0162366. doi: 10.1371/journal.pone.0162366

Marvie, P., Lisbonne, M., L'helgoualc'h, A., Rauch, M., Turlin, B., Preisser, L., et al. (2010). Interleukin-33 overexpression is associated with liver fibrosis in mice and humans. *J. Cell. Mol. Med.* 14, 1726–1739. doi: 10.1111/j.1582-4934.2009.00801.x

Mesa, R. A., Yasothan, U., and Kirkpatrick, P. (2012). Ruxolitinib. *Nat. Rev. Drug Discov.* 11, 103–104. doi: 10.1038/nrd3652

Miller, A. M. (2011). Role of IL-33 in inflammation and disease. *J. Inflamm.* 8:22. doi: 10.1186/1476-9255-8-22

Mitchell, C., and Willenbring, H. (2008). A reproducible and well-tolerated method for 2/3 partial hepatectomy in mice. *Nat. Protoc.* 3, 1167–1170. doi: 10.1038/nprot.2008.80

Moya, C., Huang, Z., Cheng, P., Jayaraman, A., and Hahn, J. (2011). Investigation of IL-6 and IL-10 signalling via mathematical modelling. *IET Syst. Biol.* 5:15. doi: 10.1049/iet-syb.2009.0060

Mueller, S., Huard, J., Waldow, K., Huang, X., D'alessandro, L. A., Bohl, S., et al. (2015). T160-phosphorylated CDK2 defines threshold for HGF-dependent proliferation in primary hepatocytes. *Mol. Syst. Biol.* 11:795. doi: 10.15252/msb.20156032

Murray, P. J. (2006). Understanding and exploiting the endogenous interleukin-10/STAT3-mediated anti-inflammatory response. *Curr. Opin. Pharmacol.* 6, 379–386. doi: 10.1016/j.coph.2006.01.010

Nakamura, K., Nonaka, H., Saito, H., Tanaka, M., and Miyajima, A. (2004). Hepatocyte proliferation and tissue remodeling is impaired after liver injury in oncostatin M receptor knockout mice. *Hepatology* 39, 635–644. doi: 10.1002/hep.20086

Navikas, V., Matusevicius, D., Soderstrom, M., Fredrikson, S., Kivisakk, P., Ljungdahl, A., et al. (1996). Increased interleukin-6 mRNA expression in blood and cerebrospinal fluid mononuclear cells in multiple sclerosis. *J. Neuroimmunol.* 64, 63–69. doi: 10.1016/0165-5728(95)00155-7

Nechemia-Arbely, Y., Shriki, A., Denz, U., Drucker, C., Scheller, J., Raub, J., et al. (2011). Early hepatocyte DNA synthetic response posthepatectomy is modulated by IL-6 trans-signaling and PI3K/AKT activation. *J. Hepatol.* 54, 922–929. doi: 10.1016/j.jhep.2010.08.017

Nelson, D. E., Ihekwaba, A. E. C., Elliott, M., Johnson, J. R., Gibney, C. A., Foreman, B. E., et al. (2004). Oscillations in NF-kappa B signaling control the dynamics of gene expression. *Science* 306, 704–708. doi: 10.1126/science.1099962

Nishina, T., Komazawa-Sakon, S., Yanaka, S., Piao, X. H., Zheng, D. M., Piao, J. H., et al. (2012). Interleukin-11 Links Oxidative Stress and Compensatory Proliferation. *Sci. Signal.* 5:ra5. doi: 10.1126/scisignal.2002056

Norrby-Teglund, A., Pauksens, K., Norgren, M., and Holm, S. E. (1995). Correlation between serum TNF alpha and IL6 levels and severity of group a streptococcal infections. *Scand. J. Infect. Dis.* 27, 125–130. doi: 10.3109/00365549509018991

Pettitt, S. J., Liang, Q., Rairdan, X. Y., Moran, J. L., Prosser, H. M., Beier, D. R., et al. (2009). Agouti C57BL/6N embryonic stem cells for mouse genetic resources. *Nat. Methods* 6, 493–495. doi: 10.1038/nmeth.1342

Piao, W., Ru, L. W., Piepenbrink, K. H., Sundberg, E. J., Vogel, S. N., and Toshchakov, V. Y. (2013). Recruitment of TLR adapter TRIF to TLR4 signaling complex is mediated by the second helical region of TRIF TIR domain. *Proc. Natl. Acad. Sci. U.S.A.* 110, 19036–19041. doi: 10.1073/pnas.1313575110

Pietrangelo, A., Dierssen, U., Valli, L., Garuti, C., Rump, A., Corradini, E., et al. (2007). STAT3 is required for IL-6-gp130-dependent activation of hepcidin *in vivo*. *Gastroenterology* 132, 294–300. doi: 10.1053/j.gastro.2006.10.018

Quintas-Cardama, A., Kantarjian, H., Cortes, J., and Verstovsek, S. (2011). Janus kinase inhibitors for the treatment of myeloproliferative neoplasias and beyond. *Nat. Rev. Drug Discov.* 10, 127–140. doi: 10.1038/nrd3264

Quintas-Cardama, A., Vaddi, K., Liu, P., Manshouri, T., Li, J., Scherle, P. A., et al. (2010). Preclinical characterization of the selective JAK1/2 inhibitor INCB018424: therapeutic implications for the treatment of myeloproliferative neoplasms. *Blood* 115, 3109–3117. doi: 10.1182/blood-2009-04-214957

Raia, V., Schilling, M., Bohm, M., Hahn, B., Kowarsch, A., Raue, A., et al. (2011). Dynamic mathematical modeling of IL13-induced signaling in Hodgkin and primary mediastinal B-cell lymphoma allows prediction of therapeutic targets. *Cancer Res.* 71, 693–704. doi: 10.1158/0008-5472.CAN-10-2987

Rao, R., Graffeo, C. S., Gulati, R., Jamal, M., Narayan, S., Zambirinis, C. P., et al. (2014). Interleukin 17-producing gamma delta T Cells promote hepatic regeneration in mice. *Gastroenterology* 147, 473–484. doi: 10.1053/j.gastro.2014.04.042

Raue, A., Steiert, B., Schelker, M., Kreutz, C., Maiwald, T., Hass, H., et al. (2015). Data2Dynamics: a modeling environment tailored to parameter estimation in dynamical systems. *Bioinformatics* 31, 3558–3560. doi: 10.1093/bioinformatics/btv405

Reich, N. C., and Liu, L. (2006). Tracking STAT nuclear traffic. *Nat. Rev. Immunol.* 6, 602–612. doi: 10.1038/nri1885

Ren, X. D., Hu, B., and Colletti, L. M. (2010). IL-22 is involved in liver regeneration after hepatectomy. *Am. J. Physiol. Gastrointest. Liver Physiol.* 298, G74–G80. doi: 10.1152/ajpgi.00075.2009

Ritchie, M. E., Phipson, B., Wu, D., Hu, Y., Law, C. W., Shi, W., et al. (2015). limma powers differential expression analyses for RNA-sequencing and microarray studies. *Nucleic Acids Res.* 43:e47. doi: 10.1093/nar/gkv007

Rote, L. (2016). *Jakavi (R) [Package Insert]; Novartis Pharma GmbH.* Nürnberg. Available online at: http://www.patienteninfo-service.de/a-z-liste/j/jakaviR-5-mg-10-mg-15-mg-20-mg-tabletten/ (Accessed February 21, 2017).

Sabat, R., Grutz, G., Warszawska, K., Kirsch, S., Witte, E., Wolk, K., et al. (2010). Biology of interleukin-10. *Cytokine Growth Factor Rev.* 21, 331–344. doi: 10.1016/j.cytogfr.2010.09.002

Sakamori, R., Takehara, T., Tatsumi, T., Shigekawa, M., Hikita, H., Hiramatsu, N., et al. (2010). STAT3 signaling within hepatocytes is required for anemia of inflammation *in vivo*. *J. Gastroenterol.* 45, 244–248. doi: 10.1007/s00535-009-0159-y

Sakamoto, T., Liu, Z., Murase, N., Ezure, T., Yokomuro, S., Poli, V., et al. (1999). Mitosis and apoptosis in the liver of interleukin-6-deficient mice after partial hepatectomy. *Hepatology* 29, 403–411. doi: 10.1002/hep.510290244

Samsonov, A., Zenser, N., Zhang, F., Zhang, H. Y., Fetter, J., and Malkov, D. (2013). Tagging of genomic STAT3 and STAT1 with fluorescent proteins and insertion of a luciferase reporter in the cyclin D1 gene provides a modified A549 cell line to screen for selective STAT3 inhibitors. *PLoS ONE* 8:e68391. doi: 10.1371/journal.pone.0068391

Sasagawa, S., Ozaki, Y., Fujita, K., and Kuroda, S. (2005). Prediction and validation of the distinct dynamics of transient and sustained ERK activation. *Nat. Cell Biol.* 7, 365–373. doi: 10.1038/ncb1233

Schilling, M., Maiwald, T., Bohl, S., Kollmann, M., Kreutz, C., Timmer, J., et al. (2005a). Computational processing and error reduction strategies for standardized quantitative data in biological networks. *FEBS J.* 272, 6400–6411. doi: 10.1111/j.1742-4658.2005.05037.x

Schilling, M., Maiwald, T., Bohl, S., Kollmann, M., Kreutz, C., Timmer, J., et al. (2005b). Quantitative data generation for systems biology: the impact of randomisation, calibrators and normalisers. *Syst. Biol.* 152, 193–200. doi: 10.1049/ip-syb:20050044

Schindelin, J., Arganda-Carreras, I., Frise, E., Kaynig, V., Longair, M., Pietzsch, T., et al. (2012). Fiji: an open-source platform for biological-image analysis. *Nat. Methods* 9, 676–682. doi: 10.1038/nmeth.2019

Schmitz, J., Owyang, A., Oldham, E., Song, Y., Murphy, E., McClanahan, T. K., et al. (2005). IL-33, an interleukin-1-like cytokine that signals via the IL-1 receptor-related protein ST2 and induces T helper type 2-associated cytokines. *Immunity* 23, 479–490. doi: 10.1016/j.immuni.2005.09.015

Schoeberl, B., Pace, E. A., Fitzgerald, J. B., Harms, B. D., Xu, L., Nie, L., et al. (2009). Therapeutically targeting ErbB3: a key node in ligand-induced activation of the ErbB receptor-PI3K axis. *Sci. Signal.* 2:ra31. doi: 10.1126/scisignal.2000352

Schust, J., Sperl, B., Hollis, A., Mayer, T. U., and Berg, T. (2006). Stattic: a small-molecule inhibitor of STAT3 activation and dimerization. *Chem. Biol.* 13, 1235–1242. doi: 10.1016/j.chembiol.2006.09.018

Schwenk, F., Baron, U., and Rajewsky, K. (1995). A cre-transgenic mouse strain for the ubiquitous deletion of loxP-flanked gene segments including deletion in germ cells. *Nucleic Acids Res.* 23, 5080–5081. doi: 10.1093/nar/23.24.5080

Shi, J. G., Chen, X., McGee, R. F., Landman, R. R., Emm, T., Lo, Y., et al. (2011). The pharmacokinetics, pharmacodynamics, and safety of orally dosed INCB018424 phosphate in healthy volunteers. *J. Clin. Pharmacol.* 51, 1644–1654. doi: 10.1177/0091270010389469

Shilling, A. D., Nedza, F. M., Emm, T., Diamond, S., McKeever, E., Punwani, N., et al. (2010). Metabolism, excretion, and pharmacokinetics of [14C]INCB018424, a selective Janus tyrosine kinase 1/2 inhibitor, in humans. *Drug Metab. Dispos.* 38, 2023–2031. doi: 10.1124/dmd.110.033787

Sick, S., Reinker, S., Timmer, J., and Schlake, T. (2006). WNT and DKK determine hair follicle spacing through a reaction-diffusion mechanism. *Science* 314, 1447–1450. doi: 10.1126/science.1130088

Simoncic, P. D., Lee-Loy, A., Barber, D. L., Tremblay, M. L., and McGlade, C. J. (2002). The T cell protein tyrosine phosphatase is a negative regulator of janus family kinases 1 and 3. *Curr. Biol.* 12, 446–453. doi: 10.1016/S0960-9822(02)00697-8

Singh, A., Jayaraman, A., and Hahn, J. (2006). Modeling regulatory mechanisms in IL-6 signal transduction in hepatocytes. *Biotechnol. Bioeng.* 95, 850–862. doi: 10.1002/bit.21026

Slotwinski, R., Olszewski, W. L., Paluszkiewicz, R., Zieniewicz, K., Hevelke, P., Zaleska, M., et al. (2002). Serum cytokine concentration after liver lobe harvesting for transplantation. *Ann. Transplant.* 7, 36–39.

Stahl, N., Farruggella, T. J., Boulton, T. G., Zhong, Z., Darnell, J. E. Jr., and Yancopoulos, G. D. (1995). Choice of STATs and other substrates specified by modular tyrosine-based motifs in cytokine receptors. *Science* 267, 1349–1353. doi: 10.1126/science.7871433

Starr, R., Willson, T. A., Viney, E. M., Murray, L. J., Rayner, J. R., Jenkins, B. J., et al. (1997). A family of cytokine-inducible inhibitors of signalling. *Nature* 387, 917–921. doi: 10.1038/43206

Steiert, B., Raue, A., Timmer, J., and Kreutz, C. (2012). Experimental design for parameter estimation of gene regulatory networks. *PLoS ONE* 7:e40052. doi: 10.1371/journal.pone.0040052

Swameye, I., Muller, T. G., Timmer, J., Sandra, O., and Klingmuller, U. (2003). Identification of nucleocytoplasmic cycling as a remote sensor in cellular signaling by databased modeling. *Proc. Natl. Acad. Sci. U.S.A.* 100, 1028–1033. doi: 10.1073/pnas.0237333100

Taga, T., Hibi, M., Hirata, Y., Yamasaki, K., Yasukawa, K., Matsuda, T., et al. (1989). Interleukin-6 triggers the association of its receptor with a possible signal transducer, gp130. *Cell* 58, 573–581. doi: 10.1016/0092-8674(89)90438-8

Tennent, G. A., Lovat, L. B., and Pepys, M. B. (1995). Serum amyloid P component prevents proteolysis of the amyloid fibrils of Alzheimer disease and systemic amyloidosis. *Proc. Natl. Acad. Sci. U.S.A.* 92, 4299–4303. doi: 10.1073/pnas.92.10.4299

Vandam, M., Mullberg, J., Schooltink, H., Stoyan, T., Brakenhoff, J. P. J., Graeve, L., et al. (1993). Structure-function analysis of interleukin-6 utilizing human murine chimeric molecules - involvement of 2 separate domains in receptor-binding. *J. Biol. Chem.* 268, 15285–15290.

Vandesompele, J., De Preter, K., Pattyn, F., Poppe, B., Van Roy, N., De Paepe, A., et al. (2002). Accurate normalization of real-time quantitative RT-PCR data by geometric averaging of multiple internal control genes. *Genome Biol.* 3:research0034. doi: 10.1186/gb-2002-3-7-research0034

Vanlier, J., Tiemann, C. A., Hilbers, P. A. J., and Van Riel, N. A. W. (2013). Parameter uncertainty in biochemical models described by ordinary differential equations. *Math. Biosci.* 246, 305–314. doi: 10.1016/j.mbs.2013.03.006

Vannucchi, A. M., Kiladjian, J. J., Griesshammer, M., Masszi, T., Durrant, S., Passamonti, F., et al. (2015). Ruxolitinib versus standard therapy for the treatment of polycythemia vera. *N. Engl. J. Med.* 372, 426–435. doi: 10.1056/NEJMoa1409002

Verstovsek, S., Mesa, R. A., Gotlib, J., Levy, R. S., Gupta, V., Dipersio, J. F., et al.

basic and clinical investigations. The JAK1/2 inhibitor Ruxolitinib/INCB018424 (Jakavi/Jakafi, Incyte Pharmaceuticals, Novartis; Lin et al., 2009; Quintas-Cardama et al., 2010) has been internationally approved for the therapy of myelofibrosis (Mesa et al., 2012; Verstovsek et al., 2012) and polycythemia vera (Vannucchi et al., 2015), which are frequently caused by the V617F gain-of-function mutation within JAK2 (Kralovics et al., 2005). According to the guidelines, the recommendation for Jakavi is a repetitive, constant dose of 10 mg twice daily (q12h) for polycythemia vera or 20 mg twice daily (q12h) for myelofibrosis (Rote, 2016). Ruxolitinib affects the hematological status of patients and therefore the platelet count should be assessed before the start of a therapy. Since low neutrophil counts have been observed in 66% of healthy volunteers treated with 100 mg Ruxolitinib daily (q24h; Shi et al., 2011), it is of great importance not to exceed the recommended daily doses. Ruxolitinib is also tested for the treatment of other malignancies as well as chronic inflammatory diseases such as rheumatoid arthritis (Williams et al., 2008; Quintas-Cardama et al., 2011).

The STAT3 inhibitor Stattic, which is not approved for clinical applications, targets the STAT3 SH2 domain, thus blocking receptor association and dimerization. Stattic treatment inhibited IL-6-induced STAT3 phosphorylation and nuclear translocation in hepatocytes (Schust et al., 2006). Moreover, increased apoptosis was observed in STAT3-dependent cancer cell lines upon Stattic treatment (Schust et al., 2006). Although the molecular mechanisms of Ruxolitinib and Stattic are well-established, their impact on the dynamics of signal transduction, expression of target genes, and cellular response is, due to the non-linear reactions, not intuitive.

Mathematical models based on ordinary differential equations (ODEs) are well-suited to study the dynamics of signal transduction and have enabled the identification of therapeutic targets within signaling networks (Schoeberl et al., 2009; Raia et al., 2011). ODEs describe concentration changes of species over time. The law of mass-action kinetics defines a reaction rate to be proportional to the concentrations of reacting biomolecules thus facilitating the translation of a pathway map into a set of ODEs. In the model, species concentrations are the state variables, while rate constants, initial conditions, or other proportionality factors are termed parameters. Although, some parameter values such as initial protein concentrations may be accessible by measurements, most parameter values remain unknown and have to be estimated based on experimental data (Aldridge et al., 2006; Chen et al., 2010). This process is called model calibration and requires highly quantitative and reproducible experimental data, as well as a sufficient number of data points and measured species (Bachmann et al., 2012).

Formulating biological hypotheses in terms of mathematical models allows to quantitatively test such hypotheses by challenging model predictions with additional experimental data. For example Swameye et al. established a dynamic pathway model for the JAK2-STAT5 signaling pathway and tested conflicting hypothesis on signal transduction from the cell surface receptor to the nucleus (Swameye et al., 2003). The mathematical model revealed that STAT5 acts as a remote sensor for receptor activation and that repeated nucleocytoplasmic cycling of STAT5 is required for effective target gene activation in the nucleus. Furthermore, by a mathematical modeling approach Sasagawa et al. showed that the transient activation of ERK depends on rapid increases in the amount of epidermal growth factor and nerve growth factor (NGF), while sustained ERK activation depends on the final NGF concentration (Sasagawa et al., 2005). Nelson et al. revealed that oscillations observed in TNFalpha induced activation of NF-kB control the dynamics of gene expression. The mathematical modeling approach revealed that two molecular species were strongly coupled to the oscillation dynamics (Nelson et al., 2004). By iteratively combining mathematical modeling with model-guided experiments, these and other studies (Alon et al., 1999; Sick et al., 2006; Borisov et al., 2009; Becker et al., 2010; Bachmann et al., 2011) demonstrated that it is possible to capture biological behavior, reject hypotheses which fail to describe data and make non-trivial predictions for validation experiments. Moreover, uncertainty analysis can give insight into how well a model is constrained and what kind of predictive power one can expect when predicting similar experiments (Kreutz et al., 2012; Vanlier et al., 2013). Additionally, validation experiments guided by well-constrained predictions can be performed to improve the confidence in the model (Steiert et al., 2012).

Although several ODE-based mathematical models of IL-6 signaling have been reported to date (Singh et al., 2006; Moya et al., 2011; Dittrich et al., 2012), only with a recently described mathematical model (Xu et al., 2015) potential effects of targeting selected pathway components on APP expression were tested *in silico*. These studies predicted that IL-6 signaling could be best targeted at the receptor level, and that reduced inhibitor dose may be achievable by applying possible inhibitor combinations (Xu et al., 2015). However, the model-based predictions reported by Xu et al. were not experimentally validated, thus limiting applicability to targeting IL-6 signaling in human disease.

Here we present an ODE model of IL-6-induced JAK1-STAT3 signaling in primary mouse hepatocytes. Based on extensive experimental data, the mathematical model describes pathway activation and key target gene induction during regenerative and inflammatory conditions, as well as the impact of the pathway inhibitors Ruxolitinib and Stattic. We combined model predictions with experimental validation to optimize the long-term Ruxolitinib-mediated reduction of APP gene expression, while maintaining gene expression levels that are present during regenerative conditions without employing excessive inhibitor concentrations. The presented approach represents a starting point for systematic clinical intervention in inflammatory or malignant diseases.

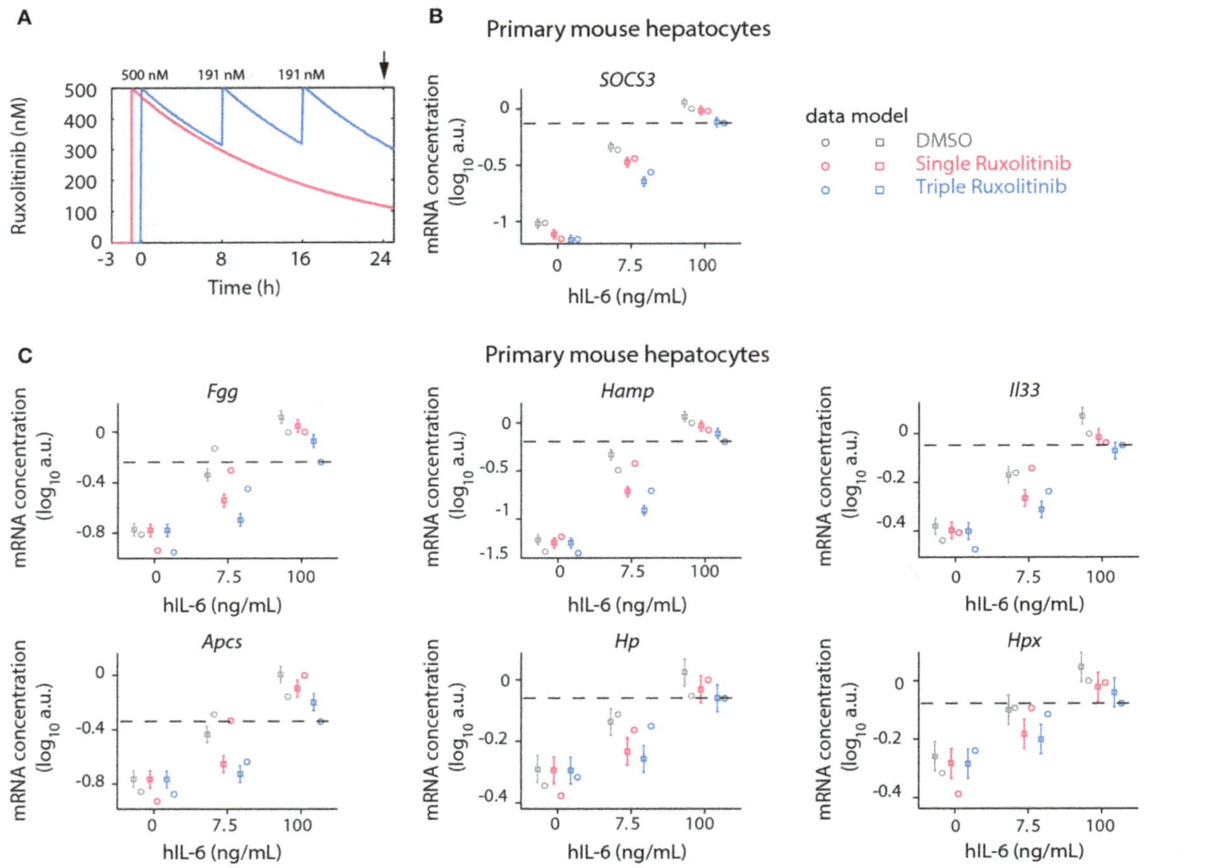

FIGURE 8 | Optimized inhibition of APP gene expression in primary mouse hepatocytes. **(A)** Model predictions for Ruxolitinib concentrations over time after single treatment with 500 nM at $t = -1$ h (Single), or using the optimized triple treatment scenario, including Ruxolitinib treatments at $t = 0$ h (500 nM), 8 h (191 nM), and 16 h (191 nM) (Triple). Arrow indicates the time point of gene expression analysis. **(B,C)** Expression of *Socs3* **(B)** and APP genes **(C)** at 24 h after inhibitor treatments as described in **(A)**. Squares represent model predictions and circles represents experimental data, while error bars indicate the measurement noise estimated by the error model. a.u., arbitrary units. Dashed lines indicate the level of gene expression after triple inhibitor dosing of the cells treated with inflammatory dose of hIL-6 (100 ng/mL). Displayed are results of one biological replicate, while two more replicates are shown in Appendix Figure S7. For additional experimental data used for model validation see Appendix Figures S89–S91.

(**Figure 1**). In hepatocytes derived from mKate2-STAT3 mice, we analyzed the nuclear mKate2-STAT3 concentration within the time frame 20–24 h (after start of IL-6 treatment) by live-cell imaging (**Figure 7C**). Comparing model predictions and experimental data for the different Ruxolitinib treatment regimens and IL-6 concentrations revealed good agreement between model and experiment (**Figure 7D** and Appendix Figure S6): Ruxolitinib-mediated suppression of mKate2-STAT3 nuclear translocation was improved when the triple treatment regime was applied, compared with single treatment. In wild type hepatocytes we measured APP gene expression at 24 h. Triple Ruxolitinib treatment lead to improved suppression of most genes, compared with single Ruxolitinib treatment (**Figure 8** and Appendix Figure S7). The effect was most obvious for *Socs3*, and also recognizable for all other genes, although error bars were partly overlapping for single and triple treatment. Importantly, triple Ruxolitinib treatment reduced gene expression observed at inflammatory IL-6 concentrations (100 ng/mL) to levels more closely resembling regenerative conditions (7.5 ng/mL, DMSO control) for all genes (**Figure 8** and Appendix Figure S7). To conclude, our mathematical model and experimental validation suggested that a triple treatment with Ruxolitinib and not a single dose is required, when an effective attenuation of IL-6-dependent responses in hepatocytes is desired.

To provide a proof-of-concept that these insights, obtained with our model based approach for primary mouse hepatocytes, are applicable to the human system, we employed primary human hepatocytes to compare a single bolus treatment with the model-suggested triple dosing strategy. To mimic the regenerative and inflammatory situation in the human system, 1.8 and 50 ng/mL hIL-6 were chosen to stimulate human hepatocytes, assuming that the potency of human IL-6 on human hepatocytes is comparable to that of mouse IL-6 on primary mouse hepatocytes and by utilizing the dose response curves shown in **Figure 1D**.

(2012). A double-blind, placebo-controlled trial of ruxolitinib for myelofibrosis. *N. Engl. J. Med.* 366, 799–807. doi: 10.1056/NEJMoa1110557

Waage, A., Brandtzaeg, P., Halstensen, A., Kierulf, P., and Espevik, T. (1989). The complex pattern of cytokines in serum from patients with meningococcal septic shock. association between interleukin 6, interleukin 1, and fatal outcome. *J. Exp. Med.* 169, 333–338. doi: 10.1084/jem.169.1.333

Wallace, D. F., and Subramaniam, V. N. (2015). Analysis of IL-22 contribution to hepcidin induction and hypoferremia during the response to LPS *in vivo*. *Int. Immunol.* 27, 281–287. doi: 10.1093/intimm/dxu144

Wegenka, U. M., Dikopoulos, N., Reimann, J., Adler, G., and Wahl, C. (2007). The murine liver is a potential target organ for IL-19, IL-20 and IL-24: type I Interferons and LPS regulate the expression of IL-20R2. *J. Hepatol.* 46, 257–265. doi: 10.1016/j.jhep.2006.08.009

Weinstein, D. A., Roy, C. N., Fleming, M. D., Loda, M. F., Wolfsdorf, J. I., and Andrews, N. C. (2002). Inappropriate expression of hepcidin is associated with iron refractory anemia: implications for the anemia of chronic disease. *Blood* 100, 3776–3781. doi: 10.1182/blood-2002-04-1260

Williams, W., Scherle, P., Shi, J., Newton, R., McKeever, E., Fridman, J., et al. (2008). *A Randomized Placebo-Controlled Study of INCB018424, A Selective Janus kinase 1& 2 (JAK1 & 2) Inhibitor in Rheumatoid Arthritis (RA)*. American College of Rheumatology - Annual Scientific Meeting.

Wisniewski, J. R., Vildhede, A., Noren, A., and Artursson, P. (2016). In-depth quantitative analysis and comparison of the human hepatocyte and hepatoma cell line HepG2 proteomes. *J. Proteomics* 136, 234–247. doi: 10.1016/j.jprot.2016.01.016

Wrighting, D. M., and Andrews, N. C. (2006). Interleukin-6 induces hepcidin expression through STAT3. *Blood* 108, 3204–3209. doi: 10.1182/blood-2006-06-027631

Xu, W., Joo, H., Clayton, S., Dullaers, M., Herve, M. C., Blankenship, D., et al. (2012). Macrophages induce differentiation of plasma cells through CXCL10/IP-10. *J. Exp. Med.* 209, 1813–1823, S1811–S1812. doi: 10.1084/jem.20112142

Xu, Z., Karlsson, J., and Huang, Z. (2015). Modeling the dynamics of acute phase protein expression in human hepatoma cells stimulated by IL-6. *Processes* 3, 50–70. doi: 10.3390/pr3010050

Yamamoto, T., Sekine, Y., Kashima, K., Kubota, A., Sato, N., Aoki, N., et al. (2002). The nuclear isoform of protein-tyrosine phosphatase TC-PTP regulates interleukin-6-mediated signaling pathway through STAT3 dephosphorylation. *Biochem. Biophys. Res. Commun.* 297, 811–817. doi: 10.1016/S0006-291X(02)02291-X

Yamanaka, Y., Nakajima, K., Fukada, T., Hibi, M., and Hirano, T. (1996). Differentiation and growth arrest signals are generated through the cytoplasmic region of gp130 that is essential for Stat3 activation. *EMBO J.* 15, 1557–1565.

Yasukawa, H., Ohishi, M., Mori, H., Murakami, M., Chinen, T., Aki, D., et al. (2003). IL-6 induces an anti-inflammatory response in the absence of SOCS3 in macrophages. *Nat. Immunol.* 4, 551–556. doi: 10.1038/ni938

Yin, S., Wang, H., Park, O., Wei, W., Shen, J., and Gao, B. (2011). Enhanced liver regeneration in IL-10-deficient mice after partial hepatectomy via stimulating inflammatory response and activating hepatocyte STAT3. *Am. J. Pathol.* 178, 1614–1621. doi: 10.1016/j.ajpath.2011.01.001

Zeremski, M., Dimova, R., Brown, Q., Jacobson, I. M., Markatou, M., and Talal, A. H. (2009). Peripheral CXCR3-associated chemokines as biomarkers of fibrosis in chronic hepatitis C virus infection. *J. Infect. Dis.* 200, 1774–1780. doi: 10.1086/646614

Zeremski, M., Petrovic, L. M., Chiriboga, L., Brown, Q. B., Yee, H. T., Kinkhabwala, M., et al. (2008). Intrahepatic levels of CXCR3-associated chemokines correlate with liver inflammation and fibrosis in chronic hepatitis C. *Hepatology* 48, 1440–1450. doi: 10.1002/hep.22500

Zimmers, T. A., Pierce, R. H., McKillop, I. H., and Koniaris, L. G. (2003). Resolving the role of IL-6 in liver regeneration. *Hepatology* 38, 1590–1591; author reply: 1591. doi: 10.1016/j.hep.2003.09.021

2

Dynamic Metabolic Zonation of the Hepatic Glucose Metabolism is Accomplished by Sinusoidal Plasma Gradients of Nutrients and Hormones

Nikolaus Berndt[1,2] *and Hermann-Georg Holzhütter*[1*]

[1] *Computational Biochemistry Group, Institute of Biochemistry, Charite—University Medicine Berlin, Berlin, Germany,*
[2] *Institute for Computational and Imaging Science in Cardiovascular Medicine, Charite—University Medicine Berlin, Berlin, Germany*

Correspondence:
Hermann-Georg Holzhütter
hergo@charite.de

Being the central metabolic organ of vertebrates, the liver possesses the largest repertoire of metabolic enzymes among all tissues and organs. Almost all metabolic pathways are resident in the parenchymal cell, hepatocyte, but the pathway capacities may largely differ depending on the localization of hepatocytes within the liver acinus-a phenomenon that is commonly referred to as metabolic zonation. Metabolic zonation is rather dynamic since gene expression patterns of metabolic enzymes may change in response to nutrition, drugs, hormones and pathological states of the liver (e.g., fibrosis and inflammation). This fact has to be ultimately taken into account in mathematical models aiming at the prediction of metabolic liver functions in different physiological and pathological settings. Here we present a spatially resolved kinetic tissue model of hepatic glucose metabolism which includes zone-specific temporal changes of enzyme abundances which are driven by concentration gradients of nutrients, hormones and oxygen along the hepatic sinusoids. As key modulators of enzyme expression we included oxygen, glucose and the hormones insulin and glucagon which also control enzyme activities by cAMP-dependent reversible phosphorylation. Starting with an initially non-zonated model using plasma profiles under fed, fasted and diabetic conditions, zonal patterns of glycolytic and gluconeogenetic enzymes as well as glucose uptake and release rates are created as an emergent property. We show that mechanisms controlling the adaptation of enzyme abundances to varying external conditions necessarily lead to the zonation of hepatic carbohydrate metabolism. To the best of our knowledge, this is the first kinetic tissue model which takes into account in a semi-mechanistic way all relevant levels of enzyme regulation.

Keywords: metabolism, metabolic zonation, kinetic model, multiscale model, gene expression

INTRODUCTION

The tightly controlled switch between hepatic uptake and release of glucose keeps the plasma glucose concentrations within a range between 4 and 10 mM despite largely varying carbohydrate intake and utilization. This homeostatic function of the liver with respect to plasma glucose is achieved by several enzyme-regulatory mechanisms acting on different time scales. On the short term, hormone-dependent reversible enzyme phosphorylation and changes of reaction rates elicited by concentration changes of reaction substrates/products and allosteric modulators enable a metabolic response within seconds or minutes. Recurrent activation of these fast regulatory modes is typically accompanied by slow changes in the abundance of metabolic enzymes on a time scale of hours to days (Hopgood et al., 1973; Weinberg and Utter, 1980). Both the fast and slow mode of enzyme regulation are important for the regulation of the glucose exchange flux between hepatocytes and blood plasma (Bulik et al., 2016), Owing to concentration gradients of oxygen, metabolites, hormones, and morphogens along the hepatic capillaries (sinusoids) the expression of metabolic enzymes may differ in various zones of the liver acinus. For example, the oxygen pressure decreases by 50% along the porto-central axis of the acinus (Jungermann and Kietzmann, 2000). This goes in line with the number and structure of mitochondria (Schmucker et al., 1978) and glycolytic capacities in the periportal and pericentral zone (Braeuning et al., 2006). Hepatocytes close to the portal pole (zone 1) experiencing the highest concentration of oxygen pressure are predestined for strong ATP-demanding anabolic pathways like gluconeogenesis and urea synthesis. Contrary, hepatocytes close to the venous pole of the acinus (zone 3) experience the lowest oxygen concentrations and thus possess a high glycolytic capacity, a typical feature of cells working under conditions of permanent oxygen deprivation. The heterogeneous allocation of gluconeogenetic and glycolytic capacities to different hepatocytes along the porto-central axis may even result in a situation where a certain fraction of glucose produced by periportal cells is used to fuel the glycolysis of pericentral cells (Berndt et al., 2018).

Several blood-born factors have been identified as regulators of zone-dependent gene expression of metabolic enzymes. Oxygen, glucose, the hormones glucagon and insulin, the morphogens Wnt and hedgehog and the growth factor HGF belong to the best studied factors. The various factors appear to act in a hierarchical fashion whereby the gradients of morphogens and growth factors create a basic expression pattern that is further modulated by nutrition-related factors such as oxygen, glucose, fatty acids and the hormones insulin and glucagon. In this work, we will focus on the latter group of modifiers, i.e., we restrict our model to the metabolic response of the liver to nutritional challenges and oxygen availability.

Metabolic adaptation of hepatocytes to varying oxygen pressures is mainly controlled by hypoxia-inducible transcription factors (HIFs), heterodimeric complexes consisting of a constitutively expressed β-subunit and an oxygen-sensitive α-subunit. In the liver, HIF-1α regulates primarily glycolytic genes whereas HIF-2α is known to primarily regulate genes involved in cell proliferation and iron metabolism (Ramakrishnan and Shah, 2017). In line with the falling oxygen pressure along the porto-central axis, HIFαs were found with higher levels in the less aerobic pericentral zone (Kietzmann et al., 2001). Besides oxygen, the pancreatic hormones insulin and glucagon are important drivers of zone-dependent differences in enzyme activities. The regulatory role of these hormones is 2-fold. They control the cellular cAMP level in an antagonistic manner and thus exert opposite effects on the reversible phosphorylation of key regulatory enzymes of glycolysis and gluconeogenesis as PFK2, PK, and PEPCK. The hepatic clearance of the two hormones by endocytic uptake into hepatocytes creates a concentration gradient along the porto-central axis which entails zone-dependent differences in the phosphorylation level of interconvertible enzymes. With respect to gene expression of metabolic enzymes, insulin and glucagon also control the efficiency of several transcription factors as ChREBP, SREBP-1c, CREB, and Foxo (Han et al., 2016). Both actions of glucagon and insulin are tightly interrelated and function in part through the same mechanisms. For example, the cAMP-activated protein kinase A (PKA) is responsible for phosphorylation of interconvertible enzymes such as FBPFK2 and PK, as well as for the phosphorylation of the transcription factors ChREBP and CREP (Uyeda and Repa, 2006). cAMP is produced by glucagon-induced activation of the adenylate cyclase and degraded by insulin-stimulated cAMP phosphodiesterase. Consequently, the protein level of key regulatory enzymes reflects the integral hormone levels over longer time periods.

In this work we included dynamic changes in the abundance of metabolic enzymes into our previously developed multi-scale tissue model of hepatic glucose metabolism (Berndt et al., 2018). The rates of protein synthesis and degradation were modeled by phenomenological rate equations which were parameterized by using experimentally determined protein levels at varying concentrations of oxygen, glucose, insulin, and glucagon. The central aims of our work were (i) to provide a proof of principle for integrating in a self-consistent manner the temporal gene expression of enzymes into kinetic models of cellular metabolism, (ii) to lend further support to the concept of post-differentiation patterning according to which metabolic zonation is driven by gradients of oxygen, nutrients and hormones in the capillary blood and (iii) to present a modeling approach that obviates the requirement to measure the cellular abundance of metabolic enzymes (e.g., by quantitative proteomics) in different physical states of the liver, a procedure burdened with many problems as, for example, invasive tissue sampling and protein quantification in cells separated from different zones.

MODEL DESCRIPTION

The model combines a mathematical model of the sinusoidal tissue unit (STU) (Berndt et al., 2018) with a kinetic model of the protein turnover of key regulatory enzymes.

Compartment Model of Metabolite and Hormone Transport in the Sinusoidal Tissue Unit (STU)

Structurally, the STU is defined by a single sinusoid, the adjacent space of Disse and a monolayer of hepatocytes flanking the space of Disse (see **Figure 1A**). Functionally, the model describes the exchange of oxygen, metabolites and hormones between the sinusoidal blood, the space of Disse and the hepatocytes and the glucose metabolism within hepatocytes. The transport of metabolite and hormones within the STU is driven by diffusion

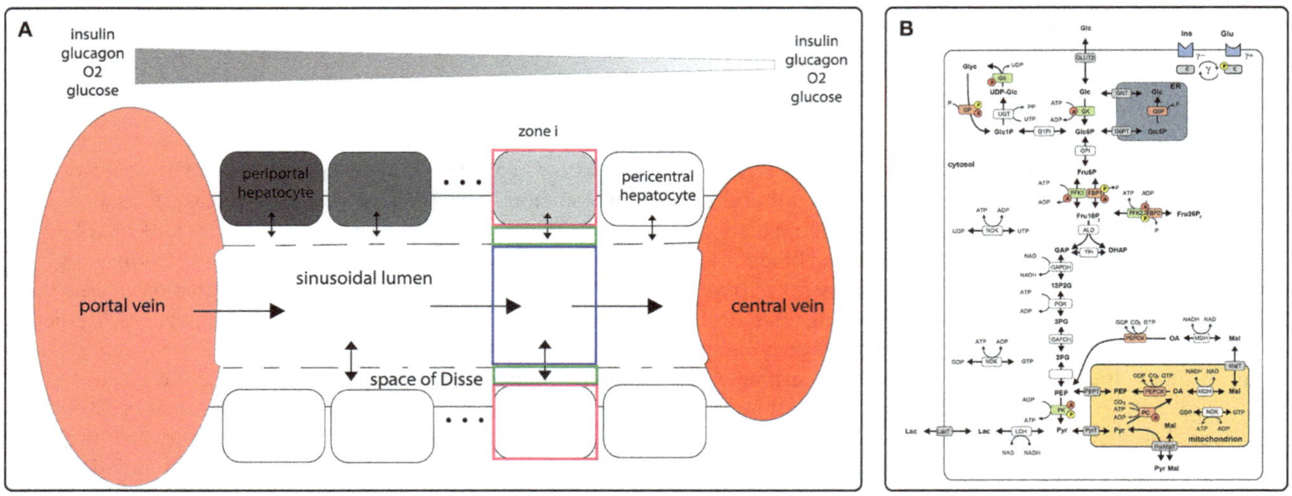

FIGURE 1 | Schematic model representation **(A)** sinusoidal blood flow model describing blood flow, nutrient and hormone distribution within the sinusoids. The model encompasses a single sinusoid, the adjacent space of Disse and the surrounding layer of hepatocytes. It is described by morphological parameters (blood vessel radius, thickness of the space of Disse, hepatocyte thickness, hepatocyte number, sinusoid length, degree of fenestration), and systemic parameters (central and portal vein hydrostatic pressure, plasma and lymph oncotic pressure, diffusion coefficients); **(B)** model of carbohydrate metabolism encompassing glycolysis, glyconeogenesis and glycogen synthesis and utilization. These pathways comprise the enzymes Glucokinase (GK), Glucose-6-phosphate isomerase (GPI), Phosphofructokinase 1 (PFK1), Aldolase (ALD), Triosephosphate isomerase (TPI), Glyceraldehydephosphate dehydrogenase (GAPDH), Phosphoglycerate kinase (PGK), Phosphoglycerate mutase (PGM), Enolase (EN), Pyruvate kinase (PK) Lactate dehydrogenase (LDH), Glucose-6-phosphate phosphatase (G6P), Phosphofructokinase 2 (PFK2), Fructose-2,6-bisphosphatase (FBP2), Fructose-1,6-bisphosphatase (FBP1), Phosphoenolpyruvate carboxykinase (PEPCK), Pyruvate carboxylase (PC), Nucleoside-diphosphate kinase (NDK), Malate dehydrogenase (MDH), Pyrophosphatase (PPASE), Glucose-1-phosphate isomerase (P1PI), Glycuronosyltransferase (UGT), Glycogen phosphorylase (GP), Glycogen synthase (GS) and transporters (ER <-> cytosol: Glucose-6-phosphate transporter (Glc6PT), Glucose transporter (GlcT); mitochondrion <-> cytosol: Pyruvate transporter (PYRT), Phosphoenolpyruvate transporter (PEPT), Malate transporter (MALT); extern <-> cytosol: Glucose transporter 2 (GLUT2), Lactate transporter (LACT). Enzymes that are phosphorylated or dephosphorylated in response to insulin (Ins) and glucagon (Glu) stimulus are marked by a yellow P, allosteric modification of enzymes is marked by a red A. The model contains the metabolites: glucose (Glc), glucose-6-phosphate (Glc6P), fructose-6-phosphate (Fru6P), fructose-1,6-bisphosphate ($Fru16P_2$), glyceraldehydephosphate (GraP), dihydroxyacetonephosphate (DHAP), 1,3-bisphosphoglycerate (13P2G), 3-phosphoglycerate (3PG), 2-phosphoglycerate (2PG), phosphoenolpyruvate (PEP), pyruvate (Pyr), lactate (Lac), malate (Mal), oxaloacetate (OA), glucose-1-phosphate (Glc1P), UDP-glucose (UDP-glc), glycogen, fructose-2,6-bisphosphate ($Fru26P_2$). The cofactors NADH, NAD, ATP, ADP, UTP and UDP are not treated as dynamic variables. All physiological metabolites produced or consumed in the hepatocyte during glycolysis and gluconeogenesis are comprised into lactate. Figures adapted from Berndt et al. (2018).

and directional transport along the flow of water and blood. Lateral blood flow in the vessel is described by Hagen-Poiseuille law for fluid flow through a cylinder, water flow in the space of Disse is described by Hagen-Poiseuille law for fluid flow in a hollow cylinder. Exchange of water between the vessel and the space of Disse is driven by hydrostatic and oncotic pressure difference between the blood vessel and the space of Disse.

Conceptually, the STU was divided into N_H zones, where N_H is the number of hepatocytes along the porto-central axis. Each zone is made up of the sinusoid volume, the space of Disse and the hepatocyte (**Figure 1A**). Within one zone, the concentration of metabolites and hormones is given by a single value. The mathematical description of the STU model and a complete list of parameters used can be found in Berndt et al. (2018).

Kinetic Model of Hepatocyte Glucose Metabolism

The reaction scheme for the glucose metabolism of a single hepatocyte is depicted in **Figure 1B**. It consists of the pathways for glycolysis, glyconeogenesis, glycogen synthesis and degradation. The time-dependent variation of metabolite concentrations is given by first-order differential equations. The liver specific enzymatic rate laws take into account substrate regulation, allosteric regulation and hormonal regulation by hormone-dependent reversible phosphorylation (Bulik et al., 2016).

Kinetic Model of Hormonal Signaling

The pancreatic hormones glucagon and insulin are released into the portal vein in response to the plasma glucose concentration and are partially cleared during their passage through the liver. Hence, there is a difference between their plasma concentrations determined in peripheral blood samples and effective intra-hepatic concentrations. This difference was taken into account by setting the concentration values of insulin and glucagon in the periportal blood to the 2-fold of their plasma values (Balks and Jungermann, 1984). The rate of intra-hepatic hormone clearance via receptor binding and subsequent endocytosis was put proportional to the binding and signaling strength of the hormone. We used empirical transfer functions to describe the relationship between glucose and hormone concentrations in the plasma and the relationship between and the phosphorylation state of interconvertible enzymes as described in Bulik et al. (2016). A detailed description of the functions and their construction can be found in Berndt et al. (2018).

Kinetic Model of Protein Turnover

The temporal change of the protein level P^{ENZ} of a metabolic enzyme (ENZ) is given by the difference between the rates of protein synthesis $v_{syn}^{ENZ}(E)$ and protein degradation $v_{deg}^{ENZ}(E)$:

$$\frac{d}{dt}P^{ENZ} = v^{ENZ}(E) = v_{syn}^{ENZ}(E) - v_{deg}^{ENZ}(E) \tag{1}$$

The right-hand side of equation (1), $v^{ENZ}(E)$, represents the turnover rate of the enzyme protein. It is controlled by modulators affecting either the synthesis or the degradation or both. Note that the enzyme level P^{ENZ} scales linearly with the maximal rate of the enzyme. The rate equations of protein synthesis and degradation both depend on the momentary concentration of at least one of the four modulators E_i, $i = 1$ (insulin), $i = 2$ (glucagon), $i = 3$ (glucose), $i = 4$ (oxygen) considered in the model. The general structure of the rate equation for the protein synthesis of enzyme ENZ reads.

$$v_{syn}^{ENZ} = k_{syn}^{ENZ} \prod_{i=1}^{4} (k_i^{ENZ} \pm f_i^{ENZ}) \tag{2}$$

where k_i^{ENZ} is a constant determining the basal synthesis rate and f_i is a nonlinear function of the i-th modulator. The "+" sign holds if E_i is an activator (inductor) of protein synthesis, the (-) sign holds If E_i is an inhibitor (repressor) . If E_i has not been reported so far to exert an effect on the protein synthesis of enzyme ENZ it holds $k_i^{ENZ} = 1$ and $f_i^{ENZ} = 0$ Numerical values for the rate constants k_{syn}^{enz} and k_{deg}^{enz} were fixed in such a manner that for a normal 24 h plasma profile (see below) the zone- and time averaged protein levels coincided with the stationary protein levels as reported in Bulik et al. (2016). Numerical values of all other kinetic parameters were obtained by adjusting the rate equations to experimentally determined protein levels at varying concentrations of the four possible modulators (see **Supplement 1**). **Table 1** depicts the rate equations for the synthesis and degradation of those enzymes of hepatic glucose metabolism possessing in the model timely variable protein levels.

In order to quantify the sensitivity of the turnover rate $v^{ENZ}(E)$ of a protein against small changes of an modulator E, we used the sensitivity (elasticity) coefficient as defined in metabolic control analysis:

$$SV^{ENZ} = \frac{E}{v^{ENZ}(E)} \frac{\partial v^{ENZ}(E)}{\partial E} \tag{3}$$

Figure 2 depicts the sensitivity coefficients for the turnover rates of the nine enzyme proteins with variable expression level as function of the four modulators oxygen (I), glucagon (II), insulin (III) and glucose (IV). Except for the sensitivities of the PEPCK and G6PP turnover with respect to glucagon and glucose, respectively, the extremum of all other sensitivity characteristics lies within the reported physiological range of the related modulators (green-shaded areas in **Figure 2**). The sensitivity of G6PP turnover with respect to glucose becomes important in the diabetic case, where glucose levels can exceed 20 mM (see below).

RESULTS

Dynamic Metabolic Zonation in a Well-Fed State of the Rat

First, we used the model to simulate the temporal variation of enzyme abundances, metabolite concentrations and fluxes within the various zones along the porto-central axis of the STU. The simulation was initiated with identical abundance of enzymes along the sinusoid which we set to the stationary mean protein abundance used in Bulik et al. (2016). We used as model input the diurnal glucose profile reported for the healthy normal liver of a fed rat (La Fleur et al., 1999) and carried out the numerical integration of the model over several 24 h cycles until there was no change in the 24 h enzyme and metabolite profiles.

Even with identical enzyme abundances across all hepatocytes, there occurs a progressive decline of hormone plasma levels from the portal to the central pole due to the ongoing hormone uptake by hepatocytes in each zone. Moreover, oxygen uptake in one zone diminishes the available oxygen pressure seen by the cells in the adjacent zone toward the pericentral pole. As oxygen is not part of the model, we assumed a linear decrease in oxygen partial pressure from 90 mmHG in the periportal zone to 35 mm HG in the pericentral zone (Jungermann and Kietzmann, 2000; Allen et al., 2005). These initial gradients of hormones, glucose and oxygen feed back to the level of metabolic enzymes so that finally zone-dependent patterns of both enzyme abundances and metabolic variables (see **Figures 3, 4**) are generated.

Figures 3A–C depicts the timely variation of glucose, insulin, glucagon in various sinusoidal compartments. Intriguingly, the highest glucose concentrations in the very portal zone (see red curve in **Figure 3A**) are paralleled by the lowest glucose concentrations in the very central zone (green curve). This seemingly paradoxical situation is due to the fact that the high level of insulin and low level of glucagon strongly increase the glucose uptake capacity of hepatocytes such that the otherwise strong zone-dependent differences in the glucose exchange flux (see **Figure 3E**) almost disappear. The simulation also reveals large zone-dependent differences in the cellular dynamics of glycogen (**Figure 3D**). The variation of the glycogen content in portal cells is much more pronounced than in central cells.

The time-dependent variation in the protein levels of key glycolytic and gluconeogenetic enzymes in different zones are depicted in **Figure 4**. The uniform overall shape of the curves reflects essentially the daily variation of the plasma glucose level. Generally, the daily fluctuations of enzyme levels around their 24 h mean hardly exceed 10%. Thus, as long as the liver is repeatedly confronted with the same 24 h plasma profile of metabolites and hormones, timely variations of protein levels should have only a marginal impact on the hepatic control of the plasma glucose level.

TABLE 1 | Synthesis and degradation rates of the regulatory enzymes of hepatic carbohydrate.

Enzyme name	v_{syn}^{ENZ}	v_{deg}^{ENZ}	References
Glucose transporter	$k_{syn}^{glcT} \cdot \left(k_1 + k_2 \frac{glc_{ext}}{glc_{ext}+K_{glc_{ext}}}\right)$ $k_{syn}^{glcT} = 6.1 \cdot 10^{-3}$ $k_1 = 0.8$ $k_2 = 6$ $K_{glc_{ext}} = 15\ mM$	k_{deg}^{glcT} $k_{\mathrm{deg}}^{glcT} = \frac{\ln(2)}{40}$	Postic et al., 1993; Weinstein et al., 1994
Glucokinase	$k_{syn}^{gk} \cdot \left(k_1 - k_2 \frac{o_2^n}{o_2^n+K_{o_2}^n}\right) \cdot \left(k_3 \frac{ins}{ins+K_{ins}}\right)$ $k_{syn}^{glcT} = 6.5 \cdot 10^{-3}$ $k_1 = 2$ $k_2 = 1$ $K_{o_2} = 80\ mmHG$ $n = 15$ $k_3 = 10$ $K_{ins} = 500\ pM$	k_{deg}^{gk} $k_{\mathrm{deg}}^{gk} = \frac{\ln(2)}{15}$	Dice and Goldberg, 1975; Sibrowski et al., 1981, 1982; Iynedjian et al., 1989; Kietzmann et al., 1997
Glucose-6-phosphatase	$k_{syn}^{g6p} \cdot \left(k_1 - k_2 \frac{glucagon^{n1}}{glucagon^{n1}+K_{glucagon}^n}\right) \cdot \left(k_3 + k_4 \cdot k_{eff} \frac{glc_{ext}^{n2}}{glc_{ext}^{n2}+K_{glc_{ext}}^{n2}}\right)$ $k_{syn}^{g6p} = 1.16 \cdot 10^{-2}$ $k_1 = 1$ $k_2 = 0.8$ $n1 = 3$ $K_{glucagon} = 100\ pM$ $k_3 = 1$ $k_4 = 15$ $k_{eff} = 0.3$ $K_{glc_{ext}} = 17\ mM$ $n2 = 20$	k_{deg}^{g6p} $k_{\mathrm{deg}}^{g6p} = \frac{\ln(2)}{48}$	Leskes et al., 1971; Argaud et al., 1996; Massillon, 2001
Phosphofructokinase 1	k_{syn}^{pfk1} $k_{syn}^{pfk1} = 7.8 \cdot 10^{-3}$	k_{deg}^{pfk1} $k_{\mathrm{deg}}^{pfk1} = \frac{\ln(2)}{22+k_2 \cdot \frac{ins^n}{ins^n+K_{ins}^n}}$ $k_2 = 80\ h$ $K_{ins} = 100\ pM$ $n = 1.5$	Dunaway and Weber, 1974; Dunaway et al., 1978
Fructosebis-phosphatase 1	$k_{syn}^{fbp1} \cdot \left(k_1 + k_2 \cdot \frac{glu^n}{glu^n+K_{glu}^n}\right)$ $k_{syn}^{fbp1} = 2.99 \cdot 10^{-2}$ $k_1 = 0.25$ $k_2 = 1$ $K_{glu} = 100\ pM$ $n = 3$	k_{deg}^{fbp1} $k_{\mathrm{deg}}^{g6p} = \frac{\ln(2)}{40}$	Dice and Goldberg, 1975; Zalitis and Pitot, 1979; el-Maghrabi et al., 1991
Phosphofructo-kinase 2/Fructosebis-phosphatase 2	$k_{syn}^{pk} \cdot \left(k_1 - k_2 \cdot \frac{o_2^n}{o_2^n+K_{o_2}^n}\right) \cdot \left(k_3 - k_4 \frac{glu}{glu+K_{glu}}\right)$ $k_{syn}^{pfk2} = 1.1 \cdot 10^{-2}$ $k_1 = 2$ $k_2 = 1$ $K_{o_2} = 75\ mmHG$ $n = 10$ $k_3 = 1$ $k_4 = 1$ $K_{glu} = 80\ pM$	k_{deg}^{pfk2} $k_{\mathrm{deg}}^{g6p} = \frac{\ln(2)}{69}$	Dunaway and Weber, 1974; Dunaway et al., 1978; Rosa et al., 1993; Minchenko et al., 2003
Pyruvate kinase	$k_{syn}^{pk} \cdot \left(k_1 - k_2 \cdot \frac{o_2^n}{o_2^n+K_{o_2}^n}\right) \cdot \left(k_3 - k_4 \frac{glu}{glu+K_{glu}}\right) \cdot \left(k_5 + k_6 \frac{ins^{n2}}{ins^{n2}+K_{ins}^{n2}}\right)$ $k_{syn}^{pk} = 1.06 \cdot 10^{-2}$ $k_1 = 3.2$ $k_2 = 1$ $K_{o_2} = 75\ mmHG$ $n = 10$ $k_3 = 1$ $k_4 = 0.5$ $K_{glu} = 150\ pM$ $k_5 = 0.2$ $k_6 = 1$ $K_{ins} = 500\ pM$ $n2 = 2$	k_{deg}^{pk} $k_{\mathrm{deg}}^{pk} = \frac{\ln(2)}{69}$	Hopkirk and Bloxham, 1979, 1980; Noguchi et al., 1985; Wölfle and Jungermann, 1985
Pyruvate carboxylase	$k_{syn}^{pc} \cdot \left(k_1 + k_2 \cdot \frac{glu}{glu+K_{glu}}\right)$ $k_{syn}^{pc} = 1.47 \cdot 10^{-2}$ $k_1 = 0.1$ $k_2 = 1$ $K_{glu} = 150\ pM$	k_{deg}^{pc} $k_{\mathrm{deg}}^{pc} = \frac{\ln(2)}{110}$	Weinberg and Utter, 1979, 1980
Phosphoenol-pyruvate Carboxykinase	$k_{syn}^{pepck} \cdot \left(k_1 + k_2 \cdot \frac{o_2^{n1}}{o_2^{n1}+K_{o_2}^{n1}}\right) \cdot \left(k_3 + k_4 \frac{glu^{n2}}{glu^{n2}+K_{glu}^{n2}}\right) \cdot \left(k_5 - k_6 \frac{ins}{ins+K_{ins}}\right)$ $k_{syn}^{pepck} = 3.43 \cdot 10^{-2}$ $k_1 = 0.5$ $k_2 = 2$ $K_{o_2} = 75\ mmHG$ $n1 = 10$ $k_3 = 1$ $k_4 = 3$ $n2 = 0.5$ $K_{glu} = 0.2\ pM$ $k_5 = 1$ $k_6 = 0.8$ $K_{ins} = 100\ pM$	k_{deg}^{pepck} $k_{\mathrm{deg}}^{pepck} = \frac{\ln(2)}{13}$	Nauck et al., 1981; Christ et al., 1988; Gabbay et al., 1996

In contrast to the modest time-dependent variations of protein levels, the computed zone-dependent differences of enzyme levels display a large scatter. The maximal differences between the enzyme endowment of hepatocytes closest to the portal and central pole lie between 0.1 [e.g., glucose transporter (glcT) and phosphofructokinase 1 (pfk1)] and 4.5 [phosphoenolpyruvate kinase (pepck)]. For the validation of these computational predictions, we calculated the 24 h-average protein levels of the first (most portal) and last (most central) hepatocyte and compared the ratio of the computed average protein levels with experimental data (see first columns for each enzyme in **Figure 5**). We further compared the ratio of 24 h- and zone-averaged mean protein levels between a fed and fasted rat and a diabetic and normal rat.

This analysis provided a good concordance between theoretical and experimental results. The only exception is the pyruvate carboxylase, a key regulatory enzyme of gluconeogenesis, were portal to central gradients could not be univocally explained by the reported oxygen dependency. Oxygen dependency accounts only for about 35% percent of the observed zonation (see **Table 1** and **Supplement 1**).

Dynamic Metabolic Zonation of the Liver During Adaptation to Fasting

Next, we studied how the zonation of metabolic enzymes is affected if the liver has to cope with a fundamentally different nutritional regime. To this end, we simulated the zone-dependent dynamic changes of protein levels and metabolites during the transition from a fed state of the rat to a fasting state. The simulation started with the stable 24 h zonated enzyme profile that is established if the liver experiences recurrently the same plasma profile of a fed rat (see above). At time $t = 24$ h, the

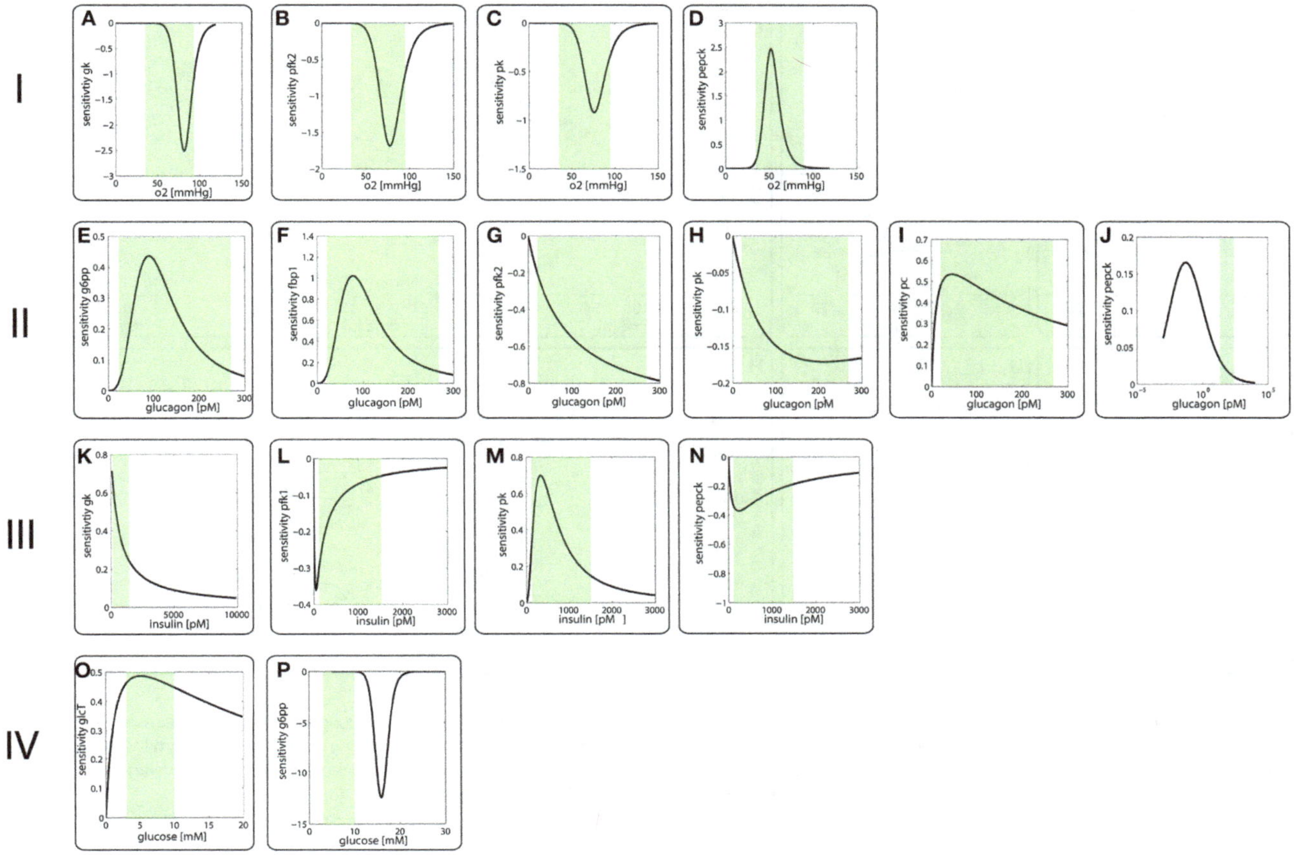

FIGURE 2 | Sensitivity coefficients of protein turnover rates defined in equation (3) as function of modulator concentrations.
I Sensitivity of protein turnover rates with respect to oxygen of **(A)** GK, **(B)** FBPFK2, **(C)** PK, **(D)** PEPCK
II Sensitivity of protein turnover rates with respect to **(E)** G6PP, **(F)** FBP1, **(G)** FBPFK2, **(H)** PK, **(I)** PC, **(J)** PEPCK
III Sensitivity of protein turnover rates with respect to **(K)** GK, **(L)** PFK1, **(M)** PK, **(N)** PEPCK
IV Sensitivity of protein turnover rates with respect to **(O)** GlcT, **(P)** G6PP
The green-shades areas indicate the reported physiological concentration range of the respective modulator.

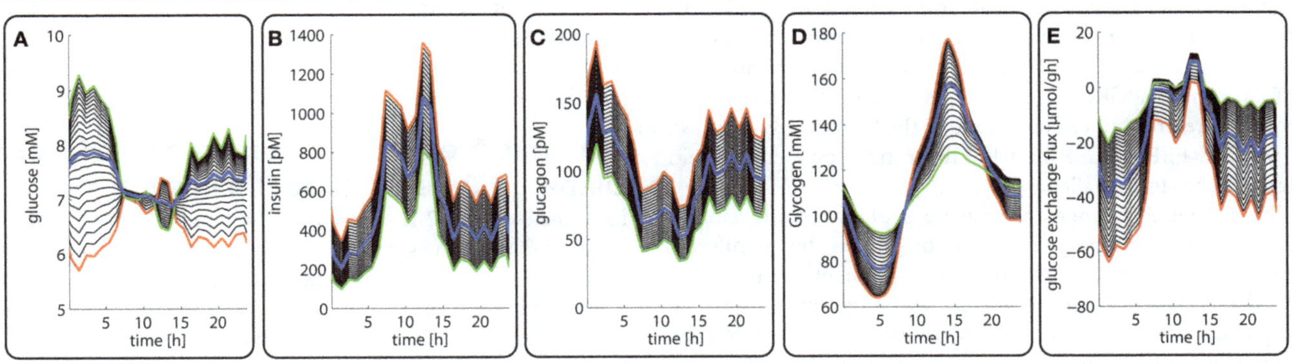

FIGURE 3 | Diurnal variations in the plasma levels of glucose **(A)**, insulin **(B)**, glucagon **(C)**, cellular glycogen **(D)** and the glucose exchange flux **(E)** in different zones along the porto-central axis. The different curves refer to different spatial positions of hepatocytes, counted from periportal (red curve) to percentral (green curve). The bold blue line refers to the means values of the shown variable. Note that the red curves (= most portal cell) for the hormones and glucose are identical with their plasma profiles.

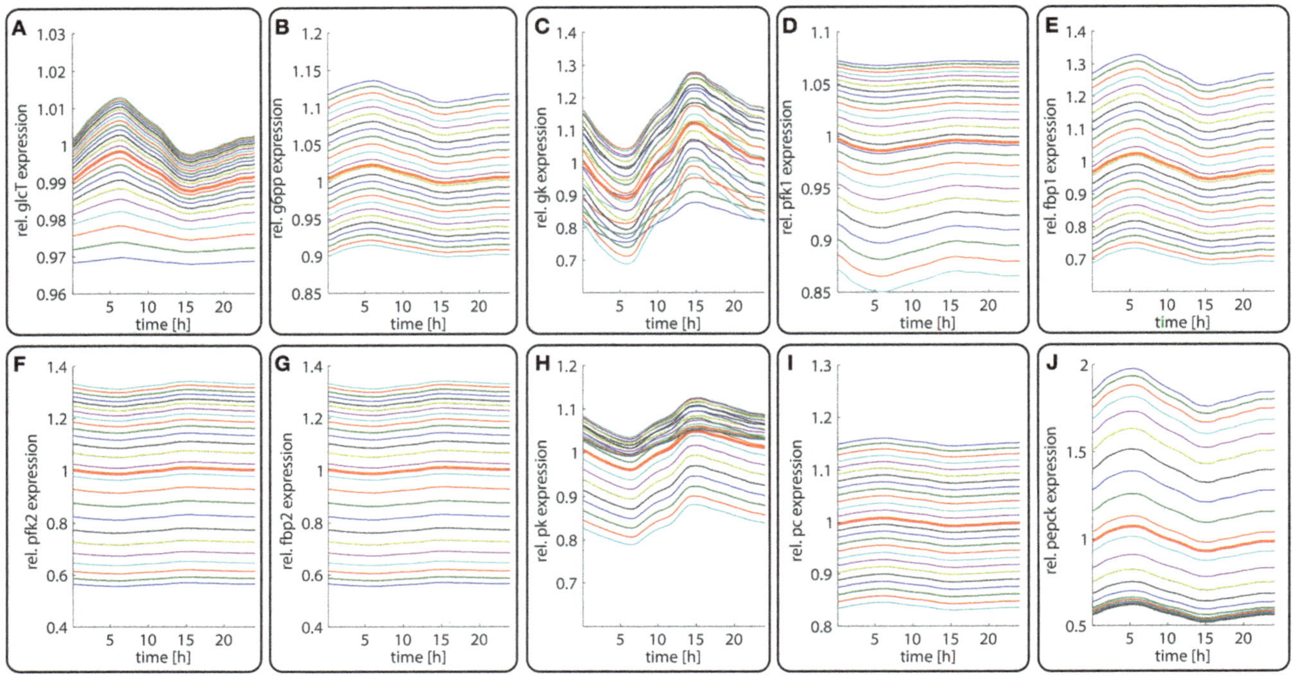

FIGURE 4 | Diurnal variations in the relative abundance of glycolytic and gluconeogenetic enzymes within hepatocytes along the porto-central axis of a well-fed rat. The curves illustrate the relative deviation of protein abundances from the overall spatial and 24h- mean (=24 h mean of the bold red curve). From the top to the bottom, the different curves refer to the spatial position of the hepatocyte counted from periportal to percentral. The bold red line refers to the average protein abundance across all cells. **(A)** GlcT, **(B)** G6PP, **(C)** GK, **(D)** PFK1, **(E)** FBPPFK1, **(F)** PFK2, **(G)** FBPPFK2, **(H)** PK, **(I)** PC, **(J)** PEPCK.

plasma profile of the fed rate was replaced by plasma profile of a fasted rat (La Fleur et al., 1999). The latter was only available for a time range of 24 h of fasting. After about 16 h of fasting, stable values of plasma metabolites were reached. Therefore, we used for time points $t > 48$ h (i.e., >24 h of fasting) for the model input a plasma profile that was composed of 6 repetitions of the last part (16–24 h) of the 24 h fasting plasma profile. As shown in **Figure 6**, the fed-to-fasting transition evokes a significant rise in the abundance of key gluconeogenetic enzymes (GlcT, FBP1, PC, PEPCK) and drop in the abundance of key glycolytic enzymes (GK, PFK1, PFK2, FBP2, PK) in all zones. For two enzymes, the GlcT and the PEPCK, the zone-dependent protein differences become more pronounced compared to the fed state. By contrast, for the GK, FBP1, GSPP, and PK the zone-dependent protein differences became smaller.

The computed changes of enzyme profiles toward a more gluconeogenetic phenotype are accompanied by significant alterations of the intra-sinusoidal glucose gradient and the zone-dependent differences in the glucose exchange rate (**Figure 7**). Compared with the fed state, the porto-venous glucose difference becomes much larger in the fasted state (**Figure 7A**). The same holds for the glucose exchange rate (**Figure 7D**).

In agreement with experimental data (Babcock and Cardell, 1974), the glycogen stores are almost depleted after about 1 day of fasting when the levels of insulin and glucagon have adopted a new stable temporal profile. Notably, also for the fasted state, the computed average protein abundance ratios are in good agreement with experimental data which further substantiates the reliability of the model (see **Figure 5**).

Figure 8 illustrates the importance of dynamic zonation for the adaptation of the porto-venous glucose difference (AVGD) to a specific nutritional regime. Regulation of interconvertible enzymes by hormone-dependent phosphorylation alone, i.e., at fixed protein levels of the fed state (blue line), would result in an AVGD of about 3.5 mM for the typical range of portal glucose concentrations in the fasted state (red shaded area). Dynamic adaption of protein levels enlarges the AVGD to about 7 mM (red line) thus rendering the liver to a strong glucose producer in the fasted state.

Dynamic Metabolic Zonation of the Liver in Diabetes Type II ("Diabetic Liver")

Late diabetes type 2 is characterized by long persistence of high postprandial plasma glucose levels, reduced insulin levels (hypo-insulinemia) and elevated glucagon levels (hyper-glucagonemia). It is mainly the shift in the insulin/glucagon ratio that renders the liver to a glucose producer which on top of the insulin-resistant muscle and adipose tissue contributes to high plasma glucose levels. We tested whether our model can also correctly describe this metabolic abnormality and the observed changes of protein abundances in different zones. To this end, we used the glucose-hormone transfer function constructed for the diabetic case (see Bulik et al., 2016) to calculate the phosphorylation state of interconvertible enzymes and confronted the model over

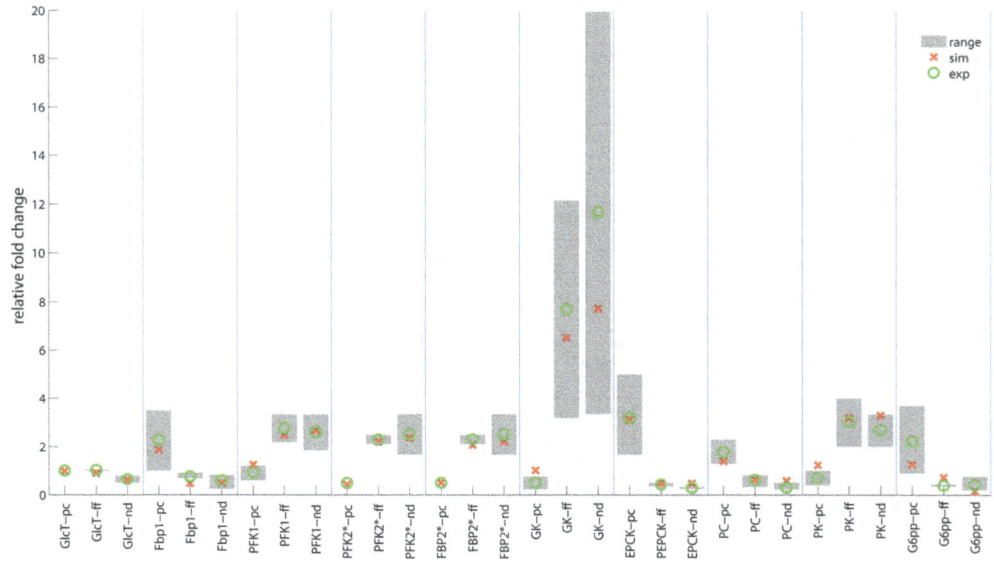

FIGURE 5 | Ratio of enzyme levels in hepatocytes. Red circles indicate the computed ratio of protein levels. Green circles and gray bars indicate the mean value and the range of variability of various experimentally determined ratios. First columns (pc): Portal-to-central ratios (= 24h-averaged protein levels between hepatocyte #1 and hepatocyte # 25) for the well-fed state of the rat. Experimental data were taken from (Sharma et al., 1964; Katz et al., 1977a,b; Trus et al., 1980; Jungermann and Katz, 1982, 1989; Probst et al., 1982; Teutsch and Lowry, 1982; Miethke et al., 1985; Quistorff, 1985; Wölfle and Jungermann, 1985; Morselt et al., 1987; Chen and Katz, 1988; Wals et al., 1988; Evans et al., 1989; Frederiks et al., 1991; Jones and Titheradge, 1996; Minchenko et al., 2003). Second columns (ff): Fed-to-fasted ratios of 24h- and zone-averaged mean enzyme levels. Experimental data taken from (Dipietro and Weinhouse, 1960; Wimhurst and Manchester, 1970b; Ballard and Hopgood, 1973; Bock et al., 1973; Zalitis and Pitot, 1979; Cladaras and Cottam, 1980; Neely et al., 1981; Bahnak and Gold, 1982; Van Schaftingen and Hers, 1983; Donofrio et al., 1984; Colosia et al., 1988; Crepin et al., 1988; Thorens et al., 1990; Giffin et al., 1993; Gannon and Nuttall, 1997). Third columns (nd): Normal-to-diabetic ratios of 24h- and zone-averaged mean enzyme levels. Experimental data taken from Dipietro and Weinhouse, 1960; Salas et al., 1963; Exton and Park, 1965; Wimhurst and Manchester, 1970a; Chang and Schneider, 1971; Dunaway et al., 1978; Weinberg and Utter, 1980; Neely et al., 1981; Donofrio et al., 1984; Miethke et al., 1985; Colosia et al., 1988; Crepin et al., 1988; Thorens et al., 1990; Miralpeix et al., 1992; Slieker et al., 1992; Gannon and Nuttall, 1997; Raju et al., 1999; Manna and Jain, 2012.

4 days repeatedly with a 24 h glucose profile of a diabetic rat until an almost stable 24 h pattern of protein abundances had established (**Figure 9**). As shown in **Figure 9D**, all hepatocytes work permanently as glucose producers, i.e., at all time points of the day the intra-sinusoidal glucose concentration increases along the portal-central axis (**Figure 9A**). The glycogen reserves are drastically diminished and the different time courses of glycogen emptying and filling between portal and central regions (see **Figure 2D**) are completely abolished. Taken together, the zonation of glucose metabolism in the diabetic liver bears a strong resemblance with that of the fasted liver. It is important to note that even in this pathophysiological case the computed average portal-to-central protein abundance ratios are in good agreement with experimental data (see **Figure 5**).

DISCUSSION

Metabolic Zonation of Hepatic Glucose Metabolism Is Driven by Concentration Gradients of Hormones and Metabolites

In this work we used a mathematical model to study the dynamic zonation of the hepatic glucose metabolism. To this end we extended our previously published multi-scale tissue model of the hepatic carbohydrate metabolism (Berndt et al., 2018) by rendering the protein levels of key regulatory enzymes of glycolysis and gluconeogenesis as dynamic model variables which are controlled by timely variable synthesis and degradation in dependence from the concentration of the four modulators glucose, insulin, glucagon and oxygen. The model correctly replicates experimentally determined protein levels in different zones of the liver acinus as well as the adaptation of the liver to a well-fed, fasted and diabetic state. From this we draw four main conclusions. (1) Zonation of the hepatic glucose metabolism is a necessary consequence of the fact that the expression of key regulatory enzymes is controlled by modulators that display a porto-central concentration gradient along the sinusoid. (2) Mechanisms controlling the adaptation of enzyme abundances to varying external conditions necessarily lead to the zonation of hepatic carbohydrate metabolism. (3) The four modulators considered in the model are sufficient to describe the dynamic zonation of the glucose metabolism of the a normal liver. (4) The use of phenomenological transfer functions which directly relate the protein turnover to known modulators of gene expression appears a promising modeling strategy to include variable protein levels in kinetic models in view of the fact that in a foreseeable future explicit kinetic modeling of complex gene-regulatory network is out of reach.

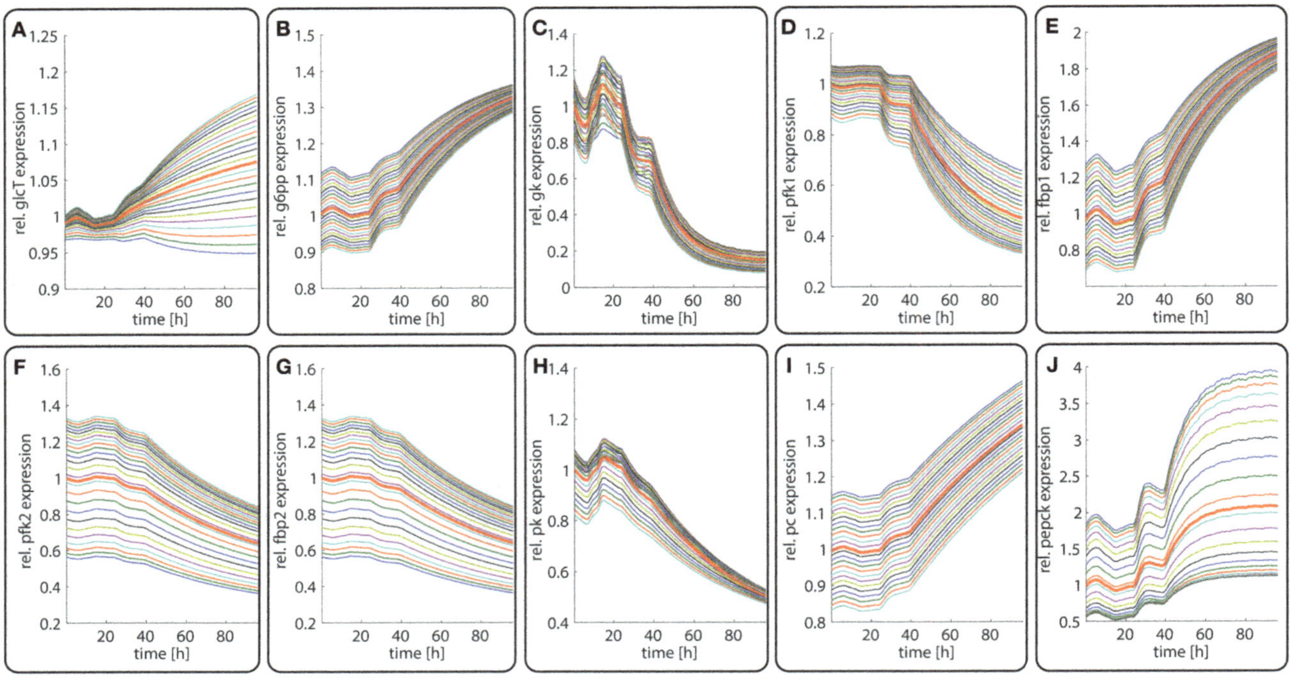

FIGURE 6 | Diurnal variations in the relative abundance of glycolytic and gluconeogenetic enzymes within hepatocytes along the porto-central axis during the transition from a fed state ($t = 0$–24 h) to a fasted state ($t > 24$ h). The curves illustrate the relative deviation of protein abundances from the overall spatial and 24 h mean (=24 h mean of the bold red curve). From the top to the bottom, the different curves refer to the spatial position of the hepatocyte counted from periportal to percentral. The bold red line refers to the average protein abundance across all cells. The vertical dotted line indicates onset of the starvation period. **(A)** GlcT, **(B)** G6PP, **(C)** GK, **(D)** PFK1, **(E)** FBPPFK1, **(F)** PFK2, **(G)** FBPPFK2, **(H)** PK, **(I)** PC, **(J)** PEPCK.

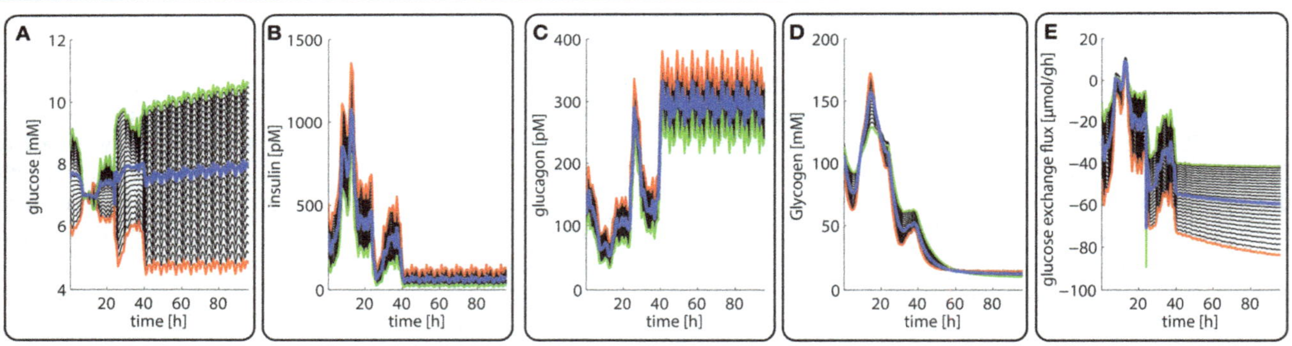

FIGURE 7 | Diurnal variations in the plasma levels of glucose **(A)**, insulin **(B)**, glucagon **(C)**, cellular glycogen **(D)** and the glucose exchange flux **(E)** in different zones along the porto-central axis during the transition from a well-fed state ($t = 0$–24 h) to a fasted state ($t > 24$ h) of the rate. The different curves refer to different spatial positions of hepatocytes, counted from periportal (red curve) to percentral (green curve). The bold blue line refers to the means values of the shown variables. Note that the red curves (= most portal cell) for the hormones and glucose are identical with their plasma profiles.

The Proposed Multi-Scale Model Encompasses All Levels of Metabolic Regulation

An important feature of the cellular metabolic network of the liver is the ability to adapt its functional output to varying external conditions such as changes in nutrient supply and varying hormone levels. These adaptive mechanisms operate at two different time scales. The short term adaptation occurs within seconds or minutes and is brought about by activity changes in the present metabolic enzymes by substrate availability, allosteric regulation and reversible phosphorylation. The second adaptive mechanism operates within hours or days and is brought about by changes in the enzyme abundances. It is already known for a long time that the total protein content of liver enzymes may largely vary owing to enhanced protein degradation during fasting (providing glucogenic amino acids as substrate for gluconeogenesis) mediated by the hormone glucagon or enhanced protein synthesis by the hormone insulin (Hopgood et al., 1980). However, such general changes of the protein content do not tell anything about the changes in the abundance of individual enzymes, whose expression by insulin and glucagon differs profoundly. Therefore, it was necessary to develop empirical rate laws for the synthesis and degradation of individual enzymes. This phenomenological approach was chosen since currently biochemical information is insufficient to establish molecular-resolved kinetic models which include, for example, the interaction of transcription factors among each other and with specific DNA promotor regions, the processing of mRNA and the regulation of mRNA translation by micro RNAs and RNA-binding proteins. For example, PEPCK, probably the best-studied gluconeogenetic enzyme, is regulated by at least a dozen transcription factors with partially unknown interactions (Yang et al., 2009). Even if it was possible to explicitly model the mRNA transcription for individual enzymes, there is still a big gap in understanding post-transcriptional regulation and the processes of post-translational modification.

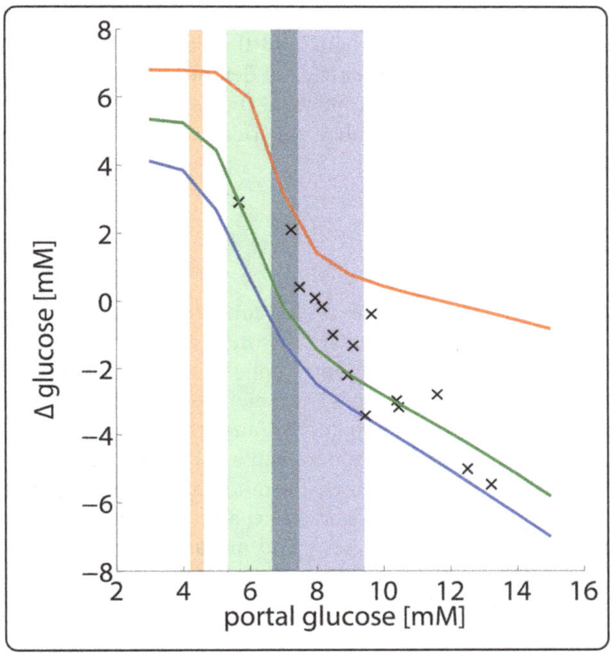

FIGURE 8 | Hepatic porto-venous glucose difference (AVGD) for the well-fed and fasted nutritional state. The daily variations of plasma glucose in the fasted, fed and well-fed state are indicated by the red-, green- and blue-shaded areas. The solid lines represent the AVGD if in the fasted state (red), fed state (green) and the well-fed state (blue). Crosses depict experimentally measured AVGD (Huang and Veech, 1988).

Metabolic Response of the Liver to Varying Nutritional Regimes

Our simulations suggest that in the presence of a constant daily nutritional regime the diurnal variation of enzyme abundances should be fairly moderate in the range of 10–20% around the mean. This is a lot less than daily variations in the abundance of the key regulatory enzyme of cholesterol synthesis, ßHMG-CoA reductase (Kirkpatrick et al., 1980), exhibiting a pronounced circadian rhythm or some enzymes of the amino acid metabolism as, for example, tyrosine transaminase the activity of which is almost four times as great several hours after nightfall as it is in the morning (Wurtman, 1974). In contrast, much larger changes of glycolytic and gluconeogenetic enzyme levels are elicited by a switch from well-fed to fasting conditions and vice versa. This metabolic adaptation occurs within a time span of several days (see **Figure 6**) and enables vertebrates to maintain the plasma glucose level in the absence of food. The slow change of enzyme concentration profiles implies that the capability of the fasted liver to clear a sudden excess of plasma glucose is diminished (impaired glucose tolerance) as the capacity of glycolytic enzymes and enzymes of the glycogen pathway a downregulated (Bulik et al., 2016). Intriguingly, there appears to be a striking similarity in the adaptive response of the liver to fasting conditions and diabetes type 2. In our modeling approach, this is mainly due to the fact that in both physiological settings the strong effect of insulin on the expression of glycolytic and gluconeogenetic

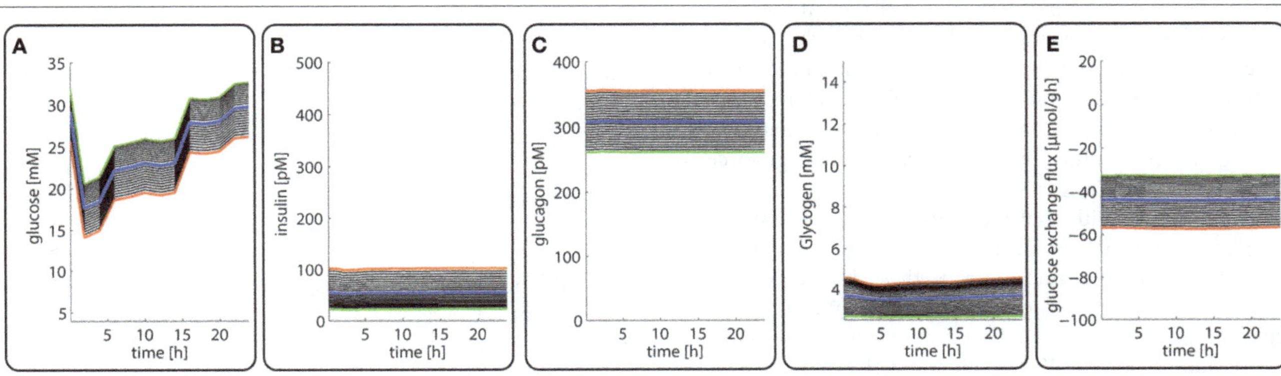

FIGURE 9 | Diurnal variations in the plasma levels of glucose **(A)**, insulin **(B)**, glucagon **(C)**, cellular glycogen **(D),** and the glucose exchange flux **(E)** in different zones along the porto-central axis of a diabetic rat.

enzymes is diminished whereas the effect of glucagon is more pronounced. As demonstrated in a previous model-based simulation study (König and Holzhütter, 2012), exposing the permanently glucose-releasing "starved" liver of the diabetic patient to a rigorous insulin treatment at persistently elevated glucagon level may increase the risk of severe hypoglycaemia. Thus, owing to the equally strong impact of both insulin and glucagon on the expression and phosphorylation state of liver enzymes, reconverting the "starved" liver of the diabetic patient into the normal metabolic phenotype requires the normalization of the plasma levels of both hormones.

Main Limitations of the Model and Outlook for Future Model Extensions

The used multiscale tissue model comprises a number of simplifications of the true anatomical structure of the liver which may impact on the simulated intra-sinusoidal concentration gradients of hormones and metabolites. For example, the blood flow rate within the pericentral zone of the sinusoid may vary if a sinusoid spreads out, forms anastomoses or merges with another sinusoid (Rappaport et al., 1954), anatomic peculiarities of liver parenchyma that are not yet considered in the STU model. Also, the number of periportal hepatocytes is higher (~2–3-fold) compared to pericentral hepatocytes. Regarding the concentration gradient of oxygen, hormones and metabolites in the sinusoid it may be of relevance that the terminal branches of the hepatic artery rarely join with the portal vein already before the blood enters the sinusoids, as presumed in our model. In the vast majority the merger of arterial blood with blood from the portal vein, occurs a few cells downstream within the sinusoid (Ekataksin and Kaneda, 1999) resulting in a local increase of the concentration of oxygen concentration at this site. Despite these limitations, the model correctly describes glucose exchange rates, gradients and indicator dilution curves for a structurally normal liver (Berndt et al., 2018). Hence, the functional implications of the above limitations and other neglected aspects of the real topology of liver tissue remain unclear. Therefore, in future work we aim to embed our metabolic cell model in a 3-D reconstructions of a mouse lobule (Hoehme et al., 2017).

The rate laws presented in this paper are effective transfer functions describing directly the relation between modulators (nutrients and hormones) and the turnover rate of a protein. Usage of effective transfer function raises the question which properties of the underlying regulatory network have to be captured. Obviously, not all known modulators of protein synthesis and degradation have been considered in the model. Ground-breaking experiments pointed initially to the oxygen gradient as the most important driving force of metabolic zonation (Jungermann and Kietzmann, 1997, 2000). Later experiments with isolated hepatocytes incubated with varying concentrations of insulin or glucagon (Probst et al., 1982) revealed an important role of these hormones for the establishment of liver zonation. Meanwhile a lot more potential modulators of metabolic zonation have been described in the literature, among them Wnt/β-catenin pathway (Torre et al., 2010; Vasilj et al., 2012), MAPK/ERK pathway (Zeller et al., 2013), Hnf4-alpha (Colletti et al., 2009), or thyroid hormones (Weinberg and Utter, 1979). However, as demonstrated in this study, the dynamic zonation of the glucose metabolism can be well described in different physiological settings by taken into account only the four modulators oxygen, glucose, glucagon and insulin. The central role of oxygen, glucose, glucagon and insulin for the dynamic zonation of the glucose metabolism does not exclude that morphogens and growth factors may have an important role in the zonation of other metabolic subsystems (Gebhardt and Matz-Soja, 2014). For example, the expression of the glutamine synthetase is restricted to last few hepatocytes close to the venous pole. Complementary, the urea cycle enzyme carbamoylphosphate synthetase I (CPS I) is present in the periportal, intermediate, and the first few layers of the perivenous zone. It has been clearly demonstrated that Wnt/ß-catenin signaling pathway plays a central role in the stable maintenance of these peculiar zonation profiles (Burke et al., 2009).

CONCLUSION

In summary, we propose a self-consistent model of liver carbohydrate metabolism that consistently takes into account variable gene expression of metabolic enzymes, regulation of metabolic pathways, exchange of metabolites and hormones between the blood and hepatocytes and microperfusion of the liver. Once the input of hormones and nutrients to the periportal region the liver acinus is known, the model allows to compute the metabolic phenotype of individual hepatocytes along the porto-central axis. The local hormone and metabolite concentrations determine the phosphorylation state of the interconvertible enzymes, hormonal clearance rates and expression level of metabolic enzymes. The metabolic phenotype in turn determines the functional output (here: glucose exchange rate) of each hepatocyte and this way the venous glucose output of the acinus. Integration across a representative set of acini yields finally the total glucose output of the liver.

AUTHOR CONTRIBUTIONS

NB developed the concept, implemented the model, carried out the simulation, wrote the manuscript. H-GH developed the concept, advised the implementation of the model, wrote the manuscript.

FUNDING

NB was funded by the German Systems Biology Program "LiSyM," grant no. 31 L0057, sponsored by the German Federal Ministry of Education and Research (BMBF). The funders had no role in study design, data collection and analysis, decision to publish, or preparation of the manuscript.

REFERENCES

Allen, J. W., Khetani, S. R., and Bhatia, S. N. (2005). *In vitro* zonation and toxicity in a hepatocyte bioreactor. *Toxicol. Sci.* 84, 110–119. doi: 10.1093/toxsci/kfi052

Argaud, D., Zhang, Q., Pan, W., Maitra, S., Pilkis, S. J., and Lange, A. J. (1996). Regulation of rat liver glucose-6-phosphatase gene expression in different nutritional and hormonal states: gene structure and 5'-flanking sequence. *Diabetes* 45, 1563–1571. doi: 10.2337/diab.45.11.1563

Babcock, M. B., and Cardell, R. R. (1974). Hepatic glycogen patterns in fasted and fed rats. *Am. J. Anat.* 140, 299–337. doi: 10.1002/aja.1001400302

Bahnak, B. R., and Gold, A. H. (1982). Effects of alloxan diabetes on the turnover of rat liver glycogen synthase. Comparison with liver phosphorylase. *J. Biol. Chem.* 257, 8775–8780.

Balks, H. J., and Jungermann, K. (1984). Regulation of peripheral insulin/glucagon levels by rat liver. *Eur. J. Biochem.*141, 645–650. doi: 10.1111/j.1432-1033.1984.tb08240.x

Ballard, F. J., and Hopgood, M. F. (1973). Phosphopyruvate carboxylase induction by L-tryptophan. Effects on synthesis and degradation of the enzyme. *Biochem. J.* 136, 259–264. doi: 10.1042/bj1360259

Berndt, N., Horger, M. S., Bulik, S., and Holzhütter, H. G. (2018). A multiscale modelling approach to assess the impact of metabolic zonation and microperfusion on the hepatic carbohydrate metabolism. *PLoS Comput. Biol.* 14:e1006005. doi: 10.1371/journal.pcbi.1006005

Bock, K. W., Fröhling, W., and Remmer, H. (1973). Influence of fasting and hemin on microsomal cytochromes and enzymes. *Biochem. Pharmacol.* 22, 1557–1564. doi: 10.1016/0006-2952(73)90021-X

Braeuning, A., Ittrich, C., Köhle, C., Hailfinger, S., Bonin, M., Buchmann, A., et al. (2006). Differential gene expression in periportal and perivenous mouse hepatocytes. *FEBS J.* 273, 5051–5061. doi: 10.1111/j.1742-4658.2006.05503.x

Bulik, S., Holzhütter, H. G., and Berndt, N. (2016). The relative importance of kinetic mechanisms and variable enzyme abundances for the regulation of hepatic glucose metabolism-insights from mathematical modeling. *BMC Biol.* 14:15. doi: 10.1186/s12915-016-0237-6

Burke, Z. D., Reed, K. R., Phesse, T. J., Sansom, O. J., Clarke, A. R., and Tosh, D. (2009). Liver zonation occurs through a beta-catenin-dependent, c-Myc-independent mechanism. *Gastroenterology* 136, 2316–2324 e2311–2313. doi: 10.1053/j.gastro.2009.02.063

Chang, A. Y., and Schneider, D. I. (1971). Hepatic enzyme activities in streptozotocin-diabetic rats before and after insulin treatment. *Diabetes* 20, 71–77. doi: 10.2337/diab.20.2.71

Chen, K. S., and Katz, J. (1988). Zonation of glycogen and glucose syntheses, but not glycolysis, in rat liver. *Biochem. J.* 255, 99–104. doi: 10.1042/bj2550099

Christ, B., Nath, A., Bastian, H., and Jungermann, K. (1988). Regulation of the expression of the phosphoenolpyruvate carboxykinase gene in cultured rat hepatocytes by glucagon and insulin. *Eur. J. Biochem.* 178, 373–379. doi: 10.1111/j.1432-1033.1988.tb14460.x

Cladaras, C., and Cottam, G. L. (1980). Turnover of Liver Pyruvate-Kinase. *Arch. Biochem. Biophys.* 200, 426–433. doi: 10.1016/0003-9861(80)90373-2

Colletti, M., Cicchini, C., Conigliaro, A., Santangelo, L., Alonzi, T., Pasquini, E., et al. (2009). Convergence of Wnt signaling on the HNF4 alpha-driven transcription in controlling liver zonation. *Gastroenterology* 137, 660–672. doi: 10.1053/j.gastro.2009.05.038

Colosia, A. D., Marker, A. J., Lange, A. J., el-Maghrabi, M. R., Granner, D. K., Tauler, A., et al. (1988). Induction of rat liver 6-phosphofructo-2-kinase/fructose-2,6-bisphosphatase mRNA by refeeding and insulin. *J. Biol. Chem.* 263, 18669–18677.

Crepin, K. M., Darville, M. I., Hue, L., and Rousseau, G. G. (1988). Starvation or diabetes decreases the content but not the mRNA of 6-phosphofructo-2-kinase in rat liver. *Febs Lett.* 227, 136–140. doi: 10.1016/0014-5793(88)80884-6

Dice, J. F., and Goldberg, A. L. (1975). Statistical-analysis of relationship between degradative rates and molecular-weights of proteins. *Arch. Biochem. Biophys.* 170, 213–219. doi: 10.1016/0003-9861(75)90112-5

Dipietro, D. L., and Weinhouse, S. (1960). Hepatic glucokinase in the fed, fasted, and alloxan-diabetic rat. *J. Biol. Chem.* 235, 2542–2545.

Donofrio, J. C., Thompson, R. S., Reinhart, G. D., and Veneziale, C. M. (1984). Quantification of liver and kidney phosphofructokinase by radioimmunoassay in fed, starved and alloxan-diabetic rats. *Biochem. J.* 224, 541–547. doi: 10.1042/bj2240541

Dunaway, G. A., Leung, G. L., Thrasher, J. R., and Cooper, M. D. (1978). Turnover of hepatic phosphofructokinase in normal and diabetic rats-role of insulin and peptide stabilizing factor. *J. Biol. Chem.* 253, 7460–7463.

Dunaway, G. A., and Weber, G. (1974). Effects of hormonal and nutritional changes on rates of synthesis and degradation of hepatic phosphofructokinase isozymes. *Arch. Biochem. Biophys.* 162, 629–637. doi: 10.1016/0003-9861(74)90225-2

Ekataksin, W., and Kaneda, K. (1999). Liver microvascular architecture: an insight into the pathophysiology of portal hypertension. *Semin. Liver Dis.* 19, 359–382. doi: 10.1055/s-2007-1007126

el-Maghrabi, M. R., Lange, A. J., Kummel, L., and Pilkis, S. J. (1991). The rat fructose-1,6-bisphosphatase gene-structure and regulation of expression. *J. Biol. Chem.* 266, 2115–2120.

Evans, J. L., Quistorff, B., and Witters, L. A. (1989). Zonation of hepatic lipogenic enzymes identified by dual-digitonin-pulse perfusion. *Biochem. J.* 259, 821–829. doi: 10.1042/bj2590821

Exton, J. H., and Park, C. R. (1965). Control of gluconeogenesis in the perfused liver of normal and adrenalectomized rats. *J. Biol. Chem.* 240, 955–957.

Frederiks, W. M., Marx, F., and van Noorden, C. J. (1991). Homogeneous distribution of phosphofructokinase in the rat liver acinus: a quantitative histochemical study. *Hepatology* 14, 634–639. doi: 10.1002/hep.1840140410

Gabbay, R. A., Sutherland, C., Gnudi, L., Kahn, B. B., O'Brien, R. M., Granner, D. K., et al. (1996). Insulin regulation of phosphoenolpyruvate carboxykinase gene expression does not require activation of the Ras/mitogen-activated protein kinase signaling pathway. *J. Biol. Chem.* 271, 1890–1897. doi: 10.1074/jbc.271.4.1890

Gannon, M. C., and Nuttall, F. Q. (1997). Effect of feeding, fasting, and diabetes on liver glycogen synthase activity, protein, and mRNA in rats. *Diabetologia* 40, 758–763. doi: 10.1007/s001250050746

Gebhardt, R., and Matz-Soja, M. (2014). Liver zonation: novel aspects of its regulation and its impact on homeostasis. *World J. Gastroenterol.* 20, 8491–8504. doi: 10.3748/wjg.v20.i26.8491

Giffin, B. F., Drake, R. L., Morris, R. E., and Cardell, R. R. (1993). Hepatic lobular patterns of phosphoenolpyruvate carboxykinase, glycogen synthase, and glycogen phosphorylase in fasted and fed rats. *J. Histochem. Cytochem.* 41, 1849–1862. doi: 10.1177/41.12.8245433

Han, H. S., Kang, G., Kim, J. S., Choi, B. H., and Koo, S. H. (2016). Regulation of glucose metabolism from a liver-centric perspective. *Exp. Mol. Med.* 48:e218. doi: 10.1038/emm.2015.122

Hoehme, S., Friebel, A., Hammad, S., Drasdo, D., and Hengstler, J. G. (2017). Creation of three-dimensional liver tissue models from experimental images for systems medicine. *Methods Mol. Biol.* 1506, 319–362. doi: 10.1007/978-1-4939-6506-9_22

Hopgood, M. F., Ballard, F. J., Reshef, L., and Hanson, R. W. (1973). Synthesis and degradation of phosphoenolpyruvate carboxylase in rat-liver and adipose-tissue-changes during a starvation-refeeding cycle. *Biochem. J.* 134, 445–453. doi: 10.1042/bj1340445

Hopgood, M. F., Clark, M. G., and Ballard, F. J. (1980). Protein-degradation in hepatocyte monolayers-effects of glucagon, adenosine 3'-5'-cyclic monophosphate and insulin. *Biochem. J.* 186, 71–79. doi: 10.1042/bj1860071

Hopkirk, T. J., and Bloxham, D. P. (1979). Studies on the biosynthesis of hepatic pyruvate-kinase and its correlation with enhanced hepatic lipogenesis in meal-trained rats. *Biochem. J.* 182, 383–397. doi: 10.1042/bj1820383

Hopkirk, T. J., and Bloxham, D. P. (1980). Biosynthesis of rat-liver pyruvate-kinase-measurement of enzyme lifetime and the rate of synthesis at weaning. *Biochem. J.* 192, 507–516. doi: 10.1042/bj1920507

Huang, M. T., and Veech, R. L. (1988). Role of the direct and indirect pathways for glycogen synthesis in rat liver in the postprandial state. *J. Clin. Invest.* 81, 872–878. doi: 10.1172/JCI113397

Iynedjian, P. B., Jotterand, D., Nouspikel, T., Asfari, M., and Pilot, P. R. (1989). Transcriptional induction of glucokinase gene by insulin in cultured liver cells and its repression by the glucagon-cAMP system. *J. Biol. Chem.* 264, 21824–21829.

Jones, C. G., and Titheradge, M. A. (1996). Measurement of metabolic fluxes through pyruvate kinase, phosphoenolpyruvate carboxykinase, pyruvate dehydrogenase, and pyruvate carboxylase in hepatocytes of different acinar origin. *Arch. Biochem. Biophys.* 326, 202–206. doi: 10.1006/abbi.1996.0066

Jungermann, K., and Katz, N. (1982). Functional hepatocellular heterogeneity. *Hepatology* 2, 385–395. doi: 10.1002/hep.1840020316

Jungermann, K., and Katz, N. (1989). Functional specialization of different hepatocyte populations. *Physiol. Rev.* 69, 708–764. doi: 10.1152/physrev.1989.69.3.708

Jungermann, K., and Kietzmann, T. (1997). Role of oxygen in the zonation of carbohydrate metabolism and gene expression in liver. *Kidney Int.* 51, 402–412. doi: 10.1038/ki.1997.53

Jungermann, K., and Kietzmann, T. (2000). Oxygen: modulator of metabolic zonation and disease of the liver. *Hepatology* 31, 255–260. doi: 10.1002/hep.510310201

Katz, N., Teutsch, H. F., Jungermann, K., and Sasse, D. (1977a). Heterogeneous reciprocal localization of fructose-1,6-bisphosphatase and of glucokinase in microdissected periportal and perivenous rat-liver tissue. *FEBS Lett.* 83, 272–276. doi: 10.1016/0014-5793(77)81021-1

Katz, N., Teutsch, H. F., Sasse, D., and Jungermann, K. (1977b). Heterogeneous distribution of glucose-6-phosphatase in microdissected periportal and perivenous rat-liver tissue. *FEBS Lett.* 76, 226–230. doi: 10.1016/0014-5793(77)80157-9

Kietzmann, T., Cornesse, Y., Brechtel, K., Modaressi, S., and Jungermann, K. (2001). Perivenous expression of the mRNA of the three hypoxia-inducible factor alpha-subunits, HIF1alpha, HIF2alpha and HIF3alpha, in rat liver. *Biochem. J.* 354, 531–537. doi: 10.1042/bj3540531

Kietzmann, T., Roth, U., Freimann, S., and Jungermann, K. (1997). Arterial oxygen partial pressures reduce the insulin-dependent induction of the perivenously located glucokinase in rat hepatocyte cultures: mimicry of arterial oxygen pressures by H_2O_2. *Biochem. J.* 321(Pt 1),17–20.

Kirkpatrick, R. B., Robinson, S. F., and Killenberg, P. G. (1980). Diurnal-variation of rat-liver enzymes catalyzing bile-acid conjugation and sulfation. *Biochim. Biophys. Acta.* 620, 627–630. doi: 10.1016/0005-2760(80)90154-X

König, M., and Holzhütter, H. G. (2012). Kinetic modeling of human hepatic glucose metabolism in type 2 diabetes mellitus predicts higher risk of hypoglycemic events in rigorous insulin therapy. *J. Biol. Chem.* 287, 36978–36989. doi: 10.1074/jbc.M112.382069

La Fleur, S. E., Kalsbeek, A., Wortel, J., and Buijs, R. M. (1999). A suprachiasmatic nucleus generated rhythm in basal glucose concentrations. *J. Neuroendocrinol.* 11, 643–652. doi: 10.1046/j.1365-2826.1999.00373.x

Leskes, A., Siekevitz, P., and Palade, G. E. (1971). Differentiation of endoplasmic reticulum in hepatocytes : II. glucose-6-phosphatase in rough microsomes. *J. Cell Biol.* 49, 288–302. doi: 10.1083/jcb.49.2.288

Manna, P., and Jain, S. K. (2012). Decreased hepatic phosphatidylinositol-3,4,5-triphosphate (PIP3) levels and impaired glucose homeostasis in type 1 and type 2 diabetic rats. *Cell. Physiol. Biochem.* 30, 1363–1370. doi: 10.1159/00034 3325

Massillon, D. (2001). Regulation of the glucose-6-phosphatase gene by glucose occurs by transcriptional and post-transcriptional mechanisms-Differential effect of glucose and xylitol. *J. Biol. Chem.* 276, 4055–4062. doi: 10.1074/jbc.M007939200

Miethke, H., Wittig, B., Nath, A., Zierz, S., and Jungermann, K. (1985). Metabolic zonation in liver of diabetic rats. Zonal distribution of phosphoenolpyruvate carboxykinase, pyruvate kinase, glucose-6-phosphatase and succinate dehydrogenase. *Biol. Chem. Hoppe. Seyler.* 366, 493–501. doi: 10.1515/bchm3.1985.366.1.493

Minchenko, O., Opentanova, I., and Caro, J. (2003). Hypoxic regulation of the 6-phosphofructo-2-kinase/fructose-2,6-bisphosphatase gene family (PFKFB-1-4) expression *in vivo*. *FEBS Lett.* 554, 264–270. doi: 10.1016/S0014-5793(03)01179-7

Miralpeix, M., Carballo, E., Bartrons, R., Crepin, K., Hue, L., and Rousseau, G. G. (1992). Oral-administration of vanadate to diabetic rats restores liver 6-phosphofructo-2-kinase content and messenger-Rna. *Diabetologia* 35, 243–248. doi: 10.1007/BF00400924

Morselt, A. F., Frederiks, W. M., Copius Peereboom-Stegeman, J. H., and van Veen, H. A. (1987). Mechanism of damage to liver cells after chronic exposure to low doses of cadmium chloride. *Arch. Toxicol. Suppl.* 11, 213–215. doi: 10.1007/978-3-642-72558-6_34

Nauck, M., Wölfle, D., Katz, N., and Jungermann, K. (1981). Modulation of the glucagon-dependent induction of phosphoenolpyruvate carboxykinase and tyrosine aminotransferase by arterial and venous oxygen concentrations in hepatocyte cultures. *Eur. J. Biochem.* 119, 657–661. doi: 10.1111/j.1432-1033.1981.tb05658.x

Neely, P., El-Maghrabi, M. R., Pilkis, S. J., and Claus, T. H. (1981). Effect of diabetes, insulin, starvation, and refeeding on the level of rat hepatic fructose 2,6-bisphosphate. *Diabetes* 30, 1062–1064. doi: 10.2337/diab.30.12.1062

Noguchi, T., Inoue, H., and Tanaka, T. (1985). Transcriptional and post-transcriptional regulation of L-type pyruvate-kinase in diabetic rat-liver by insulin and dietary fructose. *J. Biol. Chem.* 260, 4393–4397.

Postic, C., Burcelin, R., Rencurel, F., Pegorier, J. P., Loizeau, M., Girard, J., et al. (1993). Evidence for a transient inhibitory effect of insulin on GLUT2 expression in the liver: studies *in vivo* and *in vitro*. *Biochem. J.* 293(Pt 1), 119–124.

Probst, I., Schwartz, P., and Jungermann, K. (1982). Induction in primary culture of gluconeogenic and glycolytic hepatocytes resembling periportal and perivenous cells. *Eur. J. Biochem.* 126, 271–278. doi: 10.1111/j.1432-1033.1982.tb06775.x

Quistorff, B. (1985). Gluconeogenesis in periportal and perivenous hepatocytes of rat liver, isolated by a new high-yield digitonin/collagenase perfusion technique. *Biochem. J.* 229, 221–226. doi: 10.1042/bj2290221

Raju, J., Gupta, D., Rao, A. R., and Baquer, N. Z. (1999). Effect of antidiabetic compounds on glyoxalase I activity in experimental diabetic rat liver. *Ind. J. Exp. Biol.* 37, 193–195.

Ramakrishnan, S. K., and Shah, Y. M. (2017). A central role for hypoxia-inducible factor (HIF)-2alpha in hepatic glucose homeostasis. *Nutr. Healthy Aging* 4, 207–216. doi: 10.3233/NHA-170022

Rappaport, A. M., Borowy, Z. J., Lougheed, W. M., and Lotto, W. N. (1954). Subdivision of hexagonal liver lobules into a structural and functional unit - role in hepatic physiology and pathology. *Anat. Rec.* 119, 11–33. doi: 10.1002/ar.1091190103

Rosa, J. L., Ventura, F., Tauler, A., and Bartrons, R. (1993). Regulation of hepatic 6-phosphofructo-2-kinase fructose 2,6-bisphosphatase gene-expression by glucagon. *J. Biol. Chem.* 268, 22540–22545.

Salas, M., Vinuela, E., and Sols, A. (1963). Insulin-dependent synthesis of liver glucokinase in the rat. *J. Biol. Chem.* 238, 3535–3538.

Schmucker, D. L., Mooney, J. S., and Jones, A. L. (1978). Stereological analysis of hepatic fine structure in the Fischer 344 rat. Influence of sublobular location and animal age. *J. Cell Biol.* 78, 319–337. doi: 10.1083/jcb.78.2.319

Sharma, C., Manjeshwar, R., and Weinhouse, S. (1964). Hormonal and dietary regulation of hepatic glucokinase. *Adv. Enzyme Regul.* 2, 189–200. doi: 10.1016/S0065-2571(64)80013-3

Sibrowski, W., Müller, M. J., and Seitz, H. J. (1981). Effect of different thyroid states on rat-liver glucokinase synthesis and degradation *Invivo*. *J. Biol. Chem.* 256, 9490–9494.

Sibrowski, W., Staegemann, U., and Seitz, H. J. (1982). Accelerated turnover of hepatic glucokinase in starved and streptozotocin-diabetic rat. *Eur. J. Biochem.* 127, 571–574. doi: 10.1111/j.1432-1033.1982.tb06910.x

Slieker, L. J., Sundell, K. L., Heath, W. F., Osborne, H. E., Bue, J., Manetta, J., et al. (1992). Glucose transporter levels in tissues of spontaneously diabetic Zucker fa/fa rat (ZDF/drt) and viable yellow mouse (Avy/a). *Diabetes* 41, 187–193. doi: 10.2337/diab.41.2.187

Teutsch, H. F., and Lowry, O. H. (1982). Sex specific regional differences in hepatic glucokinase activity. *Biochem. Biophys. Res. Commun.* 106, 533–538. doi: 10.1016/0006-291X(82)91143-3

Thorens, B., Flier, J. S., Lodish, H. F., and Kahn, B. B. (1990). Differential regulation of two glucose transporters in rat liver by fasting and refeeding and by diabetes and insulin treatment. *Diabetes* 39, 712–719. doi: 10.2337/diab.39.6.712

Torre, C., Perret, C., and Colnot, S. (2010). Molecular determinants of liver zonation. *Prog. Mol. Biol. Transl. Sci.* 97, 127–150. doi: 10.1016/B978-0-12-385233-5.00005-2

Trus, M., Zawalich, K., Gaynor, D., and Matschinsky, F. (1980). Hexokinase and glucokinase distribution in the liver lobule. *J. Histochem. Cytochem.* 28, 579–581. doi: 10.1177/28.6.7391551

Uyeda, K., and Repa, J. J. (2006). Carbohydrate response element binding protein, ChREBP, a transcription factor coupling hepatic glucose utilization and lipid synthesis. *Cell Metab.* 4, 107–110. doi: 10.1016/j.cmet.2006.06.008

Van Schaftingen, E., and Hers, H. G. (1983). The role of fructose 2,6-bisphosphate in the long-term control of phosphofructokinase in rat liver. *Biochem. Biophys. Res. Commun.* 113, 548–554. doi: 10.1016/0006-291X(83)91760-6

Vasilj, A., Gentzel, M., Ueberham, E., Gebhardt, R., and Shevchenko, A. (2012). Tissue proteomics by one-dimensional gel electrophoresis combined with label-free protein quantification. *J. Proteome Res.* 11, 3680–3689. doi: 10.1021/pr300147z

Wals, P. A., Palacin, M., and Katz, J. (1988). The zonation of liver and the distribution of fructose 2,6-bisphosphate in rat liver. *J. Biol. Chem.* 263, 4876–4881.

Weinberg, M. B., and Utter, M. F. (1979). Effect of thyroid-hormone on the turnover of rat-liver pyruvate-carboxylase and pyruvate-dehydrogenase. *J. Biol. Chem.* 254, 9492–9499.

Weinberg, M. B., and Utter, M. F. (1980). Effect of streptozotocin-induced diabetes mellitus on the turnover of rat liver pyruvate carboxylase and pyruvate dehydrogenase. *Biochem. J.* 188, 601–608. doi: 10.1042/bj1880601

Weinstein, S. P., O'Boyle, E., Fisher, M., and Haber, R. S. (1994). Regulation of GLUT2 glucose transporter expression in liver by thyroid hormone: evidence for hormonal regulation of the hepatic glucose transport system. *Endocrinology* 135, 649–654. doi: 10.1210/endo.135.2.8033812

Wimhurst, J. M., and Manchester, K. L. (1970a). A comparison of the effects of diabetes induced with either alloxan or streptozotocin and of starvation on the activities in rat liver of the key enzymes of gluconeogenesis. *Biochem. J.* 120, 95–103. doi: 10.1042/bj1200095

Wimhurst, J. M., and Manchester, K. L. (1970b). Suppression of pyruvate carboxylase by glucose in perfused rat liver. *Febs Lett.* 8, 91–94 doi: 10.1016/0014-5793(70)80232-0

Wölfle, D., and Jungermann, K. (1985). Long-term effects of physiological oxygen concentrations on glycolysis and gluconeogenesis in hepatocyte cultures. *Eur. J. Biochem.* 151, 299–303. doi: 10.1111/j.1432-1033.1985.tb09100.x

Wurtman, R. J. (1974). Daily rhythms in tyrosine-transaminase and other hepatic enzymes that metabolize amino-acids-mechanisms and possible consequences. *Life Sci.* 15, 827–847. doi: 10.1016/0024-3205(74)90001-0

Yang, J., Reshef, L., Cassuto, H., Aleman, G., and Hanson, R. W. (2009). Aspects of the control of phosphoenolpyruvate carboxykinase gene transcription. *J. Biol. Chem.* 284, 27031–27035. doi: 10.1074/jbc.R109.040535

Zalitis, J. G., and Pitot, H. C. (1979). Synthesis and degradation of rat-liver and kidney fructose bisphosphatase *Invivo. Arch. Biochem. Biophys.* 194, 620–631. doi: 10.1016/0003-9861(79)90657-X

Zeller, E., Hammer, K., Kirschnick, M., and Braeuning, A. (2013). Mechanisms of RAS/beta-catenin interactions. *Arch. Toxicol.* 87, 611–632. doi: 10.1007/s00204-013-1035-3

3

The Potential for Circulating Tumor Cells in Pancreatic Cancer Management

*Michael Pimienta[1,2], Mouad Edderkaoui[2], Ruoxiang Wang[2] and Stephen Pandol[2]**

[1] *University of California, San Diego School of Medicine, La Jolla, CA, United States,* [2] *Cedars-Sinai Medical Center, Basic and Translational Pancreas Research, Los Angeles, CA, United States*

Correspondence:
Stephen Pandol
stephen.pandol@cshs.org

Pancreatic cancer is one the most lethal malignancies. Only a small proportion of patients with this disease benefit from surgery. Chemotherapy provides only a transient benefit. Though much effort has gone into finding new ways for early diagnosis and treatment, average patient survival has only been improved in the order of months. Circulating tumor cells (CTCs) are shed from primary tumors, including pre-malignant phases. These cells possess information about the genomic characteristics of their tumor source *in situ*, and their detection and characterization holds potential in early cancer diagnosis, prognosis, and treatment. Liquid Biopsies present an alternative to tumor biopsy that are hard to sample. Below we summarize current methods of CTC detection, the current literature on CTCs in pancreatic cancer, and future perspectives.

Keywords: circulating tumor cells, pancreatic cancer, pancreatic adenocarcinoma, metastasis, epithelial to mesenchymal transition, mesenchymal to epithelial transitions

INTRODUCTION

Virtually all cancers have the potential to metastasize, and metastatic disease comes about from a series of events involving the interplay between primary tumor cells and their microenvironment. The end result is the dissemination and growth of tumor cells in new tissue environments. First described in the literature in the nineteenth century by British surgeon James Paget, metastatic disease largely remains an unsolved worldwide public health concern today—metastasis accounts for more than 90% of cancer-related deaths (Ashworth, 1869; Spano et al., 2012).

We now know that metastasis is an "extremely complex" multistep process. Tumor cells must advance through an invasion-metastasis cascade. In order to produce clinically detectable lesions, primary tumor cells need to progressively intravasate through the basal membrane into the systemic or lymphatic circulation, survive in the circulatory environment, adhere to vessel walls, extravasate into a foreign tissue site, and adapt, survive, and proliferate in their new microenvironment (Fidler, 2003).

The potential for mobilization and invasion are critical to the process of intravasation. Cells should be able to degrade the extracellular matrix (ECM) and secrete proteolytic enzymes to facilitate migration and intravasation into the circulatory system. These epithelium-derived cancer cells are thought to undergo a morphological change of epithelial-to-mesenchymal transition (EMT; Leber and Efferth, 2009; Dhamija and Diederichs, 2016). At metastatic sites, neoplastic cells should also infiltrate the endothelium in order to colonize new tissues and be able to induce neo-angiogenesis to ensure sufficient blood supply to the newly formed tumor in order to maintain metabolic needs (Leber and Efferth, 2009; **Figure 1**). The preferred growth and survival of cancer cells at certain metastatic sites is less understood, although a reverse behavioral change, mesenchymal-to-epithelium transition (MET), is hypothesized to take place for this to occur (Dhamija and Diederichs, 2016).

Metastasis itself is a highly inefficient process, as each step in the metastasis cascade may play a limiting role in disease progression, that is—if one fails then all fails. Only few cancer cells are able to go on to form malignant secondary tumors. Animal studies on the kinetics of each step have shown that post-extravasation steps create the largest barrier to metastasis. An early report, for example, found that 80% of injected cancer cells survive in circulation and extravasate into distant tissues, but only 1 in 40 cells formed micrometastasis and 1 in 100 micrometastasis actually progressed to macroscopic tumors (Luzzi et al., 1998). Further, studies found similar results, showing the high efficiency of extravasation and survival in the circulation to be independent of cell's malignant potential (Koop et al., 1995, 1996; Cameron et al., 2000). These findings suggest that the growth of circulating tumor cells (CTCs) in a new microenvironment is a key step in metastatic tumor formation.

Materials shed from tumors are being investigated for their potential use in diagnosis, prognosis, and management of cancer. CTCs, cell-free circulating tumor DNA (ctDNA), and tumor cell produced exosomes (oncosomes) all hold promise in the current cancer research for future clinical use in diagnosis and management. Oncosomes, nanovesicles actively shed from most types of cancers in large numbers, like CTCs, are a dynamic source of information regarding the genomic characteristics from the parent tumor of which they are release (Deneve et al., 2013; Pantel and Alix-Panabieres, 2013; Speicher and Pantel, 2014). Though each has their own technical challenges, these materials are now being isolated and detected in peripheral blood of patients with many types metastatic cancers and are leading the way toward use of "liquid biopsies."

CTCS IN MODERN CANCER RESEARCH

While, it is estimated that only 0.01% of CTCs have metastatic potential, the clinical importance of CTCs in "modern cancer research" over the past two decades has become increasingly apparent (Zhe et al., 2011). Although the presence of CTCs in blood could not exclusively indicate clinically significant macro-metastases, partly due to metastatic inefficiency, it surely indicates the presence of malignant tumors *in situ*. More and more data suggests that solid tumor shedding occurs early in disease. A recent study detected disseminated tumor cells (DTCs) in bone marrow of a mouse breast cancer model during pre-malignant stages, reinforcing the idea of early spread of tumor cells to distant organs. Fast, specific, and sensitive detection of CTCs may have potential to enhance diagnosis, treatment, and cancer monitoring. CTCs may additionally be exploited for genotypic and phenotypic abnormalities representative of the tumor *in situ*.

CTC detection in peripheral blood has been reported in a number of cancer types, such as lung (Zhang et al., 2014), metastatic breast (Riethdorf et al., 2007), prostate (Hu et al., 2013), colorectal cancer (Kuboki et al., 2013), and gastrointestinal and biliary cancers (Al Ustwani et al., 2012; Tsujiura et al., 2014). Many of these cancers are diagnosed at late stages, resulting in high rates of mortality. Advancements in CTC collection, enrichment, and characterization have led to increased interest in the clinical use of CTCs. Studies in various organ systems have consistently shown that CTCs rarely exist in the blood of healthy subjects, consolidating their utility in the clinical laboratory (Sastre et al., 2008; Hou et al., 2013; Tsai et al., 2016), while supporting the premise of CTCs with the potential of a powerful biomarker.

Various available CTC detection technologies have expanded their use from simply diagnostic markers to tools to evaluate overall survival, risk of metastasis, and response to therapy. Recently, using the Veridex Cell Search System, the only FDA approved method for CTC enumeration in whole blood, Weissenstein et al., found a strong correlation between median overall survival in metastatic breast cancer patients with <5 CTC/7.5 ml vs. those with ≥ 5 CTC ($p = 0.00006$; Weissenstein et al., 2012). In a review of multicenter study of 1,358 individuals, Miller et al. found a highly significant median overall survival in favorable CTC counts vs. patients with unfavorable CTC counts with metastatic breast cancer, metastatic colorectal cancer, and prostate cancer ($p < 0.0001$). Additionally, patients enrolled in therapies that decreased CTC counts displayed improvements in overall survival, pointing to the utility that CTC analysis in the response to anti-cancer treatments holds (Miller et al., 2010). Studies have also taken advantage of the current available methods to correlate tumor dissemination and stage to CTC count. Hiraiwa et al. showed that CTC counts were higher in metastatic patients than in non-metastatic esophageal, gastric, and colorectal cancers and were significantly correlated to advanced tumor stages. High CTC count, defined as 2 or more CTCs per 7.5 ml in this study, was linked to pleural and peritoneal dissemination (Hiraiwa et al., 2008). Further, validation in clinical settings will establish CTC detection as a marker for sensitive and non-invasive cancer diagnosis, treatment evaluation and prognosis.

CTC ENRICHMENT AND DETECTION

CTCs are rare cells, detected in numbers ranging from 1 to 10 s per ml whole blood, among billions of red blood cells and millions of leukocytes. CTC detection and isolation remain being technologically challenging (Joosse and Pantel, 2013). In the infancy of this rapidly growing field, current CTC detection and analysis rely mainly on various methods of enrichment.

CTC enrichment approaches exploit the unique biological and/or physical properties of this specified tumor cell type among vast numbers of peripheral blood cells, in order to increase CTC recovery by many orders of magnitude. Immunoaffinity platforms select for CTCs based on the expression of specific surface antigens, through either positive or negative selection.

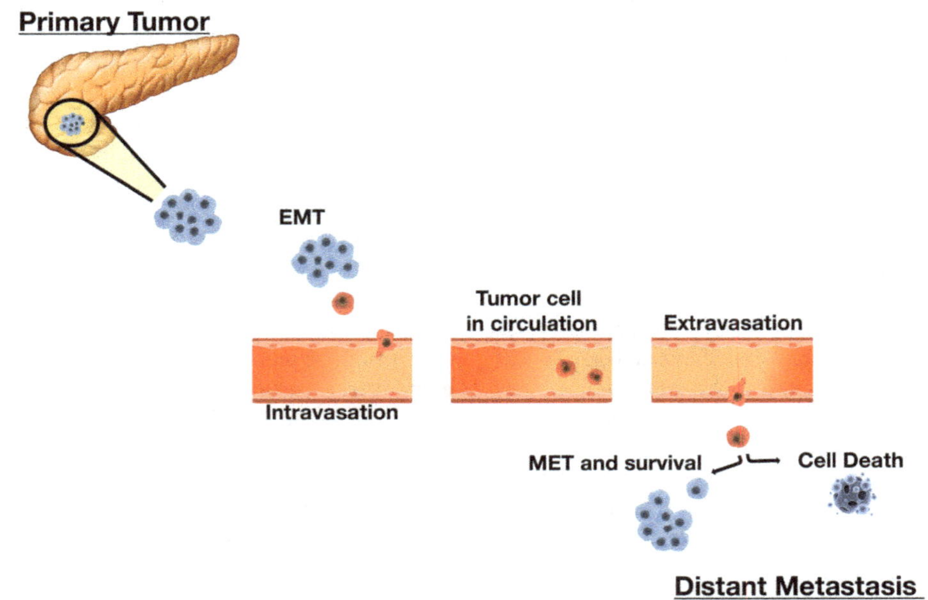

FIGURE 1 | The Sequential Process of Cancer Metastasis. Metastasis is a complex multi-step process. Tumor cells undergo remarkable morphological and phenotypical changes enabling migration and infiltration of adjacent sites as single cells or small clusters. An initial epithelial-to-mesenchymal transition (EMT) allows cells to acquire mesenchymal properties essential for motility and migration. Upon infiltrating local stroma, cancer cells intravasate into the vascular or lymphatic system and circulate throughout the body as circulating tumor cells (CTCs). In the circulation, disseminated CTCs must overcome barriers such as sheer-stress and the immune system. CTCs that survive the circulation extravasate and invade distant tissues by reestablishing characteristics of their corresponding primary tumor. CTC plasticity allows them to undergo the mesenchymal-to-epithelial transition (MET) to achieve this. Each step in this metastasis cascade is rate-limiting. Cells that successfully adapt to their microenvironment and resume proliferation successfully form overt secondary tumors. Alternately, cells that do not survive undergo cell death.

Since most carcinomas express epithelial markers, epithelial cell adhesion molecule (EpCAM) is most commonly used in antibody-based positive selection with commercial technologies. Negative selection depletes other mononucleated cells through anti-CD45 antibody use. Established collection methods have employed these proteins to attract and adhere CTCs to columns, microposts, or magnetic apparatus (Alix-Panabières and Pantel, 2014).

Two early platforms, magnetic-activate cell sorting system (MACS), and Dynabeads use magnetic fields for attract CTCs to anti-EpCAM antibody coated magnetic microbeads (Nagrath et al., 2016). Similarly, CellSearch (Janssen Diagnostics) uses anti-EpCAM conjugated ferrofluid nano-particles to immunomagnetically capture CTCs, which may then be differentiated from contaminating leukocytes based on positive cytokeratin or EpCAM staining and negative CD45 staining (Hayes et al., 2006). Despite much progress in platform development, CellSearch remains the only FDA approved method of whole blood CTC enrichment and enumeration. Another platform, MagSweeper (Stanford University), uses magnetic rods, stirred through diluted blood samples, to attract CTCs pre-labeled with EpCAM-magnetic beads (Talasaz et al., 2009). This platform was one of the first to enrich CTCs with a notably higher purity than its predecessors. Importantly, it has the ability to isolate live CTCs without perturbing gene expression throughout the enrichment process, providing viable CTCs for analysis (Krebs et al., 2014).

Microfluidic devices, which allow separation of CTCs, from small fluid volumes under laminar flow, are promising technologies. Nearly 10 years ago, Nagrath et al. was able to selectively and efficiently isolate CTCs from whole blood of 115/116 (99%) cancer patients using anti-EpCAM-coated posts with this "CTC-Chip" platform, eliminating the need for pre-labeling or sample processing (Nagrath et al., 2007). New microfluidic approaches have appeared since then, including methods taking advantage of physical properties as well, making the platform applicable to isolation of CTCs that lack or have down regulated EpCAM expression (Stott et al., 2010; Ozkumur et al., 2013).

Positive and negative CTC enrichment is also tested based on physical properties alone. Tumor cells and CTCs are generally thought to be larger (>8 μm) than hematologic cells (Vona et al., 2000, 2004; Hosokawa et al., 2013). Size-based filtration methods, such as isolation by size of epithelial tumor cells (ISET) through membrane filters with size exclusive pores, have been previously used to isolate individual CTCs and achieved higher sensitivity than CellSearch (Hofman et al., 2011; Hou et al., 2011).

As CTCs extravasate and intravastate the circulation, they undergo massive deformations in their structure due to mechanical forces which they endure. Cancer cells are known to be more deformable than normal cells, a quality that is correlated to their metastatic potential and is exploited by some enrichment platforms (Byun et al., 2013; Park et al., 2016). Additionally, platforms utilizing tumor cell property differences in electrical charge and density have been reported (Müller et al., 2005; Fabbri et al., 2013; Yoo et al., 2016).

While many of the platforms available have been able to detect CTCs in blood samples, these small peripheral blood collections, of several milliliters, may not be representative of the of the entire patient blood volume. Recently, an antibody coated medical wire (CellCollector; Gilupi GmbH) capable of detecting EpCAM and cytokeratin positive CTCs *in vivo* was introduced. In a recent study, a 30 min incubation period, in which the wire was exposed to circulating blood in the arm vein of lung cancer patients, showed over a 2-fold increase in CTC detection in comparison to CellSearch (Gorges et al., 2016b). Further, efforts to enhance the biocompatibility of these wire coatings, have been employed to maximize functionality for downstream processes such as sequencing analyses of captured cells (Scherag et al., 2017).

Once enriched, CTCs are detected/confirmed through various techniques. Immunocytological and molecular approaches are the most commonly employed. Immunocytochemistry (ICC) may differentiate CTCs from contaminating cells through biomarker detection. Such biomarkers can be specific for nuclear content, epithelial proteins (i.e., cytokeratins), and hematopoietic markers (i.e., CD45). A common immunocytological CTC definition, currently used by CellSearch and other platforms, is a $\text{Nucleus}^{+}/\text{CK}^{+}/\text{CD45}^{-}$ cell. However, it should be noted that CTC designation depending primarily on epithelial marker expression may lead to false negatives by failing to detect CTCs that have undergone EMT (Lustberg et al., 2012). As cell phenotypes can vary in different malignancies, the heterogeneity of CTCs pose barriers to efficient and thorough detection by liquid biopsies.

Reliance on epithelial markers, which most epithelial carcinomas express, for enrichment and identification, fails to capture subpopulations of CTCs, such as mesenchymal cells, that may harbor clinically important information. Currently, cancer studies in breast and prostate have already demonstrated that mesenchymal marker expression by CTCs is associated with poorer survival (Aktas et al., 2009; Yokobori et al., 2013). Recently, negative depletion strategies that enrich CTCs in phenotype-independent ways have been introduced in an effort to solve this problem and enhance detection. Immunostaining of CD45 and cell sorting with flow cytometry was used to enrich the breast cancer CTC population (Lara et al., 2004). Multi-marker Immunomagnetic Negative Depletion Enrichment of CTCs (MINDEC), relies on depletion of non-CTCs as opposed to targeting specific properties of CTCs (Lapin et al., 2016). This technique is based on a multi-marker antibody cocktail (CD45, CD16, CD19, CD163, and CD235a/GYPA) to target various contaminating blood classes. This technique has shown high enrichment efficiency of both epithelial and mesenchymal CTCs, with better hematopoietic depletion than CD45 alone. Additional, novel cell surface marker-independent techniques have been shown to effectively detect CTCs in epithelial and non-epithelial malignancies in the absence of cell surface tumor markers. For example, a novel method introduced by Zhang et al., selectively labeled CTCs through GFP expression in human samples and cancer cell lines transfected with tumor selective replicating HSV-1 with a high detection efficiency (Zhang et al., 2016).

Table 1 shows various CTC isolation methods used in the last few years.

Newer methods have employed combinations of epithelial, mesenchymal, tumor-specific, and tissue-specific marker expression (Pantel and Alix-Panabieres, 2013).

Additionally, nucleic acid-based technologies have provided an alternate avenue (Yu et al., 2011), as improvements in non-fixating enrichment procedures have allowed for the use of RT-PCR and qRT-PCR to amplify single or multiple gene transcripts for CTC detection.

Most recently, emerging single-cell sequencing techniques have shifted the field toward individual CTC analysis of genetic alterations associated with tumor mechanisms, clinical outcomes, therapy response, and drug targets and resistance. The usefulness of genomic analyses, however, is limited by heterogeneity between cancer subtypes, presenting barriers toward finding universal markers. Similarly, all the current enrichment, detection, and analysis techniques available harbor their own technical challenges and limitations. Most of these are outside the scope of this discussion.

CTCS IN PANCREATIC CANCER DIAGNOSIS

Pancreatic cancer is one of the deadliest malignancies. Pancreatic ductal carcinoma (PDAC) makes up the majority of pancreatic cancers. While advancements in the treatment of other cancer types may have led to significant improvement in patient survival, advancements in pancreatic cancer research have not been met with the same success. PDAC incidence has remained stable over the last 30 years and the lack of fruitful therapies and new/useful diagnostic methods have yet to be changed in pancreatic cancer (Ryan et al., 2014). With current therapies improving survival outcomes by only a few months, pancreatic cancer patients face a 5 year survival rate of only 7%. Gemcitabine, the first-line of PDAC therapy, only modestly improves survival in advanced pancreatic cancer, while the clinical benefit of combinational-targeted therapies (Erlotinib+Gemcitabine) has proven to have only slight benefit, increasing overall survival by less than a month (Burris et al., 1997; Moore et al., 2007). Recent work in combinational chemotherapeutics has led to a promising approach, FOLFIRINOX (Oxaliplatin, Irinotecan, Leucovorin, and 5-fluorouracil), which has almost doubled survival in metastatic pancreatic adenocarcinoma patients to 11.1 months compared to 6.8 months with single-agent gemcitabine (Conroy et al., 2011). In another promising approach, albumin bound paclitaxel (Abraxane) plus standard gemcitabine therapy increased overall survival to 8.5 months compared to standard gemcitabine therapy with an overall survival of 6.7 months (Von Hoff et al., 2013). The toxicity associated with these regimens is unfavorable and should be used in patients with good performance status. Unfortunately, 5 year survival rates remain

TABLE 1 | CTC isolation techniques.

CTC isolation method	Disease	Comment	References
Size-based filtration method: Use of membrane filters with size exclusive pores	Multiple carcinomas	Isolation of CTCs based on cell size to isolate them from leukocytes	Vona et al., 2000, 2004; Hosokawa et al., 2013
Veridex cell search system: Anti-EpCAM antibody coated microbeads	Multiple carcinomas	The only FDA approved	Allard et al., 2004
Magnetic-activated cell sorting system (MACS)	Breast cancer	Enrichment of the CTC population	Lara et al., 2004
Use of electrical charges and density properties of cancer cells	Primary breast cancer	CTCs detected in 8.3% of patients before surgery. After Chemotherapy, CTCs detected in 44% of previously negative patients	Müller et al., 2005
Cell Search System	Gastro-intestinal cancers	High CTC number corrected with metastasis and with low survival	Hiraiwa et al., 2008
MagSweeper: Magnetic rods	Metastatic breast cancer	Higher purity than the Cell search system	Talasaz et al., 2009
Microfluidic devices: Microfluid approaches taking advantage of physical properties	Metastatic prostate cancer	Isolate CTC with down regulated EpCAM	Stott et al., 2010; Ozkumur et al., 2013
Combination of epithelial and mesenchymal markers: Use combination of antibodies to select CTC with epithelial and mesenchymal properties	Localized and metastatic colorectal cancer	Avoid CTC phenotype problem	Deneve et al., 2013
MINDEC: Multi-Marker Immuno-magnetic Negative Depletion Enrichment	Metastatic pancreatic cancer	Enhanced negative depletion strategy—MINDEC-based on multi-marker (CD45, CD16, CD19, CD163, and CD235a/GYPA) depletion of blood cells	Lapin et al., 2016
GILUPI cell collector: cell Collector-Wire coating: EpCAM and Cytokeratin antibody coated medical wire	Lung cancer	Isolation of CTCs from peripheral blood to overcome the blood volume limitations	Gorges et al., 2016b
Wire coating enhanced: Enhanced wire coting to maximize functionality	Breast cancer cells	Improvement of the wire technology	Scherag et al., 2017

relatively unchanged. It is estimated that by 2030 pancreatic cancer will be the second leading cause of cancer-related deaths (Rahib et al., 2014; Dawson and Fernandez-Zapico, 2016).

The idea of a liquid biopsy, which could reveal diagnostic and prognostic information about a patient's state, has been gaining much traction in the past 10 years. In one of the earliest studies, with 12 types of metastatic carcinomas in 964 patients, CTCs were successfully detected in patients with pancreatic cancer using CellSearch, albeit in lower numbers than the other cancers (Allard et al., 2004). Below, we summarize the studies of CTCs in the diagnosis, staging, and prognosis for pancreatic cancer patients.

Pancreatic cancer is a fast progressive disease and its early diagnosis is challenging. Initial pancreatic cancer diagnosis depends largely upon symptoms, which would only appear late when tumor have fully progressed and are not specific to be recognized at early stages. Due to the pathobiology and aggressiveness of PDAC, by the time anorexia, early satiety, pain, and weight loss start present, the disease has already progressed, leaving little room for a favorable prognosis. Additionally, of the 15% of patients seeking medical care 6 months prior to diagnosis, 25% have symptoms resembling upper abdominal disease that may lead to misdiagnosis (DiMagno, 1999). Affirmative diagnosis is made by tissue biopsies obtained by surgery, image guided CT biopsy, or fine needle aspiration through endoscopic ultrasound (EUS-FNA). Despite its widespread use, EUS-FNA does have diagnostic drawbacks, specifically a sensitivity range from 75 to 94% and a specificity of 78 to 95%, with low but lethal complications such as pancreatitis and bowel perforation (Court et al., 2015; Bournet et al., 2016). For CTC detection to be adopted to pancreatic cancer diagnosis, it must be useful for early diagnosis and/or monitoring treatment responses. A key performance milestone necessary for the implementation of CTC technologies is an understanding of disease stage at which CTCs can be detected. At the same time, it should be kept in mind that CTC research in pancreatic cancer is at nascent stage, while CTC detection methods and criteria vary largely between studies. It is important to critically analyze the markers available and to characterize CTCs at different stages of cancer progression.

CTC detection has been explored in early diagnosis of various cancers and CTCs have been detected prior to tumor detection by traditional methods. A recent study, for instance, found that CTCs could be detected 1–4 years before lung cancer became detectable through CT-scan screening in the same patients (Ilie et al., 2014). For breast cancer, the American Society of Clinical Oncology (ASCO) has already approved the use of CTCs as a tumor marker, creating new directions for early breast cancer diagnosis (Harris et al., 2007).

Similar results have been obtained in pancreatic cancer. In a mouse model of PDAC, Rhim et al. found that inflicted pancreatic cells underwent EMT early during cancer development. These cells with EMT were predicted to represent early cancer cells, as the extent of EMT correlated well to invasive properties in tumor cells, facilitated their intravasation to circulating the blood and hepatic seeding, prior to the manifestation of primary tumors (Rhim et al., 2012). Additionally, blood samples from patients with pancreatic cystic lesions were detected to contain pancreas epithelial cells, at a time prior to cancer diagnosis. These findings suggested that pancreatic cell appearance in circulating blood precedes *in situ* tumor formation, and detection of CTCs could be an early biomarker for PDAC early diagnosis.

CTC-specific gene expression has been explored as surrogate markers for early cancer detection. Such studies mostly detect CTCs via detecting their expression of epithelial proteins. Reverse transcription-coupled polymerase chain reaction (RT-PCR) could be used to examine potential epithelial markers in CTCs derived from tumors of the epithelia. Soeth et al., evaluated cytokeratin 20 (CK20) detection, through RT-PCR detection from the marrow and venous blood in pancreatic ductal carcinoma patients. CK-20 positivity was detected in cells of 52 of 154 patients in venous blood, where higher CK20 level was correlated to UICC-tumor stage (Soeth et al., 2005). In a study of 34 pancreatic cancer patients prior to treatments, de Albuquerque et al used immunomagnetic enrichment for CTCs in peripheral blood based on mucin-1 and EpCAM expression. Subsequently, multi-marker RT-PCR analysis was used to detect tumor-associated transcripts, including KRT19, MUC1, EpCAM, CEACAM5, and BIRC5. CTCs with at least one marker in peripheral blood were detected in 47.1% patients prior to undergoing treatment (de Albuquerque et al., 2012). Detection efficacy was increased with the use of multiple markers as opposed to single marker use, indicating differential gene expression among CTCs from the same cancer patient.

Zhang et al., used an alternative strategy by enriching and identifying CTCs through a combination of CD45 and CK with a FISH-CEP8 probe in 22 pancreatic cancer patients. CTCs were detected from 15 of the patients, with CTCs ranging from 0 to 60 cells/3.75 ml of blood. In comparison, healthy controls, and patients with benign pancreatic tumors were negative for detection of CTCs, and sensitivity and specificity of CTC detection in pancreatic diagnosis were determined to be 68.18 and 94.87%, respectively, when using 2 cells/3.75 ml as cutoff. CTC-positive patients exhibited metastasis and poorer survival rates upon a 1.5 year follow-up. CTC positivity did not correlate significantly to CA19-9 levels of the *in situ* tumor. It is well-known that, though CA19-9 has a high sensitivity and specificity in advanced pancreatic cancers, its diagnostic usefulness is questionable to diseases at early asymptomatic stages. The combination of CA19-9 and CTC positivity in the study above increased detection rates from 68.18 to 77.3% (Zhang et al., 2015). The results from this study suggest CTCs as biomarkers for the diagnosis of early stage pancreatic cancers, in asymptomatic patients, and from patients with normal CA19-9 plasma levels. A later study by Xu et al., used a similar approach in 40 patients and dramatically high detection rates in PC patients (90%). Diagnostic rates increased to 97% when combining CTC ≥ 2 and CA19-9 > 37 μmol/L as a cutoff. Identification of chromosomal instability in CTCs, characterized as chromosome 8 triploids, showed a significantly statistic prognostic correlation. Patients with triploid CTCs < 3 displayed both higher 1 year and overall survival compared to those with ≥ 3 (Xu et al., 2017).

Doublecortin-like kinase 1 (DCLK1) may be another marker for CTC detection in early PDAC stages. Prior work suggests that Dclk1 marks stem cells, being able to differentiate cancer from normal stem cells. Interestingly, this marker protein is overexpressed in pancreatic and colorectal cancers (Nakanishi et al., 2012; Bailey et al., 2014). Qu et al., found elevated serum DCLK1 levels in stage I and II PDAC patients relative to controls and a decline in stage III and IV patients to levels similar to those seen in control patients. Diagnostic utility analysis showed both DLCK1 sensitivity and specificity to be significant in stage I and II patients. Furthermore, the investigators evaluated DCLK1 in the KPC mouse model, finding the serum DCLK1 levels to be significantly elevated as early as 5 weeks in KPC mice, compared to control mice. Over 50% of CTCs isolated from KPC mice whole blood were DLCK1^{+}, suggesting a possible biomarker to be used in conjunction with CTCs for detection of early stage pancreatic cancer (Qu et al., 2015).

Kulemann et al., investigated the usefulness of CTC detection in pancreatic cancers from both localized and advanced stages. Peripheral blood from PDAC patients was used to capture CTCs for cytological and KRAS mutational analysis using the ScreenCell isolation method (Kulemann et al., 2015). High CTC detection efficiency as low as 2 cells/ml was calibrated by spiking experiments with healthy donor blood. CTC *KRAS* mutations were identified in 8 of 11 PDAC patients (73%). This is in sharp contrast to conventional biopsy-based diagnosis for the same patients, by which 2 of 11 samples (18%) were cytologically categorized as negative/non-diagnostic, while the rest exhibited abnormal morphology (18%) or were categorized as suspicious (64%). Moreover, the authors found no difference in the detection rate between early and advanced diseases, suggesting that CTCs are disseminated from primary tumors early in disease development and can be used to diagnose pancreatic cancer at initial stages where curative surgery may be available. It should be pointed out that this finding is contrary to those shown by Soeth et al. (2005), in which significant stage dependent differences were observed in CTC detection. Further studies are needed to clarify whether the difference is due to the differences in CTC detection strategies.

CTCS IN METASTASIS AND EARLY CANCER

Early local invasion and metastasis are prominent factors in the poor prognosis of pancreatic cancer, as most patients are found with metastatic disease at diagnosis (DiMagno et al., 1999; Pandol et al., 2009). The impact of CTCs on pancreatic cancer metastasis, recurrence, and prognosis has been investigated.

A recent 9-cohort meta-analysis of separate studies using CellSearch and RT-PCR detection methods, involving 623 pancreatic cancer patients altogether, revealed associations between CTC detection and poor prognosis. Out of 623 patients, 268 (43%) were classified as CTC positive and displayed poor progression-free survival and worse overall survival than those in the non-CTC group (Han et al., 2014).

Using the CellSearch enrichment method, Kurihara et al., investigated the utility of CTCs in peripheral blood as a marker of clinical outcomes in 26 patients with pancreatic cancer. CTC positivity was found in 11 of 26 pancreatic cancer patients (42%). The authors demonstrated a significant difference in median survival times between CTC positive and negative patients, for 110.5 and 375.8 days, respectively ($P < 0.001$; Kurihara et al., 2008). Given that the detection method was shown to have 100% specificity, with no CTCs detected in the non-cancer groups, CellSearch detection strategy may not be sensitive enough, as no CTCs were detected from the other 58% pancreatic cancer patients. These results suggest the need of developing more sensitive methods to detect positive CTCs in all pancreatic cancer cases.

Similarly, de Albuquerque et al found a correlation between CTC positivity (47% of patients) and median progression-free survival (PFS). Patients with at least one tumor-associated transcript found in their CTCs, enriched from peripheral blood using immunomagnetic EpCAM and mucin 1 detection, had a PFS of 66.0 vs. 138.0 days in those who did not. Intriguingly, CTC enumeration was found to have no correlation to clinicopathological features of the disease, including metastasis status and tumor stages (de Albuquerque et al., 2012).

Bidard et al. studied CTC detection rates in a subset of 79 patients with locally advanced pancreatic carcinoma enrolled in the LAP 07 trial. The primary study (LAP 07) assessed the effect of subsequent chemotherapy vs. chemo-radiotherapy continuation on overall survival in patients whose disease was controlled after 4 months of chemotherapy alone. The patient subgroup was screened for CTCs using CellSearch technology prior to chemotherapy administration and 2 months after treatment. While the investigators found that CTC positivity was not prognostic of PFS, they found it to be an independent prognostic factor associated with poor tumor differentiation and shorter overall survival (Bidard et al., 2013).

Bissolati et al., used the same CellSearch technique with systemic and portal vein blood of 20 patients undergoing pancreatic resection. No significant differences in both overall survival and disease-free survival between CTC-positive and -negative groups. The authors did, however, find a higher incidence of liver metastasis upon a 2 and 3 year follow up in the CTC-positive portal vein group (Bissolati et al., 2015).

Similarly, an early study investigated CTC positivity in 67 intraoperative patients with biliary-cancer. Molecular detection of CEA mRNA-positive CTCs from peripheral, central, and portal veins via RT-PCR was associated with a significant incidence of hematogenous metastases compared to CTC-negative patients (37.5 vs. 11.4%; Uchikura et al., 2002). Nonetheless, whether surgical resection of the pancreas itself may contribute to tumor cell shedding remains to be addressed. Pancreaticoduodenectomy (PD), involving the pancreatic head, and distal pancreatosplenectomy (DPS), involving the pancreatic body and tail, are standard surgical procedures. Both require necessary mobilization of the pancreas, and may lead to CTC dissemination via the portal vein to increase the risk of liver metastasis (Kuroki and Eguchi, 2017).

Table 2 represents data showing association between CTC presence and pancreatic cancer stage and outcome.

Chausovsky et al., used RT-PCR to examine the usefulness of CK20 expression in CTCs in the diagnosis of metastatic lung, stomach, colon, and pancreatic cancers (Chausovsky et al., 1999), since CK20 has been shown to not be transcribed in cells of hematopoietic lineage (Burchill et al., 1995). Chausovsky concluded that CK20 is a potential biomarker for detecting metastasis, with a sensitivity of 22/28 (78.6%) in patients with metastatic pancreatic cancer. Cytokeratins are used conventionally to characterize cancer cells of epithelial origin (Cooper et al., 1985; Lane and Alexander, 1990). Combination of cytokeratin and additional gene expression may improve the efficacy of CTC detection.

Poruk et al., assessed the potential of CTCs as biomarkers in 50 patients prior to surgical resection, based on EMT-related epithelial and mesenchymal marker expression. CTCs were acquired from blood samples through the method of ISET. CTCs were further identified by immunofluorescence staining with antibodies against pan-cytokeratins and the mesenchymal cell protein, vimentin. This analysis found that 78% of patients had CTCs expressing cytokeratin and 67% co-expressed vimentin, while no CTCs were found to express vimentin only. The authors found a significant association between cytokeratin only positive CTCs and worse survival. Interestingly, co-expression of vimentin was predictive of recurrence ($p = 0.01$). Of the patients diagnosed with metastatic cancer at the time of surgery, all the CTCs were positive for dual staining (Poruk et al., 2016). These findings indicate the involvement of EMT mechanism in metastatic progression. EMT would render CTCs heterogeneous and multi-marker analysis would have to be employed in order to ensure a comprehensive detection of all CTCs in a patient blood sample.

A recent study enumerated CTCs independently of surface marker status using a GFP expressed tumor selective Herpes Simplex Virus replicated based on telomerase activity. Transfected cells of 290 samples of patients with different solid tumors were examined and CTCs were detected in patients with epithelial and non-epithelial tumors from as little as 4 ml of blood. PC patients had a positive CTC detection rate of 88.2% across various stages and had the highest average number of cells identified per samples (43.1). Additionally, CTC detection rates increased to 100% in PC patients with regional lymph node metastasis but no distant metastasis (N+M0), further supporting the use of CTCs as a biomarker in disease progression (Zhang et al., 2016). Other recent phenotypic-independent enrichment platforms have shown some success in CTC enumeration regardless of epithelial or mesenchymal surface proteins. Negative selection of hematopoietic cells in blood samples of

TABLE 2 | Association between CTC presence and disease stage and outcome.

References	Finding	Number of patients	CTC Detection method in pancreatic cancer patients
Allard et al., 2004	First detection of CTC in pancreatic cancer biopsies	16	Cell search
Soeth et al., 2005	Higher CK20 in the blood correlated with tumor stage	154	CK20 RT-PCR
Kurihara et al., 2008	Association between presence of CTC and survival	26	Cell Search
de Albuquerque et al., 2012	Association between presence of CTC and decreased PF survival. No association between presence of CTC and disease stage	34	Multi marker RT-PCR
Bidard et al., 2013	No PF survival association but association with poorer overall survival	79	Cell Search
Han et al., 2014	Association between CTC detection and poor prognosis	623	Cell Search and RT-PCR (9-cohort meta-analysis study)
Zhang et al., 2015	CT-positive patients exhibited metastasis and poorer survival	22	CD45 and CK with FISH-CEP8 probe
Xu et al., 2017	Diagnostic rate increased to 97% when combining CTC>2 and CA19-9>37	40	NE-iFISH
Kulemann et al., 2015	No correlation between CTC and stage. CTC could be used as early marker	11	Screen Cell Isolation Method
Bissolati et al., 2015	No PF or overall survival association. But higher liver metastasis incidence	20	Cell Search

PC patients using MINDEC showed a CTC detection rate of 71%. Further, characterization of the enriched cells showed the presence of both epithelial and mesenchymal CTC populations. While the high rate of positivity in this proof-of-principle study, in comparison to previous phenotype specific platforms, could be due to the authors use of patients with metastatic disease only, its ability to detect both epithelial and mesenchymal cells, in addition to CTC clusters, marks a progressive trend toward comprehensive detection of both epithelial and mesenchymal CTCs with one technique (Lapin et al., 2016). More importantly, both CTC surface marker-independent enrichment techniques allow for the viability of collected cells to be subsequently used for downstream genetic analysis without compromise from high background leukocyte levels.

Recent works characterizing EMT found CTCs positive for both epithelial and mesenchymal markers in peripheral blood of breast cancer patients (Yu et al., 2013). Studies in mouse models have provided insight into the composition of CTCs in pancreatic cancer. Single-cell RNA sequencing revealed the expression of both epithelial and mesenchymal markers in KPC *LSL-KrasG12D, Trp53flox/flox or +, Pdx1-Cre* (KPC) mouse pancreatic tumors. Moreover, the authors observed substantial loss of the classical *E-cadherin* expression, suggesting that some CTCs of epithelial lineage could indeed adopt a partial mesenchymal stromal phenotype through EMT, while retaining other epithelial features such as cytokeratin expression (Ting et al., 2014).

Different from epithelial cells, most mesenchymal stromal cells harbor certain stem cell properties, being able to be induced to differentiate into more mature cells (Zhau et al., 2011). The EMT phenotype is usually associated with expression of cancer stemness markers (Kong et al., 2011). Compared to other cancers, however, very little is known about stemness in pancreatic cancer CTCs.

In breast cancer, expression of cancer stem cell markers in CTCs is a sign of increased the metastatic ability (Papadaki et al., 2014). The expression of cancer stemness marker ALDH1 on CTCs was found to correlate to the stage of the disease and to the expression of EMT markers vimentin and fibronectin in prostate cancer patients (Raimondi et al., 2011). A study by Barrière et al. (2012) aimed at the detection of CTCs endowed with mesenchymal and/or stem cell characteristics, at the time of initial diagnosis with breast cancer, found that EMT and cancer stemness occur in the primary tumors and are associated with an enhanced ability for tumor cells to intravasate in the early phase of cancer development.

Multiplex transcriptome profiling of single CTCs revealed presence of sub-populations of CTCs expressing multiple pro-cancer transcripts including cancer stem cell markers such as CD44 and CD24 (Gorges et al., 2016a). So far multiple markers have been used to detect CTC stem cell properties in CTCs, including CD44, CD133, CXCR4, ABCG2, and ALDH1. Other markers used uniquely for pancreatic cancer CTCs include CD24 and c-Met (Yang et al., 2015). Whether CTCs with mesenchymal or stem cell characteristics may be used as a marker for aggressiveness of the disease remains to be evaluated in future studies.

CHALLENGES

There has been much progresses over the last decade to overcome the initial barriers of CTC research in the laboratory and clinic. Significant technological development has been made for CTC detection, enrichment, and molecular characterization. On the other hand, CTC research in gastrointestinal cancers had a late start relative to other human malignancies (Allard et al., 2004). Due to gastrointestinal biology, pancreatic cancer detection via CTCs has its own set of challenges. It is widely proposed that the liver sequesters CTCs as they pass into the systemic circulation via the portal vein (Jiao et al., 2009). The predominant dissemination of pancreatic cancers to the liver have supported this notion. A recent report detected CTCs in 100% (14/14) of portal vein samples of patients with pancreaticobiliary cancers as opposed to under 25% (3/14) when peripheral samples were used for detection (Catenacci et al., 2015), a result consistent with the notion that higher CTC numbers are detected in portal vein as opposed to peripheral blood (Waxman et al., 2014). Furthermore, there was a significant increase in CTC detection in portal blood vs. peripheral blood, with a mean of 125.64 CTCs/7.5 ml as opposed to 0.8 CTCs/7.5 ml ($p = 0.01$; Catenacci et al., 2015). This study further emphasizes the importance that the collection site plays in CTC detection.

While preliminary studies in various cancers are demonstrating the potential of CTCs in early cancer detection, the continuous data coming out using different platforms (exploiting size, density, charge, surface antigens, etc.) make it challenging to reach a consensus for clinical application. The diversity of methods for CTC enumeration and characterization can confuse the research and the clinical communities. There is a lack of large studies comparing enrichment and detection between CTC detection platforms. A pilot comparative study of 54 pancreatic cancer patients investigated differences between CellSearch and a marker-independent ISET CTC isolation (Khoja et al., 2012). The authors detected significantly more CTCs using ISET in comparison to CellSearch (93 vs. 40%). Similar studies in other cancers have pointed out the discrepancies between platforms (Farace et al., 2011; Hofman et al., 2011).

Discrepancies can partially be attributed to different types of carcinomas and their expression of surface markers. Furthermore, the differences in specificity and sensitivity may lead investigators to adapt different platforms for their specific study. This raises many concerns in regards to the identities of CTCs. As EMT facilitates CTCs with increased capacity for detachment and invasion, the loss of epithelial lineage marker expression makes the identification particularly difficult. We must further explore the limitations that certain platforms create in capture efficiency. For example, EpCAM expression, which CellSearch exploits, is heterogeneous and cleavage has been reported (Maetzel et al., 2009). Limitations of other epithelial cell markers have also been reported, such as the down regulation of CK20 in tumors leading to false-negatives (Vlems et al., 2002; Krebs et al., 2014). It would be ideal for platforms to detect both mesenchymal and epithelial characteristics of CTCs, and the platforms must be carefully validated.

Additionally, not only do detection rates vary by platforms, but also between cancers. There is currently no consensus on the cutoff value for CTC positivity, even within a single platform. Stringent parameters should be set for CTC use not only in detection, but also as a prognostic marker of clinical outcomes in pancreatic cancer. Although it may be difficult due to the differences in enrichment and detection between platforms, standardization across single or multiple platforms is paramount for future incorporation into the field.

Due to the complex nature of the metastatic process, disseminated cells may be clinically silent for long durations. In breast cancer, cytological assessment suggests that CTCs actively undergoing mitosis are most common in late-stage disease and have prognostic value (Adams et al., 2016). One study found that aberrant VCAM1 expression, a common complication of breast cancer, was crucial for the transition from dormancy to overt metastasis (Lu et al., 2011). We must continue to explore ways to stratify CTCs in ways that will allow us to distinguish indolent micrometastasis from aggressive CTCs prior to clinically significant metastasis in pancreatic cancer patients.

CONCLUSION AND FUTURE DIRECTIONS

Literature evaluating the diagnostic and prognostic role of CTCs in cancer is continuously being reported. Many studies in different malignancies have shown clear associations of CTCs with clinical cancer progression. Much of the current research is now shifting to CTC characterization in order to select appropriate therapies for individuals based on the gene signatures of the CTCs and to measure response to therapies. For example, CTC count now outperforms traditional response evaluation methods in patients with metastatic castration-resistant prostate cancer (Onstenk et al., 2016). With reports estimating the half-life of CTCs to be on the order of hours, their detection can provide a current representation of the malignancy (Meng et al., 2004; Stott et al., 2010).

Future investigations should thoroughly explore CTC response to pancreatic cancer treatments. Furthermore, *ex vivo* CTC culture and expansion experiments can improve our understanding of the mechanisms of dissemination and escape from dormancy. Single-cell sequencing with next-generation sequencing platforms is paving the way toward understanding the genetic makeup of CTCs and the clinical significance of their genomic alterations (Alix-Panabières and Pantel, 2014). A recent study in a pancreatic cancer mouse model used single-molecule RNA sequencing of CTCs to identify Wnt2 as an up-regulated gene in pancreatic cancer CTCs, which is implicated in cell-death suppression and cancer dissemination. In addition, the authors observed the same Wnt2 signaling aberrations in CTCs of 5/11 patients with metastatic pancreatic cancer (Yu et al., 2013). Such studies have the potential to improve our current clinical management, especially ones exploring new drug targets involved in cancer spread. CTC use as a biomarker is currently being investigated in over 360 open clinical trials registered on ClinicalTrials.gov (Alix-Panabières and Pantel, 2014).

Considering that methods have been developed that have the possibility of being used in the diagnosis, stratification of patients and monitoring of therapy, next efforts require a focus on validation of leading methods for aiding clinical care. For the methods chosen, the validation of the method for certification in clinical use followed by well-designed studies to show utility of the method in the clinical setting are necessary for approval of test for clinical application.

There are challenges in the pancreatic cancer field for development of a test that has utility in early diagnosis or choice of chemotherapy. For example, in the area of early diagnosis, a population at increased risk is needed to show performance of the method in detecting pancreatic cancer at an earlier stage than that achieved with current approaches. Currently, the Consortium on Chronic Pancreatitis, Diabetes, and Pancreatic Cancer (CPDPC) in the United States is developing a protocol for this purpose choosing patients with diabetes after age 50 as the best high risk group to use to identify early diagnostic biomarkers (http://cpdpc.mdanderson.org). Because about 1% of these patients will be found to have pancreatic cancer over 3 years after the diagnosis of diabetes, the CPDPC has determined that the study will require enrollment of 10,000 subjects. At present, the inclusion of measurement of CTCs is not being considered because of the technical difficulties involve with CTC measurements. On the other hand, once a proteomic, ctDNA and/or RNA technique is developed to identify patients with early pancreatic cancer, measurements of CTCs can be applied to this group for further characterization including choice of therapy.

Similarly, it is difficult to apply CTC technology to the choice of chemotherapy as the current therapies do not have a significant effect on long term survival. One the other hand, surgery does have significant effects on long term survival in a substantial percentage of patients. Thus, it seems that currently the best situation to develop a validated test for CTC measurements uses patients who are candidates for curative surgery. Hypotheses to be tested should focus on the role of CTC measurements in predicting the outcome of curative surgery and early demonstration of disease recurrence. Certainly, studies that show performance of CTC measurements in determining and monitoring outcome in surgical patients will have important impacts in disease management and are much more feasible than studies designed for early diagnosis.

Another area of significant importance in the field is the determination of the biology of CTCs. As these cells represent the metastatic process which is the key determinant of poor outcome in pancreatic cancer patients, a better understanding of the biology of these cells will be central to advancing our treatments. Are there unique mechanisms in pancreatic cancer that account for its high rate of metastasis? Are there properties of pancreatic cancer CTCs that account for its resistance to therapy? Exploring these questions will require advancing the methods of isolation and propagating these cells so that the biologic experiments including observing their behavior in cell culture and animal models can be performed.

AUTHOR CONTRIBUTIONS

SP provided oversight and direction for the development of the manuscript. MP did literature searches and drafting of a primary manuscript. ME and RW provided additions and editing for the manuscript.

FUNDING

Funding was provided in part by NIH grants P01 CA163200 and U01 DK108314.

REFERENCES

Adams, D. L., Adams, D. K., Stefansson, S., Haudenschild, C., Martin, S. S., Charpentier, M., et al. (2016). Mitosis in circulating tumor cells stratifies highly aggressive breast carcinomas. *Breast Cancer Res.* 18:44. doi: 10.1186/s13058-016-0706-4

Aktas, B., Tewes, M., Fehm, T., Hauch, S., Kimmig, R., and Kasimir-Bauer, S. (2009). Stem cell and epithelial-mesenchymal transition markers are frequently overexpressed in circulating tumor cells of metastatic breast cancer patients. *Breast Cancer Res.* 11:R46. doi: 10.1186/bcr2333

Al Ustwani, O., Iancu, D., Yacoub, R., and Iyer, R. (2012). Detection of circulating tumor cells in cancers of biliary origin. *J. Gastrointest. Oncol.* 3, 97–104. doi: 10.3978/j.issn.2078-6891.2011.047

Alix-Panabières, C., and Pantel, K. (2014). Challenges in circulating tumour cell research. *Nat. Rev. Cancer* 14, 623–631. doi: 10.1038/nrc3820

Allard, W. J., Matera, J., Miller, M. C., Repollet, M., Connelly, M. C., Rao, C., et al. (2004). Tumor cells circulate in the peripheral blood of all major carcinomas but not in healthy subjects or patients with nonmalignant diseases. *Clin. Cancer Res.* 10, 6897–6904. doi: 10.1158/1078-0432.CCR-04-0378

Ashworth, T. R. (1869). A case of cancer in which cells similar to those in the tumors were seen in the blood after death. *Aust. Med. J.* 14, 146–149.

Bailey, J. M., Alsina, J., Rasheed, Z. A., Mcallister, F. M., Fu, Y.-Y., Plentz, R., et al. (2014). DCLK1 marks a morphologically distinct subpopulation of cells with stem cell properties in pre-invasive pancreatic cancer. *Gastroenterology* 146, 245–256. doi: 10.1053/j.gastro.2013.09.050

Barrière, G., Riouallon, A., Renaudie, J., Tartary, M., and Rigaud, M. (2012). Mesenchymal and stemness circulating tumor cells in early breast cancer diagnosis. *BMC Cancer* 12:114. doi: 10.1186/1471-2407-12-114

Bidard, F. C., Huguet, F., Louvet, C., Mineur, L., Bouche, O., Chibaudel, B., et al. (2013). Circulating tumor cells in locally advanced pancreatic adenocarcinoma: the ancillary CirCe 07 study to the LAP 07 trial. *Ann. Oncol.* 24, 2057–2061. doi: 10.1093/annonc/mdt176

Bissolati, M., Sandri, M. T., Burtulo, G., Zorzino, L., Balzano, G., and Braga, M. (2015). Portal vein-circulating tumor cells predict liver metastases in patients with resectable pancreatic cancer. *Tumor Biol.* 36, 991–996. doi: 10.1007/s13277-014-2716-0

Bournet, B., Vignolle-Vidoni, A., Grand, D., Roques, C., Breibach, F., Cros, J., et al. (2016). Endoscopic ultrasound-guided fine-needle aspiration plus KRAS and GNAS mutation in malignant intraductal papillary mucinous neoplasm of the pancreas. *Endosc. Int. Open* 4, E1228–E1235. doi: 10.1055/s-0042-117216

Burchill, S. A., Bradbury, M. F., Pittman, K., Southgate, J., Smith, B., and Selby, P. (1995). Detection of epithelial cancer cells in peripheral blood by reverse transcriptase-polymerase chain reaction. *Br. J. Cancer* 71, 278–281. doi: 10.1038/bjc.1995.56

Burris, H. A., Moore, M. J., Andersen, J., Green, M. R., Rothenberg, M. L., Modiano, M. R., et al. (1997). Improvements in survival and clinical benefit with gemcitabine as first-line therapy for patients with advanced pancreas cancer: a randomized trial. *J. Clin. Oncol.* 15, 2403–2413. doi: 10.1200/JCO.1997.15.6.2403

Byun, S., Son, S., Amodei, D., Cermak, N., Shaw, J., Kang, J. H., et al. (2013). Characterizing deformability and surface friction of cancer cells. *Proc. Natl. Acad. Sci. U.S.A.* 110, 7580–7585. doi: 10.1073/pnas.1218806110

Cameron, M. D., Schmidt, E. E., Kerkvliet, N., Nadkarni, K. V., Morris, V. L., Groom, A. C., et al. (2000). Temporal progression of metastasis in lung: cell survival, dormancy, and location dependence of metastatic inefficiency. *Cancer Res.* 60, 2541–2546. Retrieved from: http://cancerres.aacrjournals.org

Catenacci, D. V. T., Chapman, C. G., Xu, P., Koons, A., Konda, V. J., Siddiqui, U. D., et al. (2015). Acquisition of portal venous circulating tumor cells from patients with pancreaticobiliary cancers by endoscopic ultrasound. *Gastroenterology* 149, 1794.e4–1803.e4. doi: 10.1053/j.gastro.2015.08.050

Chausovsky, G., Luchansky, M., Figer, A., Shapira, J., Gottfried, M., Novis, B., et al. (1999). Expression of cytokeratin 20 in the blood of patients with disseminated carcinoma of the pancreas, colon, stomach, and lung. *Cancer* 86, 2398–2405. doi: 10.1002/(SICI)1097-0142(19991201)86:11<2398::AID-CNCR30>3.0.CO;2-5

Conroy, T., Desseigne, F., Ychou, M., Bouché, O., Guimbaud, R., Bécouarn, Y., et al. (2011). FOLFIRINOX versus gemcitabine for metastatic pancreatic cancer. *N.Engl. J. Med.* 364, 1817–1825. doi: 10.1056/NEJMoa1011923

Cooper, D., Schermer, A., and Sun, T. T. (1985). Classification of human epithelia and their neoplasms using monoclonal antibodies to keratins: strategies, applications, and limitations. *Lab. Invest.* 52, 243–256.

Court, C. M., Ankeny, J. S., Hou, S., Tseng, H.-R., and Tomlinson, J. S. (2015). Improving pancreatic cancer diagnosis using circulating tumor cells: prospects for staging and single-cell analysis. *Expert Rev. Mol. Diagn.* 15, 1491–1504. doi: 10.1586/14737159.2015.1091311

Dawson, D. W., and Fernandez-Zapico, M. E. (2016). Gemcitabine activates natural killer cells to attenuate pancreatic cancer recurrence. *Gastroenterology.* 151, 234–237. doi: 10.1053/j.gastro.2016.06.032

de Albuquerque, A., Kubisch, I., Breier, G., Stamminger, G., Fersis, N., Eichler, A., et al. (2012). Multimarker gene analysis of circulating tumor cells in pancreatic cancer patients: a feasibility study. *Oncology* 82, 3–10. doi: 10.1159/000335479

Deneve, E., Riethdorf, S., Ramos, J., Nocca, D., Coffy, A., Daures, J.-P., et al. (2013). Capture of viable circulating tumor cells in the liver of colorectal cancer patients. *Clin. Chem.* 59, 1384–1392. doi: 10.1373/clinchem.2013.202846

Dhamija, S., and Diederichs, S. (2016). From junk to master regulators of invasion: lncRNA functions in migration, EMT and metastasis. *Int. J. Cancer* 139, 269–280. doi: 10.1002/ijc.30039

DiMagno, E. P. (1999). Pancreatic cancer: clinical presentation, pitfalls and early clues. *Ann. Oncol.* 10(Suppl. 4), 140–142. doi: 10.1093/annonc/10.suppl_4.S140

DiMagno, E. P., Reber, H. A., and Tempero, M. A. (1999). AGA technical review on the epidemiology, diagnosis, and treatment of pancreatic ductal adenocarcinoma. American Gastroenterological Association. *Gastroenterology* 117, 1464–1484. doi: 10.1016/s0016-5085(99)70298-2

Fabbri, F., Carloni, S., Zoli, W., Ulivi, P., Gallerani, G., Fici, P., et al. (2013). Detection and recovery of circulating colon cancer cells using a dielectrophoresis-based device: KRAS mutation status in pure CTCs. *Cancer Lett.* 335, 225–231. doi: 10.1016/j.canlet.2013.02.015

Farace, F., Massard, C., Vimond, N., Drusch, F., Jacques, N., Billiot, F., et al. (2011). A direct comparison of CellSearch and ISET for circulating tumour-cell detection in patients with metastatic carcinomas. *Br. J. Cancer* 105, 847–853. doi: 10.1038/bjc.2011.294

Fidler, I. J. (2003). Timeline: the pathogenesis of cancer metastasis: the "seed and soil" hypothesis revisited. *Nat. Rev. Cancer* 3, 453–458. doi: 10.1038/nrc1098

Gorges, T. M., Kuske, A., Röck, K., Mauermann, O., Müller, V., Peine, S., et al. (2016a). Accession of tumor heterogeneity by multiplex transcriptome profiling of single circulating tumor cells. *Clin. Chem.* 62, 1504–1515. doi: 10.1373/clinchem.2016.260299

Gorges, T. M., Penkalla, N., Schalk, T., Joosse, S. A., Riethdorf, S., Tucholski, J., et al. (2016b). Enumeration and molecular characterization of tumor cells in lung cancer patients using a novel *in vivo* device for capturing circulating tumor cells. *Clin. Cancer Res.* 22, 2197–2206. doi: 10.1158/1078-0432.CCR-15-1416

Han, L., Chen, W., and Zhao, Q. (2014). Prognostic value of circulating tumor cells in patients with pancreatic cancer: a meta-analysis. *Tumor Biol.* 35, 2473–2480. doi: 10.1007/s13277-013-1327-5

Harris, L., Fritsche, H., Mennel, R., Norton, L., Ravdin, P., Taube, S., et al. (2007). American society of clinical oncology 2007 update of recommendations for the use of tumor markers in breast cancer. *J. Clin. Oncol.* 25, 5287–5312. doi: 10.1200/JCO.2007.14.2364

Hayes, D. F., Cristofanilli, M., Budd, G. T., Ellis, M. J., Stopeck, A., Miller, M. C., et al. (2006). Circulating tumor cells at each follow-up time point during therapy of metastatic breast cancer patients predict progression-free and overall survival. *Clin. Cancer Res.* 12(14 Pt 1), 4218–4224. doi: 10.1158/1078-0432.CCR-05-2821

Hiraiwa, K., Takeuchi, H., Hasegawa, H., Saikawa, Y., Suda, K., Ando, T., et al. (2008). Clinical significance of circulating tumor cells in blood from patients with gastrointestinal cancers. *Ann. Surg. Oncol.* 15, 3092–3100. doi: 10.1245/s10434-008-0122-9

Hofman, V., Ilie, M. I., Long, E., Selva, E., Bonnetaud, C., Molina, T., et al. (2011). Detection of circulating tumor cells as a prognostic factor in patients undergoing radical surgery for non-small-cell lung carcinoma: comparison of the efficacy of the CellSearch Assay^{TM} and the isolation by size of epithelial tumor cell method. *Int. J. Cancer* 129, 1651–1660. doi: 10.1002/ijc.25819

Hosokawa, M., Kenmotsu, H., Koh, Y., Yoshino, T., Yoshikawa, T., Naito, T., et al. (2013). Size-based isolation of circulating tumor cells in lung cancer patients using a microcavity array system. *PLoS ONE* 8:e67466. doi: 10.1371/journal.pone.0067466

Hou, H. W., Warkiani, M. E., Khoo, B. L., Li, Z. R., Soo, R. A., Tan, D. S.-W., et al. (2013). Isolation and retrieval of circulating tumor cells using centrifugal forces. *Sci. Rep.* 3:1259. doi: 10.1038/srep01259

Hou, J.-M., Krebs, M., Ward, T., Sloane, R., Priest, L., Hughes, A., et al. (2011). Circulating tumor cells as a window on metastasis biology in lung cancer. *Am. J. Pathol.* 178, 989–996. doi: 10.1016/j.ajpath.2010.12.003

Hu, B., Rochefort, H., and Goldkorn, A. (2013). Circulating tumor cells in prostate cancer. *Cancers* 5, 1676–1690. doi: 10.3390/cancers5041676

Ilie, M., Hofman, V., Long-Mira, E., Selva, E., Vignaud, J.-M., Padovani, B., et al. (2014). "Sentinel" circulating tumor cells allow early diagnosis of lung cancer in patients with chronic obstructive pulmonary disease. *PLoS ONE* 9:e111597. doi: 10.1371/journal.pone.0111597

Jiao, L. R., Apostolopoulos, C., Jacob, J., Szydlo, R., Johnson, N., Tsim, N., et al. (2009). Unique localization of circulating tumor cells in patients with hepatic metastases. *J. Clin. Oncol.* 27, 6160–6165. doi: 10.1200/JCO.2009.24.5837

Joosse, S. A., and Pantel, K. (2013). Biologic challenges in the detection of circulating tumor cells. *Cancer Res.* 73, 8–11. doi: 10.1158/0008-5472.CAN-12-3422

Khoja, L., Backen, A., Sloane, R., Menasce, L., Ryder, D., Krebs, M., et al. (2012). A pilot study to explore circulating tumour cells in pancreatic cancer as a novel biomarker. *Br. J. Cancer* 106, 508–516. doi: 10.1038/bjc.2011.545

Kong, D., Li, Y., Wang, Z., and Sarkar, F. H. (2011). Cancer stem cells and epithelial-to-mesenchymal transition (EMT)-phenotypic cells: are they cousins or twins? *Cancers* 3, 716–729. doi: 10.3390/cancers30100716

Koop, S., MacDonald, I. C., Luzzi, K., Schmidt, E. E., Morris, V. L., Grattan, M., et al. (1995). Fate of melanoma cells entering the microcirculation: over 80% survive and extravasate. *Cancer Res.* 55, 2520–2523.

Koop, S., Schmidt, E. E., Macdonald, I. C., Morris, V. L., Khokha, R., GRATTANt, M., et al. (1996). Independence of metastatic ability and extravasation: metastatic ras-transformed and control fibroblasts extravasate equally well (metastasis/invasion/*in vivo* videomicroscopy). *Med. Sci.* 93, 11080–11084.

Krebs, M. G., Metcalf, R. L., Carter, L., Brady, G., Blackhall, F. H., and Dive, C. (2014). Molecular analysis of circulating tumour cells—biology and biomarkers. *Nat. Rev. Clin. Oncol.* 11, 129–144. doi: 10.1038/nrclinonc.2013.253

Kuboki, Y., Matsusaka, S., Minowa, S., Shibata, H., Suenaga, M., Shinozaki, E., et al. (2013). Circulating tumor cell (CTC) count and epithelial growth factor receptor expression on CTCs as biomarkers for cetuximab efficacy in advanced colorectal cancer. *Anticancer Res.* 33, 3905–3910. Retrieved from: http://ar.iiarjournals.org

Kulemann, B., Pitman, M. B., Liss, A. S., Valsangkar, N., Fernández-del Castillo, C., Lillemoe, K. D., et al. (2015). Circulating tumor cells found in patients with localized and advanced pancreatic cancer. *Pancreas* 44, 547–550. doi: 10.1097/MPA.0000000000000324

Kurihara, T., Itoi, T., Sofuni, A., Itokawa, F., Tsuchiya, T., Tsuji, S., et al. (2008). Detection of circulating tumor cells in patients with pancreatic cancer: a preliminary result. *J. Hepatobiliary. Pancreat. Surg.* 15, 189–195. doi: 10.1007/s00534-007-1250-5

Kuroki, T., and Eguchi, S. (2017). No-touch isolation techniques for pancreatic cancer. *Surg. Today* 47, 8–13. doi: 10.1007/s00595-016-1317-5

Lane, E. B., and Alexander, C. M. (1990). Use of keratin antibodies in tumor diagnosis. *Semin. Cancer Biol.* 1, 165–179.

Lapin, M., Tjensvoll, K., Oltedal, S., Buhl, T., Gilje, B., Smaaland, R., et al. (2016). MINDEC-an enhanced negative depletion strategy for circulating tumour cell enrichment. *Sci. Rep.* 6:28929. doi: 10.1038/srep2892955.

Lara, O., Tong, X., Zborowski, M., and Chalmers, J. J. (2004). Enrichment of rare cancer cells through depletion of normal cells using density and flow-through, immunomagnetic cell separation. *Exp. Hematol.* 32, 891–904. doi: 10.1016/j.exphem.2004.07.007

Leber, M. F., and Efferth, T. (2009). Molecular principles of cancer invasion and metastasis (review). *Int. J. Oncol.* 34, 881–895. doi: 10.3892/ijo_00000214

Lu, X., Mu, E., Wei, Y., Riethdorf, S., Yang, Q., Yuan, M., et al. (2011). VCAM-1 Promotes osteolytic expansion of indolent bone micrometastasis of breast cancer by engaging α4β1-positive osteoclast progenitors. *Cancer Cell* 20, 701–714. doi: 10.1016/j.ccr.2011.11.002

Lustberg, M., Jatana, K. R., Zborowski, M., and Chalmers, J. J. (2012). Emerging technologies for CTC detection based on depletion of normal cells. Recent Results in Cancer Research. Fortschritte Der Krebsforschung. *Prog. Dans Recher. Cancer* 195, 97–110. doi: 10.1007/978-3-642-28160-0_9

Luzzi, K. J., MacDonald, I. C., Schmidt, E. E., Kerkvliet, N., Morris, V. L., Chambers, A. F., et al. (1998). Multistep nature of metastatic inefficiency. *Am. J. Pathol.* 153, 865–873. doi: 10.1016/S0002-9440(10)65628-3

Maetzel, D., Denzel, S., Mack, B., Canis, M., Went, P., Benk, M., et al. (2009). Nuclear signalling by tumour-associated antigen EpCAM. *Nat. Cell Biol.* 11, 162–171. doi: 10.1038/ncb1824

Meng, S., Tripathy, D., Frenkel, E. P., Shete, S., Naftalis, E. Z., Huth, J. F., et al. (2004). Circulating tumor cells in patients with breast cancer dormancy. *Clin. Cancer Res.* 10, 8152–8162. doi: 10.1158/1078-0432.CCR-04-1110

Miller, M. C., Doyle, G. V., and Terstappen, L. W. M. M. (2010). Significance of circulating tumor cells detected by the cellsearch system in patients with metastatic breast colorectal and prostate cancer. *J. Oncol.* 2010:617421. doi: 10.1155/2010/617421

Moore, M. J., Goldstein, D., Hamm, J., Figer, A., Hecht, J. R., Gallinger, S., et al. (2007). Erlotinib plus gemcitabine compared with gemcitabine alone in patients with advanced pancreatic cancer: a phase III Trial of the National Cancer Institute of Canada Clinical Trials Group. *J. Clin. Oncol.* 25, 1960–1966. doi: 10.1200/JCO.2006.07.9525

Müller, V., Stahmann, N., Riethdorf, S., Rau, T., Zabel, T., Goetz, A., et al. (2005). Circulating tumor cells in breast cancer: correlation to bone marrow micrometastases, heterogeneous response to systemic therapy and low proliferative activity. *Clin. Cancer Res.* 11, 3678–3685. doi: 10.1158/1078-0432.CCR-04-2469

Nagrath, S., Jack, R. M., Sahai, V., and Simeone, D. M. (2016). Opportunities and challenges for pancreatic circulating tumor cells. *Gastroenterology* 151, 412–426. doi: 10.1053/j.gastro.2016.05.052

Nagrath, S., Sequist, L. V., Maheswaran, S., Bell, D. W., Irimia, D., Ulkus, L., et al. (2007). Isolation of rare circulating tumour cells in cancer patients by microchip technology. *Nature* 450, 1235–1239. doi: 10.1038/nature06385

Nakanishi, Y., Seno, H., Fukuoka, A., Ueo, T., Yamaga, Y., Maruno, T., et al. (2012). Dclk1 distinguishes between tumor and normal stem cells in the intestine. *Nat. Genet.* 45, 98–103. doi: 10.1038/ng.2481

Onstenk, W., de Klaver, W., de Wit, R., Lolkema, M., Foekens, J., and Sleijfer, S. (2016). The use of circulating tumor cells in guiding treatment decisions for patients with metastatic castration-resistant prostate cancer. *Cancer Treat. Rev.* 46, 42–50. doi: 10.1016/j.ctrv.2016.04.001

Ozkumur, E., Shah, A. M., Ciciliano, J. C., Emmink, B. L., Miyamoto, D. T., Brachtel, E., et al. (2013). Inertial focusing for tumor antigen-dependent and -independent sorting of rare circulating tumor cells. *Sci. Transl. Med.* 5, 179ra47. doi: 10.1126/scitranslmed.3005616

Pandol, S., Edderkaoui, M., Gukovsky, I., Lugea, A., and Gukovskaya, A. (2009). Desmoplasia of pancreatic ductal adenocarcinoma. *Clin. Gastroenterol. Hepatol.* 7, S44–S47. doi: 10.1016/j.cgh.2009.07.039

Pantel, K., and Alix-Panabieres, C. (2013). Real-time liquid biopsy in cancer patients: fact or fiction? *Cancer Res.* 73, 6384–6388. doi: 10.1158/0008-5472.CAN-13-2030

Papadaki, M. A., Kallergi, G., Zafeiriou, Z., Manouras, L., Theodoropoulos, P. A., Mavroudis, D., et al. (2014). Co-expression of putative stemness and epithelial-to-mesenchymal transition markers on single circulating tumour cells from patients with early and metastatic breast cancer. *BMC Cancer* 14:651. doi: 10.1186/1471-2407-14-651

Park, E. S., Jin, C., Guo, Q., Ang, R. R., Duffy, S. P., Matthews, K., et al. (2016). Continuous flow deformability-based separation of circulating tumor cells using microfluidic ratchets. *Small* 12, 1909–1919. doi: 10.1002/smll.201503639

Poruk, K. E., Valero, V., Saunders, T., Blackford, A. L., Griffin, J. F., Poling, J., et al. (2016). Circulating tumor cell phenotype predicts recurrence and survival in pancreatic adenocarcinoma. *Ann. Surg.* 264, 1073–1081. doi: 10.1097/SLA.0000000000001600

Qu, D., Johnson, J., Chandrakesan, P., Weygant, N., May, R., Aiello, N., et al. (2015). Doublecortin-like kinase 1 is elevated serologically in pancreatic ductal adenocarcinoma and widely expressed on circulating tumor cells. *PLoS ONE* 10:e0118933. doi: 10.1371/journal.pone.0118933

Rahib, L., Smith, B. D., Aizenberg, R., Rosenzweig, A. B., Fleshman, J. M., and Matrisian, L. M. (2014). Projecting cancer incidence and deaths to 2030: the unexpected burden of thyroid, liver, and pancreas cancers in the United States. *Cancer Res.* 74, 2913–2921. doi: 10.1158/0008-5472.CAN-14-0155

Raimondi, C., Gradilone, A., Naso, G., Vincenzi, B., Petracca, A., Nicolazzo, C., et al. (2011). Epithelial-mesenchymal transition and stemness features in circulating tumor cells from breast cancer patients. *Breast Cancer Res. Treat.* 130, 449–455. doi: 10.1007/s10549-011-1373-x

Rhim, A. D., Mirek, E. T., Aiello, N. M., Maitra, A., Bailey, J. M., McAllister, F., et al. (2012). EMT and dissemination precede pancreatic tumor formation. *Cell* 148, 349–361. doi: 10.1016/j.cell.2011.11.025

Riethdorf, S., Fritsche, H., Muller, V., Rau, T., Schindlbeck, C., Rack, B., et al. (2007). Detection of circulating tumor cells in peripheral blood of patients with metastatic breast cancer: a validation study of the cellsearch system. *Clin. Cancer Res.* 13, 920–928. doi: 10.1158/1078-0432.CCR-06-1695

Ryan, D. P., Hong, T. S., and Bardeesy, N. (2014). Pancreatic adenocarcinoma. *N.Engl. J. Med.* 371, 1039–1049. doi: 10.1056/NEJMra1404198

Sastre, J., Maestro, M. L., Puente, J., Veganzones, S., Alfonso, R., Rafael, S., et al. (2008). Circulating tumor cells in colorectal cancer: correlation with clinical and pathological variables. *Ann. Oncol.* 19, 935–938. doi: 10.1093/annonc/mdm583

Scherag, F. D., Niestroj-Pahl, R., Krusekopf, S., Lücke, K., Brandstetter, T., and Rühe, J. (2017). Highly selective capture surfaces on medical wires for fishing tumor cells in whole blood. *Anal. Chem.* 89, 1846–1854. doi: 10.1021/acs.analchem.6b04219

Soeth, E., Grigoleit, U., Moellmann, B., Röder, C., Schniewind, B., Kremer, B., et al. (2005). Detection of tumor cell dissemination in pancreatic ductal carcinoma patients by CK 20 RT-PCR indicates poor survival. *J. Cancer Res. Clin. Oncol.* 131, 669–676. doi: 10.1007/s00432-005-0008-1

Spano, D., Heck, C., De Antonellis, P., Christofori, G., and Zollo, M. (2012). Molecular networks that regulate cancer metastasis. *Semin. Cancer Biol.* 22, 234–249. doi: 10.1016/j.semcancer.2012.03.006

Speicher, M. R., and Pantel, K. (2014). Tumor signatures in the blood. *Nat. Biotechnol.* 32, 441–443. doi: 10.1038/nbt.2897

Stott, S. L., Lee, R. J., Nagrath, S., Yu, M., Miyamoto, D. T., Ulkus, L., et al. (2010). Isolation and characterization of circulating tumor cells from patients with localized and metastatic prostate cancer. *Sci. Transl. Med.* 2, 25ra23. doi: 10.1126/scitranslmed.3000403

Talasaz, A. H., Powell, A. A., Huber, D. E., Berbee, J. G., Roh, K.-H., Yu, W., et al. (2009). Isolating highly enriched populations of circulating epithelial cells and other rare cells from blood using a magnetic sweeper device. *Proc. Natl. Acad. Sci. U.S.A.* 106, 3970–3975. doi: 10.1073/pnas.0813188106

Ting, D. T., Wittner, B. S., Ligorio, M., Vincent Jordan, N., Shah, A. M., Miyamoto, D. T., et al. (2014). Single-cell RNA sequencing identifies extracellular matrix gene expression by pancreatic circulating tumor cells. *Cell Rep.* 8, 1905–1918. doi: 10.1016/j.celrep.2014.08.029

Tsai, W.-S., Chen, J.-S., Shao, H.-J., Wu, J.-C., Lai, J.-M., Lu, S.-H., et al. (2016). Circulating tumor cell count correlates with colorectal neoplasm progression and is a prognostic marker for distant metastasis in non-metastatic patients. *Sci. Rep.* 6:24517. doi: 10.1038/srep24517

Tsujiura, M., Ichikawa, D., Konishi, H., Komatsu, S., Shiozaki, A., and Otsuji, E. (2014). Liquid biopsy of gastric cancer patients: circulating tumor cells and cell-free nucleic acids. *World J. Gastroenterol.* 20, 3265–3286. doi: 10.3748/wjg.v20.i12.3265

Uchikura, K., Takao, S., Nakajo, A., Miyazono, F., Nakashima, S., Tokuda, K., et al. (2002). Intraoperative molecular detection of circulating tumor cells by reverse transcription-polymerase chain reaction in patients with biliary-pancreatic cancer is associated with hematogenous metastasis. *Ann. Surg. Oncol.* 9, 364–370. doi: 10.1007/BF02573871

Vlems, F. A., Diepstra, J. H. S., Cornelissen, I. M. H. A., Ruers, T. J. M., Ligtenberg, M. J. L., Punt, C. J. A., et al. (2002). Limitations of cytokeratin 20 RT-PCR to detect disseminated tumour cells in blood and bone marrow of patients with colorectal cancer: expression in controls and downregulation in tumour tissue. *Mol. Pathol.* 55, 156–163. doi: 10.1136/mp.55.3.156

Von Hoff, D. D., Ervin, T., Arena, F. P., Chiorean, E. G., Infante, J., Moore, M., et al. (2013). Increased survival in pancreatic cancer with nab-paclitaxel plus gemcitabine. *N.Engl. J. Med.* 369, 1691–1703. doi: 10.1056/NEJMoa1304369

Vona, G., Estepa, L., Béroud, C., Damotte, D., Capron, F., Nalpas, B., et al. (2004). Impact of cytomorphological detection of circulating tumor cells in patients with liver cancer. *Hepatology* 39, 792–797. doi: 10.1002/hep.20091

Vona, G., Sabile, A., Louha, M., Sitruk, V., Romana, S., Schütze, K., et al. (2000). Isolation by size of epithelial tumor cells. *Am. J. Pathol.* 156, 57–63. doi: 10.1016/S0002-9440(10)64706-2

Waxman, I., Koons, A., Konda, V. J., Siddiqui, U. D., Gelrud, A., Xu, P., et al. (2014). Detection of Portal Vein (PV) Circulating Tumor Cells (CTCs) in Pancreatic Cancer (PC) patients obtained by EUS guided Pv sampling. a safety and feasibility trial. *Gastrointest. Endosc.* 79, AB173–AB174. doi: 10.1016/j.gie.2014.02.187

Weissenstein, U., Schumann, A., Reif, M., Link, S., Toffol-Schmidt, U. D., and Heusser, P. (2012). Detection of circulating tumor cells in blood of metastatic breast cancer patients using a combination of cytokeratin and EpCAM antibodies. *BMC Cancer* 12:206. doi: 10.1186/1471-2407-12-206

Xu, Y., Qin, T., Li, J., Wang, X., Gao, C., Xu, C., et al. (2017). Detection of circulating tumor cells using negative enrichment immunofluorescence and an *in situ* hybridization system in pancreatic cancer. *Int. J. Mol. Sci.* 18:622. doi: 10.3390/ijms18040622

Yang, M.-H., Imrali, A., and Heeschen, C. (2015). Circulating cancer stem cells: the importance to select. *Chin. J. Cancer Res.* 27, 437–449. doi: 10.3978/j.issn.1000-9604.2015.04.08

Yokobori, T., Iinuma, H., Shimamura, T., Imoto, S., Sugimachi, K., Ishii, H., et al. (2013). Plastin3 is a novel marker for circulating tumor cells undergoing the epithelial-mesenchymal transition and is associated with colorectal cancer prognosis. *Cancer Res.* 73, 2059–2069. doi: 10.1158/0008-5472.CAN-12-0326

Yoo, C. E., Park, J.-M., Moon, H.-S., Joung, J.-G., Son, D.-S., Jeon, H.-J., et al. (2016). Vertical magnetic separation of circulating tumor cells for somatic genomic-alteration analysis in lung cancer patients. *Sci. Rep.* 6:37392. doi: 10.1038/srep37392

Yu, M., Bardia, A., Wittner, B. S., Stott, S. L., Smas, M. E., Ting, D. T., et al. (2013). Circulating breast tumor cells exhibit dynamic changes in epithelial and mesenchymal composition. *Science* 339, 580–584. doi: 10.1126/science.1228522

Yu, M., Stott, S., Toner, M., Maheswaran, S., and Haber, D. A. (2011). Circulating tumor cells: approaches to isolation and characterization. *J. Cell Biol.* 192, 373–382. doi: 10.1083/jcb.201010021

Zhang, W., Bao, L., Yang, S., Qian, Z., Dong, M., Yin, L., et al. (2016). Tumor-selective replication herpes simplex virus-based technology significantly improves clinical detection and prognostication of viable circulating tumor cells. *Oncotarget* 7, 39768–39783. doi: 10.18632/oncotarget.9465

Zhang, Y., Wang, F., Ning, N., Chen, Q., Yang, Z., Guo, Y., et al. (2015). Patterns of circulating tumor cells identified by CEP8, CK and CD45 in pancreatic cancer. *Int. J. Cancer* 136, 1228–1233. doi: 10.1002/ijc.29070

Zhang, Z., Shiratsuchi, H., Lin, J., Chen, G., Reddy, R. M., Azizi, E., et al. (2014). Expansion of CTCs from early stage lung cancer patients using a microfluidic co-culture model. *Oncotarget* 5, 12383–12397. doi: 10.18632/oncotarget.2592

Zhau, H. E., He, H., Wang, C. Y., Zayzafoon, M., Morrissey, C., Vessella, R. L., et al. (2011). Human prostate cancer harbors the stem cell properties of bone marrow mesenchymal stem cells. *Clin. Cancer Res.* 17, 2159–2169. doi: 10.1158/1078-0432.CCR-10-2523

Zhe, X., Cher, M. L., and Bonfil, R. D. (2011). Circulating tumor cells: finding the needle in the haystack. *Am. J. Cancer Res.* 1, 740–751. Retrieved from: http://www.ajcr.us

4

A Combined Metabolomic and Proteomic Study Revealed the Difference in Metabolite and Protein Expression Profiles in Ruminal Tissue from Goats Fed Hay or High-Grain Diets

Changzheng Guo[1]*, Daming Sun*[1]*, Xinfeng Wang*[2] *and Shengyong Mao*[1]*

[1] Jiangsu Key Laboratory of Gastrointestinal Nutrition and Animal Health, Laboratory of Gastrointestinal Microbiology, National Experimental Teaching Demonstration Center of Animal Science, National Center for International Research on Animal Gut Nutrition, Joint International Research Laboratory of Animal Health and Food Safety, College of Animal Science and Technology, Nanjing Agricultural University, Nanjing, China, [2] *College of Animal Science and Technology, Shihezi University, Shihezi, China*

***Correspondence:**
Shengyong Mao
maoshengyong@163.com

Currently, knowledge about the impact of high-grain (HG) feeding on metabolite and protein expression profiles in ruminal tissue is limited. In this study, a combination of proteomic and metabolomic approaches was applied to evaluate metabolic and proteomic changes of the rumen epithelium in goats fed a hay diet (Hay) or HG diet. At the metabolome level, results from principal component analysis (PCA) and PLS-DA revealed clear differences in the biochemical composition of ruminal tissue of the control (Hay) and the grain-fed groups, demonstrating the evident impact of HG feeding on metabolite profile of ruminal epithelial tissues. As compared with the Hay group, HG feeding increased the levels of eight metabolites and decreased the concentrations of seven metabolites in ruminal epithelial tissues. HG feeding mainly altered starch and sucrose metabolism, purine metabolism, glyoxylate and dicarboxylate metabolism, glycerolipid metabolism, pyruvate metabolism, glycolysis or gluconeogenesis, galactose metabolism, glycine, serine and threonine metabolism, and arginine and proline metabolism in ruminal epithelium. At the proteome level, 35 differentially expressed proteins were found in the rumen epithelium between the Hay and HG groups, with 12 upregulated and 23 downregulated proteins. The downregulated proteins were related to fatty acid metabolism, carbohydrate metabolic processes and nucleoside metabolic processes, while most of upregulated proteins were involved in oxidative stress and detoxification. In general, our findings revealed that HG feeding resulted in differential proteomic and metabolomic profiles in the rumen epithelia of goats, which may contribute to better understanding how rumen epithelium adapt to HG feeding.

Keywords: goat, metabolomics, proteomic, rumen epithelium, high grain feeding

INTRODUCTION

In modern intensive animal production, feeding high-grain (HG) diets to feedlot goats has become a common practice to meet the energy requirements for the maintenance of the production performance (Penner et al., 2011). However, although HG feeding can increase energy available to the animal, there is a risk of developing acidotic ruminal epithelial damage, thus affecting nutrient absorption. The rumen epithelium is well known to play an important role in maintaining the host's energy balance and health (Gabel et al., 2002). Previous studies revealed that the short chain volatile fatty acids (SCVFAs) absorbed by the rumen epithelium can meet up to 70% of the energy requirement of ruminants (Bergman, 1990; Penner et al., 2011). In addition, rumen epithelial cells also are the first line of defense against hostile rumen conditions such as acidic pH, high osmotic pressure, and harmful microbial-derived metabolites, such as lipopolysaccharide (LPS) and histamine (Penner et al., 2011). In recent years, the effect of HG feeding on rumen epithelial morphology (Bannink et al., 2008) and physiological functions (Uppal et al., 2003) have been widely investigated, and the results revealed that HG feeding increased length and surface of rumen papilla (Shen et al., 2004) and also impact rumen epithelial absorption, barrier, and immune function (Liu et al., 2013). Undoubtedly, these findings improved our understanding of the adaptative mechanism of the ruminal epithelium in response to HG diet feeding. However, to our knowledge, previous studies are only focused on one level (gene, metabolite or morphology) to investigate the response of rumen epithelial function to HG feeding, which is limited to understand the global change in physiological functions of rumen epithelium during HG feeding.

In recent years, omics technologies have been widely used in understanding the biological mechanism of ruminant (Ametaj et al., 2010; Bondzio et al., 2011), and this also makes it possible to investigate the changes in the physiological functions of rumen epithelium to HG diet comprehensively, therefore it will be beneficial for modulating the animal performance and minimizing the negative effect of HG feeding on rumen health. Up to now, only a few studies have attempted to investigate the effect of HG feeding on rumen epithelium based on the omics technologies. For example, Bondzio et al. (2011) used two dimensional-differential in gel electrophoresis (2D-DIGE) based proteome analysis methods and identified differentially expressed proteins related to morphological alterations of the ruminal epithelium adapting to HG feeding. However, 2D-DIGE does not allow for the detection of regulatory proteins (Gerber et al., 2003). As compared with the 2D-DIGE proteomics methods, label-free liquid chromatography–tandem mass spectrometry (LC–MS/MS) approach is reported to be particularly effective for large-scale protein identification (Lin et al., 2003). Thus, a label-free based proteomic method would provide more information on the alternation in function of the rumen epithelial during HG feeding.

In addition to its role in SCVFA absorption and as a selective barrier, the ruminal epithelium also plays an important role in the metabolism of SCVFA (Bannink et al., 2016). Until now, the effect of different dietary strategy on metabolic function of ruminal epithelial tissue has rarely been studied, and the knowledge of how the epithelial tissue responds to an HG diet feeding is very limited. Accordingly, it is of great interest to gain further insight into how HG diet feeding strategies affect metabolite profiles and function of rumen epithelial tissue. Metabolomics, one of omics technology, has been reported to be a useful approach to characterize the global metabolites of rumen fluid in goats and dairy cows (Ametaj et al., 2010; Mao et al., 2016), and thereby it will be possible to enable a more quantitative characterization of the biochemical composition of this tissue and thereby provide a method to investigate the metabolic activity of the ruminal epithelial tissue. However, until now, few studies have been conducted on investigating the changes in metabolic characterization of ruminal epithelium during HG feeding.

In the present study, we hypothesized that goats fed HG diet or hay diet had differences in profile of metabolomics and proteomics. Therefore, a gas chromatography–mass spectrometry (GC–MS) based metabolomics method and a label-free LC-MS/MS proteomics method was used to characterize the proteomic and metabolic response of rumen papillae to HG diets.

MATERIALS AND METHODS

Animals, Diets, and Experimental Design

The experimental design and procedures for this study were approved by the Animal Care and Use Committee of Nanjing Agricultural University following the requirements of the Regulations for the Administration of Affairs Concerning Experimental Animals (The State Science and Technology Commission of P. R. China, 1988). The current study is a continuation of previous research, where the effect of HG diets on the function and health of the rumen by traditional research methods was investigated (Liu et al., 2013). In the current study, we mainly paid attention to the effect of HG feeding on metabolic and proteomic profiles of rumen epithelium in goats. The experiment design and treatments are described in detail (Liu et al., 2013). Briefly, a total of 10 rumen-cannulated male goats of 2–3 years old were used in the experiment. A pure hay diet was provided for all the goats *ad libitum* for 5 weeks before the experiment treatment, and then, all animals were placed in individual pens (1.2 × 1.2 m) and randomly allocated into two groups. The body weights of the goats between the two groups had no significant difference (29.8 ± 0.86 vs. 30.0 ± 1.05 kg; $P = 0.886$) at the beginning of the feeding trial. One was the Hay group that was fed a hay diet (Hay; 81% *Leymus chinensis*, 15% lucerne, 0.5% $CaCO_3$, 0.8% NaCl, 1.7% $CaHPO_4$, and 1% mineral and vitamin supplement; 101 g crude protein/kg DM, and 570 g neutral-detergent fiber/kg DM; $n = 5$), and the other was the HG group that was fed an HG diet (HG; 30% *Leymus chinensis*, 45% maize meal, 20% wheat meal, 1.1% soybean meal, 0.95% $CaCO_3$, 0.65% NaCl, 1.2% $CaHPO_4$, 1% mineral and vitamin supplement, and 0.1% $NaHCO_3$; 101 g crude protein/kg DM, 252 g neutral-detergent fiber/kg DM, and 582 g starch/kg DM; $n = 5$). The diets (750 g DM/animal per day) were offered in equal amounts at 08:30 and 16:30 h daily for 7 weeks.

Sample Collection

The animals were slaughtered for sampling after 7 weeks. A segment of the rumen wall from the ventral sac was collected, and the ruminal epithelium was separated from the muscular and serosal layers by blunt dissection and immediately washed three times in ice-cold PBS and frozen immediately in liquid nitrogen. The ruminal epithelium (2 cm × 2 cm) was used for extracting proteins and metabolomics analysis.

Protein Extraction and Sample Preparation

The total proteins were extracted with RIPA Lysis Buffer (Cat. P0013B, Beyotime Institute of Biotechnology, Shanghai, China). Proteins were dissolved in 50 mM Tris-HCl (pH 8.0) with 8 M urea and incubated for 60 min in a 60°C water bath and alkylated with 1 M iodoacetamide. Subsequently, the samples were incubated for 45 min at room temperature. Finally, proteins on the membrane were dissolved in 50 mM NH_4HCO_3 (pH 7.8). The digested protein by trypsin was desalted using a C18 column and then freeze-dried before sample injection.

Mass Spectrometry

The peptides were first dissolved in buffer A (0.1% formic acid). A 15-cm analytical C18 column (C18, 3 μm, 100 Å) was used for LC separation. The peptides were eluted by a 2–95% gradient of buffer B (aqueous 80% acetonitrile in 0.08% formic acid) at a flow rate of 300 nL/min. The peptides were ionized by nano-electrospray and subsequent tandem mass spectrometry (MS/MS) on a Q Exactive^{TM} Plus (Thermo Fisher Scientific, San Jose, CA, United States) with the electrospray voltage was 2.2 kV. The Orbitrap was performed with full scan MS spectra with a resolution of 60,000 from m/z 350 to 1800.

Protein Identification and Quantification

The original data was analyzed by Proteome Discoverer (version 1.4, Thermo Fisher Scientific, Waltham, MA, United States). Based on the *Q*-value, we verified the results of protein identification to ensure that the error detection rate was less than 1%. The SIEVE software (Version 2.1 Thermo Scientific, San Jose, CA, United States) was used to analyze two original files for each group by ChromAlign. When alignment scores aligned by retention time and mass is higher than 0.75, it is regarded as a further quantitative analysis. The area under the curve for each group was calculated.

Metabolite Profiling of the Ruminal Epithelium

The GC-MS analysis has been described previously (Sun et al., 2016). Briefly, 30 mg of the ruminal epithelium was mixed with 900 μL methanol containing ^{13}C2-myristic acid (12.5 μg/mL). The mixed liquor were grounded and centrifuged at 20,000 × *g* for 10 min at 4°C. Then, 100 μL of the supernatant was dried in a SpeedVac evaporator (Savant Instruments, Farmingdale, NY, United States). The dried analytes were methoximated with methoxyamine pyridine solution and trimethylsilylated with methyl-trimethyl-silyltrifluoroacetamide.

Thirty microliters of *n*-heptane and methyl stearate (30 μg/mL) were mixed with samples and then the 0.5 μL of mixture was performed by an RTx-5MS column (30 m × 0.25 mm i.d. and film thickness of 0.25 μm; Restek Corporation, Bellefonte, PA, United States). After the raw data were collected, identification of the compounds was achieved by comparison of the mass spectra and retention index of all the detected compounds with authentic reference standards and those available in the National Institute of Standards and Technology Library 2.0.

Data Analysis

Statistical calculations of metabolomic and proteomic data were carried out by conducting tests using the SPSS software package (SPSS version 18.0.1 for Windows; SPSS Inc., Chicago, IL, United States). The normality of the distribution of the variables was tested using the Shapiro–Wilk test. The independent samples *t*-test procedure was used to analyze the variables found to have a normal distribution. The Kruskal–Wallis test was used to analyze the variables found to have a non-normal distribution. Significance was set at $P < 0.05$.

Principal component analysis (PCA), PLS-DA, and loading plot were carried out using SIMCA-P + 13.0 software (Umetrics, Umeå, Sweden). Variable importance in projection (VIP) was obtained from PLS-DA analysis. Differentially expressed metabolites (VIP > 1.2) and proteins (FC > 1.5) were selected according to VIP and statistical analysis ($P < 0.05$). The differentially expressed metabolites has been analyzed using the MetaboAnalyst web server[1] for the pathway enrichment analysis.

Bioinformatic Analysis of Differential Abundance Proteins

The differentially expressed proteins (**Table 2**) has been analyzed using the OmicsBean[2] for the protein–protein interaction analysis (PPI) based on gene ontology (GO) enrichment and Kyoto Encyclopedia of Genes and Genomes (KEGG) pathway.

RESULTS

Effects of HG Diet Feeding on Ruminal pH and Concentrations of SCVFAs, Lactate, and LPS

It is helpful to briefly describe the data of rumen fermentation published previously (**Supplementary Table S1**). Briefly, HG feeding decreased the ruminal pH ($P < 0.001$) and increased the concentrations of propionate, butyrate, valerate, isovalerate, total SCVFA, and lactate ($P < 0.001$ to $P = 0.019$).

Multivariate Analysis of Rumen Tissue Metabolites

A total of 158 valid peaks were detected by the GC-MS that were unique and non-overlapping in the rumen epithelium

[1]http://www.metaboanalyst.ca
[2]http://www.omicsbean.cn/

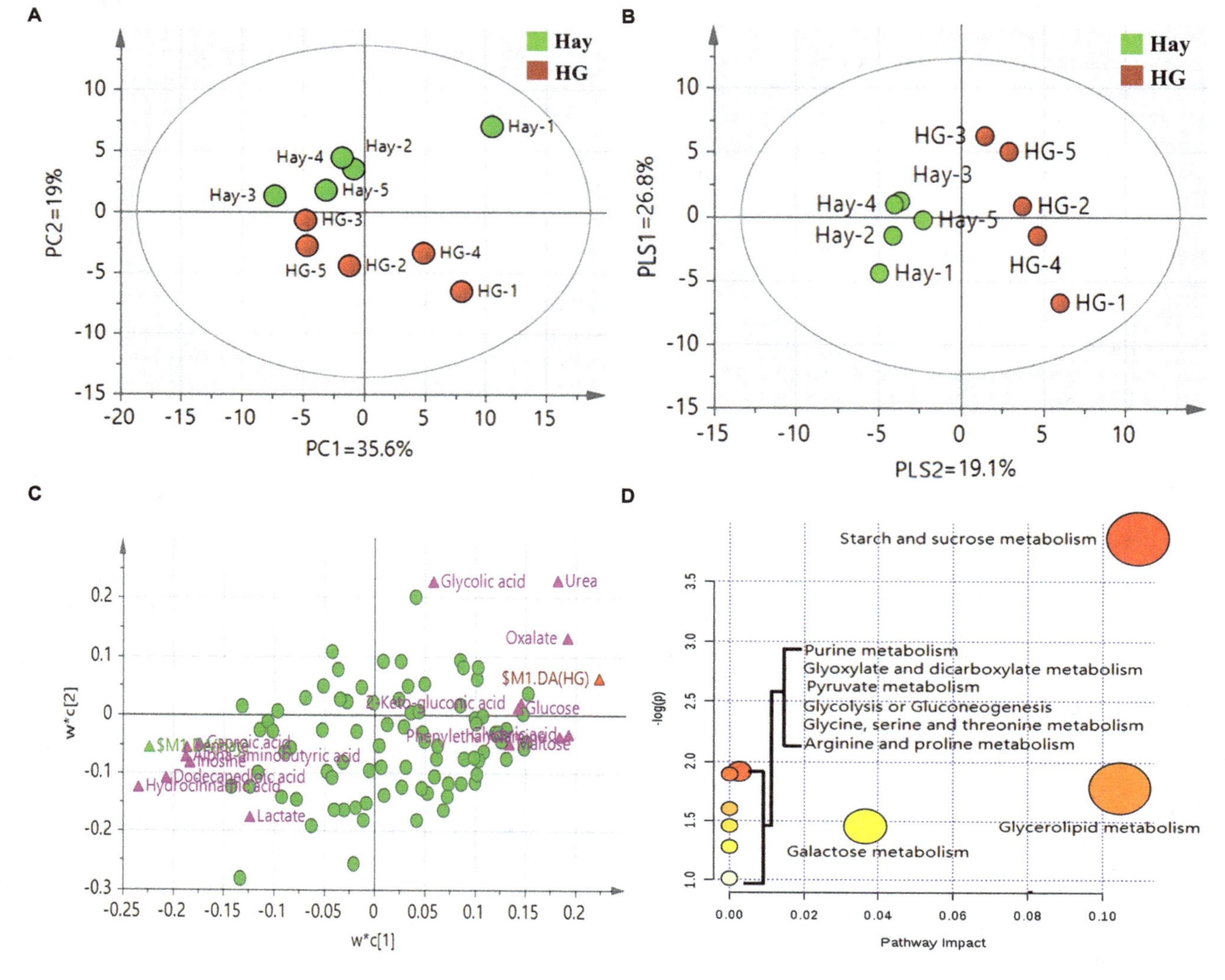

FIGURE 1 | (A) Principal component analysis (PCA) of metabolites in rumen epithelium in goats fed hay (Hay) and high grain (HG) diets. PC, the principal component that distinguish the Hay group and the HG group. PC1 is the first principal component; PC2 is the second principal component; PC1 could explained 35.6% of the variation; PC2 explained 19% of the variation. **(B)** Partial least squares discriminant analysis (PLS-DA) of metabolites in rumen epithelium in goats fed hay (Hay) and high grain (HG) diets. PLS, the principal component that distinguish the Hay group and the HG group. PLS1 is the first principal component; PLS2 is the second principal component. **(C)** Loading plot of the 91 commonly detected compounds projected into the PLS-DA model, the most important compounds (VIP > 1.2) responsible for the discrimination are labeled and colored in pink, and the other compounds were colored in green. Compounds are labeled by the names used in **Table 1**. Variables with the same distance from 0 with similar positions are positively correlated. Those in the opposite direction are negatively correlated.
(D) Pathway analysis. Plots depicting computed metabolic pathways as a function of $-\log(p)$ and pathway impact for the key differential metabolites. The impact is the pathway impact value calculated from pathway topology analysis. The larger size indicates higher pathway enrichment, and the darker color indicates higher pathway impact values.

samples. After rigorous quality control and identification, we obtained 101 metabolites across all samples. The metabolites mainly included amino acids, carbohydrates, lipids, nucleoside and organic chemicals. PCA was carried out to explore the differences of the metabolites between the two dietary treatments. As shown in **Figure 1A**, the first two principal components (PCs) can explain 54.6% of the variation. The separation of the two groups in PC 2 revealed significant differences of rumen tissue metabolites in goats fed the HG diet and hay diet, which is particularly apparent in **Figure 1B**, as analyzed by PLS-DA. PLS-DA scores plots discriminating between the rumen tissue of goats fed Hay and HG diet [predictive ability parameter (Q^2) (cum) = 0.978, goodness-of-fit parameter (R^2) (Y) = 0.997]. To investigate the individual rumen tissue metabolites responsible for the variation of the first two PCs, loading plots were used (**Figure 1C**). The loading plot revealed a statistically significant elevation of glyceric acid, urea, oxalate, 2-keto-gluconic acid, glucose, phenylethanolamine, allonic acid and maltose in the HG group compared with the Hay group. Conversely, the metabolic

TABLE 1 | Candidate compounds in rumen epithelium that differed between hay (Hay) and high grain (HG) groups.

Compounds	Chemical class	VIP[1]	FC[2]	*P*-value
Alpha-aminobutyric acid	Amino acids	1.86	0.45	0.009
Maltose	Carbohydrates	1.34	6.53	0.047
Allonic acid	Carbohydrates	1.47	2.14	0.028
Glyceric acid	Carbohydrates	1.93	2.11	0.016
Glucose	Carbohydrates	1.43	2.00	0.028
2-Keto-gluconic acid	Carbohydrates	1.45	1.85	0.047
Caproic acid	Lipids	1.72	0.52	0.047
Inosine	Nucleoside	1.82	0.50	0.016
Phenylethanolamine	Organic chemicals	1.84	2.18	0.009
Urea	Organic chemicals	1.82	1.76	0.016
Oxalate	Organic chemicals	1.91	1.70	0.016
Lactate	Organic chemicals	1.23	0.76	0.047
Dodecanedioic acid	Organic chemicals	2.06	0.29	0.009
Hydrocinnamic acid	Organic chemicals	2.32	0.20	0.009
Benzoate	Organic chemicals	1.85	0.50	0.016

[1]VIP, variable importance in the projection. [2]FC, fold change, mean value of peak area obtained from HG group/mean value of peak area obtained from Hay group. If the FC value less than 1, it means that metabolites are less in HG group than in Hay group.

signature of rumen epithelium tissue in the Hay group consisted of a higher concentration of alpha-aminobutyric acid, caproic acid, inosine, lactate, dodecanedioic acid, hydrocinnamic acid and benzoate. To identify which compounds were responsible for this difference, the following parameters were used as criteria: VIP $>$ 1.2 and $P < 0.05$. As shown in **Table 1**, eight of the compounds (allonic acid, glyceric acid, glucose, 2-keto-gluconic acid, phenylethanolamine, urea, oxalate, and maltose) were enriched while seven (alpha-aminobutyric acid, caproic acid, inosine, lactate, dodecanedioic acid, hydrocinnamic acid, and benzoate) were reduced in the HG group compared with the Hay group. Through the enrichment analysis, the results showed that starch and sucrose metabolism, purine metabolism, glyoxylate and dicarboxylate metabolism, pyruvate metabolism, glycolysis or gluconeogenesis, glycerolipid metabolism, and galactose metabolism were significantly enriched ($P < 0.05$) with different diets. Through the pathway topology analysis, the results showed that the pathway impact values of 3 metabolic pathways, which included starch and sucrose metabolism, glycerolipid metabolism, and galactose metabolism were higher than 0.03. Based on both the enrichment analysis and impact value, starch and sucrose metabolism, glycerolipid metabolism, and galactose metabolism were closely related with HC diet (**Figure 1D**).

Identification and Comparison of Proteins of Differential Abundance

Using label-free LC–MS/MS analysis, a total of 2,150 proteins were identified within the false discovery rate of 1%. Following statistical analysis, 35 proteins were found to be differentially expressed in the rumen epithelium between Hay and HG groups, with 12 upregulated and 23 downregulated (**Table 2**) in the HG group compared with the Hay group. The upregulated proteins were mainly related to oxidative stress, detoxification, immune system processes and anabolism of fatty acid, while the downregulated proteins were mainly related to cell growth and proliferation, protein metabolic processes, and catabolism of fatty acids.

Gene Ontology Annotations of Proteins With Different Abundance

In the cellular component group, the differentially expressed proteins were concentrated in the cytoplasmic part and cytoplasm (**Figure 2**). In the molecular functional group, the differentially expressed proteins that work as binding proteins and catalytic activity were ranked at the top of the category (**Figure 2**). In the biological process category, the proteins that participate in single-organism metabolic process and response to chemical had the highest ratios among the differentially expressed proteins (**Figure 2**).

The PPI of the differentially expressed proteins allow us better understand the key proteins and pathways affected by HG feeding in the rumen epithelium (**Figure 3**). The PPI network indicated that the protein changes in rumen epithelium were mainly involved in synthesis and degradation of ketone bodies, butanoate metabolism and valine, leucine and isoleucine degradation pathways (**Figures 3, 4**).

DISCUSSION

Here, we investigated the relationships among diet, rumen epithelial metabolome and proteome. In the present study, results from PCA and PLS-DA reveal clear differences in the biochemical composition of ruminal tissue of the Hay and the HG fed groups (**Figures 1A,B**), also demonstrating the evident impact of HG feeding on metabolites of rumen epithelium. This alteration in the composition of compounds in ruminal epithelial tissues may be due to the alternation in the ruminal parameters such as ruminal pH and ruminal metabolites concentration caused by the high grain feeding (Asma et al., 2013).

TABLE 2 | List of differentially expressed proteins in rumen epithelium from HG group and Hay group.

Protein ID	Gene symbol	Protein name	Ration (HG/Hay)	*P*-value
Fatty acid metabolism				
B6UV59	HADHA	Long-chain 3-hydroxyacyl-CoA dehydrogenase	0.38	0.020
W5PGM1	OXCT1	Succinyl-coa:3-ketoacid-coenzyme a transferase	0.01	0.035
K9LQQ8	FABP3	Fatty acid binding protein 3	0.04	0.011
W5QGP1	BDH1	Uncharacterized protein	1.81	0.010
W5Q740	ABCD3	ATP binding cassette subfamily d member 3	0.01	0.044
W5PAS5	HMGCL	Uncharacterized protein	3.03	0.014
Cell growth and proliferation				
M4WED3	CDC42	Cell division cycle 42	0.26	0.041
W5PPT6	TUBB	Uncharacterized protein	0.31	0.020
W5QJ02	DHRS7	Uncharacterized protein	1.74	0.024
W5PXP2	SDPR	Uncharacterized protein	0.32	0.032
W5P043	NPM1	Nucleophosmin 1	0.23	0.007
Carbohydrate metabolic processes				
D7R7V6	GAPDH	Glyceraldehyde-3-phosphate dehydrogenase	0.56	0.016
W5PK04	PGAM1	Phosphoglycerate mutase family member 1	0.57	0.041
Oxidative stress and detoxification				
L0CSP6	PRDX5	Peroxiredoxin-5	2.35	0.038
W5PH14	LOC101117764	UDP-glucuronosyltransferase	2.06	0.037
W5NZJ1	SULT1A1	Sulfotransferase	1.55	0.036
W5PJJ7	LOC101109421	Uncharacterized protein	2.71	0.017
W5P382	ZADH2	Uncharacterized protein	0.02	0.050
W5PHN8	LOC101107119	Uncharacterized protein	3.56	0.014
Protein metabolic processes				
W5NS93	PSMA4	Proteasome subunit alpha type	2.39	0.034
W5NSG2	TMEM43	Transmembrane protein 43	0.02	0.025
W5PVT6	UBA1	Ubiquitin-activating enzyme E1	0.60	0.031
W5Q834	ERO1A	Endoplasmic reticulum oxidoreductase 1 alpha	0.55	0.040
W5PAG0	KARS	Lysine–trna ligase	0.02	0.025
W5QB61	FKBP1A	Peptidyl-prolyl *cis–trans* isomerase	0.04	0.049
W5Q1N8	RPS23	Small subunit ribosomal protein S23E	0.10	0.025
W5PHW0	HSP90AB1	Heat shock protein 90 alpha family class b member 1	0.59	0.007
Immune system processes				
W5Q5H8	FGA	Fibrinogen alpha chain	2.89	0.031
W5PCN2	ANXA7	Annexin	12.29	0.020
Nucleoside metabolic processes				
W5PR48	HPRT1	Hypoxanthine phosphoribosyltransferase	0.08	0.035
W5Q3H9	UPP1	Uridine phosphorylase	0.19	0.026
Ion transport				
W5PVJ0	N/A	Ferritin	45.13	0.013
W5QGG0	TFRC	Transferrin receptor	0.09	<0.001
W5PK33	EFHD2	Uncharacterized protein	0.43	0.026
W5PP37	ATP5H	Uncharacterized protein	0.18	0.04

In the current study, our data revealed that HG diet supports a greater level of maltose in the ruminal epithelial tissues compared with the Hay group (**Table 1**). As mentioned above, rumen epithelial tissue has many functions including metabolism, nutrient absorption, as well as barrier functions. Normally, maltose cannot be absorbed intact from the lumen of the rumen, however, a decreased ruminal pH, combined with a high LPS level, may impair the ruminal epithelial barrier function (Gäbel et al., 1987; Penner et al., 2011) and further increase the permeability of the epithelium. A possible explanation for this result is that HG feeding resulted in an increase in the permeability of the epithelium. Similarly, a greater abundance of glucose was also detected in the rumen epithelium of goats that were fed an HG diet. In the present study, our data also showed that oxalate level in rumen tissue were significantly greater in HG group (**Table 1**). A previous study showed that acidification of the caecum in rats enhanced the intestinal oxalate absorption (Diamond et al., 1988). A possible explanation could be the fact

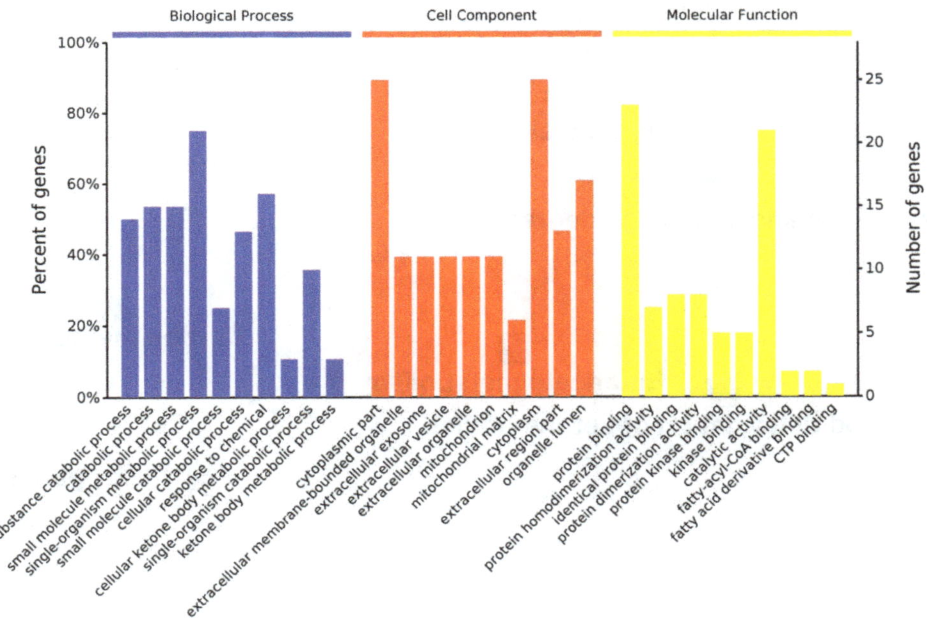

FIGURE 2 | Gene ontology distribution analysis of differentially expressed proteins in the rumen epithelium in goats from the high grain (HG) group and the hay (Hay) group.

that lower luminal pH induced by HG diets may cause more influx of oxalate from the lumen to epithelium.

Hydrocinnamic acid (3-phenylpropionic acid) is derived from the ruminal metabolism of *p*-coumaric and ferulic acids in cellulose (Chesson et al., 1982). Significant down-regulation of hydrocinnamic acid in the HG group was probably due to a lower ruminal cellulose degradation ability than in the Hay group, which is evidenced by the incidence that greater numbers of cellulolytic bacteria existed in hay-fed animals (Fernando et al., 2010). The above findings demonstrated that the cellulose metabolism was affected in rumen of goats fed HG diet. Mao et al. (2016) found that the lower dodecanedioic acid concentrations in rumen fluid in goats fed an HG diet may be caused by acid inhibition of biohydrogenation. Lower levels of dodecanedioic acid in the rumen fluid may result in decreased absorption by the ruminal epithelium. In line with this assumption, in the present study, a significant decrease in dodecanedioic acid level was found in extracts of ruminal epithelium in the HG group (**Table 1**). Caproic acid, a six-carbon straight-chain fatty acid, is found in trace amounts in rumen fluid. A previous study revealed that a greater ratio of corn starch led to a lower concentration of caproic acid in the rumen (Orskov et al., 1967). The decrease in caproic acid levels in the extracts of ruminal epithelium of the HG group probably can be attributed to the greater ratio of grain in their diet. Phenylethanolamine is a type of biogenic amine detected in the serum of rats and pigs, and it is known to play an important role in mammalian nervous system function (Shannon et al., 1981). Previous studies revealed that HG feeding increased the biogenic amine concentration in rumen fluid of cattle (Wang et al., 2013), thus, in the present study, the increased phenylethanolamine detected in extracts of ruminal epithelium of animal fed HG group may be due to the greater level of phenylethanolamine in rumen fluid of these animals.

Urea is quantitatively the most important end product of nitrogen metabolism in ruminants. Previous studies showed that part of the endogenous urea that is utilized moves into the rumen interior with saliva, but most of it moves from the blood directly through the rumen epithelium (Abdoun et al., 2006). Huntington (1989) reported that feeding a high-starch diet increased the transfer of urea from the blood into the rumen in beef steers, indicating that dietary carbohydrate has a marked effect on urea transfer. Thus, in the present study, a greater urea content in the rumen epithelium in the HG group is reasonable. The current study also revealed that the level of lactate in rumen epithelium tissues in the HG group was lower than that in the Hay group (**Table 1**). Lactate can be directly absorbed through the rumen wall to the blood and partially converted into ketone bodies in the rumen epithelium (Pennington and Sutherland, 1956). Our results are contrary to a report from a previous study that showed increasing concentrate intake had increased the net portal absorption of lactate in lambs (Huntington et al., 1980). The reason behind this observation is not clear and needs further investigation. Inosine is an endogenous purine nucleoside, which is formed during the breakdown of adenosine by adenosine deaminase (Barankiewicz and Cohen, 1985). The changes in inosine content could indicate a greater amount of metabolic active tissue by a concomitant increased HG intake.

As mentioned earlier, protein expression patterns of the ruminal epithelium of bovine in response to various feeding regimes have been explored using two-dimensional electrophoresis, and differentially expressed proteins that were mainly related to functions involved cellular stress and

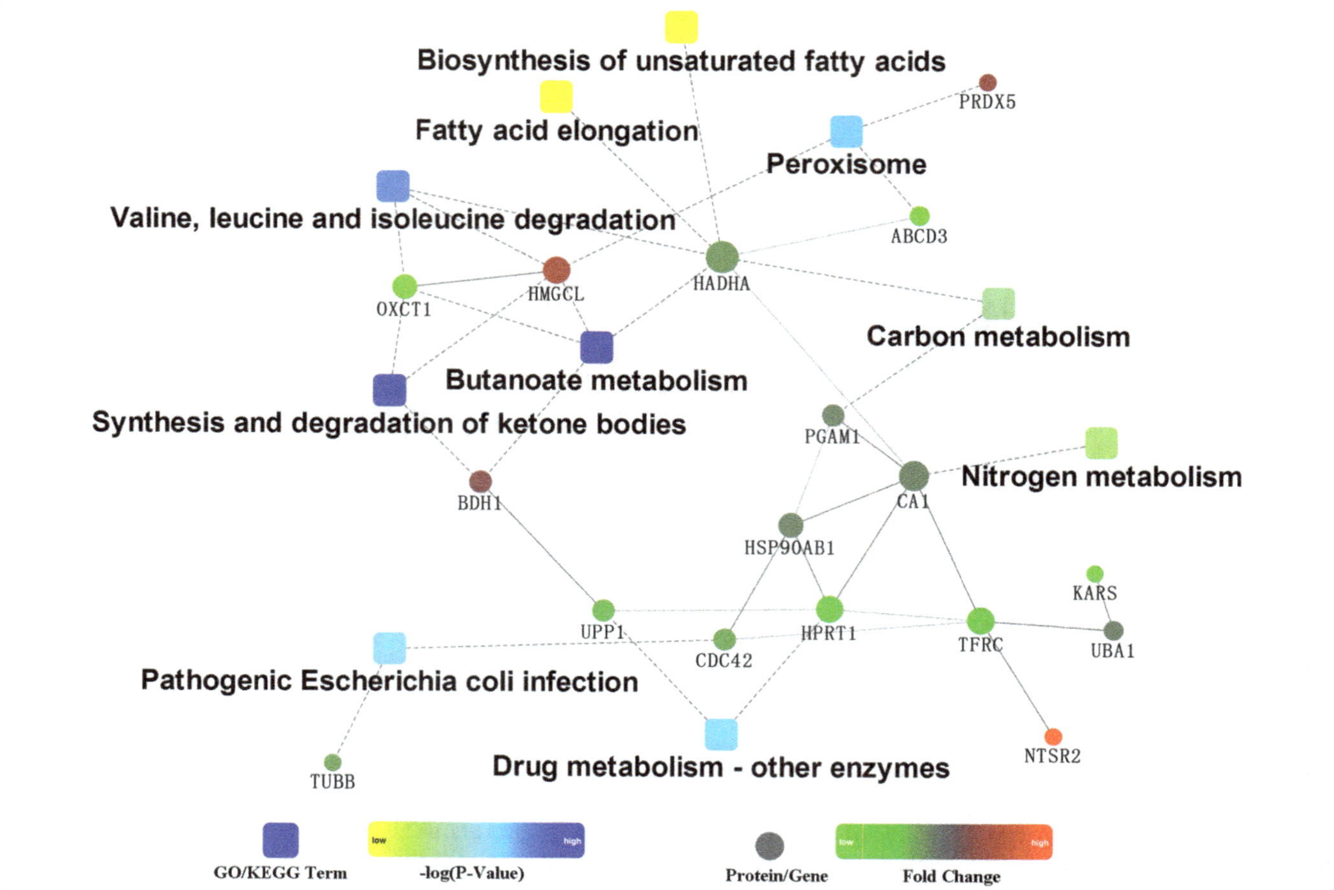

FIGURE 3 | Protein–protein interaction analysis by the OmicsBean.

metabolism (Bondzio et al., 2011). Until now, little information has been available to characterize the goat rumen tissue proteome. In the present study, a total of 34 differentially expressed proteins related to fatty acid metabolism, cell growth and proliferation, carbohydrate metabolic processes, oxidative stress and detoxification, protein metabolic processes, immune system processes, nucleoside metabolic processes and ion transport were detected between the two groups in goats (**Table 2**). Of these differentially expressed proteins, our data revealed that HG diet feeding decreased the expression of proteins involved in fatty acid metabolism, such as long-chain 3-hydroxyacyl-CoA dehydrogenase (**HADHA**), succinyl-coa:3-ketoacid-coenzyme a transferase (**OXCT1**), and FABP3. Among these downregulated expression of proteins, HADHA protein can catalyze the third step of mitochondrial beta-oxidation (Haglind et al., 2015), FABP3 protein act as a transport of fatty acids to the mitochondria or peroxisome for beta-oxidation (Furuhashi and Hotamisligil, 2008), ATP binding cassette subfamily d member 3 (**ABCD3**) functions as a transporter for moving the fatty acids into peroxisome for beta-oxidation (van Roermund et al., 2014), and OXCT1 was a key enzyme for ketone body utilization (Song et al., 1997). Thus, the downregulated expression of these proteins indicates a decreased catabolism of fatty acids in the HG group. In addition, the present study also revealed that HG diet feeding resulted in a decreased expression of proteins related to the carbohydrate metabolic process, including GAPDH and phosphoglycerate mutase family member 1 (**PGAM1**). It is well known that GAPDH and PGAM1 can catalyze the sixth and eighth step of glycolysis, respectively, and play an important in glucose metabolism. Thus, the reduced expressions of these two proteins in the HG group indicate that HG feeding may result in a decrease in glycolysis in ruminal epithelial tissues.

Our study also demonstrated that seven differentially regulated proteins related to protein metabolism, including lysine–tRNA ligase (**KARS**), endoplasmic reticulum oxidoreductase 1 alpha (**ERO1A**), proteasome subunit alpha type (**PSMA4**), peptidyl-prolyl *cis–trans* isomerase (**FKBP1A**), small subunit ribosomal protein S23E (**RPS23**), HSP90AB1, and UBA1, were affected by HG feeing in goats. Of these proteins mentioned earlier, ERO1A is reported to be involved in the essential step of correct protein folding for the formation of disulfide bonds by reoxidizing protein disulfide isomerase (Gess et al., 2003). In the present study, the downregulation of ERO1A might relate to the decrease in the protein disulfide-isomerase, as Hollmann et al. (2013) reported that HG feeding decreased the protein disulfide-isomerase which plays a synergistic

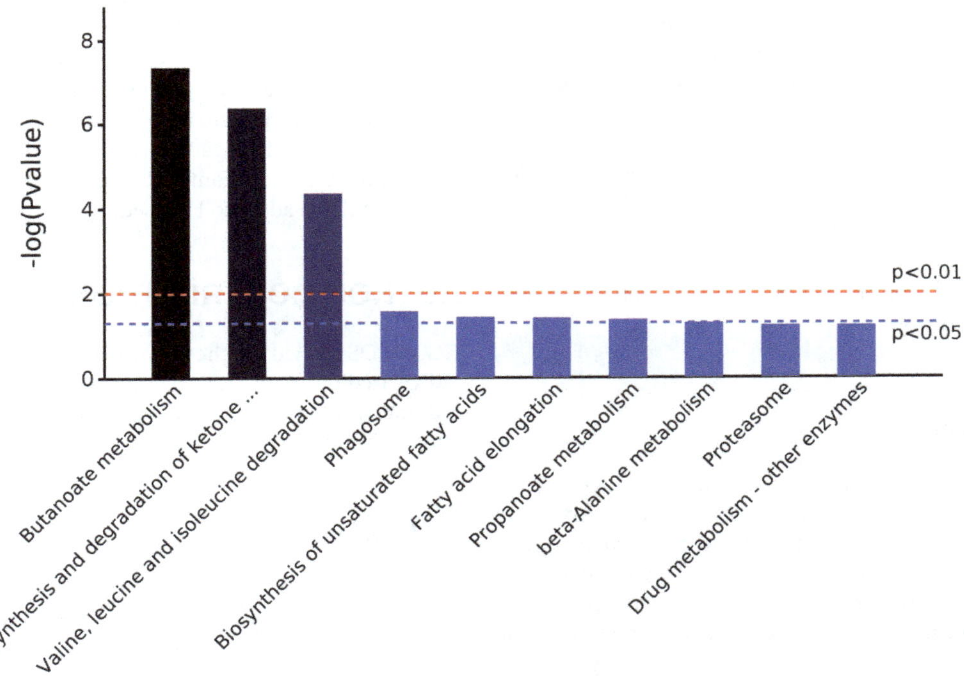

FIGURE 4 | The *p*-value of enriched KEGG pathway.

effect on protein folding with ERO1A (Santos et al., 2009). Regarding other differentially regulated proteins involved in protein metabolism, RPS23 is reported to be involved in protein synthesis, while KARS plays an important role in the process of inserting lysine into proteins (Freist and Gauss, 1995). FKBP1A is believed to play an important role in accelerating the rate at which proteins fold into their native conformation (Siekierka et al., 1990), and PSMA4 and UBA1 are involved in the ubiquitin-proteasome proteolytic pathway (Ciechanover, 1994). HSP90AB1 plays a key role in protein folding, degradation, and morphological evolution. Generally, the findings of these differentially regulated proteins suggest that HG feeding affected the synthesis, correct folding, and breaking down of proteins in rumen epithelium.

Interestingly, in the present study, six proteins, PRDX5, UDP-glucuronosyltransferase (LOC101117764), sulfotransferase (SULT1A1), ZADH2, LOC101107119, and LOC101109421, related to oxidative stress and detoxification were upregulated in response to an HG diet. Of these upregulated expression of protein, SULT1A1 and LOC101117764 are key components of the body's chemical defense system and these two enzymes protein are believed to play an important role in maintaining host health (Rubin et al., 1996; Xu et al., 2005). In the present study, the increase in the relative expression of these two enzymes protein probably indicates the HG feeding may result in an enhancement in host deference in response to more toxic substances such as endotoxin and biogenic amine translocating from the rumen into the rumen epithelium (Eisenhofer et al., 1997). In the present study, we also found HG feeding upregulated immune system processes-related ANXA7 proteins, and this is consistent with the report by Bondzio et al. (2011) who found increased expression of ANXA7 in the rumen epithelium in response to HG diets. As ANXA7 is one of the annexin family members that is upregulated in inflammatory myopathies (Probst-Cousin et al., 2004), thus, the upregulation of ANXA7 imply that HG feeding may trigger an inflammatory response in rumen epithelium, and this peculations corresponds well to the findings in our previous report that HG feeding caused local inflammation of the rumen epithelium (Liu et al., 2013).

Several proteins related to ion transportation were also different between the two groups. Transferrin receptor (**TFRC**) is present on the surface of cells and binds to transferrin to transport iron into the cell. A previous work showed decreased TFRC combined with increased ferritin, which may indicate a disorder of iron metabolism in the HG group. In line with our findings, Hollmann et al. (2013) found downregulation of transferrin in the rumen epithelium in response to HG diets. The previous study has already reported that HG diets decrease the duration time of the cell cycle in the ruminal epithelium, and the rates of cell division and turnover are considered to be related to the pathological conditions, including hyperkeratosis, parakeratosis, and ruminitis (Goodlad, 1981). In the present study, six differentially regulated proteins related to cell growth and proliferation were observed. Given that the inhibition of CDC42 and Nucleophosmin 1 (**NPM1**) could induce cell apoptosis (Ambrogio et al., 2008), the downregulation of them in response to HG diets may be attributed to accelerated turnover by promoting cell apoptosis in the ruminal epithelium.

PPI showed that three pathways were enriched in the KEGG, including butanoate metabolism, synthesis and degradation of ketone bodies, and valine, leucine and isoleucine degradation. Although it was well established that rumen epithelium plays a crucial role in SCVFA absorption and metabolism (Bannink et al., 2016), no other differentially expressed protein related to other SCVFAs uptake and metabolism was detected except for the protein related to butyrate metabolism. This may be because butyrate is more readily absorbed and metabolized in the rumen epithelium than other SCVFAs (Pennington, 1952). Interestingly, in line with our research, only gene expression related to butyrate metabolism was upregulated in lower risk of SARA cows compared to higher risk of SARA cows (Gao and Oba, 2016), indicating butyrate metabolism in the rumen epithelium could be more crucial for SCVFA metabolism and rumen epithelial function.

CONCLUSION

In general, our data showed that long-term feeding of an HG diet discriminatively altered the protein expression (with 12 upregulated and 23 downregulated proteins) and metabolites profiles (with 8 increased metabolites and 7 decreased metabolites). The downregulated proteins were related to fatty acid metabolism, carbohydrate metabolic processes and nucleoside metabolic processes, while most of upregulated proteins were related to oxidative stress and detoxification. The enrichment analysis of different metabolites indicated that HG diet mainly affected starch and sucrose metabolism, purine metabolism, glyoxylate and dicarboxylate metabolism, glycerolipid metabolism, pyruvate metabolism, glycolysis or gluconeogenesis, galactose metabolism, glycine, serine and threonine metabolism, and arginine and proline metabolism. These findings may contribute to better understanding how rumen epithelia adapt to HG feeding.

AUTHOR CONTRIBUTIONS

CG and DS carried out the majority of the animal studies. CG and SM carried out data interpretation and manuscript preparation. SM and XW were responsible for the conception of the project and the oversight of the experiments.

FUNDING

This work was supported by the National Natural Science Foundation of China (Grant No. 31572436) and the Jiangsu Agriculture Science and Technology Innovation Fund (CX(18)2003).

REFERENCES

Abdoun, K., Stumpff, F., and Martens, H. (2006). Ammonia and urea transport across the rumen epithelium: a review. *Anim. Health Res. Rev.* 7, 43–59. doi: 10.1017/S1466252307001156

Ambrogio, C., Voena, C., Manazza, A. D., Martinengo, C., Costa, C., Kirchhausen, T., et al. (2008). The anaplastic lymphoma kinase controls cell shape and growth of anaplastic large cell lymphoma through Cdc42 activation. *Cancer Res.* 68, 8899–8907. doi: 10.1158/0008-5472.CAN-08-2568

Ametaj, B. N., Zebeli, Q., Saleem, F., Psychogios, N., Lewis, M. J., Dunn, S. M., et al. (2010). Metabolomics reveals unhealthy alterations in rumen metabolism with increased proportion of cereal grain in the diet of dairy cows. *Metabolomics* 6, 583–594. doi: 10.1007/s11306-010-0227-6

Asma, Z., Sylvie, C., Laurent, C., Jérôme, M., Christophe, K., Olivier, B., et al. (2013). Microbial ecology of the rumen evaluated by 454 GS FLX pyrosequencing is affected by starch and oil supplementation of diets. *FEMS Microbiol. Ecol.* 83, 504–514. doi: 10.1111/1574-6941.12011

Bannink, A., France, J., Lopez, S., Gerrits, W., Kebreab, E., Tamminga, S., et al. (2008). Modelling the implications of feeding strategy on rumen fermentation and functioning of the rumen wall. *Anim. Feed Sci. Technol.* 143, 3–26. doi: 10.1016/j.anifeedsci.2007.05.002

Bannink, A., van Lingen, H. J., Ellis, J. L., France, J., and Dijkstra, J. (2016). The contribution of mathematical modeling to understanding dynamic aspects of rumen metabolism. *Front. Microbiol.* 7:1820. doi: 10.3389/fmicb.2016.01820

Barankiewicz, J., and Cohen, A. (1985). Purine nucleotide-metabolism in resident and activated rat macrophages *invitro*. *Eur. J. Immunol.* 15, 627–631. doi: 10.1002/eji.1830150618

Bergman, E. N. (1990). Energy contributions of volatile fatty-acids from the gastrointestinal-tract in various species. *Physiol. Rev.* 70, 567–590. doi: 10.1152/physrev.1990.70.2.567

Bondzio, A., Gabler, C., Badewien-Rentzsch, B., Schulze, P., Martens, H., and Einspanier, R. (2011). Identification of differentially expressed proteins in ruminal epithelium in response to a concentrate-supplemented diet. *Am. J. Physiol. Gastrointest. Liver Physiol.* 301, G260–G268. doi: 10.1152/ajpgi.00304.2010

Chesson, A., Stewart, C. S., and Wallace, R. J. (1982). Influence of plant phenolic acids on growth and cellulolytic activity of rumen bacteria. *Appl. Environ. Microbiol.* 44, 597–603.

Ciechanover, A. (1994). The ubiquitin-proteasome proteolytic pathway. *Cell* 79, 13–21. doi: 10.1016/0092-8674(94)90396-4

Diamond, K. L., Fox, C. C., and Barch, D. H. (1988). Role of cecal pH in intestinal oxalate absorption in the rat. *J. Lab. Clin. Med.* 112, 352–356.

Eisenhofer, G., Aneman, A., Friberg, P., Hooper, D., Fandriks, L., Lonroth, H., et al. (1997). Substantial production of dopamine in the human gastrointestinal tract. *J. Clin. Endocrinol. Metab.* 82, 3864–3871.

Fernando, S. C., Purvis, H. T. II, Najar, F. Z., Sukharnikov, L. O., Krehbiel, C. R., Nagaraja, T. G., et al. (2010). Rumen microbial population dynamics during adaptation to a high-grain diet. *Appl. Environ. Microbiol.* 76, 7482–7490. doi: 10.1128/AEM.00388-10

Freist, W., and Gauss, D. H. (1995). Lysyl-tRNA synthetase. *Biol. Chem. Hoppe Seyler* 376, 451–472.

Furuhashi, M., and Hotamisligil, G. S. (2008). Fatty acid-binding proteins: role in metabolic diseases and potential as drug targets. *Nat. Rev. Drug Discov.* 7, 489–503. doi: 10.1038/nrd2589

Gabel, G., Aschenbach, J. R., and Muller, F. (2002). Transfer of energy substrates across the ruminal epithelium: implications and limitations. *Anim. Health Res. Rev.* 3, 15–30. doi: 10.1079/AHRR200237

Gäbel, G., Martens, H., Sündermann, M., and Galfi, P. (1987). The effect of diet, intraruminal pH and osmolarity on sodium, chloride and magnesium absorption from the temporarily isolated and washed reticulo-rumen of sheep. *Q. J. Exp. Physiol.* 72, 501–511. doi: 10.1113/expphysiol.1987.sp003092

Gao, X., and Oba, M. (2016). Characteristics of dairy cows with a greater or lower risk of subacute ruminal acidosis: volatile fatty acid absorption, rumen digestion, and expression of genes in rumen epithelial cells. *J. Dairy Sci.* 99, 8733–8745. doi: 10.3168/jds.2016-11570

Gerber, S. A., Rush, J., Stemman, O., Kirschner, M. W., and Gygi, S. P. (2003). Absolute quantification of proteins and phosphoproteins from cell lysates by tandem MS. *Proc. Natl. Acad. Sci. U.S.A.* 100, 6940–6945. doi: 10.1073/pnas.0832254100

Gess, B., Hofbauer, K. H., Wenger, R. H., Lohaus, C., Meyer, H. E., and Kurtz, A. (2003). The cellular oxygen tension regulates expression of the endoplasmic oxidoreductase ERO1-L alpha. *Eur. J. Biochem.* 270, 2228–2235. doi: 10.1046/j.1432-1033.2003.03590.x

Goodlad, R. A. (1981). Some effects of diet on the mitotic index and the cell cycle of the ruminal epithelium of sheep. *Q. J. Exp. Physiol.* 66, 487–499. doi: 10.1113/expphysiol.1981.sp002590

Haglind, C. B., Nordenstrom, A., Ask, S., von Dobeln, U., Gustafsson, J., and Stenlid, M. H. (2015). Increased and early lipolysis in children with long-chain 3-hydroxyacyl-CoA dehydrogenase (LCHAD) deficiency during fast. *J. Inherit. Metab. Dis.* 38, 315–322. doi: 10.1007/s10545-014-9750-3

Hollmann, M., Miller, I., Hummel, K., Sabitzer, S., Metzler-Zebeli, B. U., Razzazi-Fazeli, E., et al. (2013). Downregulation of cellular protective factors of rumen epithelium in goats fed high energy diet. *PLoS One* 8:e81602. doi: 10.1371/journal.pone.0081602

Huntington, G. B. (1989). Hepatic urea synthesis and site and rate of urea removal from blood of beef steers fed alfalfa hay or a high concentrate diet. *Can. J. Anim. Sci.* 69, 215–223. doi: 10.4141/cjas89-025

Huntington, G. B., Prior, R. L., and Britton, R. A. (1980). Glucose and lactate absorption and metabolic interrelationships in lambs switched from low to high concentrate diets. *J. Nutr.* 110, 1904–1913. doi: 10.1093/jn/110.9.1904

Lin, D., Tabb, D. L., and Yates, J. R. (2003). Large-scale protein identification using mass spectrometry. *Biochim. Biophys. Acta* 1646, 1–10. doi: 10.1016/S1570-9639(02)00546-0

Liu, J. H., Xu, T. T., Liu, Y. J., Zhu, W. Y., and Mao, S. Y. (2013). A high-grain diet causes massive disruption of ruminal epithelial tight junctions in goats. *Am. J. Physiol. Regul. Integr. Comp. Physiol.* 305, R232–R241. doi: 10.1152/ajpregu.00068.2013

Mao, S. Y., Huo, W. J., and Zhu, W. Y. (2016). Microbiome-metabolome analysis reveals unhealthy alterations in the composition and metabolism of ruminal microbiota with increasing dietary grain in a goat model. *Environ. Microbiol.* 18, 525–541. doi: 10.1111/1462-2920.12724

Orskov, E. R., Flatt, W. P., Moe, P. W., and Oltjen, R. R. (1967). Caproic acid and ethanol in ruminal ingesta of cattle receiving purified diets. *J. Dairy Sci.* 50, 239–242. doi: 10.3168/jds.S0022-0302(67)87398-3

Penner, G. B., Steele, M. A., Aschenbach, J. R., and McBride, B. W. (2011). Ruminant nutrition symposium: molecular adaptation of ruminal epithelia to highly fermentable diets. *J. Anim. Sci.* 89, 1108–1119. doi: 10.2527/jas.2010-3378

Pennington, R. J. (1952). The metabolism of short-chain fatty acids in the sheep. 1. Fatty acid utilization and ketone body production by rumen epithelium and other tissues. *Biochem. J.* 51, 251. doi: 10.1042/bj0510251

Pennington, R. J., and Sutherland, T. M. (1956). Ketone-body production from various substrates by sheep-rumen epithelium. *Biochem. J.* 63, 353. doi: 10.1042/bj0630353

Probst-Cousin, S., Berghoff, C., Neundorfer, B., and Heuss, D. (2004). Annexin expression in inflammatory myopathies. *Muscle Nerve.* 30, 102–110. doi: 10.1002/mus.20077

Rubin, G. L., Sharp, S., Jones, A. L., Glatt, H., Mills, J. A., and Coughtrie, M. W. H. (1996). Design, production and characterization of antibodies discriminating between the phenol- and monoamine-sulphating forms of human phenol sulphotransferase. *Xenobiotica* 26, 1113–1119. doi: 10.3109/00498259609050256

Santos, C. X. C., Tanaka, L. Y., Wosniak, J., and Laurindo, F. R. M. (2009). Mechanisms and implications of reactive oxygen species generation during the unfolded protein response: roles of endoplasmic reticulum oxidoreductases, mitochondrial electron transport, and NADPH oxidase. *Antioxid. Redox Signal.* 11, 2409–2427. doi: 10.1089/ARS.2009.2625

Shannon, H. E., Cone, E. J., and Yousefnejad, D. (1981). Physiologic effects and plasma kinetics of phenylethanolamine and its N-methyl homolog in the dog. *J. Pharmacol. Exp. Ther.* 217, 379–385.

Shen, Z., Seyfert, H. M., Lohrke, B., Schneider, F., Zitnan, R., Chudy, A., et al. (2004). An energy-rich diet causes rumen papillae proliferation associated with more IGF type 1 receptors and increased plasma IGF-1 concentrations in young goats. *J. Nutr.* 134, 11–17. doi: 10.1093/jn/134.1.11

Siekierka, J. J., Wiederrecht, G., Greulich, H., Boulton, D., Hung, S. H. Y., Cryan, J., et al. (1990). The cytosolic-binding protein for the immunosuppressant Fk-506 Is both a ubiquitous and highly conserved peptidyl-prolyl cis-trans isomerase. *J. Biol. Chem.* 265, 21011–21015.

Song, X. Q., Fukao, T., Mitchell, G. A., KassovskaBratinova, S., Ugarte, M., Wanders, R. J. A., et al. (1997). Succinyl-CoA:3-ketoacid coenzyme A transferase (SCOT): development of an antibody to human SCOT and diagnostic use in hereditary SCOT deficiency. *Biochim. Biophys. Acta* 1360, 151–156. doi: 10.1016/S0925-4439(96)00074-9

Sun, Y., Yu, K., Zhou, L., Fang, L., Su, Y., and Zhu, W. (2016). Metabolomic and transcriptomic responses induced in the livers of pigs by the long-term intake of resistant starch. *J. Anim. Sci.* 94, 1083–1094. doi: 10.2527/jas.2015-9715

Uppal, S. K., Wolf, K., Khahra, S. S., and Martens, H. (2003). Modulation of Na+ transport across isolated rumen epithelium by short-chain fatty acids in hay- and concentrate-fed sheep. *J. Anim. Physiol. Anim. Nutr.* 87, 380–388. doi: 10.1046/j.1439-0396.2003.00448.x

van Roermund, C. W. T., Ijlst, L., Wagemans, T., Wanders, R. J. A., and Waterham, H. R. (2014). A role for the human peroxisomal half-transporter ABCD3 in the oxidation of dicarboxylic acids. *Biochim. Biophys. Acta* 1841, 563–568. doi: 10.1016/j.bbalip.2013.12.001

Wang, D. S., Zhang, R. Y., Zhu, W. Y., and Mao, S. Y. (2013). Effects of subacute ruminal acidosis challenges on fermentation and biogenic amines in the rumen of dairy cows. *Livest. Sci.* 155, 262–272. doi: 10.3168/jds.2011-4671

Xu, C. J., Li, C. Y. T., and Kong, A. N. T. (2005). Induction of phase I, II and III drug metabolism/transport by xenobiotics. *Arch. Pharm. Res.* 28, 249–268. doi: 10.1007/BF02977789

5

Discovery of a Potential Plasma Protein Biomarker Panel for Acute-on-Chronic Liver Failure Induced by Hepatitis B Virus

Ni Zhou [1†], Kuifeng Wang [1†], Shanhua Fang [2,3†], Xiaoyu Zhao [1], Tingting Huang [1], Huazhong Chen [1], Fei Yan [1], Yongzhi Tang [1], Hu Zhou [2,3] and Jiansheng Zhu [1*]*

[1] Department of Infectious Diseases, Affiliated Taizhou Hospital of Wenzhou Medical University, Taizhou, China, [2] E-Institute of Shanghai Municipal Education Committee, Shanghai University of Traditional Chinese Medicine, Shanghai, China, [3] Department of Analytical Chemistry and CAS Key Laboratory of Receptor Research, Shanghai Institute of Materia Medica, Chinese Academy of Sciences, Shanghai, China

***Correspondence:**
Hu Zhou
zhouhu@simm.ac.cn
Jiansheng Zhu
zhujs@enzemed.com*

[†] These authors have contributed equally to this work.

Hepatitis B virus (HBV)-associated acute-on-chronic liver failure (HBV-ACLF), characterized by an acute deterioration of liver function in the patients with chronic hepatitis B (CHB), is lack of predicting biomarkers for prognosis. Plasma is an ideal sample for biomarker discovery due to inexpensive and minimally invasive sampling and good reproducibility. In this study, immuno-depletion of high-abundance plasma proteins followed by iTRAQ-based quantitative proteomic approach was employed to analyze plasma samples from 20 healthy control people, 20 CHB patients and 20 HBV-ACLF patients, respectively. As a result, a total of 427 proteins were identified from these samples, and 42 proteins were differentially expressed in HBV-ACLF patients as compared to both CHB patients and healthy controls. According to bioinformatics analysis results, 6 proteins related to immune response (MMR), inflammatory response (OPN, HPX), blood coagulation (ATIII) and lipid metabolism (APO-CII, GP73) were selected as biomarker candidates. Further ELISA analysis confirmed the significant up-regulation of GP73, MMR, OPN and down-regulation of ATIII, HPX, APO-CII in HBV-ACLF plasma samples ($p < 0.01$). Moreover, receiver operating characteristic (ROC) curve analysis revealed high diagnostic value of these candidates in assessing HBV-ACLF. In conclusion, present quantitative proteomic study identified 6 novel HBV-ACLF biomarker candidates and might provide fundamental information for development of HBV-ACLF biomarker.

Keywords: HBV-ACLF, CHB, iTRAQ, proteomics, biomarker

INTRODUCTION

Acute-on-chronic liver failure (ACLF) is increasingly recognized as an acute deterioration of liver function combining with liver and multi-organ failures in patients with pre-existing chronic liver disease, although there is no consensus about its definition (Bernal et al., 2015; Anand and Dhiman, 2016; Arroyo and Jalan, 2016). Hepatitis B virus (HBV) associated ACLF, as a subtype of ACLF, can develop at any stage in the progression of chronic hepatitis B (CHB) (Zamora Nava et al., 2014). It is estimated that about 70% of liver failure is caused by HBV infections in the Eastern countries

(Sarin et al., 2009), and there are approximately 97 million people suffering from HBV infection in China alone (Cui and Jia, 2013). HBV-ACLF has a poor prognosis with high mortality rate (>70%), if emergency liver transplantation is not available (Marrero et al., 2003). Therefore, it is believed that predicting and stopping the progression of CHB to ACLF at an early stage may be the most effective strategy of reducing the mortality of patients with HBV-ACLF.

Despite a number of scoring systems such as Child-Pugh score have been used for diagnosis of end-stage liver diseases, not all of these scores are specifically designed for HBV-ACLF. So far, various biochemical molecules (e.g., Prealbumin, Serum ferritin), cytokines (e.g., Interleukin 17, Fibroleukin) and chemokines (e.g., Macrophage inflammatory protein-3α) have been evaluated to be novel indicators for HBV-ACLF as reviewed by Chen et al. (2015). Wan et al. (2015) performed a particle-enhanced immunonephelometry assay on serum samples from ACLF patients, and they found that the level of cystain C (CysC) was significantly higher in the ACLF with kidney failure group than those in the healthy controls and CHB patients. Their results suggested that CysC could be considered as a biomarker for renal dysfunction in ACLF patients. However, no protein biomarker has reached the clinical setting yet. Considering the complexity and heterogeneity of HBV-ACLF pathology, it has been suggested that integrated panel of biomarkers with specific and complementary functions rather than a single biomarker be useful in diagnosis of patients with HBV-ACLF.

Unbiased proteomic analysis of plasma samples holds the promise to discover clinically effective disease biomarkers. Plasma proteomics is an appealing concept in medicine due to inexpensive and minimally invasive sampling and good reproducibility (Harel et al., 2015). Plasma proteins comprise not only actual plasma proteins that maintain physiological homeostasis but also low abundance "leakage" proteins from damaged tissues, which may provide direct information about the pathology of disease and may serve as clinical biomarkers for diagnosis and treatment (Lv et al., 2007). Several studies have successfully applied this strategy to identify biomarkers of liver disease, including Hepatitis B (He et al., 2003), Hepatitis C (HCV) associated hepatic fibrosis (Yang et al., 2011) and HBV-associated hepatocellular carcinoma (HCC) (Niu et al., 2010).

With regard to HBV-ACLF, a study using matrix-assisted laser desorption/ionization time-of-flight (MALDI-TOF) mass spectrometry (MS) approach showed that protein profiling was markedly changed during the progression of CHB to liver failure and suggested that these dynamic changes can distinguish different stages of the CHB (Han et al., 2010). Another study employed two-dimensional gel electrophoresis (2-DE) MS/MS approach to compared serum samples collected from normal individuals, CHB patients and HBV-ACLF patients, which proposed that Alpha-1-acid glycoprotein (A1-AGF) might be a potential biomarker of ACLF diagnosis for CHB patients (Ren et al., 2010). Currently, with the advent of quantitative proteomic technology, isobaric tagging for relative and absolute quantitation (iTRAQ) technology makes it possible to quantify several proteins in a single experiment with improved accuracy and reproducibility of quantitation (Pierce et al., 2008). Using this technology, Peng et al. (2013) has identified total of 16 significantly differential proteins in serum from patients with CHB and patients with HBV-ACLF compared to healthy controls, and suggested five of those proteins were potentially associated with progression of hepatitis B and ACLF.

In this study, iTRAQ coupled with LC-MS/MS approach was utilized to construct the plasma proteome in healthy controls, patients with CHB and HBV-ACLF to explore disease-associated alterations of plasma proteins. In addition, we sought to validate several potential biomarkers that could distinguish ACLF from both CHB and healthy control by ELISA analysis and subsequent receiver operating characteristic (ROC) curves analysis. The six candidates identified in present study can aid clinical biomarker discovery for HBV-ACLF.

Abbreviations: HBV-ACLF, HBV induced acute-on-chronic liver failure; MMR, mannose receptor; OPN, osteopontin; HPX, hemopexin; GP73, golgi membrane protein 1; ATIII, antithrombin-III; APO-CII, apolipoprotein CII; CHB, chronic hepatitis B; CHC, Chronic hepatitis C.

MATERIALS AND METHODS

Human Plasma Sample Collection

Blood samples from healthy people (CON), patients with chronic hepatitis B (CHB) and patients with HBV induced acute-on-chronic liver failure (HBV-ACLF) were provided by Department of Infectious Diseases of Taizhou Hospital of Zhejiang Province, China ($n = 20$ per group). The study was approved by scientific ethics committee (Taizhou hospital of Zhejiang Province, China). Written informed consent was given from all participants and legal guardians before commencement of this study. The diagnoses of HBV-ACLF were based on criteria previously described (Sarin et al., 2009). Exclusion criteria included: pregnant or lactating women; liver cancer or suspected liver cancer; recent infection; use of immune-suppressive agents; anti-viral therapy, immune disease or malignant tumor; other types of hepatitis infection and HIV infection patients. Rejection criteria included: died within 7 days after enrollment, liver transplantation after enrollment. Information of clinical and demographic characteristics of patients with CHB, HBV-ACLF and healthy controls were shown in **Table 1**. HBV-ACLF samples were referred to as ACLF in the figure captions. The collected blood samples were then centrifuged at 3,000 rpm for 10 min at room temperature to remove any cells and debris. Twenty clarified plasma samples of each group were pooled into 4 samples that contained equal volume of 5 individual plasma samples from each group. As a result, a total of 60 samples were randomly pooled into 12 pooled samples.

Plasma Sample Preparation for Proteomic Analysis

Since disease biomarkers in the plasma are usually covered by high-abundance proteins, and their signals are weak in the mass spectrum, removal of high-abundant proteins was performed using Agilent High-Capacity Human-14 Multiple Affinity Removal System (MARS Human-14, Agilent, USA) according

TABLE 1 | Clinical and demographic characteristics of subjects enrolled in this study.

Variation	ACLF ($n = 23$)	CHB ($n = 45$)	CON ($n = 20$)	p-value
Age (year)	45.8 ± 13.3	40.9 ± 10.7	42.7 ± 10.9	0.250
Gender: male (%)	14 (60.9)	30 (66.7)	12 (60)	0.833
ALT (U/L)	427.2 ± 27.5	422.6 ± 16.4	30.2 ± 1.2	0.042
AST (U/L)	316.4 ± 13.5	189.3 ± 4.4	24.8 ± 0.4	<0.001
TB (μmol/L)	267.2 ± 3.8	37.6 ± 1.4	11.0 ± 0.2	<0.001
HBV-DNA (log_{10}/mL)	5.4 ± 1.6	5.7 ± 1.4	ND	–
HBsAg: positive (%)	23 (100)	45 (100)	ND	–
HBeAg: positive (%)	16 (69.6)	33 (73.3)	ND	–

ALT, alanine transaminase; AST, glutamic-oxalacetic transaminase; TB, total bilirubin; ND, not determined.

to the manufacturer's instructions. Protein concentrations were determined by tryptophan fluorescence emission at 350 nm using an excitation wave length of 295 nm (Geiger et al., 2010). Removal effect was verified by Coomassie-stained gel. Then 100 μg of protein from each pooled sample was processed by the Filter Assisted Sample Preparation (FASP) method as previously described (Wiśniewski et al., 2010). Briefly, each sample was transferred to a 10 kDa filter (Millipore Corporation) and centrifuged at 14,000 g for 40 min at 20°C. Then, 200 μL of urea buffer (8 M urea, 0.1 M Tris-HCl, pH 8.5) was added and followed by another centrifugation at 15,000 g for 40 min. This step was repeated one more time. The concentrate was then mixed with 100 μL of 50 mM iodoacetamide (IAA) in urea buffer and incubated for an additional 40 min at room temperature in darkness. After that, IAA was removed by centrifugation at 14,000 g for 40 min. Next, the sample was diluted with 200 μL of urea buffer and centrifuged two more times. Then, 200 μL of 50 mM tetraethyl ammonium bromide (TEAB) was added and the sample was centrifuged at 14,000 g for 40 min. This step was repeated twice. Finally, samples were digested with trypsin (1:50, enzyme to protein in 50 mM TEAB) by incubating at 37°C for 16 h.

iTRAQ Labeling of Plasma Samples

Peptides were labeled with iTRAQ reagents according to the manufacturer's instructions (AB Sciex, Foster City, CA). To quantify 12 samples, 2 batches of 8-plex iTRAQ labeling experiment were performed, with a mixture of 12 samples in equal amount as a bridge for comparison among different batches. Each aliquot (50 μg of peptide equivalent) was reacted with one tube of iTRAQ reagent. After the sample was dissolved in 15 μL of 0.5 M TEAB solution, pH 8.5, the iTRAQ reagent was dissolved in 50 μL of isopropanol. The mixture was incubated at room temperature for 2 h. The 8-plex labeled samples in the same experiment branch was pooled together and lyophilized.

High pH Reverse Phase Fractionation (HPRP)

iTRAQ-labeled peptides mixture was fractionated using a Waters XBridge BEH130 C18 3.5 μm 2.1 × 150 mm column on a Agilent 1260 HPLC operating at 0.2 mL/min. Buffer A consisted of 10 mM ammonium formate and buffer B consisted of 10 mM ammonium formate with 90% acetonitrile; both buffers were adjusted to pH 10 with ammonium hydroxide as described previously (Wang et al., 2011). A CBS-B programed multifunction automatic fraction collecting instrument (Huxi instrument, Shanghai, China) was coupled to the HPLC and used to collect eluted peptides. A total of 28 fractions were collected for each peptides mixture, and then concatenated to 14 (pooling equal interval RPLC fractions). The fractions were dried for nano LC-MS/MS analysis.

LC-MS/MS Analysis

The reverse phase high-performance liquid chromatography (RP-HPLC) separation was achieved on the Easy nano-LC system (Thermo Fisher Scientific) using a self-packed column (75 μm × 150 mm; 3 μm ReproSil-Pur C18 beads, 120 Å, Dr. Maisch GmbH, Ammerbuch, Germany) at a flow rate of 300 nL/min. The mobile phase A of RP-HPLC was 0.1% formic acid in water, and B was 0.1% formic acid in acetonitrile. The peptides were eluted using a gradient (2–90% mobile phase B) over a 90 min period into a nano-ESI Orbitrap Elite mass spectrometer (Thermo Fisher Scientific). The mass spectrometer was operated in data-dependent mode with each full MS scan (m/z 300–1,500) followed by MS/MS for the 12 most intense ions with the parameters: $\geq +2$ precursor ion charge, 2 Da precursor ion isolation window, 80 first mass and 38 normalized collision energy of HCD. Dynamic Exclusion™ was set for 30 s. The full mass and the subsequent MS/MS analyses were scanned in the Orbitrap analyzer with $R = 60{,}000$ and $R = 15{,}000$, respectively.

Database Searching and Analysis

Data were processed by search against the UniProt/SwissProt Human database (IPI.human.v3.87) using Maxquant (version 1.5.1.0), with default settings including the allowance of one missed cleavage and 8-plex iTRAQ fixed modifications. Minimum 7 amino acids for peptide, >2 peptides were required per protein. For peptide and protein identification, false discovery rate (FDR) was set to 1%. iTRAQ reporter ion intensity were used for quantification. By setting the median of intensity for each channel to equal and matching the distributions of each treatment iTRAQ reporter group (114, 115, 116, 118, 119, and 121) to those of the control iTRAQ reporter group (113, which corresponded to the mixture sample), we able to make consistent comparisons across different samples obtained from different iTRAQ 8-plex experiments. The ratio was restored to the intensity by multiplying the median of intensity of the first channel 113 (MIX1).

Bioinformatics Analysis

Functional enrichment analysis of Gene Ontology (GO) of biological process, molecular function, and cellular component was performed using DAVID Bioinformatics Resources version

6.7. The protein-protein interaction (PPI) network analysis of differentially expressed proteins was performed using STRING (https://www.string-db.org/). And the PPI network was further processed by Cytoscape software.

Elisa Assay

The expression levels of selected biomarkers were measured in plasma samples from 20 healthy controls, 45 CHB patients and 23 HBV-ACLF patients using ELISA quantitation kits (APO-CII, GP73, OPN, MMR, HPX purchased from RayBiotech; ATIII purchased from R&D systems, UK). The experimental methods were carried out according to the manufacturer's instructions.

Evaluation of the Diagnostic Accuracy

Mathematical models for separation of HBV-ACLF from CHB patients were performed on ELISA results of 6 candidate biomarkers using SPSS 19.0 software (Chicago, IL, USA). The diagnostic score of CHB patient was set as "0," while that of ALCF patient was set as "1." The forward stepwise multivariate regression analysis was conducted to determine which proteins should be included or excluded from the diagnostic model. The global performances of the model and individual biomarkers were evaluated by constructing receiver operating characteristic (ROC) curves and calculating the area under the curve (AUC) values.

Statistical Analysis

One way analysis of variance (ANOVA) and Tukey's honestly significant difference (HSD) test was performed with language R. p-value <0.05 was defined as statistically significant. Clinical chemistry data are expressed as mean ± SEM. Hierarchical clustering of proteins was performed on logarithmized data, using Euclidean distances and Ward clustering method using Package of "pheatmap" in language R. Correlation between samples was analyzed using Spearman's rank correlation coefficient.

RESULTS

Identification of Significantly Changed Proteins in CHB and HBV-ACLF Groups

In this study, plasma samples from healthy control, CHB and HBV-ACLF patients were subjected to LC-MS/MS analysis following removal of high abundance protein, FASP preparation, tryptic digestion and iTRAQ labeling. The experimental workflow is illustrated in **Figure 1**. iTRAQ 113 and 117 were used to label the mixture of all samples as a reference pool in different sets, thus allowing for cross-set comparison (Song et al., 2008).

With the false discovery rate (FDR) <1%, 397 and 396 proteins were identified in the 8-plex iTRAQ data set 1 and 2, respectively, resulting in a total of 427 proteins identified (Table S1). Of which, 364 non-redundant proteins were commonly identified across all samples by these two iTRAQ experiments. The quality of the proteomic dataset and instrumental reproducibility was evaluated. As shown in **Figure 2A**, the box plot analysis showed that the $\log_2$ protein intensity medians of all 12 pooled samples were about 1.25, almost at the same levels across all the samples, suggesting that there were no biases toward any samples. In addition, correlation analysis was performed on intensities between biological replicates inside each cohort or between different cohorts. **Figure 2B** showed that all of correlation coefficients between each two samples were higher than 0.86, demonstrating good reproducibility of biological replicates. Taken together, these results suggest that the iTRAQ-MS/MS analysis yielded a high quality reproducible dataset.

Filtering the iTRAQ data set using criteria of p-value < 0.05 and fold change >2, we identified a total of 149 significantly changed proteins through comparing each two groups. A full list of all significantly differential proteins is given in Table S2.

A heatmap analysis of 149 differential proteins using an unsupervised hierarchical clustering and correlation distance metric was generated to depict the change of expression level in different groups (**Figure 2C**). As the dendrogram indicated, CON, CHB and HBV-ACLF group samples formed three distinct clusters and the individuals within each group displayed the closest relationship.

Venn diagrams displayed unique and overlapping differential proteins in CHB and HBV-ACLF as compared to CON. As shown in **Figure 2D**, 3 overlapping differential proteins were identified by comparison of each two groups. There were 143 proteins differentially expressed between HBV-ACLF and CON, of which 42 were significantly changed when HBV-ACLF was compared to both CON and CHB. There were only 13 proteins differentially expressed between CHB and CON.

Bioinformatics Analysis of Differentially Expressed Proteins

To understand biological significance regarding to differentially expressed proteins in HBV-ACLF patients, the cellular component, molecular function and biological process of the 143 proteins were explored by Gene Ontology (GO) annotation (Table S3). In the cellular component category of GO, the most over-represented term is high-density lipoprotein particle (**Figure 3A**) and the most significant molecular function is endopeptidase inhibitor activity (**Figure 3B**). The top 3 biological processes terms were regulation of endopeptidase activity, platelet degranulation and regulation of complement activation. Other important biological processes such as regulation of fibrinolysis, complement activation, immune response and inflammatory response were also over-represented (**Figure 3C**).

To understand functional relationship among the 42 differential proteins between CHB and HBV-ACLF groups, protein protein interaction (PPI) network based on STRING action scores was illustrated. The annotations of biological processes based on GO analysis were also indicated in this view. PPI analysis showed a complex network with several distinct biological subgroups that contained highly connected proteins. As shown in **Figure 3D**, proteins involved in immune response, inflammatory response, blood coagulation and lipid metabolism were highly connected with each other, indicating that functional network of these processes contribute to

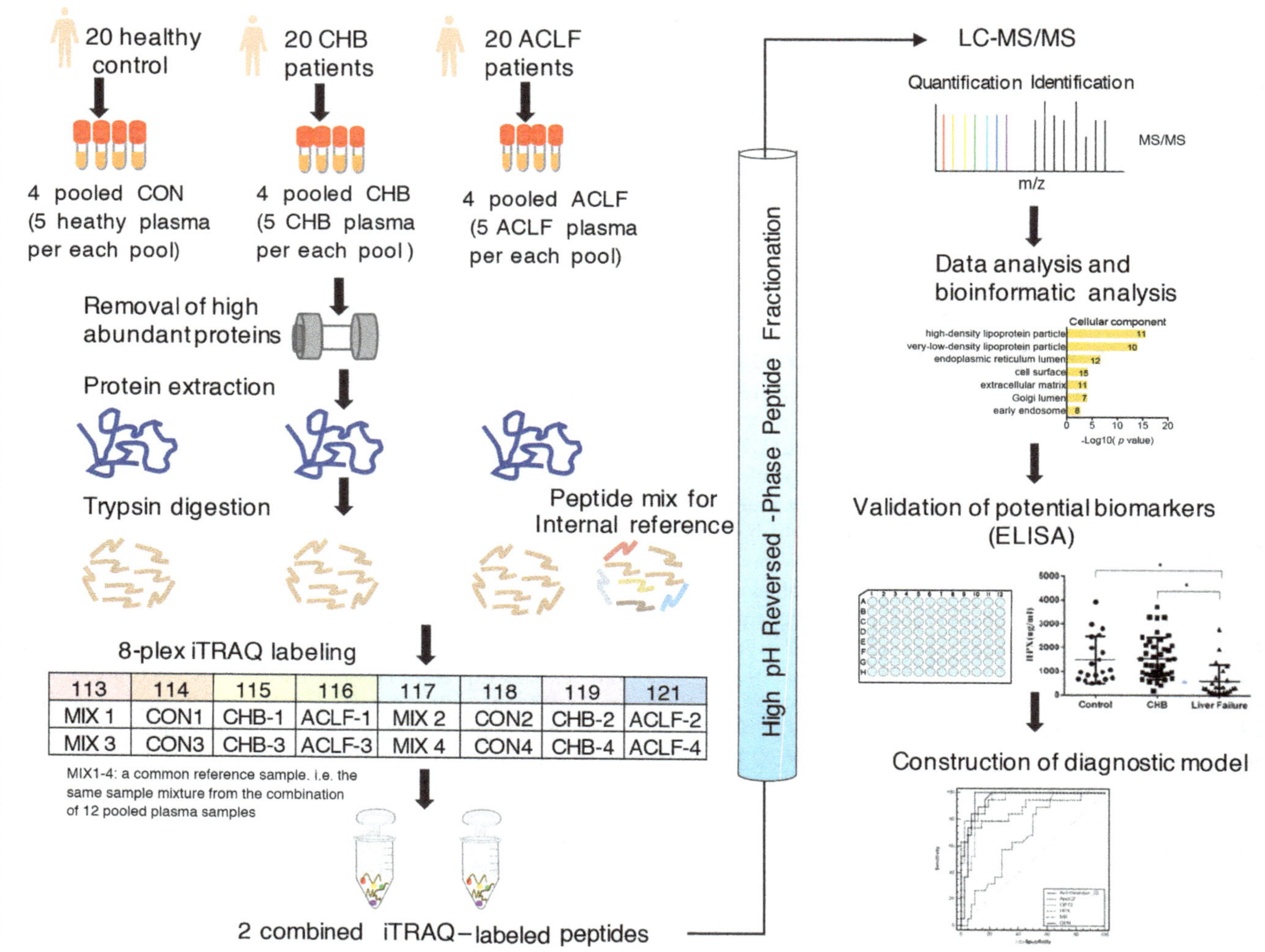

FIGURE 1 | Workflow chart of the proteomic study. Twelve pooled plasma samples (pooled from $n = 5$) from 20 healthy controls, 20 CHB patients and 20 ACLF patients were subjected to removal of high abundant proteins. Then equal amounts of proteins from each sample were digested with trypsin. Resultant peptides were processed 8-plex iTRAQ labeling, HPRP fractionation and subsequent LC-MS/MS analysis. Bioinformatics analysis was performed using Uniprot and STRING database. The plasma levels of candidate proteins were further verified by ELISA assay and diagnostic value of these biomarkers were assessed by forward stepwise logistic regression analysis and ROC curve analysis.

HBV-ACLF pathophysiology. Based on promising reports from literature, 6 proteins antithrombin-III (ATIII), mannose receptor (MMR), golgi membrane protein 1 (GP73), osteopontin (OPN), apolipoprotein CII (APO-CII), hemopexin (HPX) involved in biological processes mentioned above were selected for further verification.

Evaluation of Six Selected Proteins as Biomarker Candidates

To verify whether alterations of 6 selected candidates are reliably presented in clinical samples, we performed an ELISA assay to measure protein levels in plasma samples from healthy controls (CON, $n = 20$), CHB patients (CHB, $n = 45$), HBV-ACLF patients (ACLF, $n = 23$). The results showed significant elevation of GP73, MMR, and OPN ($p < 0.01$) and significant reduction of ATIII, HPX, APO-CII expression levels ($p < 0.01$) in the HBV-ACLF group as compared to both CHB and CON groups. In addition, significant differences in GP73 and MMR levels were also observed between the CHB and CON groups ($p < 0.01$). These results are consistent with the data obtained from the proteomic studies (**Figure 4A**).

Subsequently, the diagnostic values of 6 candidates were analyzed by forward stepwise multivariate regression. The result showed that MMR and ATIII were included in this logistic regression model as below (e is the mathematical constant and base value of natural logarithms):

$$P = \mathrm{e}^{-0.0496+0.006\mathrm{MMR}-0.176\mathrm{ATIII}}/1 + \mathrm{e}^{-0.0496+0.006\mathrm{MMR}-0.176\mathrm{ATIII}}$$

Odds ratios of MMR and ATIII in the diagnostic model were 1.006 and 0.839 respectively. Furthermore, receiver operating

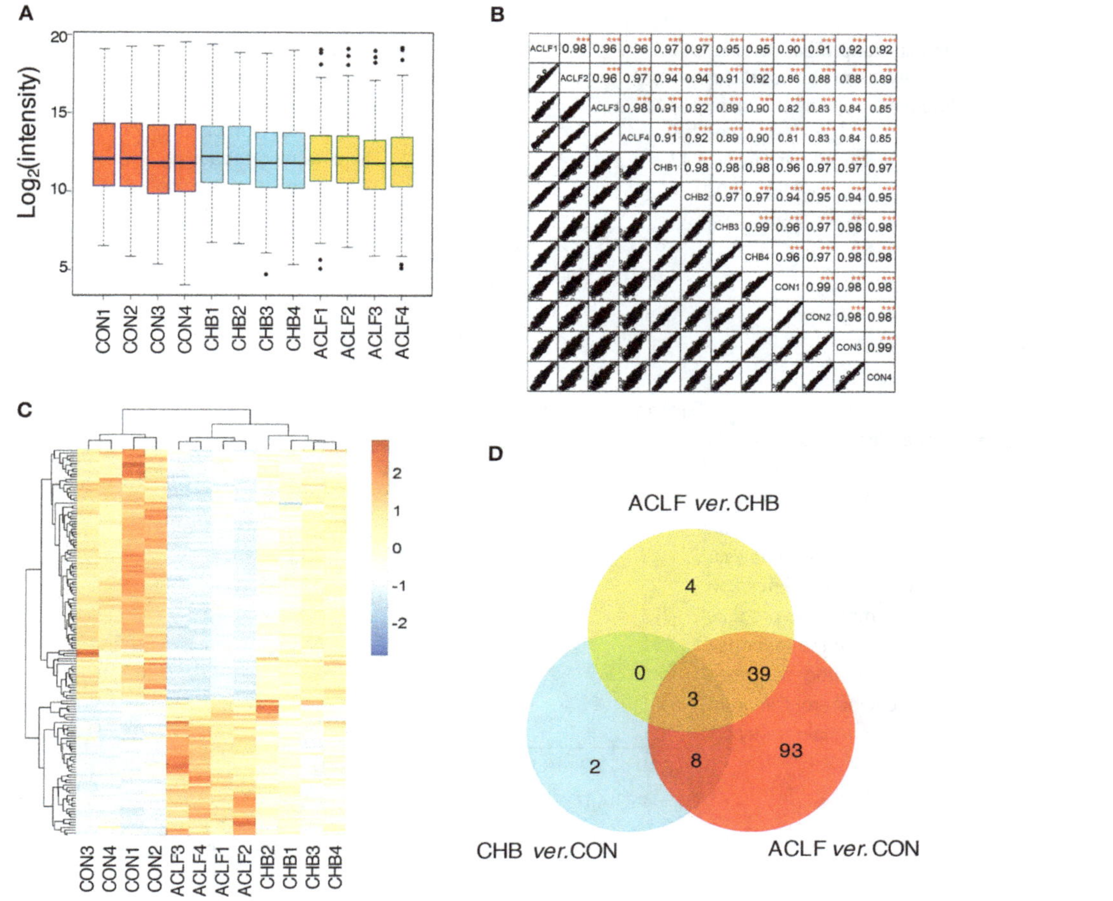

FIGURE 2 | Identification of total proteins and differentially expressed proteins. **(A)** Box plots of $\log_2$ protein intensity average for each sample. **(B)** Correlation analysis between each two samples. Rows and columns represent samples, and each square shows the correlation coefficients between two samples. $^{***}p < 0.001$ comparing intensity of each two samples. **(C)** Heatmap of the significantly changed proteins. Rows represent proteins and columns represent different samples. Color of each cell represents expression change of proteins, red is increased and blue is decreased relative to control group. **(D)** Venn diagram shows the overlap of differential proteins between comparison of each two groups.

characteristic (ROC) curve was exploited based on the results of the area under the curve (AUC), sensitivity and specificity. **Figures 4B,C** and **Table 2** showed the results of ROC analysis of individual biomarkers and the combined biomarker model for discriminating liver failure patients from CHB patients. The AUC of the combined biomarker model ATIII+MMR was 0.993, higher than any other individual biomarkers, indicating the combination of ATIII and MMR can effectively discriminate the HBV-ACLF patients from CHB patients.

DISCUSSION

To our knowledge, there are two representative ACLF definitions proposed by the Asia-Pacific Association for the Study of the Liver (APASL) and the American Association for the Study of Liver Disease and the European Association for the Study of the Liver (AASLD/EASL) (Kim and Kim, 2013). The APASL focused on the occurrence of complication such as ascites and encephalopathy within 4 weeks in patients with chronic liver disease (Sarin et al., 2009), whereas the other one emphasized the occurrence of multi-organ failure and 3 months mortality (Olson and Kamath, 2011). However, most researchers agree that the concept of ACLF should include: acute deterioration of pre-existing chronic liver disease, multi-system organ failure and with a mortality ≥15% at day 28 (Kim and Kim, 2013; Blasco-Algora et al., 2015). Unfortunately, there is a lack of biomarker highly sensitive and minimally invasive to predict ACLF in CHB patients. In this study, plasma proteome profiling of healthy controls, CHB patients and HBV-ACLF patients was established by iTRAQ-based proteomic analysis, aiming to search novel diagnostic biomarkers of HBV-ACLF. We identified 6 candidates with strong biological relevance to HBV-ACLF pathogenesis and further confirmed their change of plasma levels in 68 subjects using ELISA assay.

Demographic information exhibited that approximately 60% patients are male in either CHB or ACLF group as shown in **Table 1**. This result was consistent with the study from Rifai et al. (2012). They found that significantly more males than females

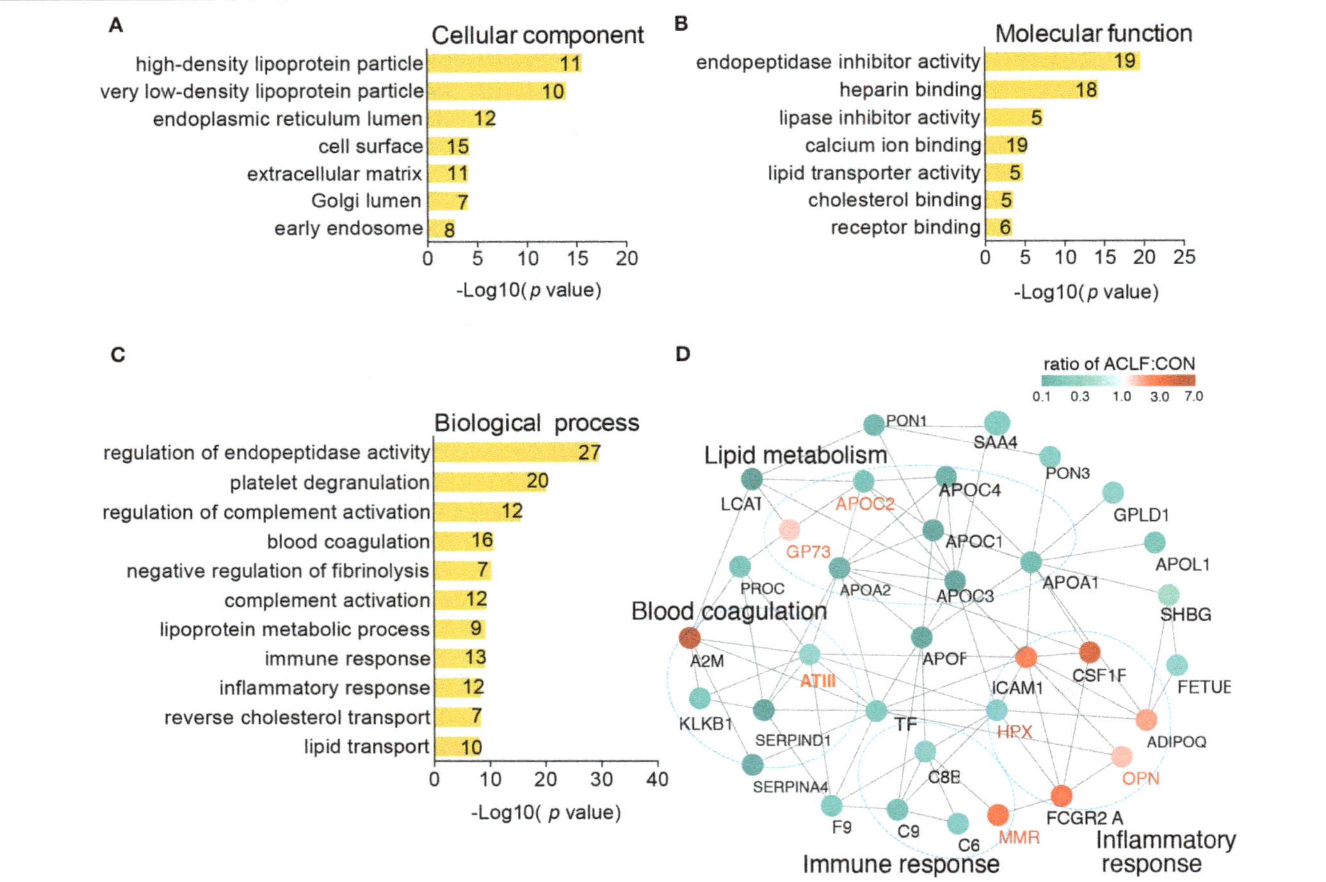

FIGURE 3 | Bioinformatics analysis of differentially expressed proteins. All of 147 proteins were functionally annotated in according to their cellular component **(A)**, molecular function **(B)**, and biological process **(C)**. The x axis represent the negative log of *p*-value. Digits mentioned inside each bar represent the number of proteins involved in each GO term. **(D)** Protein-protein interaction analysis of 42 differential proteins between CHB and HBV-ACLF using STRING database. Interactions between two proteins were indicated with gray edges. Color of node indicates fold change in ACLF. Green represents down-regulated protein and red represents up-regulated protein. Manual functional annotations based on GO analysis were shown.

underwent liver transplantation for CHB. There may be a gender difference with more men susceptible to HBV infection and developing to end-stage liver disease, which could be attribute to sex hormone effects on HBV transcription and immune response to HBV infection (Wang et al., 2015).

Individual variations among patients make a big challenge for applications of conventional proteomics. This issue has been addressed in plasma proteomic studies (Zhou et al., 2012). In the present study, particularly, each 5 plasma samples in the same group were randomly pooled to minimize the individual variations (Schisterman and Vexler, 2008). Plasma has been widely used in proteomic study for biomarker discover. However, the large dynamic range of protein concentrations in plasma samples exceeds the analytical capabilities of traditional proteomic methods, making those lower abundance plasma proteins undetectable (Pernemalm and Lehtiö, 2014). Therefore, we firstly conducted removal of high-abundance proteins (such as Albumin and IgG) using immune affinity-based depletion method to improve depth of detection in plasma sample. In doing so, a total of 427 proteins were identified across all samples. We found that more extensive molecular response was occurred in progression of ACLF (143 altered proteins as compared to healthy control) than in that of CHB (13 altered proteins as compared to healthy control).

Accurate diagnostic prediction is critical for distinguishing CHB patients who require transplantation from those who will survive following intensive medical care alone. Current Venn diagram revealed that expression of 42 proteins were changed significantly when HBV-ACLF group were compared with both healthy control and CHB groups, indicating these proteins may be helpful in identifying biomarkers for discriminating HBV-ACLF from CHB patients. Analysis of the protein-protein interaction of 42 proteins revealed that these proteins connected each other to regulate distinct biological process, including immune response, inflammatory response, blood coagulation, and lipid metabolic process.

It is well accepted that ACLF is an exaggerated systemic inflammatory response in context of immune dysregulation.

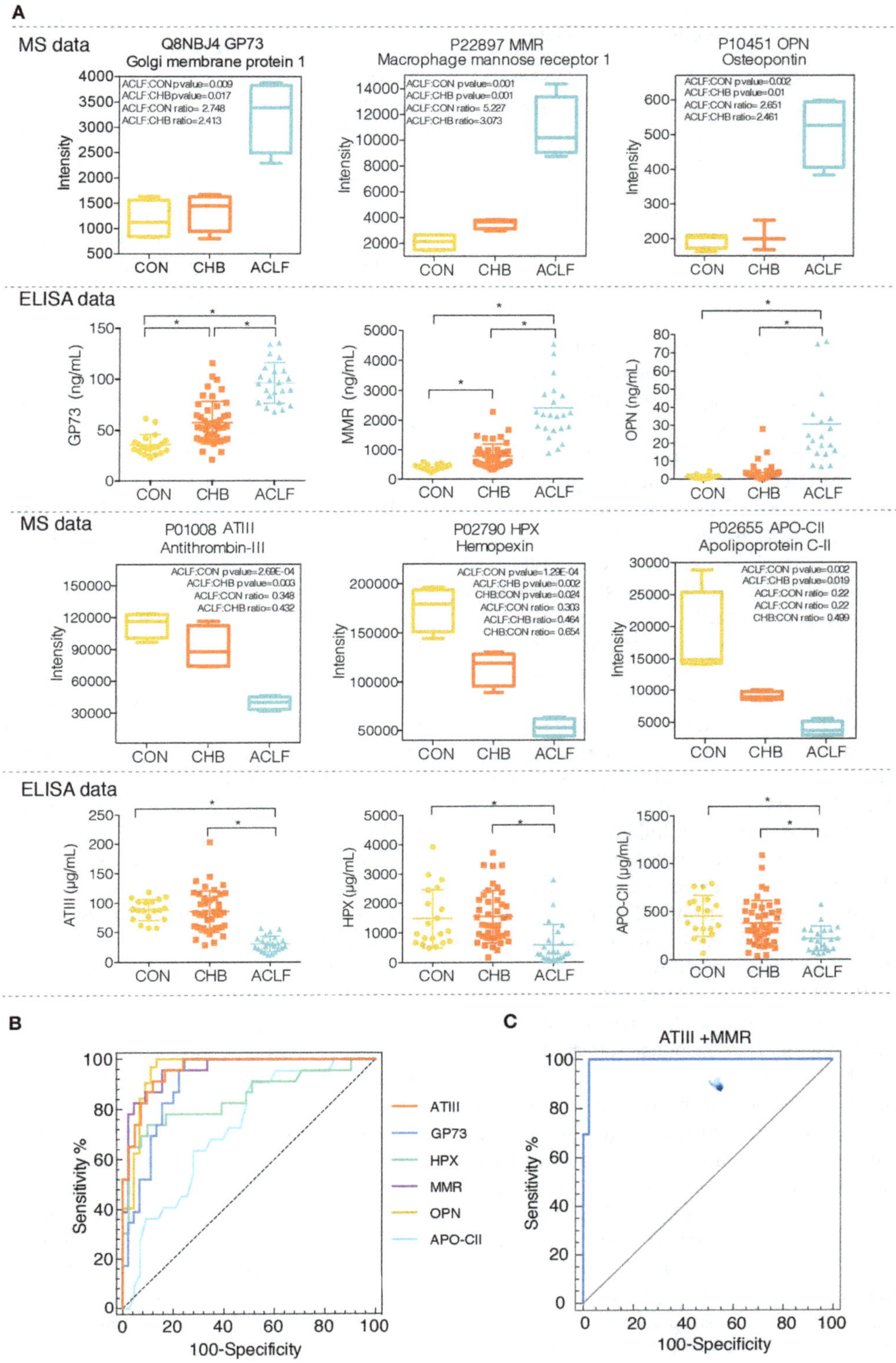

FIGURE 4 | Evaluation of plasma levels of 6 candidate proteins in healthy controls, CHB patients and HBV-ACLF patients using ELISA assay. **(A)** Plasma levels of six candidates (ATIII, HPX, APO-CII, GP73, MMR, and OPN) in different groups were analysis by ELISA assay. Median values were shown with a horizontal line. $^{*}p < 0.01$, Upper panel indicates protein intensity of each candidate obtained from iTRAQ-proteomic analysis. **(B)** ROC curve analysis of the 6 individual biomarkers. **(C)** ROC curve analysis of the combination of ATIII and MMR.

TABLE 2 | ROC analysis of individual biomarkers and combined diagnostic model.

Proteins	AUC	95% CI	Sensitivity (%)	Specificity (%)
GP73	0.91	0.81–0.96	100.00	75.56
HPX	0.86	0.75–0.93	73.91	90.91
MMR	0.96	0.88–0.99	82.61	95.56
OPN	0.96	0.87–0.99	100.00	88.64
ATIII	0.96	0.89–0.99	91.30	88.89
APO-CII	0.72	0.60–0.82	90.91	50.00
MMR+ATIII	0.99	0.93–1.00	100.00	97.78

The inflammation may also result in the unbalance of pro-thrombotic and anti-thrombotic states that may be manifested by either bleeding or thrombotic complications (Blasco-Algora et al., 2015). Since these biological processes are closely related to ACLF pathology, we considered 6 proteins (MMR, OPN, HPX, GP73, ATIII, and APO-CII) involved in these processes as potential biomarkers for diagnosis of HBV-ACLF and the clinical relevance of these proteins was further confirmed by ELISA assay. Subsequent ROC analysis indicated that these candidates, especially combination of MMR and ATIII, have good sensitivity and specificity in predicting HBV-ACLF.

Mannose receptor (MMR) locates on the surface of various cell types such as macrophages and dendritic cells (Martinez-Pomares, 2012). As a pattern recognition receptor, MMR binds and internalizes the glycoproteins from various pathogens (e.g., virus, bacteria and parasites) (Stahl and Ezekowitz, 1998), thus playing an important role in innate and adaptive immune response (Apostolopoulos and McKenzie, 2001). Another function of the MMR is to eliminate inflammatory agents released into the circulation during the inflammatory response (Lee et al., 2002). It has been reported that the concentration of soluble MMR (sMR) in serum from CHC patients with cirrhosis was higher than that with mild hepatic fibrosis patients (Andersen et al., 2014). Similarly, our study showed that levels of plasma MMR in HBV-ACLF patients were higher than CHB patients and healthy controls. It can be speculated that MMR-mediated immune and inflammatory response was dramatically triggered in context of HBV-ACLF.

Osteopontin (OPN), as a phosphorylated integrin-binding protein, has been implicated in many distinct pathophysiological processes including wound healing, bone turnover and tumorigenesis. Particularly, its roles in immune response and inflammation have been extensively studied (Rittling and Singh, 2015). OPN contributes to development of immune-mediated and inflammatory disease by promoting inflammatory cells recruitment (Apte et al., 2005), enhancing B cell proliferation (Wang and Denhardt, 2008) and suppressing apoptosis of immune cells (Denhardt et al., 2001). Several studies have shown that expression level of OPN was positively associated with CHB, CHC, alcoholic liver disease, fibrosis and HCC (Nagoshi, 2014; Fouad et al., 2015; Duarte-Salles et al., 2016). Recent studies reported remarkable elevation of serum OPN concentration in fulminant hepatic failure (FHF) patients and acute liver failure patients (Arai et al., 2006; Srungaram et al., 2015). Consistent with these findings, this study showed that level of plasma OPN was significantly elevated in HBV-ACLF groups as compared to CHB and healthy control groups, and this up-regulation of OPN may aggravate hepatic inflammation of CHB patients in progression to ACLF.

Hemopexin (HPX), as an acute phase glycoprotein, can bind heme with high affinity (Paoli et al., 1999), and the resultant Heme-HPX complex can be taken up by liver, protecting the body against free heme-induced oxidative damage (Hvidberg et al., 2005). Recent study reported anti-inflammatory function of HPX through its ability to regulate the pro-inflammatory cytokines and infiltration of Th17 cell (Liang et al., 2009). Xu et al. (2014) concluded that serum HPX concentration is negatively associated with severity of rat acute rejection after liver allograft. In addition, decrease of of HPX level was also observed in rat model of liver fibrosis induced by carbon tetrachloride (CCl_4) (Zhang et al., 2015). In present study, plasma HPX level was significantly reduced in HBV-ACLF patients compared to CHB patients and healthy controls. Low HPX level may be attribute to impaired function of hepatocyte that is principal site of HPX synthesis, and decreased HPX may further aggravate liver damage. However, the role of HPX in pathogenesis of HBV-ACLF remains elusive to contradictory results reported by Lu et al. (2010), where up-regulation of HPX level was observed in plasma sample from HBV infected patients with liver fibrosis.

Golgi membrane protein 1 (GP73), as a type II Golgi membrane protein with unknown function, mainly presents in biliary epithelial cell and is rarely expressed in normal hepatocytes (Ba et al., 2012). However, serum GP73 levels are dramatically elevated in context of various types of liver disease such as viral infection (HBV, HCV), alcohol-induced liver disease (Kladney et al., 2002), cirrhosis (Iftikhar et al., 2004), or HCC (Gao et al., 2015; Sai et al., 2015; Zhang et al., 2016). Wei et al. (2014) revealed that expression level of serum GP73 was significantly up-regulated in patient with HBV-ACLF compared to HCC patients, CHB patients, and healthy controls, supporting our present result. Biological significance of GP73 elevation requires further study.

One of the typical clinical characteristics of liver failure is coagulation dysfunction because of the dysregulated production of coagulation factors and anti-coagulation factors. Antithrombin-III (ATIII), exclusively synthesized by hepatocytes, is a natural anticoagulant that inactivates several enzymes of coagulation system (Castelino and Salem, 1997). It was reported that ATIII levels are reduced in various liver disorders, such as cirrhosis, hepatitis and the fatty liver of pregnancy (Castelino and Salem, 1997). Tischendorf et al. (2016) suggested that reduced activity of ATIII was independent predictors of hepatic encephalopathy in patients with liver cirrhosis. Evaluating 158 HCC patients subjected to hepatectomy, Mizuguchi et al. (2012) demonstrated the decrease of serum ATIII as a useful predictor for postoperative liver dysfunction post hepatectomy. Similar conclusion was also yielded by Kuroda et al. (2015). In line with these findings, plasma ATIII level was significantly reduced in HBV-ACLF patients group.

Liver is the primary site of production for apolipoproteins that is responsible for the maintenance of lipoproteins and lipid metabolism (Bell, 1979). Apolipoprotein CII (APO-CII), together with APO-CI and APO-CIII are constituents of chylomicrons, very low-density lipoprotein (VLDL), and high-density lipoprotein (HDL) in blood circulation. APO-CII regulates triglyceride metabolism through interact with lipoprotein lipase (LPL), a enzyme for hydrolysis and clearance of triglycerides from VLDL and chylomicrons (Jong et al., 1999). However, both an excess and a lack of APO-CII inhibit LPL activity and thus result in hypertriglyceridemia (Kei et al., 2012). Song et al. (2012) concluded that reduced serum APO-CII and APO-CIII were associated with aberrant biliary cycle, and considered APO-CII and APO-CIII as potential biomarker for diagnosis of biliary atresia. Trieb et al. (2016) found that decrease of serum APO-CIII level was associated with cirrhosis mortality. However, the relationship between APO-CII and liver damage such as ACLF has not been reported. Previous study has suggested that APO-CII levels would not be affected in most patients with liver disease, despite a down-regulation of APO-CIII levels (Koga et al., 1984). Our study showed that the plasma concentration of APO-CII was reduced in HBV-ACLF patients compared to both CHB patients and healthy controls, which may reflect impairment of lipid metabolism in HBV-ACLF disease.

According to the previous proteomic study reported by Peng et al. (2013), there were 16 proteins differentially expressed in CHB and ACLF patients. We did the comparison of our differentially expressed proteins with their 16 proteins, and three proteins were overlapped, including vitronectin (VTN), C-reactive protein (CRP) and platelet factor 4 (PF4). In their study, vitronectin (VTN) showed 1.23- and 2.14-fold down-regulation in CHB and ACLF patients, respectively, and this protein was also down-regulated in our dataset with the ratio of CHB/CON = 0.73 in CHB patients and the ratio of ACLF/CON = 0.48 in ACLF patients (Table S2). As a cell adhesion and spreading factor found in serum and tissues, VTN was reported that its plasma level dramatically decreased in chronic liver disease (Tomihira, 1991; Kobayashi et al., 1994). In Peng et al.'s study, pro-inflammatory protein C-reactive protein (CRP) was 2.46-fold down-regulated and 4.59-fold up-regulated in CHB and ACLF patients, respectively, and our data demonstrated that CRP was up-regulated with the ratio of CHB/CON = 1.97 in CHB patients and the ratio of ACLF/CON = 5.43 in ACLF patients. Platelet factor 4 (PF4) was down-regulated with 1.15- and 1.87-fold in CHB and ACLF patients respectively, and our data is consistent with theirs with the ratio of CHB/CON = 0.21 in CHB patients and the ratio of ACLF/CON = 0.12 in ACLF patients. Thus, the similar tendency of these three proteins between Peng et al.'s study and ours suggested that the potential clinical application of these proteins for HBV-ACLF diagnosis can be further investigated.

In summary, this study employed an iTRAQ-based quantitative proteomic approach to identify plasma biomarkers for HBV-ACLF diagnosis. Based on protein-protein interaction analysis, we focused on 6 differentially expressed proteins involved in inflammation, immune response, blood coagulation and lipid metabolism. And the following ELISA analysis of plasma samples from patient cohorts further confirmed the up-regulation of GP73, MMR, OPN and the down-regulation of ATIII, HPX, APO-CII in HBV-ACLF patients. These proteins were involved in the key pathological processes on acute occurrence of complication or multi-organ failure in the progression of ACLF. So we believed that these proteins can be considered as the potential biomarkers for HBV-ACLF diagnosis. However, more confirmatory studies are required with hope that theses candidate biomarkers can be applied to routine clinical practice.

AUTHOR CONTRIBUTIONS

NZ, KW, SF, HZ and JZ designed the experiments and wrote the manuscript. NZ, KW and SF performed the experiments with the support and help from FY and YT. NZ and XZ performed the clinic sample collection and ELISA experiments and statistical data analysis with the assistance of TH and HC. All authors critically reviewed content and approved final version for publication.

FUNDING

This work was financially supported by the Zhejiang Province Major Science and Technology Programs (No. 2012C13018-3), Zhejiang Provincial Natural Science Foundation (No. LY15H030003), National Natural Science Foundation of China (Grant No. 21375138 and 81500469) and by the Strategic Priority Research Program of the Chinese Academy of Science, "Personalized Medicines-Molecular Signature-based Drug Discovery and Development" (No. XDA12030203).

ACKNOWLEDGMENTS

We thank Dr. Jing Gao and Han He for their technical assistance. The authors declare no competing financial interest. The mass spectrometry proteomics data have been deposited to the ProteomeXchange Consortium via the PRIDE partner repository with the data set identifier PXD007975 (http://www.ebi.ac.uk/pride).

REFERENCES

Anand, A. C., and Dhiman, R. K. (2016). Acute on chronic liver failure-what is in a 'definition'? *J. Clin. Exp. Hepatol.* 6, 233–240. doi: 10.1016/j.jceh.2016.08.011

Andersen, E. S., Rødgaard-Hansen, S., Moessner, B., Christensen, P. B., Møller, H. J., and Weis, N. (2014). Macrophage-related serum biomarkers soluble CD163 (sCD163) and soluble mannose receptor (sMR) to differentiate mild liver fibrosis from cirrhosis in patients with chronic hepatitis C: a pilot study.

Eur. J. Clin. Microbiol. Infect. Dis. 33, 117–122. doi: 10.1007/s10096-013-1936-3

Apostolopoulos, V., and McKenzie, I. F. (2001). Role of the mannose receptor in the immune response. *Curr. Mol. Med.* 1, 469–474. doi: 10.2174/1566524013363645

Apte, U. M., Banerjee, A., McRee, R., Wellberg, E., and Ramaiah, S. K. (2005). Role of osteopontin in hepatic neutrophil infiltration during alcoholic steatohepatitis. *Toxicol. Appl. Pharmacol.* 207, 25–38. doi: 10.1016/j.taap.2004.12.018

Arai, M., Yokosuka, O., Kanda, T., Fukai, K., Imazeki, F., Muramatsu, M., et al. (2006). Serum osteopontin levels in patients with acute liver dysfunction. *Scand. J. Gastroenterol.* 41, 102–110. doi: 10.1080/00365520510024061

Arroyo, V., and Jalan, R. (2016). Acute-on-Chronic Liver Failure: definition, diagnosis, and clinical characteristics. *Semin. Liver Dis.* 36, 109–116. doi: 10.1055/s-0036-1583202

Ba, M. C., Long, H., Tang, Y. Q., and Cui, S. Z. (2012). GP73 expression and its significance in the diagnosis of hepatocellular carcinoma: a review. *Int. J. Clin. Exp. Pathol.* 5, 874–881.

Bell, A. W. (1979). Lipid metabolism in liver and selected tissues and in the whole body of ruminant animals. *Prog. Lipid Res.* 18, 117–164.

Bernal, W., Jalan, R., Quaglia, A., Simpson, K., Wendon, J., and Burroughs, A. (2015). Acute-on-chronic liver failure. *Lancet* 386, 1576–1587. doi: 10.1016/S0140-6736 (15)00309-8

Blasco-Algora, S., Masegosa-Ataz, J., Gutiérrez-García, M. L., Alonso-López, S., and Fernández-Rodríguez, C. M. (2015). Acute-on-chronic liver failure: pathogenesis, prognostic factors and management. *World J. Gastroenterol.* 21, 12125–12140. doi: 10.3748/wjg.v21.i42.12125

Castelino, D. J., and Salem, H. H. (1997). Natural anticoagulants and the liver. *J. Gastroenterol. Hepatol.* 12, 77–83.

Chen, E. Q., Zeng, F., Zhou, L. Y., and Tang, H. (2015). Early warning and clinical outcome prediction of acute-on-chronic hepatitis B liver failure. *World J. Gastroenterol.* 21, 11964–11973. doi: 10.3748/wjg.v21.i42.11964

Cui, Y., and Jia, J. (2013). Update on epidemiology of hepatitis B and C in China. *J. Gastroenterol. Hepatol.* 28 (Suppl. 1), 7–10. doi: 10.1111/jgh.12220

Denhardt, D. T., Noda, M., O'Regan, A. W., Pavlin, D., and Berman, J. S. (2001). Osteopontin as a means to cope with environmental insults: regulation of inflammation, tissue remodeling, and cell survival. *J. Clin. Invest.* 107, 1055–1061. doi: 10.1172/JCI12980

Duarte-Salles, T., Misra, S., Stepien, M., Plymoth, A., Muller, D., Overvad, K., et al. (2016). Circulating osteopontin and prediction of hepatocellular carcinoma development in a large european population. *Cancer Prev. Res. (Phila)* 9, 758–765. doi: 10.1158/1940-6207.CAPR-15-0434

Fouad, S. A., Mohamed, N. A., Fawzy, M. W., and Moustafa, D. A. (2015). Plasma osteopontin level in chronic liver disease and Hepatocellular Carcinoma. *Hepat. Mon.* 15:e30753. doi: 10.5812/hepatmon.30753

Gao, G., Dong, F., Xu, X., Hu, A., and Hu, Y. (2015). Diagnostic value of serum Golgi protein 73 for HBV-related primary hepatic carcinoma. *Int. J. Clin. Exp. Pathol.* 8, 11379–11385.

Geiger, T., Cox, J., Ostasiewicz, P., Wisniewski, J. R., and Mann, M. (2010). Super-SILAC mix for quantitative proteomics of human tumor tissue. *Nat. Methods* 7, 383–385. doi: 10.1038/nmeth.1446

Han, T., Liu, H., Yu, Z. L., Li, J., Wang, L., Xiao, S. X., et al. (2010). Serum peptide profiles during progression of chronic hepatitis B virus infection to liver failure. *J. Viral Hepat.* 17 (Suppl 1), 18–23. doi: 10.1111/j.1365-2893.2010.01267.x

Harel, M., Oren-Giladi, P., Kaidar-Person, O., Shaked, Y., and Geiger, T. (2015). Proteomics of microparticles with SILAC Quantification (PROMIS-Quan): a novel proteomic method for plasma biomarker quantification. *Mol. Cell. Proteomics.* 14, 1127–1136. doi: 10.1074/mcp.M114.043364

He, Q. Y., Lau, G. K., Zhou, Y., Yuen, S. T., Lin, M. C., Kung, H. F., et al. (2003). Serum biomarkers of hepatitis B virus infected liver inflammation: a proteomic study. *Proteomics* 3, 666–674. doi: 10.1002/pmic.200300394

Hvidberg, V., Maniecki, M. B., Jacobsen, C., Højrup, P., Møller, H. J., and Moestrup, S. K. (2005). Identification of the receptor scavenging hemopexin-heme complexes. *Blood* 106, 2572–2579. doi: 10.1182/blood-2005-03-1185

Iftikhar, R., Kladney, R. D., Havlioglu, N., Schmitt-Gräff, A., Gusmirovic, I., Solomon, H., et al. (2004). Disease- and cell-specific expression of GP73 in human liver disease. *Am. J. Gastroenterol.* 99, 1087–1095. doi: 10.1111/j.1572-0241.2004.30572.x

Jong, M. C., Hofker, M. H., and Havekes, L. M. (1999). Role of ApoCs in lipoprotein metabolism: functional differences between ApoC1, ApoC2, and ApoC3. *Arterioscler. Thromb. Vasc. Biol.* 19, 472–484.

Kei, A. A., Filippatos, T. D., Tsimihodimos, V., and Elisaf, M. S. (2012). A review of the role of apolipoprotein C-II in lipoprotein metabolism and cardiovascular disease. *Metabolism* 61, 906–921. doi: 10.1016/j.metabol.2011.12.002

Kim, T. Y., and Kim, D. J. (2013). Acute-on-chronic liver failure. *Clin. Mol. Hepatol.* 19, 349–359. doi: 10.3350/cmh.2013.19.4.349

Kladney, R. D., Cui, X., Bulla, G. A., Brunt, E. M., and Fimmel, C. J. (2002). Expression of GP73, a resident Golgi membrane protein, in viral and nonviral liver disease. *Hepatology* 35, 1431–1440. doi: 10.1053/jhep.2002.32525

Kobayashi, J., Yamada, S., and Kawasaki, H. (1994). Distribution of vitronectin in plasma and liver tissue: relationship to chronic liver disease. *Hepatology* 20, 1412–1417.

Koga, S., Yamamoto, K., and Ibayashi, H. (1984). Alterations in levels of apolipoprotein C-III and C-II/C-III ratios in patients with liver disease. *Gastroenterol. Jpn.* 19, 65–71.

Kuroda, S., Tashiro, H., Kobayashi, T., Hashimoto, M., Mikuriya, Y., and Ohdan, H. (2015). Administration of antithrombin III attenuates posthepatectomy liver failure in hepatocellular carcinoma. *Dig. Surg.* 32, 173–180. doi: 10.1159/000379759

Lee, S. J., Evers, S., Roeder, D., Parlow, A. F., Risteli, J., Risteli, L., et al. (2002). Mannose receptor-mediated regulation of serum glycoprotein homeostasis. *Science* 295, 1898–1901. doi: 10.1126/science.1069540

Liang, X., Lin, T., Sun, G., Beasley-Topliffe, L., Cavaillon, J. M., and Warren, H. S. (2009). Hemopexin down-regulates LPS-induced proinflammatory cytokines from macrophages. *J. Leukoc. Biol.* 86, 229–235. doi: 10.1189/jlb.1208742

Lu, Y., Liu, J., Lin, C., Wang, H., Jiang, Y., Wang, J., et al. (2010). Peroxiredoxin 2: a potential biomarker for early diagnosis of hepatitis B virus related liver fibrosis identified by proteomic analysis of the plasma. *BMC Gastroenterol.* 10:115. doi: 10.1186/1471-230X-10-115

Lv, S., Wei, L., Wang, J. H., Wang, J. Y., and Liu, F. (2007). Identification of novel molecular candidates for acute liver failure in plasma of BALB/c murine model. *J. Proteome Res.* 6, 2746–2752. doi: 10.1021/pr0701759

Marrero, J., Martinez, F. J., and Hyzy, R. (2003). Advances in critical care hepatology. *Am. J. Respir. Crit. Care Med.* 168, 1421–1426. doi: 10.1164/rccm.200303-361UP

Martinez-Pomares, L. (2012). The mannose receptor. *J. Leukoc. Biol.* 92, 1177–1186. doi: 10.1189/jlb.0512231

Mizuguchi, T., Kawamoto, M., Meguro, M., Son, S., Nakamura, Y., Harada, K., et al. (2012). Serum antithrombin III level is well correlated with multiple indicators for assessment of liver function and diagnostic accuracy for predicting postoperative liver failure in hepatocellular carcinoma patients. *Hepatogastroenterology* 59, 551–557. doi: 10.5754/hge10052

Nagoshi, S. (2014). Osteopontin: versatile modulator of liver diseases. *Hepatol. Res.* 44, 22–30. doi: 10.1111/hepr.12166

Niu, D., Feng, H., and Chen, W. N. (2010). Proteomic analysis of HBV-associated HCC: insights on mechanisms of disease onset and biomarker discovery. *J. Proteomics* 73, 1283–1290. doi: 10.1016/j.jprot.2010.02.016

Olson, J. C., and Kamath, P. S. (2011). Acute-on-chronic liver failure: concept, natural history, and prognosis. *Curr. Opin. Crit. Care* 17, 165–169. doi: 10.1097/MCC. 0b013e328344b42d

Paoli, M., Anderson, B. F., Baker, H. M., Morgan, W. T., Smith, A., and Baker, E. N. (1999). Crystal structure of hemopexin reveals a novel high-affinity heme site formed between two beta-propeller domains. *Nat. Struct. Biol.* 6, 926–931. doi: 10.1038/13294

Peng, L., Liu, J., Li, Y. M., Huang, Z. L., Wang, P. P., Gu, Y. R., et al. (2013). Serum proteomics analysis and comparisons using iTRAQ in the progression of hepatitis B. *Exp. Ther. Med.* 6, 1169–1176. doi: 10.3892/etm.2013.1310

Pernemalm, M., and Lehtiö, J. (2014). Mass spectrometry-based plasma proteomics: state of the art and future outlook. *Expert Rev. Proteomics* 11, 431–448. doi: 10.1586/14789450.2014.901157

Pierce, A., Unwin, R. D., Evans, C. A., Griffiths, S., Carney, L., Zhang, L., et al. (2008). Eight-channel iTRAQ enables comparison of the activity of six leukemogenic tyrosine kinases. *Mol. Cell. Proteomics* 7, 853–863. doi: 10.1074/mcp.M700251-MCP200

Ren, F., Chen, Y., Wang, Y., Yan, Y., Zhao, J., Ding, M., et al. (2010). Comparative serum proteomic analysis of patients with acute-on-chronic liver failure: alpha-1-acid glycoprotein maybe a candidate marker for prognosis of hepatitis B virus infection. *J. Viral Hepat.* 17, 816–824. doi: 10.1111/j.1365-2893.2009. 01242.x

Rifai, K., Hadem, J., Wiegand, J., Potthoff, A., Pischke, S., Klempnauer, J., et al. (2012). Gender differences in patient receiving liver transplantation for viral hepatitis. *Z. Gastroenterol.* 50, 760–765. doi: 10.1055/s-0031-1281631

Rittling, S. R., and Singh, R. (2015). Osteopontin in immune-mediated diseases. *J. Dent. Res.* 94, 1638–1645. doi: 10.1177/0022034515605270

Sai, W., Wang, L., Zheng, W., Yang, J., Pan, L., Cai, Y., et al. (2015). Abnormal expression of Golgi Protein 73 in clinical values and their role in HBV-Related hepatocellular carcinoma diagnosis and prognosis. *Hepat. Mon.* 15:e32918. doi: 10.5812/hepatmon.32918

Sarin, S. K., Kumar, A., Almeida, J. A., Chawla, Y. K., Fan, S. T., Garg, H., et al. (2009). Acute-on-chronic liver failure: consensus recommendations of the Asian Pacific Association for the study of the liver (APASL). *Hepatol. Int.* 3, 269–282. doi: 10.1007/s12072-008-9106-x

Schisterman, E. F., and Vexler, A. (2008). To pool or not to pool, from whether to when: applications of pooling to biospecimens subject to a limit of detection. *Paediatr. Perinat. Epidemiol.* 22, 486–496. doi: 10.1111/j.1365-3016.2008. 00956.x

Song, X., Bandow, J., Sherman, J., Baker, J. D., Brown, P. W., McDowell, M. T., et al. (2008). iTRAQ experimental design for plasma biomarker discovery. *J. Proteome Res.* 7, 2952–2958. doi: 10.1021/pr800072x

Song, Z., Dong, R., Fan, Y., and Zheng, S. (2012). Identification of serum protein biomarkers in biliary atresia by mass spectrometry and enzyme-linked immunosorbent assay. *J. Pediatr. Gastroenterol. Nutr.* 55, 370–375. doi: 10.1097/MPG.0b013e31825bb01a

Srungaram, P., Rule, J. A., Yuan, H. J., Reimold, A., Dahl, B., Sanders, C., et al. (2015). Plasma osteopontin in acute liver failure. *Cytokine* 73, 270–276. doi: 10.1016/j.cyto.2015.02.021

Stahl, P. D., and Ezekowitz, R. A. (1998). The mannose receptor is a pattern recognition receptor involved in host defense. *Curr. Opin. Immunol.* 10, 50–55.

Tischendorf, M., Miesbach, W., Chattah, U., Chattah, Z., Maier, S., Welsch, C., et al. (2016). Differential kinetics of coagulation factors and natural anticoagulants in patients with liver cirrhosis: potential clinical implications. *PLoS ONE* 11:e0155337. doi: 10.1371/journal.pone.0155337

Tomihira, M. (1991). Changes in plasma vitronectin, fibronectin, and serum laminin P1 levels and immunohistochemical study of vitronectin in the liver of patients with chronic liver diseases. *Fukuoka Igaku Zasshi* 82, 21–30.

Trieb, M., Horvath, A., Birner-Gruenberger, R., Spindelboeck, W., Stadlbauer, V., Taschler, U., et al. (2016). Liver disease alters high-density lipoprotein composition, metabolism and function. *Biochim. Biophys. Acta.* 1861, 630–638. doi: 10.1016/j.bbalip.2016.04.013

Wan, Z., Wu, Y., Yi, J., You, S., Liu, H., Sun, Z., et al. (2015). Combining serum cystatin C with total bilirubin improves shot-term mortality prediction in patients with HBV-related acute-on-chronic liver failure. *PLoS ONE* 10, 1–14. doi: 10.1371/journal.pone.0116968

Wang, K. X., and Denhardt, D. T. (2008). Osteopontin: role in immune regulation and stress responses. *Cytokine Growth Factor Rev.* 19, 333–345. doi: 10.1016/j.cytogfr.2008.08.001

Wang, S. H., Chen, P. J., and Yeh, S. H. (2015). Gender disparity in chronic hepatitis B: mechanisms of sex hormones. *J. Gastroenterol. Hepatol.* 30, 1237–1245. doi: 10.1111/jgh.12934

Wang, Y., Yang, F., Gritsenko, M. A., Wang, Y., Clauss, T., Liu, T., et al. (2011). Reversed-phase chromatography with multiple fraction concatenation strategy for proteome profiling of human MCF10A cells. *Proteomics* 11, 2019–2026. doi: 10.1002/pmic.201000722

Wei, H., Zhang, J., Li, H., Ren, H., Hao, X., and Huang, Y. (2014). GP73, a new marker for diagnosing HBV-ACLF in population with chronic HBV infections. *Diagn. Microbiol. Infect. Dis.* 79, 19–24. doi: 10.1016/j.diagmicrobio.2014.01.008

Wiśniewski, J. R., Nagaraj, N., Zougman, A., Gnad, F., and Mann, M. (2010). Brain phosphoproteome obtained by a FASP-based method reveals plasma membrane protein topology. *J. Proteome Res.* 9, 3280–3289. doi: 10.1021/pr1002214

Xu, M., Tan, C., Hu, J., Alwahsh, S. M., Yan, J., Hu, J., et al. (2014). Expression of hemopexin in acute rejection of rat liver allograft identified by serum proteomic analysis. *Shock* 42, 65–74. doi: 10.1097/SHK.00000000000 00171

Yang, L., Rudser, K. D., Higgins, L., Rosen, H. R., Zaman, A., Corless, C. L., et al. (2011). Novel biomarker candidates to predict hepatic fibrosis in hepatitis C identified by serum proteomics. *Dig. Dis. Sci.* 56, 3305–3315. doi: 10.1007/s10620-011-1745-4

Zamora Nava, L. E., Aguirre Valadez, J., Chávez-Tapia, N. C., and Torre, A. (2014). Acute-on-chronic liver failure: a review. *Ther. Clin. Risk Manag.* 10, 295–303. doi: 10.2147/TCRM.S59723

Zhang, X., Xu, L., Yin, L., Qi, Y., Xu, Y., Han, X., et al. (2015). Quantitative chemical proteomics for investigating the biomarkers of dioscin against liver fibrosis caused by CCl4 in rats. *Chem. Commun. (Camb)* 51, 11064-7. doi: 10.1039/c4cc09160d

Zhang, Y., Xi, Y., Fang, J., Luo, S., Wilson, J. J., and Huang, R. P. (2016). Identification and characterization of monoclonal antibodies against GP73 for use as a potential biomarker in liver cancer screening and diagnosis. *J. Immunoassay Immunochem.* 37, 390–406. doi: 10.1080/15321819.2016.1154866

Zhou, C., Simpson, K. L., Lancashire, L. J., Walker, M. J., Dawson, M. J., Unwin, R. D., et al. (2012). Statistical considerations of optimal study design for human plasma proteomics and biomarker discovery. *J. Proteome Res.* 11, 2103–2113. doi: 10.1021/pr200636x

6

IL-1β and TNFα Differentially Influence NF-κB Activity and FasL-Induced Apoptosis in Primary Murine Hepatocytes During LPS-Induced Inflammation

Julia Rex[1*], *Anna Lutz*[2], *Laura E. Faletti*[3], *Ute Albrecht*[4], *Maria Thomas*[5], *Johannes G. Bode*[4], *Christoph Borner*[2,6,7], *Oliver Sawodny*[1] *and Irmgard Merfort*[2,6]

[1] *Institute for System Dynamics, University of Stuttgart, Stuttgart, Germany,* [2] *Department of Pharmaceutical Biology and Biotechnology, Albert Ludwigs University Freiburg, Freiburg, Germany,* [3] *Institute of Molecular Medicine and Cell Research, Albert Ludwigs University Freiburg, Freiburg, Germany,* [4] *Clinic of Gastroenterology, Hepatology and Infection Diseases, Heinrich-Heine-University, Duesseldorf, Germany,* [5] *Dr. Margarete Fischer-Bosch Institute of Clinical Pharmacology, Stuttgart and University of Tuebingen, Tuebingen, Germany,* [6] *Spemann Graduate School of Biology and Medicine, Albert Ludwigs University Freiburg, Freiburg, Germany,* [7] *BIOSS Centre for Biological Signaling Studies, Albert Ludwigs University Freiburg, Freiburg, Germany*

Correspondence:
Julia Rex
julia.rex@isys.uni-stuttgart.de

Macrophage-derived cytokines largely influence the behavior of hepatocytes during an inflammatory response. We previously reported that both TNFα and IL-1β, which are released by macrophages upon LPS stimulation, affect Fas ligand (FasL)-induced apoptotic signaling. Whereas TNFα preincubation leads to elevated levels of caspase-3 activity and cell death, pretreatment with IL-1β induces increased caspase-3 activity but keeps cells alive. We now report that IL-1β and TNFα differentially influence NF-κB activity resulting in a differential upregulation of target genes, which may contribute to the distinct effects on cell viability. A reduced NF-κB activation model was established to further investigate the molecular mechanisms which determine the distinct cell fate decisions after IL-1β and TNFα stimulation. To study this aspect in a more physiological setting, we used supernatants from LPS-stimulated bone marrow-derived macrophages (BMDMs). The treatment of hepatocytes with the BMDM supernatant, which contains both IL-1β and TNFα, sensitized to FasL-induced caspase-3 activation and cell death. However, when TNFα action was blocked by neutralizing antibodies, cell viability after stimulation with the BMDM supernatant and FasL increased as compared to single FasL stimulation. This indicates the important role of TNFα in the sensitization of apoptosis in hepatocytes. These results give first insights into the complex interplay between macrophages and hepatocytes which may influence life/death decisions of hepatocytes during an inflammatory reaction of the liver in response to a bacterial infection.

Keywords: primary murine hepatocytes, macrophages, signaling, apoptosis, LPS-induced inflammation

1. INTRODUCTION

Liver diseases represent a major burden on health care in the European Union. Approximately 29 million people suffer from chronic liver diseases. The end-stage, liver cirrhosis with organ transplantation as single treatment option, accounts for 170,000 deaths per year (Blachier et al., 2013). Pathogenesis of most liver diseases is associated with sustained inflammation, causing enhanced cell death of hepatocytes and, finally, leading to chronic liver diseases (Malhi and Gores, 2008). Alcohol consumption, for example, increases permeability of the intestinal epithelial barrier resulting in the translocation of bacterial products such as lipopolysaccharide (LPS) from the intestinal lumen to surrounding lymph nodes and the liver. In the liver, LPS leads to the activation of Kupffer cells, the liver resident macrophages, via stimulation of the Toll-like receptor 4 (TLR4) and the induction of an inflammatory response contributing to the progression of alcoholic liver disease (Seki and Schnabl, 2012). Among many cytokines and chemokines, interleukin 1 beta (IL-1β) and tumor necrosis factor alpha (TNFα) are the most prominent pro-inflammatory cytokines released by LPS-activated macrophages (Tacke et al., 2009; Bode et al., 2012; Rex et al., 2016). Moreover, they have both been reported to exert cell death protective and promoting effects dependent on the cell type and the environmental conditions (Takehara et al., 1999; Malhi and Gores, 2008; Verma and Datta, 2010; Szabo and Csak, 2012). This is why we concentrated our work on these two cytokines.

As previously reported, TNFα sensitizes primary murine hepatocytes to Fas ligand (FasL)-induced caspase-3/7 activation and apoptosis (Schmich et al., 2011). Normally, TNFα signaling does not lead to cell death in hepatocytes (Varfolomeev and Ashkenazi, 2004) due to the inhibition of the caspase-8 containing TNF receptor complex II by the FADD-like apoptosis regulator (c-FLIP) as well as the induction of pro-survival pathways by activation of the transcription factor NF-κB (Irmler et al., 1997; Karin and Lin, 2002). Under certain circumstances, such as low c-FLIP levels or blockage of the NF-κB signaling pathway, TNFα can however trigger apoptotic signaling via caspase-8 activation in complex II (Micheau and Tschopp, 2003). TNFα also activates the c-Jun N-terminal kinase (JNK1/2) leading to the phosphorylation of the apoptosis facilitator Bim that is subsequently sequestered by the anti-apoptotic B cell leukemia/lymphoma 2 (Bcl-2) protein (Schmich et al., 2011; Geissler et al., 2013). Stimulation with FasL and generation of the truncated version of the BH3 interacting domain death agonist (tBid) by activated caspase-8 additionally depletes the anti-apoptotic Bcl-2 pool rendering hepatocytes more susceptible to caspase-3/7 activation and cell death (Schlatter et al., 2011; Schmich et al., 2011). In contrast to TNFα, IL-1β has been reported to protect mice from FasL-induced apoptosis (Takehara et al., 1999). We observed that IL-1β sensitizes hepatocytes to FasL-induced caspase-3/7 activation in a JNK/Bim- and Bid-dependent manner comparable to TNFα, but partially protects from cell death (Lutz et al., 2014). Surprisingly, increased caspase-3/7 activity after IL-1β and FasL stimulation did not result in the cleavage of the poly (ADP-ribose) polymerase (PARP) explaining why the cells did not die. The protection from FasL-induced cell death was associated with increased NF-κB DNA binding and the transcriptional upregulation of the caspase-8 inhibitor A20. The seemingly contradictious occurrence of increased caspase-3/7 activity and cell viability was further investigated by mathematical modeling, which revealed different hepatocyte subpopulations. While a fraction of cells survived the IL-1β/FasL co-treatment, others died via the type I or the type II apoptosis signaling pathway. This was dependent on a heterogeneous distribution of Bcl-2 proteins and variations in Fas signaling among the cell population. Therefore, IL-1β exerts two effects on the life-death balance in hepatocytes: It shifts hepatocytes to a mitochondrial type II apoptosis and increased caspase-3/7 activity following Fas activation and it activates NF-κB and induces upregulation of anti-apoptotic proteins, such as A20 that negatively regulates caspase-8 activation. Obviously, in the end more cells are able to escape apoptosis induction following IL-1β and FasL stimulation as compared to FasL alone.

NF-κB dimers are held inactive in the cytosol by binding to their inhibitors, the IκB proteins. Stimulation with either IL-1β or TNFα activates the IκB kinase (IKK) complex which then mediates phosphorylation, ubiquitination and degradation of IκBs allowing translocation of the free NF-κB dimer into the nucleus to initiate transcription (Karin and Ben-Neriah, 2000). The most prominent NF-κB dimer is the heterodimer containing the p50 and p65 subunits (Wang and Baldwin, 1998; Tak and Firestein, 2001) and we refer to this dimer whenever stating NF-κB hereafter. NF-κB induces transcription of a variety of target genes involved in inflammatory responses and cell survival (Baltimore, 2011). Furthermore, NF-κB induces the expression of its own inhibitor IκBα which then binds to NF-κB dimers and triggers translocation into the cytosol (Sun et al., 1993). This time delayed autoregulatory negative feedback loop causes the observed oscillatory behavior of NF-κB activation (Nelson et al., 2004; Covert et al., 2005).

FasL binds to its cognate receptor Fas/CD95 which is constitutively expressed on the cell surface of hepatocytes and induces the apoptotic pathway (Galle et al., 1995). Receptor activation leads to the formation of the death inducing signaling complex (DISC) and activation of caspase-8 (Hughes et al., 2009; Kallenberger et al., 2014). Processed caspase-8 can either directly activate the effector caspase-3 (type I pathway) or process Bid into its truncated version tBid which induces mitochondrial outer membrane permeabilization (MOMP) and release of pro-apoptotic factors such as cytochrome c and Smac/DIABLO into the cytosol (type II pathway) (Scaffidi et al., 1998; Krammer, 2000). Cytochrome c release induces formation of the apoptosome leading to activation of caspase-9 that can further process procaspase-3 (Zou et al., 1999). Smac/DIABLO inhibits the anti-apoptotic X-linked inhibitor of apoptosis protein (XIAP) that is an inhibitor of caspase-3 and caspase-9 (Verhagen et al., 2000). Thus, the release of pro-apoptotic factors from mitochondria leads to increased caspase-3 activity. FasL has been suggested to mediate hepatic cell death in experimental models of hepatitis (Galle et al., 1995; Streetz et al., 2000) and blocking FasL signaling pathways indeed ameliorates liver disease to various degrees (Kondo et al., 1997; Ksontini et al., 1998). FasL is primarily expressed on activated T lymphocytes as well as on natural killer (NK) cells (Arase et al., 1995; Suda et al., 1995) and upregulation is associated with pathogenesis of liver diseases such as viral hepatitis or alcoholic cirrhosis (Galle et al., 1995). However, the source of FasL during hepatic injury remains unclear and seems to depend on the experimental models used. Natural killer T (NKT) cells were previously reported to be key effector cells in Concanavalin A-mediated liver damage. Unlike NK cells that kill target cells by releasing TRAIL and granzyme B, NKT cells kill hepatocytes by expressing and/or releasing FasL in this model (Takeda et al., 2000). Other studies using α-galactosylceramide (α-GalCer)-induced liver injury as a murine model for autoimmune hepatitis showed that TNFα is involved in α-GalCer-induced upregulation of FasL on NKT cells (Biburger and Tiegs, 2005). In other scenarios, FasL expression was also attributed to macrophages or hepatocytes (Tsutsui et al., 1996; Luo et al., 1997; Mita et al., 2005).

In this study, we analyzed the influence of supernatant from LPS-treated bone marrow-derived macrophages (BMDMs) on FasL-induced apoptosis or survival of primary mouse hepatocytes under more physiological conditions. We show that TNFα mediates the apoptosis sensitization effect of the supernatant while IL-1β is more death protective. This is partly due to the fact that IL-1β and TNFα activate NF-κB differently. Surprisingly, the supernatant from unstimulated BMDMs protects from FasL-induced caspase-3/7 activation.

2. RESULTS

2.1. IL-1β and TNFα Differentially Influence NF-κB Target Gene Expression

As previously reported, both IL-1β and TNFα sensitized primary murine hepatocytes to FasL-induced caspase-3/7 activation (Schlatter et al., 2011; Schmich et al., 2011; Lutz et al., 2014). However, while TNFα triggered increased apoptosis (Schmich et al., 2011), IL-1β partially protected from FasL-induced death, possibly via a NF-κB-dependent upregulation of survival factors such as A20, an inhibitor of caspase-8 activation (Daniel et al., 2004; Lutz et al., 2014). To uncover differences in NF-κB activity and induction of respective target genes that may be responsible for the distinct effects of these cytokines on cell viability, the mRNA levels of 46 genes involved in apoptotic and inflammatory processes were measured. For that purpose, primary murine hepatocytes were treated with IL-1β or TNFα for 1, 4, 6, 18, and 30 h and mRNA levels were determined using the high-throughput Taqman® Fluidigm Technology. Data were analyzed using the ddCT method (Livak and Schmittgen, 2001), normalized to untreated controls and results are displayed in a heat map (**Figure 1**).

The expression pattern following stimulation with either IL-1β or TNFα appeared rather similar. mRNA of the chemokine ligand *Cxcl2* and the receptor-interacting serine-threonine kinase *Ripk2* showed the strongest upregulation. Genes involved in the NF-κB signaling pathway, i.e., the NF-κB inhibitors *IκBα* (also named *Nfkbia*) and *IκBζ* (also named *Nfkbiz*), as well as the zinc finger protein *A20*, were highly upregulated after both stimuli, whereas the Bcl-2 family members *Bcl2A1* and *Bid*, as well as *Fas* and the cellular inhibitor of apoptosis proteins 1 and 2 (*cIAP1/2*) were increased to a lesser extent. Despite an apparently similar expression pattern after both treatments, we noted some important differences. The induction of several genes such as *A20*, *COX2*, *IκBα/Nfkbia*, and *IκBζ/Nfkbiz* during the first hour of stimulation as well as their oscillations thereafter were more pronounced for IL-1β as compared to TNFα (**Figure 2**). The expression of *IκBζ* was even 62 times higher after IL-1β as compared to an upregulation of only 2.7 fold after TNFα stimulation. The Bcl-2 family members *Bcl-2*, *Bmf*, and *BclxL* showed the strongest downregulation after IL-1β and TNFα stimulation. Fas ligand (FasL) was not expressed at all time points after both stimuli.

2.2. Model-Based Investigation of NF-κB Dynamics and Cell Fate Following IL-1β and TNFα Stimulation

The dynamics of NF-κB have not yet been investigated in detail, although a NF-κB module has been part of our previously published models for the IL-1β/FasL (Lutz et al., 2014) and TNFα/FasL (Schlatter et al., 2011) sensitization regimens. The NF-κB model originally described by Lipniacki et al. (2004) has been integrated in our models to allow description of cytokine-mediated transcriptional effects on the FasL-induced apoptotic pathway. But the model is rather comprehensive with 14 species and 26 parameters and extensively describes the induced signaling events and complex formation between IKK, IκBα and/or NF-κB. However, for the observed effects within this study, mainly the dynamics of NF-κB activity and longer-term upregulation of NF-κB target genes are decisive. We therefore reduced the model to 8 states and 10 parameters, as described in detail in the **Supplementary Material** (**Presentation 1**). The reduced model (**Figure 3A**) still shows a comparable behavior to the original model regarding the aforementioned aspects (**Figure 3B**). Investigations revealed that a change of parameters influencing the activation of NF-κB, i.e., the parameters for the activation and deactivation of IKK (k_1, k_2), for A20 synthesis (k_{smrna2}, k_8) or for direct NF-κB activation (k_3) mainly influence the amplitude of the first peak of NF-κB activity. By contrast, changing the parameters of the reactions which deactivate NF-κB, i.e., complex formation of NF-κB and IκBα (k_4) or degradation of IκBα (k_{d5}), mainly affected the frequency of NF-κB activity (**Figure S1**). Especially the alteration of more than one parameter such as one for activation and one for deactivation of NF-κB, e.g., k_3 and k_4, resulted in a more pronounced oscillatory behavior of NF-κB in response to IL-1β. Indeed, as mentioned above, *A20* mRNA is more upregulated after IL-1β than after TNFα. This difference was already confirmed on the protein level in the preceding study (Lutz et al., 2014). Accordingly, a 5-fold increase of the parameters k_3 and k_4 in combination with an increase of the mRNA synthesis rate of *A20* (k_{smrna2}) and a 2-fold reduction of the A20 protein degradation rate (k_{d8}) may well explain the different biological responses after IL-1β and TNFα stimulation. All other parameter values were identical for both

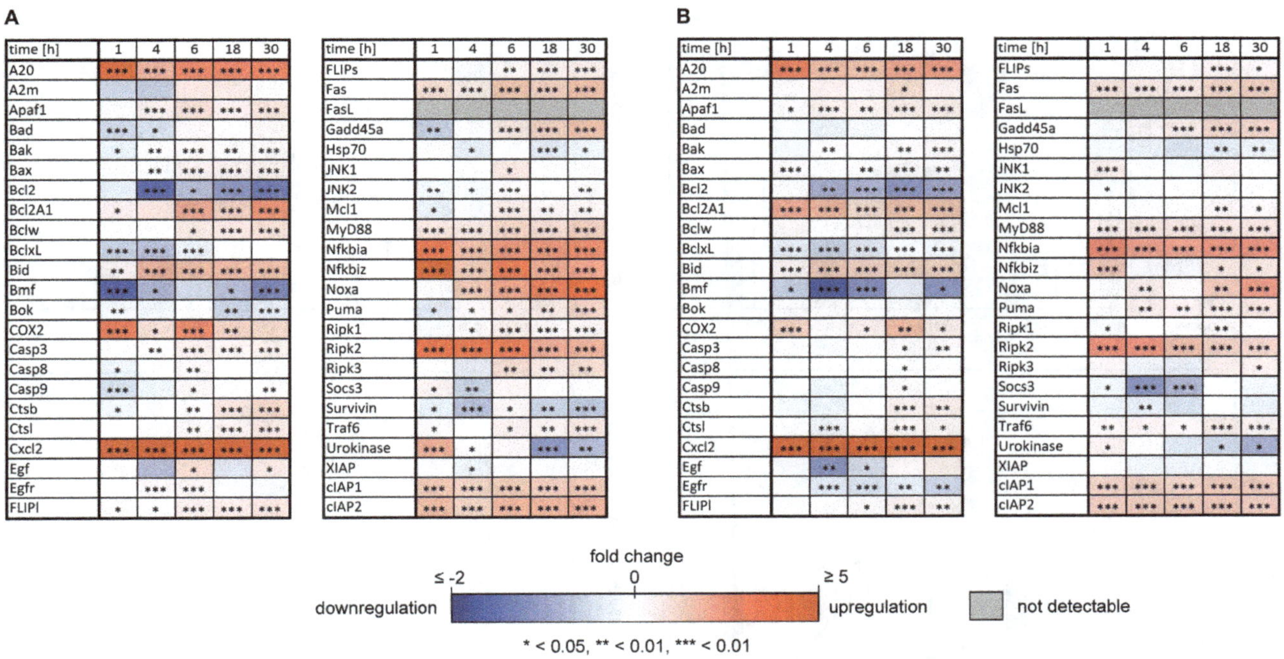

FIGURE 1 | Changes of mRNAs of apoptotic and inflammatory genes after IL-1β or TNFα stimulation of hepatocytes. Gene expression pattern of primary murine hepatocytes stimulated with **(A)** IL-1β (20 ng/ml) and **(B)** TNFα (25 ng/ml) for 1, 4, 6, 18, and 30 h measured via the high-throughput Taqman® Fluidigm system. Data are analyzed using the ddCT method, normalized to untreated controls and represent 4 independent experiments. Genes marked in red and blue represent upregulated and downregulated genes, respectively ($^{*}p < 0.05$, $^{**}p < 0.01$, $^{***}p < 0.001$).

treatments. The parameter values are given in **Table S1** and the simulated time courses of NF-κB and its target genes as well as A20 are presented in **Figure 4**, time courses of all species are shown in **Figure S2**.

The reduced NF-κB module was implemented and the influence of increased A20 expression following IL-1β stimulation on cell fate decisions was investigated. As reported earlier (Lutz et al., 2014), a cell population does not respond homogeneously to cell death stimuli; some cells die, others can escape apoptosis induction. This could result from differences in gene expression levels among different cells. In agreement with our earlier studies, we analyzed two key molecules in the apoptotic pathway and how they influence cell fate: Fas as a representative of the death-receptor signaling pathway and Bcl-2 as a representative of the mitochondrial pathway. We analyzed the influence of small differences in protein expression by varying the initial conditions of these proteins for the simulations by 10%. The majority of cells died via the type I apoptotic pathway following FasL stimulation, but a few with high levels of Fas and low Bcl-2 expression used type II apoptosis signaling (**Figure 5A**). By contrast, those with low amounts of Fas survived the treatment as reported previously (Lutz et al., 2014). When IL-1β and FasL were combined two distinct effects were observed (**Figure 5B**). On the one hand, the preincubation with IL-1β depletes the anti-apoptotic pool of Bcl-2 proteins, rendering cells more susceptible to type II apoptotic signaling leading to MOMP. On the other hand, IL-1β induced NF-κB activation mediating pro-survival effects. When considering the upregulation of A20 which interfered with caspase-8 activation at the DISC, the IL-1β-induced protective effect (**Figure 5B**, light blue fraction) becomes more pronounced as compared to our previous studies (Lutz et al., 2014). In contrast, preincubation with TNFα not only favors MOMP via depletion of Bcl-2, but also directly activates caspase-8. Since A20 is less upregulated in this case, the cells treated with TNFα all die via type II apoptosis (**Figure 5C**).

2.3. Supernatant From LPS-Stimulated Macrophages Sensitizes Hepatocytes to FasL-Induced Apoptosis

To study the differential sensitization effects of IL-1β and TNFα on FasL-induced apoptosis in a more physiological setting, the influence of supernatants from murine BMDMs stimulated with 100 ng/ml LPS for 24 h on apoptotic signaling in hepatocytes was investigated. Primary murine hepatocytes were cultured on collagen and, after starvation, incubated for 4 h with the same DMEM medium that was also used for BMDMs. Then, hepatocytes were preincubated with BMDM-derived supernatant conditioned with or without LPS for 12 h followed by incubation with 50 ng/ml FasL for further 6 h. Similar to the sensitizing effect of the single cytokines, a significant increase in caspase-3/7 activity (**Figure 6A**) and cell death (**Figure 6B**) was

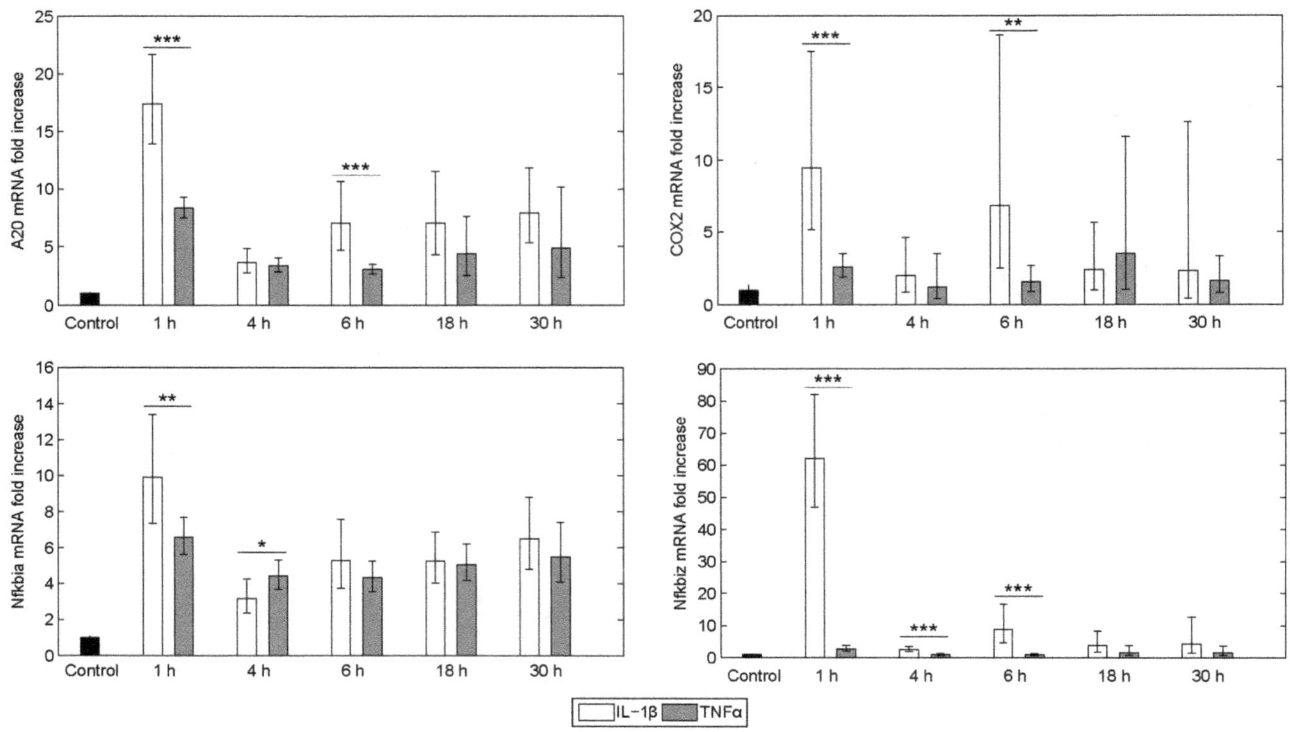

FIGURE 2 | Differential gene regulation by IL-1β and TNFα. mRNA from selected genes of primary murine hepatocytes stimulated with IL-1β (20 ng/ml) or TNFα (25 ng/ml) for 0, 1, 4, 6, 18, and 30 h. Gene expression was measured via the high-throughput Taqman® Fluidigm system. Data are analyzed using the ddCT method and normalized to untreated controls. Means of 4 independent experiments ± s.d. are displayed (***$p < 0.001$, **$p < 0.01$, *$p < 0.05$, IL-1β vs. TNFα treated cells at the corresponding time point).

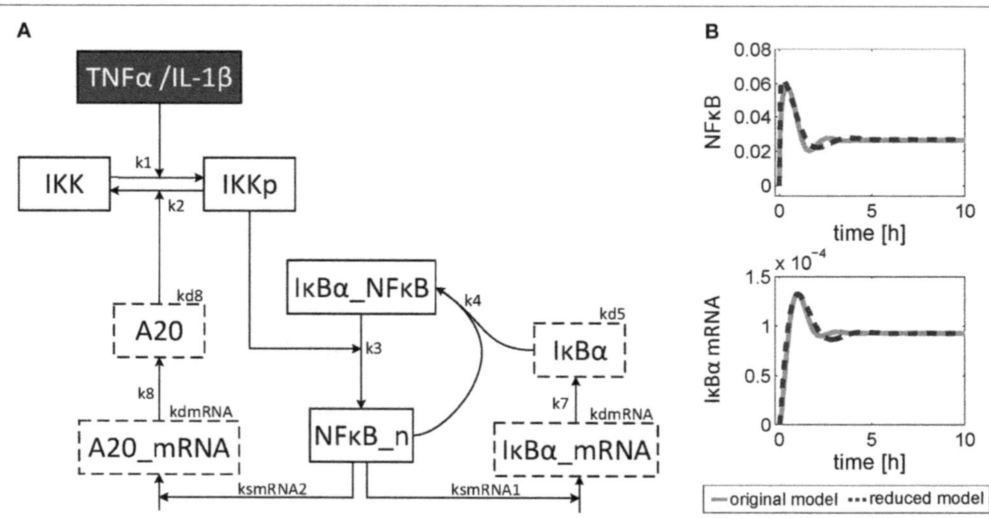

FIGURE 3 | Reduced NF-κB model. **(A)** Structure of the reduced NF-κB module. The model consists of 8 species and 10 parameters. Input of the model is either TNFα or IL-1β. The model is based on ordinary differential equations and mass action kinetics. Degradation of species is indicated by boxes with dashed border. **(B)** Simulated time courses of NF-κB and IκBα mRNA of the reduced model (dashed line) compared to the original one (solid line) in response to TNFα stimulation.

detected when using the LPS-conditioned supernatant together with FasL as compared to treatment with supernatant from untreated BMDMs in the presence of FasL. Surprisingly, the caspase-3/7 activity in hepatocytes treated with BMDM-derived supernatant without LPS stimulation and FasL (**Figures 6A,B**, dark gray bars) was even lower than after treatment with FasL

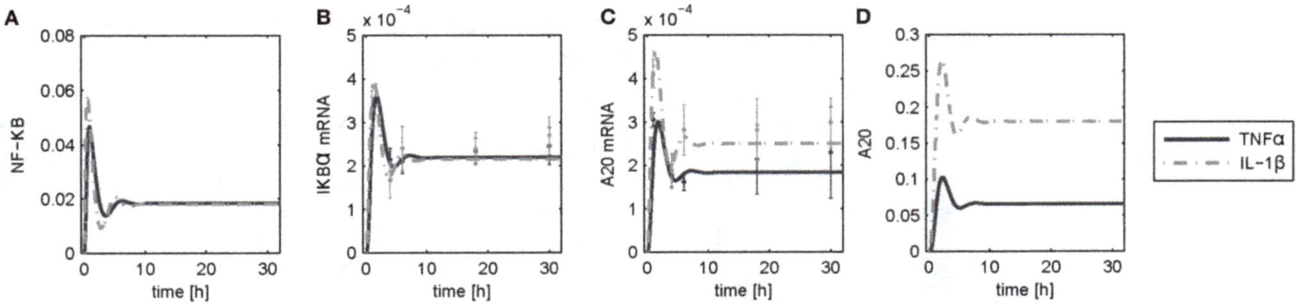

FIGURE 4 | Simulation results following TNFα and IL-1β stimulation. Simulated time courses of the reduced model of NF-κB **(A)** and measured levels of mRNA **(B,C)** as well as protein **(D)** expression after stimulation with TNFα or IL-1β.

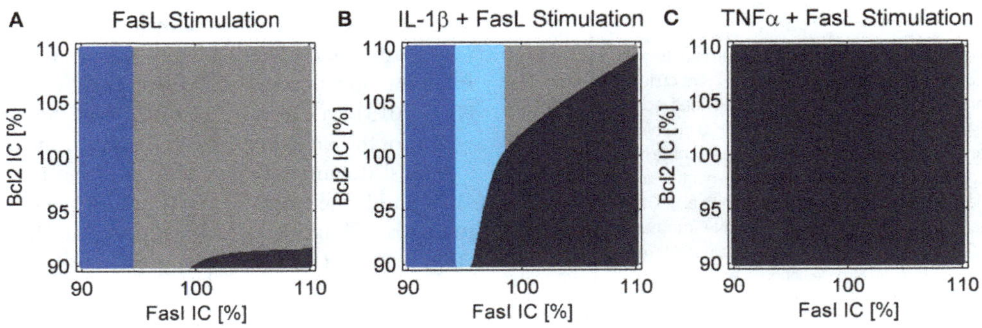

FIGURE 5 | Cell fate in dependency of the initial conditions of Fas and Bcl-2. Simulations for treatment with **(A)** FasL, **(B)** IL-1β + FasL or **(C)** TNFα + FasL for different initial conditions (IC) of Fas and anti-apoptotic Bcl-2 proteins. The nominal initial conditions are 100% for both proteins and were altered ± 10%. The cells are classified as apoptotic for caspase-3 activity values above 1.5%. If cytochrome c is released during the simulation, the cells are categorized type II apoptotic and depicted in dark gray. Otherwise they are classified as type I apoptotic and illustrated in light gray. Cells with minor levels of caspase-3 activity below 1.5% are designated as survivors depicted in blue. The light blue fraction illustrates conditions for which cells survive the combined treatment with IL-1β + FasL but would die after a single FasL stimulation.

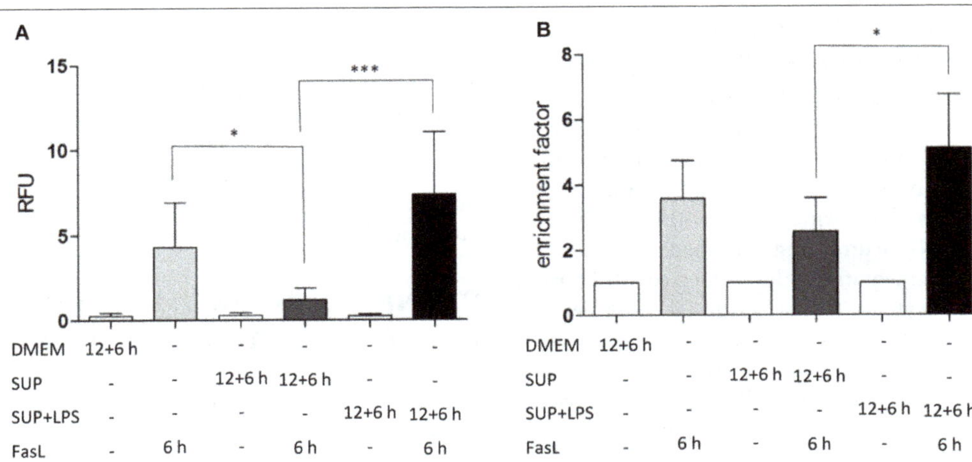

FIGURE 6 | LPS-conditioned BMDM-derived supernatant sensitizes hepatocytes to FasL-induced caspase-3/7 activity and cell death. **(A)** Caspase-3/7 activity in relative fluorescent units (RFU) determined by fluorogenic DEVDase assay of hepatocytes treated with FasL (50 ng/ml) for 6 h with or without pretreatment with BMDM-derived supernatants for 12 + 6 h. Supernatants were obtained from BMDMs stimulated with LPS (100 ng/ml) for 24 h (SUP+LPS) and from untreated BMDMs (SUP). **(B)** Cell death ELISA detecting DNA fragmentation (expressed as enrichment factor) in cells treated as described above. Values are normalized to untreated controls and represent three independent experiments. Mean and standard deviation is shown (*$p < 0.05$, ***$p < 0.001$).

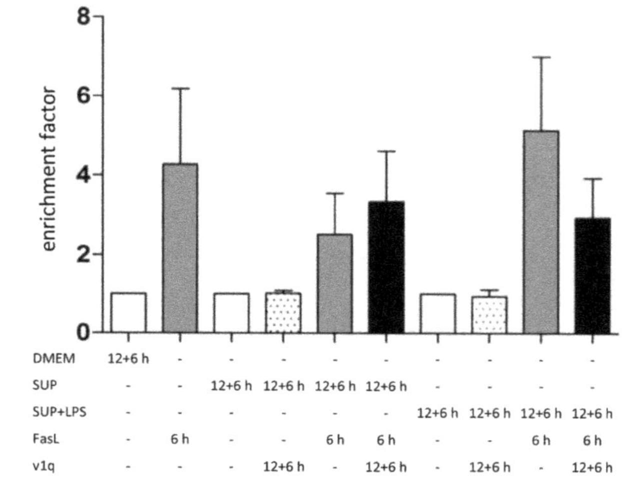

FIGURE 7 | Influence of TNFα in BMDM-derived supernatants on FasL-induced apoptosis. Primary murine hepatocytes were cultured on collagen and, after starvation, preincubated with BMDM-derived supernatant conditioned with (SUP+LPS) and without (SUP) LPS (100 ng/ml) for 24 h as well as with supernatant from cultures of the v1q cell line containing TNF-neutralizing antibodies (Quantification of v1q TNF-neutralizing antibodies is described in Echtenacher et al. (1990) and Schmich et al. (2011). Cells were stimulated with FasL (50 ng/ml) for another 6 h and DNA fragmentation was measured using the cell death ELISA Kit plus. Mean value of three independent experiments with standard deviation is shown.

alone (**Figures 6A,B**, light gray bars), indicating that untreated macrophages may secrete factors which protect against FasL-induced cell death.

2.4. Sensitization of Hepatocytes to FasL-Induced Apoptosis by the Supernatant From LPS-Treated Macrophages Is Mainly Mediated by TNFα

To investigate the role of TNFα in the apoptosis sensitization effect of BMDM-derived supernatants, hepatocytes were stimulated as described above in the absence and presence of TNF-neutralizing antibodies. Cells treated solely with BMDM-derived supernatant with and without LPS in the presence of TNF-neutralizing antibodies did not show any DNA fragmentation, as expected (**Figure 7**, dotted bars). Hepatocytes treated with BMDM-derived supernatant without LPS showed similar cell death rates after stimulation with FasL alone irrespective of the presence of the TNF-neutralizing antibodies. However, cells treated with LPS-conditioned BMDM-derived supernatant and FasL displayed a reduction in DNA fragmentation in the presence of the neutralizing antibodies as compared to their absence **Figure 7**). This finding indicates that TNFα is the cytokine secreted by macrophages which exerts the main sensitizing effect on FasL-induced apoptosis in hepatocytes. Although the data ($n = 3$) were not significant, they showed a clear tendency.

2.5. Supernatant From Unstimulated Macrophages Protects From FasL-Induced Caspase-3 Activation

Similar to the protective effect of IL-1β (Lutz et al., 2014), supernatants from resting BMDMs also appeared to protect from FasL-induced caspase-3/7 activation in hepatocytes (**Figure 6**). We therefore reinvestigated the effects of stimulation with conditioned BMDM-derived supernatant on the 46 genes involved in apoptosis and inflammation. Hepatocytes were treated with supernatant from BMDMs (18 h) that was conditioned with LPS (24 h, 100 ng/ml) and/or with FasL (6 h, 50 ng/ml) and mRNA levels were determined using the high-throughput Taqman® Fluidigm Technology. Data were analyzed using the ddCT method (Livak and Schmittgen, 2001), normalized to untreated controls (18 h DMEM) and results are displayed in a heat map (**Figure 8**). The strongest upregulation after most treatments is shown with the mRNAs of *COX2*, *Cxcl2*, and *Socs3*. These are genes typically expressed at sites of inflammation (Vane et al., 1994; Bode et al., 1999; De Filippo et al., 2013). In contrast, the mRNAs of the growth factor *Egf* as well as of the Bcl-2 proteins *Bcl-2*, *Noxa*, and *Puma* exhibited the strongest downregulation. Most of the other genes investigated also exhibit the tendency to reduced expression levels compared to controls. Stimulation with supernatant from resting BMDMs (**Figure 8**, 2nd column) abrogated the upregulation of *COX2*, *Cxcl2* and *Socs3* compared to the other treatments. The scenario that varies the most was the stimulation with supernatant from untreated BMDMs and FasL (**Figure 8**, 4th column). The inhibitors of NF-κB activation, *Iκbα/Nfkbia* and *A20*, as well as *IκBς/Nfkbiz* and *Ripk2* were strongly upregulated as compared to controls and treatment with LPS-conditioned supernatant and FasL (**Figure 9**). In addition, mRNAs of the Bcl-2 protein *Bcl2A1* and *Bid*, cathepsin B (*Ctsb*), *FLIPl*, *Fas*, and *cIAP2* were upregulated by treatment with supernatant from untreated BMDMs and FasL compared to all other stimulations. Again, the regulators of FasL-mediated apoptosis, the long splice variant of c-FLIP (*FLIPl*) and *cIAP2* were significantly higher expressed after treatment with supernatant from resting BMDMs and FasL compared to controls and stimulation with LPS-conditioned supernatant and FasL (**Figure 9**). In summary, the supernatant from resting macrophages in combination with FasL treatment induces differential expression of NF-κB target genes which could favor the observed reduction in caspase-3/7 activation.

2.6. NKT Cells Are the Source of FasL in the Liver During an Inflammatory Response

The endogenous production of FasL has been supposed to mediate hepatic cell death in the context of inflammatory disease (Galle et al., 1995; Streetz et al., 2000), but the source of FasL in the liver following LPS stimulation has remained unclear. In isolated primary murine hepatic stellate cells (HSCs) and BMDMs no LPS-mediated mRNA expression of FasL could be detected (own unpublished results). Hepatocytes also did not appear to be the source of FasL (**Figure 1**). Therefore, we investigated in our *in vivo* model whether NK and/or NKT cells express FasL. Mice were injected with 1 μg LPS/g of body weight

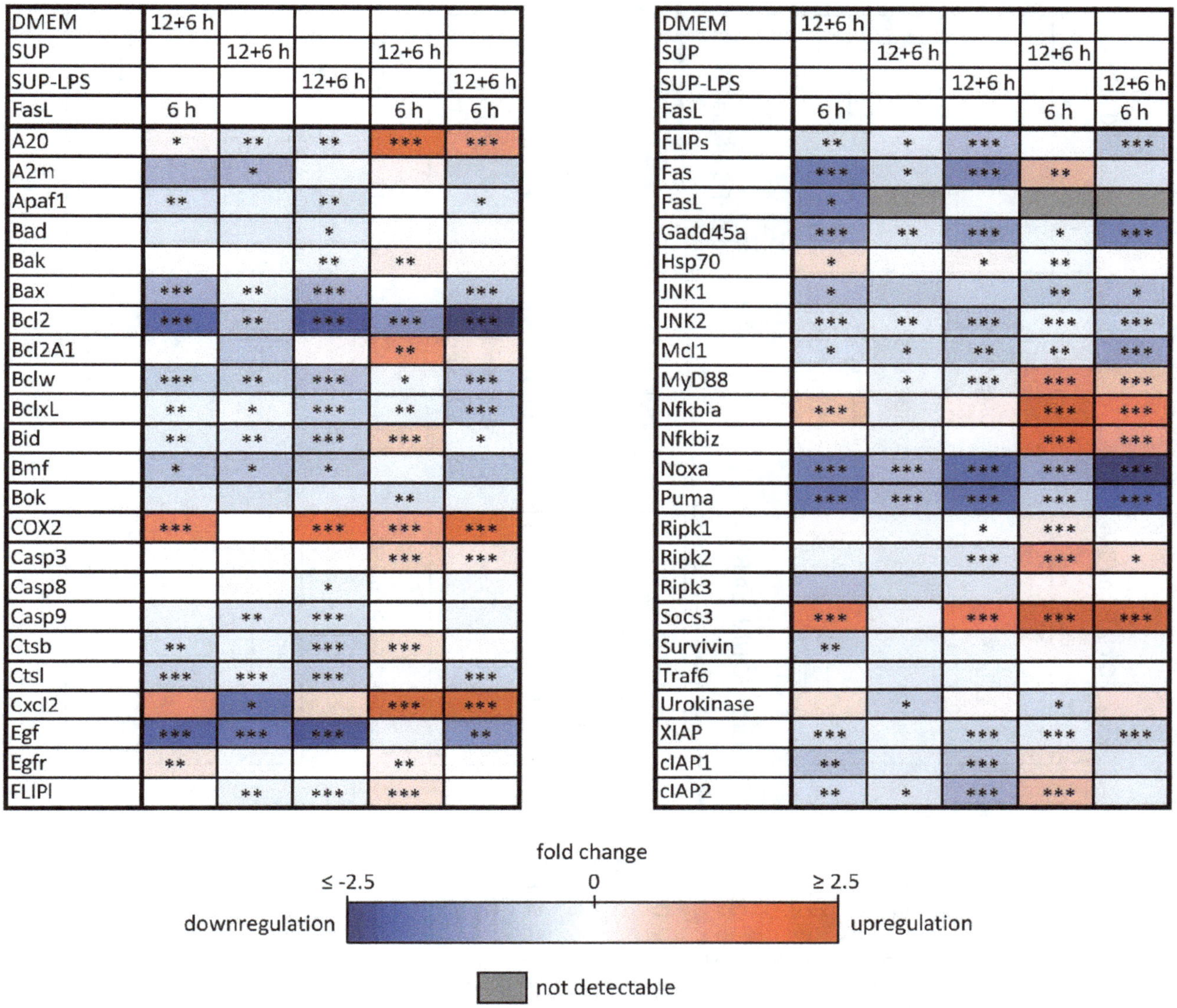

FIGURE 8 | Influence of BMDM-derived supernatant on mRNA expression of apoptotic and inflammatory genes. Primary murine hepatocytes were stimulated with supernatant from murine BMDMs for 12 h that was conditioned with (SUP-LPS) and without (SUP) LPS (100 ng/ml for 24 h). Subsequently, cells were treated with FasL (50 ng/ml) for further 6 h and mRNA was analyzed with the high-throughput Taqman® Fluidigm system. Hepatocytes treated with unconditioned DMEM and FasL (50 ng/ml) served as control. Data are analyzed using the ddCT method, normalized to untreated controls (hepatocytes treated with DMEM only) and represent 4 independent experiments. mRNAs marked in red and blue are upregulated and downregulated, respectively (*$p < 0.05$, **$p < 0.01$, ***$p < 0.001$).

and sacrificed after 6 h to obtain the NK and NKT liver cell population. Using cytometric analysis it could be demonstrated that in control mice FasL is expressed mainly on the surface of NK cells but not NKT cells. Upon LPS stimulation, however, the expression of FasL significantly increased on NKT, but not on NK cells (**Figure 10**).

3. DISCUSSION

Pro-inflammatory cytokines are involved in various aspects of liver pathogenesis such as sustained inflammation, hepatocyte cell death as well as the chronification of liver disease (Malhi and Gores, 2008; Tacke et al., 2009). We previously reported that both IL-1β as well as TNFα sensitized primary murine hepatocytes toward FasL-induced caspase-3/7 activation (Schlatter et al., 2011; Lutz et al., 2014). While this resulted in enhanced hepatocyte apoptosis in the case of TNFα, a death protective effect was noted for IL-1β (Lutz et al., 2014). Both cytokines potently activate NF-κB (Luedde and Schwabe, 2011), which is supposed to mediate the majority of anti-apoptotic effects in hepatocytes (Tak and Firestein, 2001).

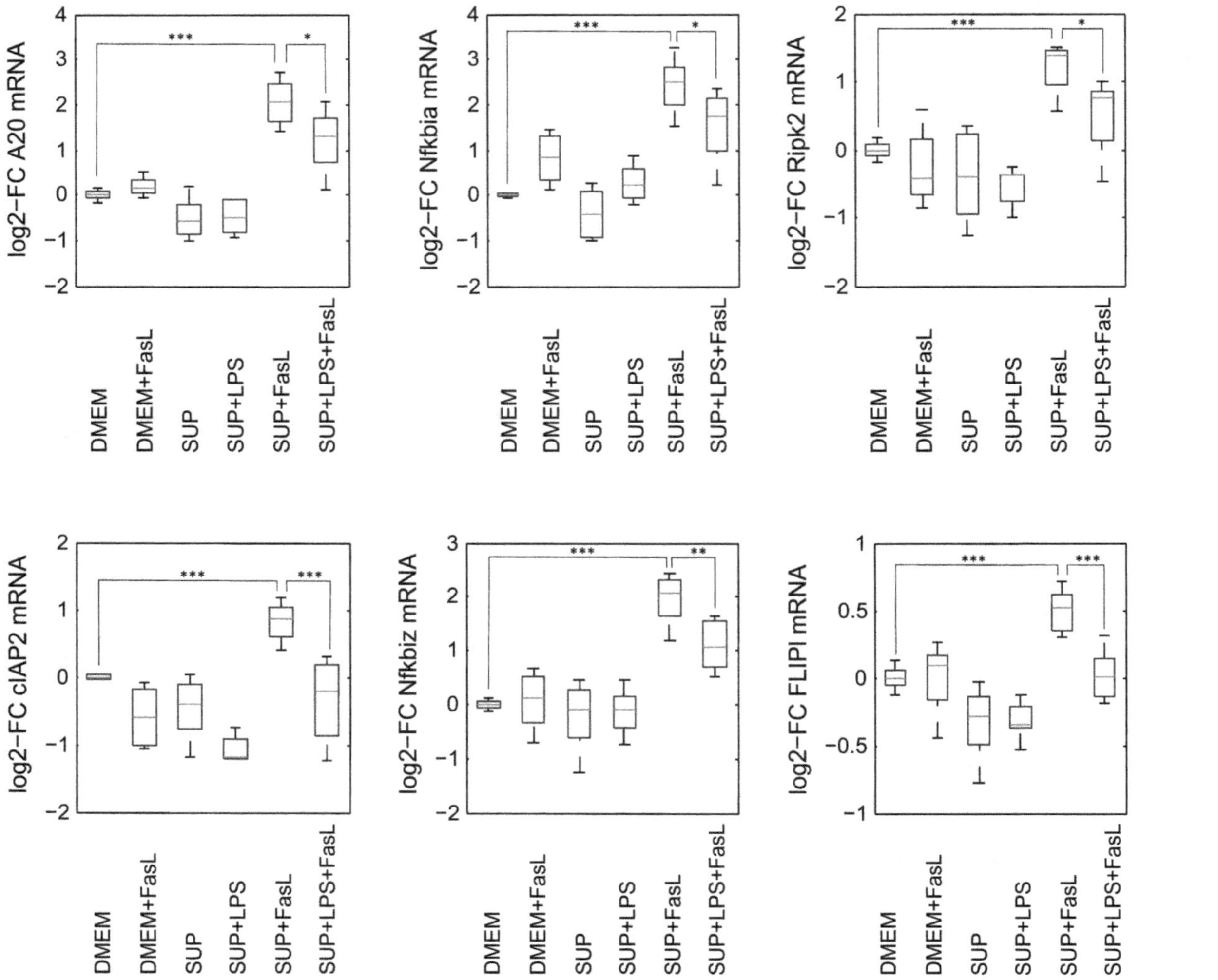

FIGURE 9 | mRNA expression levels of selected genes after stimulation with BMDM supernatant and/or FasL. mRNA expression of primary murine hepatocytes stimulated with supernatant from murine BMDMs that was conditioned with (SUP+LPS/SUP+LPS+FasL) and without LPS (SUP/SUP+FasL) and/or FasL as indicated. Gene expression was measured via the high-throughput Taqman® Fluidigm system. Data are analyzed using the ddCT method, normalized to untreated controls (DMEM) and represent 4 independent experiments. Values are expressed as log2-fold change (FC) of untreated control cells and differential expression was assessed using the two-sample Student's *t*-test (**p* < 0.05, ***p* < 0.01, ****p* < 0.001).

In this study, we uncovered a differential influence on the transcriptional activity of NF-κB as the possible explanation for the distinct effect of IL-1β and TNFα on hepatocyte survival. We investigated the transcriptional profile of 46 inflammatory and apoptotic NF-κB target genes after treatment of primary murine hepatocytes with these two cytokines. As expected, the gene expression pattern was qualitatively quite similar, especially regarding the inflammatory mediators (**Figure 1**). For example, we noted the induction of the chemokine ligand *Cxcl2*, which is known to recruit neutrophils for a hepatic inflammatory response (Krohn et al., 2009; Van Sweringen et al., 2011; Marques et al., 2012). Also high levels of *Ripk2* are expected to contribute to inflammation (Scott et al., 2010) because Ripk2 mediates innate immune signaling (Madrigal et al., 2012) and is involved in Fas-mediated NF-κB activation (Vallabhapurapu and Karin, 2009) and pro-survival signaling (Hughes et al., 2009). Similarly, mRNA of *COX2* is usually upregulated at sites of inflammation (Willoughby et al., 2000) and was reported to induce pro-survival signaling, e.g. via activation of Akt (Leng et al., 2003), and to impair apoptosis in liver cells (Fernández-Martínez et al., 2006; Casado et al., 2007). Finally, it makes sense that the mRNAs of the negative feedback inhibitors of NF-κB signaling, *IκBα* and *A20* were upregulated in response to IL-1β and TNFα (Krikos et al., 1992; Sun et al., 1993). IκBα is part of the well-known NF-κB-induced autoregulatory feedback mechanism, whereas A20 interferes with both activation of NF-κB by inhibiting IKK (Skaug et al., 2011) and of caspase-8 at the DISC (Daniel et al., 2004).

Besides these similarities, we noted differences in the dynamics of how some of the NF-κB target genes were

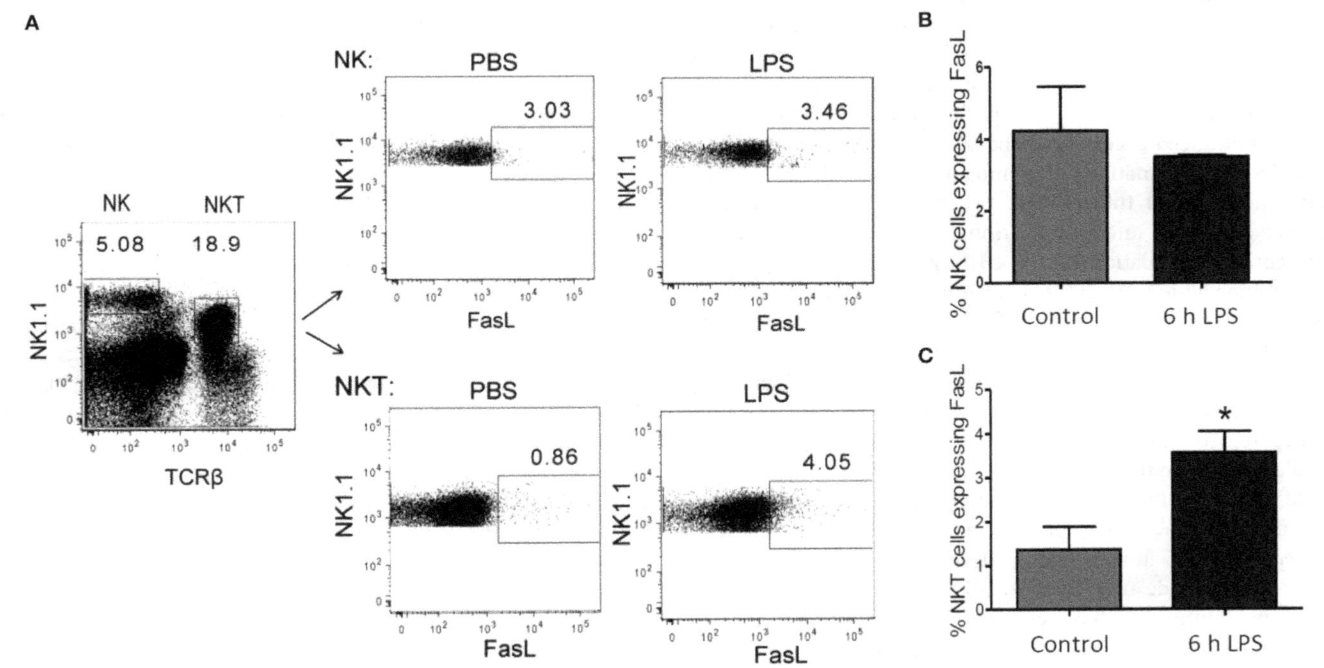

FIGURE 10 | FasL expression in NK and NKT cells after LPS injection. Mice were treated with LPS or PBS for control. After 6 h the liver was perfused using collagenase to obtain a single-cell suspension. Lymphocytes were isolated using density gradient centrifugation, as described in the materials and methods section. **(A)** Representative density plots showing gate in NK (NK1.1 positive) and in NKT (NK1.1 and TCRβ double positive) cells. Number of FasL positive cells in **(B)** the NK cell- and **(C)** NKT cell-pool from LPS-treated mice (black bar) and control mice (gray bar). Mean and standard deviation is shown (*$p < 0.05$).

transcriptionally upregulated in response to IL-1β or TNFα. The levels of *COX2*, *IκBα/Nfkbia* and *A20* mRNAs were significantly higher after IL-1β than after TNFα stimulation for various time points. Especially the first peak in gene expression after 1 h as well as the oscillations seemed more pronounced after IL-1β stimulation (**Figure 2**). Both COX2 and A20 have been shown to impair apoptosis in hepatocytes (Daniel et al., 2004; Fernández-Martínez et al., 2006). The biggest difference was noted for *IκBζ/Nfkbiz* (20-fold higher expression with IL-1β). In contrast to other IκB proteins, IκBζ localizes to the nucleus (Yamazaki et al., 2001; Totzke et al., 2006). The precise signaling roles of IκBζ have not yet been identified. IκBζ-deficient mice exhibit defective development of IL-17-producing helper T (TH17) cells and IκBζ was reported as possible transcription factor for IL-17 induction (Okamoto et al., 2010). In other studies IκBζ was described to influence NF-κB-dependent transcriptional regulation both positively and negatively (Motoyama et al., 2005). IκBζ preferably associates with p50/p50 and p65/p50 NF-κB dimers and inhibits DNA binding in the nucleus (Yamazaki et al., 2001). In this respect IκBζ may function in a pro-apoptotic manner. Indeed, transfection of IκBζ renders peritoneal macrophages more susceptible to TNFα-induced apoptosis (Yamazaki et al., 2001) and the silencing of IκBζ renders HeLa cells more resistant to apoptosis (Totzke et al., 2006). However, this pro-apoptotic property may depend on the cellular system or the type of death stimuli used. In our scenario, IκBζ is more likely to function as an anti-apoptotic factor in response to IL-1β, since this cytokine confers death protection rather than enhanced apoptosis in response to FasL treatment.

Model reduction significantly diminished the number of parameters while maintaining a very similar time course of NFκB activity and target gene expression compared to the original model. This facilitated model parametrization and allowed studying the impact of parameter variations on NF-κB activation. These investigations revealed that the amplitude and the frequency of NF-κB activity can be influenced by changing the parameter values for NF-κB activation (degradation of IκBα and liberation of NF-κB) and deactivation (reassociation of NF-κB with newly synthesized IκBα), respectively. Many posttranscriptional modifications have been described that may account different kinetics of these steps (Karin and Ben-Neriah, 2000; Perkins, 2006; Luedde and Schwabe, 2011). While the phosphorylation of two conserved serine residues of IκBα (S32/S36) target the protein for proteasomal degradation, phosphorylation of lysine residues by casein kinase II is associated with increased protein stability (DiDonato et al., 1996; Lin et al., 1996). Besides, p65 phosphorylation sites have been described to either contribute to enhanced (Zhong et al., 1997) or diminished NF-κB activity (Lawrence et al., 2005). Further posttranscriptional modifications were shown to terminate NF-κB activity (Ruland, 2011). For example, methylation of p65 at K314/K315 seemed to inhibit NF-κB activity by targeting NF-κB to proteasomal degradation (Yang et al., 2009), while acetylation of p65 prolonged NF-κB activity by preventing its binding to the inhibitory IκBα and thus nuclear export (Chen et al., 2001). All these modifications depend on the cellular stimulus and change the kinetics and dynamics of NF-κB as previously discussed (Hoffmann et al., 2002; Nelson et al., 2004; Smale, 2011). We hypothesize that IL-1β induces a more pronounced oscillatory behavior of NF-κB in hepatocytes than TNFα. Our mathematical model supports the hypothesis that differences in the oscillatory behavior of NF-κB due to distinct activation and deactivation kinetics can result in the differential upregulation of NF-κB target genes depending on the cytokine added. Whereas IL-1β induced both pro- and anti-apoptotic effects via activation of JNK and increased induction of A20, respectively, TNFα predominantly favors apoptosis induction. However, the precise regulation of the NF-κB pathway and its implication in pro-survival vs. pro-apoptotic signaling in hepatocytes during inflammatory reactions requires more detailed studies in the future.

Besides its pivotal role in inflammation, NF-κB is also described as a central player in the regulation of liver homeostasis, liver fibrosis and the development of hepatocellular carcinoma (Luedde and Schwabe, 2011; Sunami et al., 2012). The liver innate immune cell population comprises Kupffer cells, the liver-located macrophages, which are crucial for inflammatory responses (Zimmermann et al., 2012) as well as NK and NKT cells (Tacke et al., 2009). Although IL-1β and TNFα are the most important cytokines secreted by activated macrophages during an LPS-induced inflammatory response (Ulich et al., 1991; Bode et al., 2012) others such as IL-6 or IL-10 as well as the Ccl- and Cxcl-type chemokines and the type I interferon IFNβ are crucial for liver homeostasis or pathogenesis, too (Rex et al., 2016). To identify which cytokine was most important for the sensitizing effect on hepatocytes, we incubated the cells with the supernatant from LPS-treated BMDM macrophages *in vitro*. We found that the treatment of the supernatant with TNF-neutralizing antibodies tended to prevent the increase in cell death indicating that TNFα plays an important role as sensitizing mediator for apoptosis induction in hepatocytes. This is in accordance with our previous finding that macrophages secrete TNFα in much higher amounts than IL-1β (Rex et al., 2016). Therefore, TNFα should be more decisive on the fate of the cells. However, further studies are needed for final conclusions on the role of TNFα and IL-1β.

To our surprise, we observed that the supernatant from resting macrophages, i.e. without LPS conditioning, protected cells from FasL-induced caspase-3/7 activation similar to IL-1β. Investigation of the gene expression pattern revealed that FasL stimulation after preincubation with unconditioned supernatant also resulted in a differential regulation of specific NF-κB target genes such as *IκBα/NFkbia*, *A20* and *IκBζ/Nfkbiz* (**Figure 9**). In addition, we noted the upregulation of *cIAP2*, *FLIPl*, and *Ripk2*, which are all modulators of apoptosis signaling. Ripk2 favors pro-survival signaling downstream of the DISC through induction of NF-κB activity (Festjens et al., 2007; Hughes et al., 2009). cIAP2 can directly inhibit the active forms of the caspase-3 and -7 (Roy et al., 1997) and potentiate NF-κB signaling by destabilizing IκBα (Chu et al., 1997). Both pro- and anti-apoptotic roles of $FLIP_L$ have been reported (Chang et al., 2002). A few studies demonstrated that $FLIP_L$ inhibits FasL-mediated apoptosis at high concentrations (Chang et al., 2002; Sharp et al., 2005) which would be in accordance with the observed effects in this study. The initial steps in apoptosis induction, formation of the DISC and the degree of caspase-8 activation has been shown to determine cell fate (Lavrik et al., 2007; Hughes et al., 2009; Kallenberger et al., 2014). It seems that after preincubation with unconditioned BMDM supernatant less apoptotic and more anti-apoptotic signaling occurs in hepatocytes after stimulation with FasL. Fas signaling usually induces the apoptotic pathway but it is also able to trigger NF-κB activation. Studies have demonstrated that the ratio of $FLIP_L$ to caspase-8 at the DISC is decisive for apoptotic vs. pro-survival signaling (Golks et al., 2006; Fricker et al., 2010; Lavrik and Krammer, 2012). We therefore hypothesize that resting macrophages secrete protective factors that modify the balance toward pro-survival conditions such that NF-κB activation and upregulation of respective target genes prevails apoptosis induction downstream of Fas.

We finally investigated the sources of endogenous FasL in our scenario of LPS-induced inflammation since various possible sources have been reported depending on the experimental model used (Tsutsui et al., 1999; Takeda et al., 2000). NKT cells are quite abundant in the liver constituting 20–30% of the liver T cells (Bendelac et al., 1997). They have previously been implicated in liver damage during hepatitis (Takeda et al., 2000). Furthermore, FasL expression has been implicated in liver damage (Galle et al., 1995) and was associated to NK cells (Arase et al., 1995). Indeed, we could demonstrate that FasL is expressed on NK cells but strongly induced in NKT cells in our *in vivo* model of LPS-induced inflammation in mice. This suggests that endogenous production of FasL by NKT cells plays an important role in the observed hepatic cell death in inflammatory diseases (Galle et al., 1995; Streetz et al., 2000).

In summary, our study shows that it is important to investigate the aforementioned mediators and the crosstalk of pro-inflammatory cytokines released by macrophages and FasL-induced apoptotic signaling in hepatocytes in more detail. We find that macrophages modulate the hepatocytes both in the unstimulated and stimulated state. Without an inflammatory stimulus, macrophages exert a protective effect on hepatocytes, attenuate apoptosis induction and shift the balance toward pro-survival signaling. However, they sensitize hepatocytes to apoptosis induction during LPS-induced inflammation, probably to rapidly remove damaged cells.

4. MATERIALS AND METHODS

4.1. Mice Strains and Primary Cell Isolation

Wild type (C57BL/6N and C57BL/6J) mice were purchased from Jackson Laboratories. Primary hepatocytes were isolated from 8 to 14 week old BL6 mice using the collagenase perfusion technique and cultivated as previously described (Klingmüller et al., 2006; Schmich et al., 2011) (see also **Supplementary Material**, **Presentation 1**). The whole study, including the isolation procedure, was approved by the animal experimental committee (ethical permission number: X-12/22D, University of Freiburg). For generation of bone marrow-derived macrophages (BMDMs) 8–12 week old male mice were sacrificed. The animal applications were reviewed and approved by the appropriate authorities and were performed in accordance with the German animal protection law (AZ: 84-02.04.2012.A175; Landesamt für Natur, Umwelt und Verbraucherschutz Nordrhein-Westfalen, Recklinghausen). All animals were handled and housed according to specific pathogen free (SPF) conditions.

4.2. Preparation of BMDM Supernatants

The preparation and cultivation of primary murine BMDMs has been carried out according to the standard operating procedure (SOP) as previously described (Rex et al., 2016). Summarizing, after 8 days of BMDM differentiation/cultivation (DMEM: Biochrom, Berlin, Germany; FCS (Cat.: 10099141, Lot: 769367): Invitrogen, Karlsruhe, Germany; Penicillin G/Streptomycin: Cytogen, Wetzlar, Germany), adherent cells were harvested by gentle trypsinization: Cells were washed twice with prewarmed PBS (Biochrom, Berlin, Germany) and treated with 3 ml trypsin/EDTA solution (Cytogen, Wetzlar, Germany) for approximately 5–10 min. Cells were centrifuged and adjusted in M-CSF (5 ng/ml; recombinant murine M-CSF: Peprotech, Rocky Hill, NJ, USA) containing culture medium: 1.4×10^6 cells/3.5 ml per 60 mm tissue culture dish. After 6 h of cultivation, cells were stimulated with 100 ng/ml LPS (using LPS/DMEM solution; LPS from *Escherichia coli* (# L3012, Sigma-Aldrich, Munich, Germany) or were treated with the corresponding volume of Dulbecco modified Eagle medium (DMEM) as control, respectively. After 24 h, cell culture supernatant was collected under sterile conditions by centrifugation (20 min, 4°C, 5.500 rpm). Aliquots were prepared and tempered gently up to −80°C for storage.

4.3. Quantification of N2A FasL

Quantification of FasL in the Neuro2A supernatant was carried out as described before (Walter et al., 2008). Briefly, the human T cells Jurkat E6 were treated or untreated with Neuro2A supernatant diluted 1:4 (25%) in medium for 1 h. Defined concentrations of recombinant Fc-FasL served as the standard and apoptosis was quantified by GFP-annexin-V/PI FACS analysis.

4.4. Treatment of Isolated Primary Murine Hepatocytes

To investigate the influence of IL-1β and TNFα on the gene expression profile primary murine hepatocytes (1×10^6 cells) were stimulated with 20 ng/ml IL-1β or 25 ng/ml TNFα (both from R&D Systems, Minneapolis, USA) for 1, 4, 6, 18, and 30 h or left untreated as control. To study the influence of macrophage-derived mediators on FasL-induced caspase-3/7 activity and cell death, hepatocytes (2×10^6) were pre-incubated with the supernatant from LPS-stimulated BMDMs (SUP+LPS) or with the supernatant from untreated BMDMs (SUP) for 12 h and subsequently with 50 ng/ml FasL (generated by Neuro2A cells) for further 6 h. Additionally, hepatocytes were only stimulated with FasL for 6 h, with the supernatant from unstimulated (SUP), LPS-treated BMDMs (SUP+LPS), or the medium DMEM for 18 h as controls.

4.5. DEVDase Assay

The activity of the executioner caspase-3/7 in hepatocytes (1×10^6) was measured by the fluorogenic DEVDase assay as previously described (Schlatter et al., 2011; Lutz et al., 2014). See also the **Supplementary Material (Presentation 1)**.

4.6. Cell Death Detection ELISA

To quantify the amount of DNA fragmentation in hepatocytes (1×10^6) after treatment with the different stimuli the cell death detection ELISAPLUS Kit (Roche, Mannheim, Germany) was used and performed according to the manufacturer instruction (Lutz et al., 2014) (for detailed information see the **Supplementary Material (Presentation 1)**.

4.7. RNA Isolation, cDNA Synthesis and qRT-PCR

Total RNA was isolated using the RNeasyPlus Kit (Qiagen, Hilden, Germany) according to the manufacturer instruction. The quantity and purity of RNA was determined by measuring the optical density at 260 and 280 nm. 600 ng total RNA was reverse transcribed to cDNA with TaqMan Reverse Transcription Reagents (Applera GmbH, Darmstadt, Germany). For qRT-PCR the Fluidigm Biomark high throughput qPCR chip platform (Fluidigm Corporation, San Francisco, CA, USA) with pre-designed gene expression assays from Applied Biosystems was used according to the manufacturer instructions (Spurgeon et al., 2008). Data were analyzed using the ddCT method (Livak and Schmittgen, 2001) and expression values were normalized to the expression levels of the β-actin gene. All TaqMan assays are listed in the **Supplementary Material** in **Data Sheets 1**, **2** for stimulation with IL-1β/TNFα and BMDM supernatant, respectively.

4.8. FACS Analysis/ *in vivo* Experiments

C57BL/6 mice (8–14 weeks old) were injected i.p. with 1 μg LPS/g of body weight and sacrificed after 6 h. The livers were extracted and homogenized with a plunger rod over a 70 μm cell strainer in a 50 ml falcon. Hepatic lymphocytes were further isolated by density gradient centrifugation using 60% and 40% percoll. Cells were labeled with APC-conjugated anti-mouse NK 1.1, PerCP-conjugated anti-mouse TCRb and PE-anti mouse conjugated FasL. Background staining was determined using a PE-anti mouse IgG isotype control. All antibodies were used at a concentration of 1 μg/ml and purchased from BD Biosciences. Flow cytometry analysis was performed using FACSdiva (BD Bioscience).

4.9. Isolation of NK and NKT Liver Cell Populations

Single-cell suspensions were prepared from the liver by collagenase-based perfusion via the portal vein. Total liver cells were homogenized in a 40% isotonic percoll solution and slowly passed to a 60% isotonic percoll solution without mixing the layers. After centrifugation for 20 min at 900 g, the upper layer was discarded (debris and hepatocytes) and the mononuclear cells were collected from the interface. The cells were washed once with PBS (300 g, 7 min, room temperature) and then 1 ml red blood cell lysis buffer was added for 3 min. After other washing step the cells were incubated with Fc-blocking buffer for 15 min and afterwards incubated for 30 min with the following antibodies: NK1.1-APC, TCRβ-FITC and CD178-PE or Arm hamster isotype control-PE (eBioscience).

4.10. Statistical Analysis

Values are expressed as means ± standard deviation (s.d.). Differences in expression, caspase-3/7 activity and DNA fragmentation were assessed using the two-sample Student *t*-test. *P*-values were calculated and $p \leq 0.05$ was considered as significant.

4.11. Mathematical Modeling and Simulation

The model is based on ordinary differential equations and mass action kinetics and was implemented using MATLAB R2014a. The model setup and reduction is explained and all model equations can be found in the **Supplementary Material** (**Presentation 1**).

AUTHOR CONTRIBUTIONS

JR, AL, LF, UA, JB, CB, and IM: conceived and designed the experiments; AL, LF, and UA: performed the experiments; JR, AL, LF, MT, and IM: analyzed the data; MT, JB, CB, OS, and IM: contributed reagents, materials, analysis tools; JR and OS: performed the mathematical modeling; JR, LF, UA, CB, and IM: wrote the paper.

FUNDING

This work was supported by the German Federal Ministry of Education and Research (BMBF) within the research network Virtual Liver (grants FKZ 0315731, FKZ 0315751, FKZ 0315755, FKZ 0315766) and by the Robert Bosch Foundation, Stuttgart, Germany.

ACKNOWLEDGMENTS

We would like to thank Carina Franek (Clinic of Gastroenterology, Hepatology and Infectious Diseases, Heinrich-Heine-University, Dsseldorf, Germany) and Igor Liebermann (Institute of Clinical Pharmacology, Stuttgart) for technical assistance. We are grateful to Sabine MacNelly, Department of Internal Medicine II, University Hospital, Freiburg for the isolation of primary murine hepatocytes.

REFERENCES

Arase, H., Arase, N., and Saito, T. (1995). Fas-mediated cytotoxicity by freshly isolated natural killer cells. *J. Exp. Med.* 181, 1235–1238. doi: 10.1084/jem.181.3.1235

Baltimore, D. (2011). NF-κB is 25. *Nat. Immunol.* 12, 683–685. doi: 10.1038/ni.2072

Bendelac, A., Rivera, M. N., Park, S. H., and Roark, J. H. (1997). Mouse CD1-specific NK1 T cells: development, specificity, and function. *Annu. Rev. Immunol.* 15, 535–562. doi: 10.1146/annurev.immunol.15.1.535

Biburger, M., and Tiegs, G. (2005). -Galactosylceramide-induced liver injury in mice is mediated by TNF- but independent of kupffer cells. *J. Immunol.* 175, 1540–1550. doi: 10.4049/jimmunol.175.3.1540

Blachier, M., Leleu, H., Peck-Radosavljevic, M., Valla, D.-C., and Roudot-Thoraval, F. (2013). The burden of liver disease in Europe: a review of available epidemiological data. *J. Hepatol.* 58, 593–608. doi: 10.1016/j.jhep.2012.12.005

Bode, J. G., Ehlting, C., and Häussinger, D. (2012). The macrophage response towards LPS and its control through the p38 MAPK-STAT3 axis. *Cell. Signal.* 24, 1185–1194. doi: 10.1016/j.cellsig.2012.01.018

Bode, J. G., Nimmesgern, A., Schmitz, J., Schaper, F., Schmitt, M., Frisch, W., et al. (1999). LPS and TNFalpha induce SOCS3 mRNA and inhibit IL-6-induced activation of STAT3 in macrophages. *FEBS Lett.* 463, 365–370. doi: 10.1016/S0014-5793(99)01662-2

Casado, M., Mollá, B., Roy, R., Fernández-Martínez, A., Cucarella, C., Mayoral, R., et al. (2007). Protection against Fas-induced liver apoptosis in transgenic mice expressing cyclooxygenase 2 in hepatocytes. *Hepatology* 45, 631–638. doi: 10.1002/hep.21556

Chang, D. W., Xing, Z., Pan, Y., Algeciras-Schimnich, A., Barnhart, B. C., Yaish-Ohad, S., et al. (2002). c-FLIP(L) is a dual function regulator for caspase-8 activation and CD95-mediated apoptosis. *EMBO J.* 21, 3704–3714. doi: 10.1093/emboj/cdf356

Chen, L. F., Fischle, W., Verdin, E., and Greene, W. C. (2001). Duration of nuclear NF-kappaB action regulated by reversible acetylation. *Science (New York, N.Y.)* 293, 1653–1657. doi: 10.1126/science.1062374

Chu, Z. L., McKinsey, T. A., Liu, L., Gentry, J. J., Malim, M. H., and Ballard, D. W. (1997). Suppression of tumor necrosis factor-induced cell death by inhibitor of apoptosis c-IAP2 is under NF-kappaB control. *Proc. Natl. Acad. Sci. U.S.A.* 94, 10057–10062. doi: 10.1073/pnas.94.19.10057

Covert, M. W., Leung, T. H., Gaston, J. E., and Baltimore, D. (2005). Achieving stability of lipopolysaccharide-induced NF-kappaB activation. *Science (New York, N.Y.)* 309, 1854–1857. doi: 10.1126/science.11 12304

Daniel, S., Arvelo, M. B., Patel, V. I., Longo, C. R., Shrikhande, G., Shukri, T., et al. (2004). A20 protects endothelial cells from TNF-, Fas-, and NK-mediated cell death by inhibiting caspase 8 activation. *Blood* 104, 2376–2384. doi: 10.1182/blood-2003-02-0635

De Filippo, K., Dudeck, A., Hasenberg, M., Nye, E., van Rooijen, N., Hartmann, K., et al. (2013). Mast cell and macrophage chemokines CXCL1/CXCL2 control the early stage of neutrophil recruitment during tissue inflammation. *Blood* 121, 4930–4937. doi: 10.1182/blood-2013-02-4 86217

DiDonato, J., Mercurio, F., Rosette, C., Wu-Li, J., Suyang, H., Ghosh, S., et al. (1996). Mapping of the inducible IkappaB phosphorylation sites that signal its ubiquitination and degradation. *Mol. Cell. Biol.* 16, 1295–1304. doi: 10.1128/MCB.16.4.1295

Echtenacher, B., Falk, W., Männel, D. N., and Krammer, P. H. (1990). Requirement of endogenous tumor necrosis factor/cachectin for recovery from experimental peritonitis. *J. Immunol.* 145, 3762–3766.

Fernández-Martínez, A., Mollá, B., Mayoral, R., Boscá, L., Casado, M., and Martín-Sanz, P. (2006). Cyclo-oxygenase 2 expression impairs serum-withdrawal-induced apoptosis in liver cells. *Biochem. J.* 398, 371–380. doi: 10.1042/BJ20060780

Festjens, N., Vanden Berghe, T., Cornelis, S., and Vandenabeele, P. (2007). RIP1, a kinase on the crossroads of a cell's decision to live or die. *Cell Death Different.* 14, 400–410. doi: 10.1038/sj.cdd.4402085

Fricker, N., Beaudouin, J., Richter, P., Eils, R., Krammer, P. H., and Lavrik, I. N. (2010). Model-based dissection of CD95 signaling dynamics reveals both a pro- and antiapoptotic role of c-FLIPL. *J. Cell Biol.* 190, 377–389. doi: 10.1083/jcb.201002060

Galle, P. R., Hofmann, W. J., Walczak, H., Schaller, H., Otto, G., Stremmel, W., et al. (1995). Involvement of the CD95 (APO-1/Fas) receptor and ligand in liver damage. *J. Exp. Med.* 182, 1223–1230. doi: 10.1084/jem.182.5.1223

Geissler, A., Haun, F., Frank, D. O., Wieland, K., Simon, M. M., Idzko, M., et al. (2013). Apoptosis induced by the fungal pathogen gliotoxin requires a triple phosphorylation of Bim by JNK. *Cell Death Different.* 20, 1317–1329. doi: 10.1038/cdd.2013.78

Golks, A., Brenner, D., Krammer, P. H., and Lavrik, I. N. (2006). The c-FLIP-NH2 terminus (p22-FLIP) induces NF-kappaB activation. *J. Exp. Med.* 203, 1295–1305. doi: 10.1084/jem.20051556

Hoffmann, A., Levchenko, A., Scott, M. L., and Baltimore, D. (2002). The IkappaB-NF-kappaB signaling module: temporal control and selective gene activation. *Science (New York, N.Y.)* 298, 1241–1245. doi: 10.1126/science.1071914

Hughes, M. A., Harper, N., Butterworth, M., Cain, K., Cohen, G. M., and MacFarlane, M. (2009). Reconstitution of the death-inducing signaling complex reveals a substrate switch that determines CD95-mediated death or survival. *Mol. Cell* 35, 265–279. doi: 10.1016/j.molcel.2009.06.012

Irmler, M., Thome, M., Hahne, M., Schneider, P., Hofmann, K., Steiner, V., et al. (1997). Inhibition of death receptor signals by cellular FLIP. *Nature* 388, 190–195. doi: 10.1038/40657

Kallenberger, S. M., Beaudouin, J., Claus, J., Fischer, C., Sorger, P. K., Legewie, S., et al. (2014). Intra- and interdimeric caspase-8 self-cleavage controls strength and timing of CD95-induced apoptosis. *Sci. Signal.* 7:ra23. doi: 10.1126/scisignal.2004738

Karin, M., and Ben-Neriah, Y. (2000). Phosphorylation meets ubiquitination: the control of NF-κB activity. *Annu. Rev. Immunol.* 18, 621–663. doi: 10.1146/annurev.immunol.18.1.621

Karin, M., and Lin, A. (2002). NF-kappaB at the crossroads of life and death. *Nat. Immunol.* 3, 221–227. doi: 10.1038/ni0302-221

Klingmüller, U., Bauer, A., Bohl, S., Nickel, P. J., Breitkopf, K., Dooley, S., et al. (2006). Primary mouse hepatocytes for systems biology approaches: a standardized *in vitro* system for modelling of signal transduction pathways. *Syst. Biol.* 153, 433–447.

Kondo, T., Suda, T., Fukuyama, H., Adachi, M., and Nagata, S. (1997). Essential roles of the Fas ligand in the development of hepatitis. *Nat. Med.* 3, 409–413. doi: 10.1038/nm0497-409

Krammer, P. H. (2000). CD95's deadly mission in the immune system. *Nature* 407, 789–795. doi: 10.1038/35037728

Krikos, A., Laherty, C. D., and Dixit, V. M. (1992). Transcriptional activation of the tumor necrosis factor alpha-inducible zinc finger protein, A20, is mediated by kappa B elements. *J. Biol. Chem.* 267, 17971–17976.

Krohn, N., Kapoor, S., Enami, Y., Follenzi, A., Bandi, S., Joseph, B., et al. (2009). Hepatocyte transplantation-induced liver inflammation is driven by cytokines-chemokines associated with neutrophils and Kupffer cells. *Gastroenterology* 136, 1806–1817. doi: 10.1053/j.gastro.2009.01.063

Ksontini, R., Colagiovanni, D. B., Josephs, M. D., Edwards, C. K., Tannahill, C. L., Solorzano, C. C., et al. (1998). Disparate roles for TNF-alpha and Fas ligand in concanavalin A-induced hepatitis. *J. Immunol. (Baltimore, Md. : 1950)* 160, 4082–4089.

Lavrik, I. N., Golks, A., Riess, D., Bentele, M., Eils, R., and Krammer, P. H. (2007). Analysis of CD95 threshold signaling: triggering of CD95 (FAS/APO-1) at low concentrations primarily results in survival signaling. *J. Biol. Chem.* 282, 13664–13671. doi: 10.1074/jbc.M700434200

Lavrik, I. N., and Krammer, P. H. (2012). Regulation of CD95/Fas signaling at the DISC. *Cell Death Different.* 19, 36–41. doi: 10.1038/cdd.2011.155

Lawrence, T., Bebien, M., Liu, G. Y., Nizet, V., and Karin, M. (2005). IKK alpha limits macrophage NF-kappa B activation and contributes to the resolution of inflammation. *Nature* 434, 1138–1143. doi: 10.1038/nature03491

Leng, J., Han, C., Demetris, A. J., Michalopoulos, G. K., and Wu, T. (2003). Cyclooxygenase-2 promotes hepatocellular carcinoma cell growth through Akt activation: evidence for Akt inhibition in celecoxib-induced apoptosis. *Hepatology (Baltimore, Md.)* 38, 756–768. doi: 10.1053/jhep.2003.50380

Lin, R., Beauparlant, P., Makris, C., Meloche, S., and Hiscott, J. (1996). Phosphorylation of IkappaBalpha in the C-terminal PEST domain by casein kinase II affects intrinsic protein stability. *Mol. Cell. Biol.* 16, 1401–1409. doi: 10.1128/MCB.16.4.1401

Lipniacki, T., Paszek, P., Brasier, A. R. A. R., Luxon, B., and Kimmel, M. (2004). Mathematical model of NF-kappaB regulatory module. *J. Theor. Biol.* 228, 195–215. doi: 10.1016/j.jtbi.2004.01.001

Livak, K. J., and Schmittgen, T. D. (2001). Analysis of relative gene expression data using real-time quantitative PCR and the $2^{-\Delta\Delta CT}$ Method. *Methods (San Diego, Calif.)* 25, 402–408. doi: 10.1006/meth.2001.1262

Luedde, T., and Schwabe, R. F. (2011). NF-κB in the liver–linking injury, fibrosis and hepatocellular carcinoma. *Nat. Rev. Gastroenterol. Hepatol.* 8, 108–118. doi: 10.1038/nrgastro.2010.213

Luo, K. X., Zhu, Y. F., Zhang, L. X., He, H. T., Wang, X. S., and Zhang, L. (1997). *In situ* investigation of Fas/FasL expression in chronic hepatitis B infection and related liver diseases. *J. Viral Hepat.* 4, 303–307. doi: 10.1046/j.1365-2893.1997.00053.x

Lutz, A., Sanwald, J., Thomas, M., Feuer, R., Sawodny, O., Ederer, M., et al. (2014). Interleukin-1β enhances FasL-induced caspase-3/-7 activity without increasing apoptosis in primary mouse hepatocytes. *PLoS ONE* 9:e115603. doi: 10.1371/journal.pone.0115603

Madrigal, A. G., Barth, K., Papadopoulos, G., and Genco, C. A. (2012). Pathogen-mediated proteolysis of the cell death regulator RIPK1 and the host defense modulator RIPK2 in human aortic endothelial cells. *PLoS Pathog.* 8:e1002723. doi: 10.1371/journal.ppat.1002723

Malhi, H., and Gores, G. J. (2008). Cellular and molecular mechanisms of liver injury. *Gastroenterology* 134, 1641–1654. doi: 10.1053/j.gastro.2008.03.002

Marques, P. E., Amaral, S. S., Pires, D. A., Nogueira, L. L., Soriani, F. M., Lima, B. H. F., et al. (2012). Chemokines and mitochondrial products activate neutrophils to amplify organ injury during mouse acute liver failure. *Hepatology (Baltimore, Md.)* 56, 1971–1982. doi: 10.1002/hep.25801

Micheau, O., and Tschopp, J. (2003). Induction of TNF receptor I-mediated apoptosis via two sequential signaling complexes. *Cell* 114, 181–190. doi: 10.1016/S0092-8674(03)00521-X

Mita, A., Hashikura, Y., Tagawa, Y.-I., Nakayama, J., Kawakubo, M., and Miyagawa, S.-i. (2005). Expression of fas ligand by hepatic macrophages in patients with fulminant hepatic failure. *Am. J. Gastroenterol.* 100, 2551–2559. doi: 10.1111/j.1572-0241.2005.00265.x

Motoyama, M., Yamazaki, S., Eto-Kimura, A., Takeshige, K., and Muta, T. (2005). Positive and negative regulation of nuclear factor-κB-mediated transcription by IκB-ζ, an inducible nuclear protein. *J. Biol. Chem.* 280, 7444–7451. doi: 10.1074/jbc.M412738200

Nelson, D. E., Ihekwaba, A. E. C., Elliott, M., Johnson, J. R., Gibney, C. A., Foreman, B. E., et al. (2004). Oscillations in NF-kappaB signaling control the dynamics of gene expression. *Science (New York, N.Y.)* 306, 704–708. doi: 10.1126/science.1099962

Okamoto, K., Iwai, Y., Oh-Hora, M., Yamamoto, M., Morio, T., Aoki, K., et al. (2010). IkappaBzeta regulates T(H)17 development by cooperating with ROR nuclear receptors. *Nature* 464, 1381–1385. doi: 10.1038/nature08922

Perkins, N. D. (2006). Post-translational modifications regulating the activity and function of the nuclear factor kappa B pathway. *Oncogene* 25, 6717–6730. doi: 10.1038/sj.onc.1209937

Rex, J., Albrecht, U., Ehlting, C., Thomas, M., Zanger, U. M., Sawodny, O., et al. (2016). Model-based characterization of inflammatory gene expression patterns of activated macrophages. *PLoS Comput. Biol.* 12:e1005018. doi: 10.1371/journal.pcbi.1005018

Roy, N., Deveraux, Q. L., Takahashi, R., Salvesen, G. S., and Reed, J. C. (1997). The c-IAP-1 and c-IAP-2 proteins are direct inhibitors of specific caspases. *EMBO J.* 16, 6914–6925. doi: 10.1093/emboj/16.23.6914

Ruland, J. (2011). Return to homeostasis: downregulation of NF-κB responses. *Nat. Immunol.* 12, 709–714. doi: 10.1038/ni.2055

Scaffidi, C., Fulda, S., Srinivasan, A., Friesen, C., Li, F., Tomaselli, K. J., et al. (1998). Two CD95 (APO-1/Fas) signaling pathways. *EMBO J.* 17, 1675–1687. doi: 10.1093/emboj/17.6.1675

Schlatter, R., Schmich, K., Lutz, A., Trefzger, J., Sawodny, O., Ederer, M., et al. (2011). Modeling the TNFα-induced apoptosis pathway in hepatocytes. *PLoS ONE* 6:e18646. doi: 10.1371/journal.pone.0018646

Schmich, K., Schlatter, R., Corazza, N., Sá Ferreira, K., Ederer, M., Brunner, T., et al. (2011). Tumor necrosis factor α sensitizes primary murine hepatocytes to Fas/CD95-induced apoptosis in a Bim- and Bid-dependent manner. *Hepatology (Baltimore, Md.)* 53, 282–292. doi: 10.1002/hep.23987

Scott, M. J., Chen, C., Sun, Q., and Billiar, T. R. (2010). Hepatocytes express functional NOD1 and NOD2 receptors: a role for NOD1 in hepatocyte CC and CXC chemokine production. *J. Hepatol.* 53, 693–701. doi: 10.1016/j.jhep.2010.04.026

Seki, E., and Schnabl, B. (2012). Role of innate immunity and the microbiota in liver fibrosis: crosstalk between the liver and gut. *J. Physiol.* 590(Pt 3), 447–458. doi: 10.1113/jphysiol.2011.219691

Sharp, D. A., Lawrence, D. A., and Ashkenazi, A. (2005). Selective knockdown of the long variant of cellular FLICE inhibitory protein augments death receptor-mediated caspase-8 activation and apoptosis. *J. Biol. Chem.* 280, 19401–19409. doi: 10.1074/jbc.M413962200

Skaug, B., Chen, J., Du, F., He, J., Ma, A., and Chen, Z. J. (2011). Direct, noncatalytic mechanism of IKK inhibition by A20. *Mol. Cell* 44, 559–571. doi: 10.1016/j.molcel.2011.09.015

Smale, S. T. (2011). Hierarchies of NF-κB target-gene regulation. *Nat. Immunol.* 12, 689–694. doi: 10.1038/ni.2070

Spurgeon, S. L., Jones, R. C., and Ramakrishnan, R. (2008). High throughput gene expression measurement with real time PCR in a microfluidic dynamic array. *PLoS ONE* 3:e1662. doi: 10.1371/journal.pone.0001662

Streetz, K., Leifeld, L., Grundmann, D., Ramakers, J., Eckert, K., Spengler, U., et al. (2000). Tumor necrosis factor α in the pathogenesis of human and murine fulminant hepatic failure. *Gastroenterology* 119, 446–460. doi: 10.1053/gast.2000.9364

Suda, T., Okazaki, T., Naito, Y., Yokota, T., Arai, N., Ozaki, S., et al. (1995). Expression of the Fas ligand in cells of T cell lineage. *J. Immunol. (Baltimore, Md. : 1950)* 154, 3806–3813.

Sun, S. C., Ganchi, P. A., Ballard, D. W., and Greene, W. C. (1993). NF-kappa B controls expression of inhibitor I kappa B alpha: evidence for an inducible autoregulatory pathway. *Science (New York, N.Y.)* 259, 1912–1915. doi: 10.1126/science.8096091

Sunami, Y., Leithäuser, F., Gul, S., Fiedler, K., Güldiken, N., Espenlaub, S., et al. (2012). Hepatic activation of IKK/NFκB signaling induces liver fibrosis via macrophage-mediated chronic inflammation. *Hepatology (Baltimore, Md.)* 56, 1117–1128. doi: 10.1002/hep.25711

Szabo, G., and Csak, T. (2012). Inflammasomes in liver diseases. *J. Hepatol.* 57, 642–654. doi: 10.1016/j.jhep.2012.03.035

Tacke, F., Luedde, T., and Trautwein, C. (2009). Inflammatory pathways in liver homeostasis and liver injury. *Clin. Rev. Allergy Immunol.* 36, 4–12. doi: 10.1007/s12016-008-8091-0

Tak, P. P., and Firestein, G. S. (2001). NF-kappaB: a key role in inflammatory diseases. *J. Clin. Invest.* 107, 7–11. doi: 10.1172/JCI11830

Takeda, K., Hayakawa, Y., Van Kaer, L., Matsuda, H., Yagita, H., and Okumura, K. (2000). Critical contribution of liver natural killer T cells to a murine model of hepatitis. *Proc. Natl. Acad. Sci. U.S.A.* 97, 5498–5503. doi: 10.1073/pnas.040566697

Takehara, T., Hayashi, N., Tatsumi, T., Kanto, T., Mita, E., Sasaki, Y., et al. (1999). Interleukin 1beta protects mice from Fas-mediated hepatocyte apoptosis and death. *Gastroenterology* 117, 661–668. doi: 10.1016/S0016-5085(99)70460-9

Totzke, G., Essmann, F., Pohlmann, S., Lindenblatt, C., Jänicke, R. U., and Schulze-Osthoff, K. (2006). A novel member of the IκB family, human IκB-ζ, inhibits transactivation of p65 and Its DNA binding. *J. Biol. Chem.* 281, 12645–12654. doi: 10.1074/jbc.M511956200

Tsutsui, H., Kayagaki, N., Kuida, K., Nakano, H., Hayashi, N., Takeda, K., et al. (1999). Caspase-1-independent, Fas/Fas ligand-mediated IL-18 secretion from macrophages causes acute liver injury in mice. *Immunity* 11, 359–367. doi: 10.1016/S1074-7613(00)80111-9

Tsutsui, H., Nakanishi, K., Matsui, K., Higashino, K., Okamura, H., Miyazawa, Y., et al. (1996). IFN-gamma-inducing factor up-regulates Fas ligand-mediated cytotoxic activity of murine natural killer cell clones. *J. Immunol.* 157, 3967–3973.

Ulich, T. R., Watson, L. R., Yin, S. M., Guo, K. Z., Wang, P., Thang, H., et al. (1991). The intratracheal administration of endotoxin and cytokines. I. Characterization of LPS-induced IL-1 and TNF mRNA expression and the LPS-, IL-1-, and TNF-induced inflammatory infiltrate. *Am. J. Pathol.* 138, 1485–1496.

Vallabhapurapu, S., and Karin, M. (2009). Regulation and function of NF-kappaB transcription factors in the immune system. *Annu. Rev. Immunol.* 27, 693–733. doi: 10.1146/annurev.immunol.021908.132641

Van Sweringen, H. L., Sakai, N., Tevar, A. D., Burns, J. M., Edwards, M. J., and Lentsch, A. B. (2011). CXC chemokine signaling in the liver: impact on repair and regeneration. *Hepatology (Baltimore, Md.)* 54, 1445–1453. doi: 10.1002/hep.24457

Vane, J. R., Mitchell, J. A., Appleton, I., Tomlinson, A., Bishop-Bailey, D., Croxtall, J., et al. (1994). Inducible isoforms of cyclooxygenase and nitric-oxide synthase in inflammation. *Proc. Natl. Acad. Sci. U.S.A.* 91, 2046–2050. doi: 10.1073/pnas.91.6.2046

Varfolomeev, E. E., and Ashkenazi, A. (2004). Tumor necrosis factor: an apoptosis JuNKie? *Cell* 116, 491–497. doi: 10.1016/S0092-8674(04)00166-7

Verhagen, A. M., Ekert, P. G., Pakusch, M., Silke, J., Connolly, L. M., Reid, G. E., et al. (2000). Identification of DIABLO, a mammalian protein that promotes apoptosis by binding to and antagonizing IAP proteins. *Cell* 102, 43–53. doi: 10.1016/S0092-8674(00)00009-X

Verma, G., and Datta, M. (2010). IL-1beta induces ER stress in a JNK dependent manner that determines cell death in human pancreatic epithelial MIA PaCa-2 cells. *Apoptosis* 15, 864–876. doi: 10.1007/s10495-010-0498-4

Walter, D., Schmich, K., Vogel, S., Pick, R., Kaufmann, T., Hochmuth, F. C., et al. (2008). Switch from type II to I Fas/CD95 death signaling on *in vitro* culturing of primary hepatocytes. *Hepatology (Baltimore, Md.)* 48, 1942–1953. doi: 10.1002/hep.22541

Wang, D., and Baldwin, a. S. (1998). Activation of nuclear factor-kappaB-dependent transcription by tumor necrosis factor-alpha is mediated through phosphorylation of RelA/p65 on serine 529. *J. Biol. Chem.* 273, 29411–29416. doi: 10.1074/jbc.273.45.29411

Willoughby, D. A., Moore, A. R., and Colville-Nash, P. R. (2000). COX-1, COX-2, and COX-3 and the future treatment of chronic inflammatory disease. *Lancet* 355, 646–648. doi: 10.1016/S0140-6736(99)12031-2

Yamazaki, S., Muta, T., and Takeshige, K. (2001). A novel IkappaB protein, IkappaB-zeta, induced by proinflammatory stimuli, negatively regulates nuclear factor-kappaB in the nuclei. *J. Biol. Chem.* 276, 27657–27662. doi: 10.1074/jbc.M103426200

Yang, X.-D., Huang, B., Li, M., Lamb, A., Kelleher, N. L., and Chen, L.-F. (2009). Negative regulation of NF-kappaB action by Set9-mediated lysine methylation of the RelA subunit. *EMBO J.* 28, 1055–1066. doi: 10.1038/emboj.2009.55

Zhong, H., SuYang, H., Erdjument-Bromage, H., Tempst, P., and Ghosh, S. (1997). The transcriptional activity of NF-kappaB is regulated by the IkappaB-associated PKAc subunit through a cyclic AMP-independent mechanism. *Cell* 89, 413–424. doi: 10.1016/S0092-8674(00)80222-6

Zimmermann, H. W., Trautwein, C., and Tacke, F. (2012). Functional role of monocytes and macrophages for the inflammatory response in acute liver injury. *Front. Physiol.* 3:56. doi: 10.3389/fphys.2012.00056

Zou, H., Li, Y., Liu, X., and Wang, X. (1999). An APAf-1/cytochrome C multimeric complex is a functional apoptosome that activates procaspase-9. *J. Biol. Chem.* 274, 11549–11556. doi: 10.1074/jbc.274.17.11549

7

Ion Imbalance is Involved in the Mechanisms of Liver Oxidative Damage in Rats Exposed to Glyphosate

*Juan Tang[1], Ping Hu[1], Yansen Li[1], Tin-Tin Win-Shwe[2] and Chunmei Li[1]**

[1] Jiangsu Province Key Laboratory of Gastrointestinal Nutrition and Animal Health, College of Animal Science and Technology, Nanjing Agricultural University, Nanjing, China, [2] Health Effect Assessment Section Center for Health and Environmental Risk Research, National Institute for Environmental Studies, Tsukuba, Japan

***Correspondence:**
Chunmei Li
chunmeili@njau.edu.cn;
lichunmei74@gmail.com

Glyphosate (N-phosphonomethyl-glycine, GLP) is the most popular herbicide used worldwide. This study aimed to investigate the effects of glyphosate on rats' liver function and induction of pathological changes in ion levels and oxidative stress in hepatic tissue. Sprague-Dawley rats were treated orally with 0, 5, 50, and 500 mg/kg body weight of the GLP. After 5 weeks of treatment, blood and liver samples were analyzed for biochemical and histomorphological parameters. The various mineral elements content in the organs of the rats were also measured. Significant decreases were shown in the weights of body, liver, kidney and spleen between the control and treatment groups. Changes also happened in the histomorphology of the liver and kidney tissue of GLP-treated rats. The GLP resulted in an elevated level of glutamic-oxalacetic transaminase (GOT), glutamic-pyruvic transaminase (GPT) and IL-1β in the serum. Besides, decreased total superoxide dismutase (T-SOD) activity and increased malondialdehyde (MDA) contents in the serum, liver, and kidney indicated the presence of oxidative stress. Moreover, increase of hydrogen peroxide (H_2O_2) level and catalase (CAT) activity in the serum and liver and decrease of glutathione (GSH) and lutathione peroxidase (GSH-Px) activity in the kidney tissue further confirmed the occurrence of oxidative stress. The results of RT-PCR showed that the mRNA expressions of *IL-1α*, *IL-1β*, *IL-6*, *MAPK3*, *NF-κB*, *SIRT1*, *TNF-α*, *Keap1*, *GPX2,* and *Caspase-3* were significantly increased in the GLP-treated groups compared to the control group. Furthermore, *PPARα*, *DGAT*, *SREBP1c,* and *SCD1* mRNA expressions were also remarkably increased in the GLP-treated groups compared to the control group. In addition, aluminum (Al), iron (Fe), copper (Cu), zinc (Zn), and magnesium (Mg) levels were showed a significant difference reduction or increase in rat liver, kidney, spleen, lung, heart, muscle, brain, and fat tissues. These results suggested that glyphosate caused obvious damage to rats' liver and caused various mineral elements content imbalances in various organs of rats. Ion imbalance could weaken antioxidant capacity and involve in the mechanism of liver oxidative damage caused by GLP.

Keywords: ion, oxidative stress, liver, glyphosate, rat

INTRODUCTION

Glyphosate (GLP) is a non-selective, post-emergence herbicide used for weed control in various crops, especially in rice, maize and soybean (Coutinho et al., 2005). Eighty percent of genetically modified crops were GLP-resistant plants, such as corn, soy, cotton and canola and so on (Williams et al., 2000). American farmers have widely used anti-GLP crops since 1996 (Frisvold et al., 2010). It means there will be much more glyphosate in soil and water environment. Study has reported that GLP and its metabolite such as aminomethylphosphonic acid (AMPA) and formaldehyde were found in the soil and rivers (Temple and Smith, 1992). It has been extensively demonstrated that exposure to GLP leads to oxidative stress in several tissue, including the livers and kidneys (Beuret et al., 2005; El-Shenawy, 2009; Modesto and Martinez, 2010; Larsen et al., 2012; Cattani et al., 2014).

GLP can chelate the iron (Fe) and aluminum (Al), which interferes with ion assimilation in the plant (Eker et al., 2006; Bellaloui et al., 2009). GLP also change the ion levels in fish by chelated with them (Ayoola, 2008; Samsel and Seneff, 2013). Al is widespread in soil, water, and air, and is also the most widely used metal by humans (Kumar and Gill, 2009). Al is mainly absorbed by the gastrointestinal tract and easily accumulates in liver cells and organelles (e.g., macrophages and lysosomes) (Krewski et al., 2007; Kumar and Gill, 2009). Some scholars believe that Al accumulation does not causes significant hepatotoxicity, because it can be eliminated by hepatocytes (Li et al., 2011). However, most studies reported that Al causes central nervous system toxicity, hepatotoxicity, nephrotoxicity, cardiotoxicity and osteoporosis to body tissue (Crisponi et al., 2013; Geyikoglu et al., 2013). Iron (Fe) is not only an important micronutrient, but also a redox reaction of the biocatalyst, and when the transition metal reaches the transition level, is conducive to the production of reactive oxygen species (Aust et al., 1985). Zinc (Zn) as an antioxidant, involved in cell membrane stabilization, copper/zinc superoxide dismutase (Cu/Zn SOD) structure and metallothionein induction. Zn deficiency can damage the oxidant defense system and cause oxidative damage to cells or tissue (Oteiza et al., 1999). Therefore, it is important to study whether GLP can effects the ion content in the liver and other organs of rats.

The aim of this study was designed to evaluate liver histomorphological changes, oxidant/antioxidant status, levels of inflammatory markers, lipid metabolism factors, and to investigate ion levels of Al, Fe, Cu, Zn, and Mg ion levels in GLP-exposed rats' liver tissues. The specific mechanism between liver and other organs damage and ion imbalance need to be further studied.

MATERIALS AND METHODS

Chemicals

Glyphosate, N-(phosphonomethy) glycine (GLP), was purchased from Shanghai Ryon Biological Technology Co. Ltd (Shanghai, China).

Animals and Ethic Statement

Eight week-of-age male Sprague-Dawley rats weighting 180–220 g were purchased from the Nanjing Qinglongshan Experimental Animal Center (Nanjing, China). Prior to experiment, all rats were allowed to acclimate for at least 1 week. All rats were housed in separate cages under environmental conditions (23 ± 2°C, 50 ± 10% relative humidity, 12-h light: dark cycle) and had unrestricted access to food and water throughout the period of the study. Animal care and use were conducted in accordance with the National Institute of Health Guidelines for Animal Care and the Committee of Animal Research Institute, Nanjing Agricultural University, China. At the same time, the study also received ethical approval from the committee.

Animal Treatment and Sample Collection

Rats were randomly assigned to 4 groups (n = 8/group). The rats were orally administered with glyphosate (5, 50, and 500 mg/kg body weight) daily for 35 days at 9 AM. Glyphosate dose selection was according to GLP no-observed adverse effect level (NOAEL) of 1,000 mg/kg/day for developmental toxicity (Williams et al., 2000) and equivalent to 1/1,000, 1/100, and 1/10 of LD 50 in rats (Larini, 1999; Benedetti et al., 2004). GLP was orally administered at a volume of 0.5 ml/kg. Rats orally administered with distilled water were used as the control group. Twenty four hours after the last gavage, rats were weighed and decapitated. Blood samples were collected from the jugular vein and placed at 37°C for 1 h before being centrifuged (3,500 rpm, 15 min, 4°C) for biochemical assays. The liver, kidney, spleen, heart, lungs, brain, adrenal glands, muscle and fat tissue were collected, rinsed twice in phosphate-buffered saline (PBS pH 7.4), use the filter paper to dry the PBS and then accurately weigh and weighed for further examinations. One piece of liver and right kidney was used for morphometric analysis and another piece was used to prepare homogenates for analyses of tissue oxidative indexes, or frozen in liquid nitrogen for subsequent qualitative reverse transcription polymerase chain reaction (RT-PCR). The organ index is calculated as follows:

$$\text{Organ index (g/gBW)} = \text{Organ absolute weight (g)/Body weight (g)} \times 100\%$$

Histological Preparation

Samples of tissue (livers and kidneys) were obtained from the animals and fixed in 4% formaldehyde solution for 24 h then dehydrated in an ascending series of alcohol, clarified using xylene, and embedded in paraffin. Paraffin were sectioned into 5 μm slices and stained with hematoxylin-eosin (HE) for microscopic examination. The score system was used to evaluate the hepatic and renal damages (Ishak et al., 1995; Zheng et al., 2005; Klopfleisch, 2013). Briefly, the scores of liver sections graded on a 0–4 scale for lobular inflammation, focal necrosis and mononuclear cell infiltration, and kidney graded on a 0–4 scale for proximal and distal tubular necrosis, glomerular cellularity, and glomerular necrosis (where 0 represents no abnormality, and 1, 2, 3, and 4 represent mild, moderate, moderately severe, and severe abnormalities, respectively).

Biochemical Evaluation

For enzymes determination, the suspension of liver, kidney and the blood samples were centrifuged at 3,500 rpm for 15 min. The homogenate and serum were collected and used for liver function assessment including measurements of the enzymes glutamic-oxalacetic transaminase (GOT), glutamic-pyruvic transaminase (GPT), total superoxide dismutase (T-SOD), malondialdehyde (MDA), hydrogen peroxide (H_2O_2), catalase (CAT), glutathione (GSH), glutathione peroxidase (GSH-Px). The activities of SOD, H_2O_2, CAT, GSH, GSH-Px, and the content of MDA were assayed using commercial reagent kits obtained from the Institute of Biological Engineering of Nanjing Jiancheng (Nanjing, China) following the manufacturer's instructions. All operations were done at 4°C.

Analyses of the SOD activity was based on SOD-mediated inhibition of nitrite formation from hydroxyammonium in the presence of O^{2-}generators (xanthine/xanthine oxidase) (Elstner and Heupel, 1976). The total SOD activity expressed as U/mg protein. MDA was evaluated by thiobarbituric acid reactive substances method (TBARS) and expressed as nmol/mg protein (Draper and Hadley, 1990). GSH-PX activity was estimated by the analysis of reduced GSH in the enzymatic reaction (Sedlak and Lindsay, 1968). GSH-PX activity was expressed as U/mg protein. CAT activity was assayed by the method developed by Aebi (Aebi, 1984), and calculated as nM H2O2 consumed/min/mg of tissue protein. Protein concentrations in the supernatant were measured according to the Coomassie Brilliant Blue method. The activity of serum GOT and GPT was assayed according to the method that usually used in clinical examination (Reitman and Frankel, 1957).

Serum Cytokine Measures

Serum levels of IL-1β and IL-6 were determined using a commercially available enzyme-linked immunosorbent assay (ELISA) kit purchased from R&D Systems (Shanghai, China). The results were expressed as pg/mL.

Quantitative RT-PCR (qRT-PCR) Analysis

Total RNA was extracted from the tissue using the reagent box of Total RNA Kit (Invitrogen, Carlsbad, CA, US), according to the manufacturer's instructions. The concentration of RNA was measured by using a spectrophotometer and the purity was ascertained by the A 260/A 280 ratio with a Nanodrop® 8000. Total RNA from each sample was reverse transcribed to cDNA with an Omniscript® Reverse Transcription kit (Takara) with Oligo-dT primers (Takara) according to the manufacturer's instructions and used for RT-PCR. The target fragments were quantified by real-time PCR using a QuantiTectTMSYBR Green® PCR Kit (Roche) with 100 ng of the cDNA template. Each sample was tested in duplicate. The gene expression data were normalized to β-actin expression. The primers used correspond to the rat sequences shown in **Table 1**; primer design was done using Amplify software (TaKaRa, Nanjing, China). For each real-time PCR assay, the threshold cycle Ct was determined for each reaction. Ct values for each gene of interest were normalized to the housekeeping gene (β-action); PCR amplification efficiencies were taken into account by amplifying various amounts of target cDNA for each reaction. The fold differences in mRNA expression of samples were relative to the internal control sample, which was included in all runs.

Ion Concentration

The concentrations of Al, Fe, Cu, Zn, and Mg in the liver, kidney, spleen, lung, heart, muscle, brain, and fat tissue were determined by inductively coupled plasma optical emission spectrometry (Optima 2100 DV; Perkin Elmer, Waltham, MA) using nitric acid–perchloric acid-based wet digestion. Approximately 200 μl or 0.5 g of each sample was digested with nitric acid (75%) and perchloric acid (25%) in a microwave digester (MDS- 81D; CEM Corp., Matthews, NC). We have used the same part of organ from the control and treated animals and accurately weighed.

Statistical Analysis

The data were expressed as mean ± standard error of the mean (SEM) and were analyzed by one-way analysis of variance (ANOVA), followed by Dunnett's multiple comparison tests, which was performed with GraphPad Prismsoftware (GraphPad Software, San Diego, CA, USA). Differences were considered to be statistically significant when the p level was less than 0.05.

RESULTS

Body and Organ Weights

After administration of GLP, there was a significant distinction in rat body weight between the control group and the 500 mg/kg GLP group ($p < 0.05$, **Table 2**). The body weight gain decreased significantly in 50 mg/kg and 500 mg/kg GLP treatment groups compared with the control group ($p < 0.05$). Significant difference was also observed in the average-day-gain and average daily feed intake in GLP treatment groups compared with the control group ($p < 0.05$). Both of the absolute organ weight or the relative organ weight for liver, spleen and kidney showed a significant decrease in the 500 mg/kg GLP group ($p < 0.05$, **Table 2**), which suggested that GLP manifest toxicity principally toward growth and development at the studied dosages.

Histopathologic Evaluation

The liver and kidney histopathological changes were showed in **Figure 1**. The control rats showed hepatic lobules consisting of a central vein surrounded by radiating hepatocytes which were separated and did not exhibit any damage in the tissue (**Figure 1A**). By contrast, the liver sections of GLP-treated rats showed apoptosis of some hepatocyte, focal necrosis and mononuclear cell infiltration in liver tissue. Compared with the control group, after 5 mg/kg of GLP exposure, the rats showed mild periportal expansion and apoptosis of some hepatocyte (**Figure 1B**). In comparison, the livers of rats in the 50 mg/kg and 500 mg/kg GLP-treated groups demonstrated greater levels of structural disorder, apoptosis of some hepatocyte and monocyte infiltration (**Figures 1C,D**).

The HE staining of renal tissue in control rats demonstrated overall integrity of glomerulus surrounded by Bowman capsule

TABLE 1 | Primers used for quantitative real-time PCR.

Gene symbol	Accession No.	Primer sequence (5′ to 3′)	Product size (bp)	40 PCR cycles
IL-1α	NM_017019.1	F: GAGTCGGCAAAGAAATCAAGA R: TTCAGAGACAGATGGTCAATGG	112	95°C for 15 s 60°C for 30 s 72°C for 30 s
IL-1β	NM_031512.2	F: GCCAACAAGTGGTATTCTCCA R: TGCCGTCTTTCATCACACAG	120	95°C for 15 s 60°C for 30 s 72°C for 30 s
IL-6	NM_012589.2	F: AGTTGCCTTCTTGGGACTGA R: ACTGGTCTGTTGTGGGTGGT	102	95°C for 15 s 60°C for 30 s 72°C for 30 s
MAPK3	NM_017347.2	F: CTACACGCAGCTGCAGTACATC R: GTGCGCTGACAGTAGGTTTGA	153	95°C for 15 s 60°C for 30 s 72°C for 30 s
NF-kB	NM_001276711.1	F: CGACGTATTGCTGTGCCTTC R: TTGAGATCTGCCCAGGTGGTA	198	95°C for 15 s 60°C for 30 s 72°C for 30 s
SIRT1	NC_005119.4	F: GAAACCCTCAATTTCTGTTCTGCT R: AATGCGATGCTGACTTCCTTCT	226	95°C for 15 s 60°C for 30 s 72°C for 30 s
TNF-α	NM_012675.3	F: TTCCGTCCCTCTCATACACTG R: AGACACCGCCTGGAGTTCT	149	95°C for 15 s 60°C for 30 s 72°C for 30 s
Keap1	NM_057152.2	F: CATCGGCATCGCCAACTTC R: GCTGGCAGTGTGACAGGTTGA	278	95°C for 15 s 60°C for 30 s 72°C for 30 s
GPx2	NM_183403.2	F: CCGTGCTGATTGAGAATGTG R: AGGGAAGCCGAGAACCACTA	113	95°C for 15 s 60°C for 30 s 72°C for 30 s
Caspase-3	NM_012922	F: AAGCCGAAACTCTTCATC R: TGAGCATTGACACAATACAC	349	95°C for 15 s 60°C for 30 s 72°C for 30 s
PPARα	NM_001145367.1	F: CTCGTGCAGGTCATCAAGAA R: CAGCCCTCTTCATCTCCAAG	158	95°C for 15 s 60°C for 30 s 72°C for 30 s
DGAT	NM_053437.1	F: TCTTCCTACCGGGATGTCAATC R: TCCCTGCAGACACAGCTTG	204	95°C for 15 s 60°C for 30 s 72°C for 30 s
SREBP1c	NM_001271207.1	F: GCCATGGATTGCACATTG R: TGTGTCTCCTGTCTCACCCC	187	95°C for 15 s 60°C for 30 s 72°C for 30 s
SCD1	NM_009127.4	F: CCTTAACCCTGAGATCCCGTAGA R: AGCCCATAAAAGATTTCTGCAAA	237	95°C for 15 s 60°C for 30 s 72°C for 30 s
FAS	NM_139194.2	F: GGACATGGTCACAGACGATGAC R: GGAGGCGTCGAACTTGGA	279	95°C for 15 s 60°C for 30 s 72°C for 30 s
β-actin	NM_031144.3	F:AGCCATGTACGTAGCCATCC R:CTCTCAGCTGTGGTGGTGAA	227	95°C for 15 s 60°C for 30 s 72°C for 30 s

and convoluted tubules (**Figure 1E**). In comparison with control kidney, GLP administration induced markable histological changes, including proximal and distal tubular necrosis and glomerular toxicity (**Figures 1F–H**). And the histologic score of hepatic and renal damages was significantly increased in the both GLP-treated groups compared with the control group ($p < 0.01$) (**Figures 1I,J**).

Assessment of Liver Function

To confirm the damage of GLP to liver, the serum GOT and GPT levels, the main enzymes of liver function, were determined. The results showed that the levels of the GOT and GPT were increased in GLP-treated groups compared with the control rats. Furthermore, there was a significant increase in GOT and GPT levels with 500 mg/kg of glyphosate compared with the control group ($p < 0.05$) as shown in **Figures 2A,B**. These results showed that glyphosate can affect hepatic metabolism, causing oxidative damage to the hepatic tissue.

Assessment of Enzyme Levels in the Serum to Test Oxidative Stress

To determine whether the GLP could induce the oxidative stress *in vivo*, we first examined the SOD, CAT, GSH, and GSH-PX activities as well as the level of MDA in the serum. The results showed that SOD activity significantly decreased in the 500 mg/kg GLP-treated group compared to the control ($p < 0.05$). The MDA content showed significant increase in the 50 mg/kg GLP-treated group compared with the control ($p < 0.05$), and significantly increased CAT activity than the control in the 500 mg/kg GLP-treated group compared with the control ($p < 0.05$) (**Table 3**).

Assessment of Enzyme Levels in the Liver and Kidney to Test Oxidative Stress

Liver and kidney are two major organs that suffer from the oxidative stress, since GLP metabolism mainly occurs in the liver and the metabolites discharge in the kidney. After GLP

TABLE 2 | Body weights and organ weights of rats treated with Glyphosate for 5 weeks.

	Control	GLP (mg/kg body weight)		
	0	5	50	500
Number of animals	8	8	8	8
Initial body weight (g)	298.60 ± 5.17	323.30 ± 4.94	313.40 ± 7.12	311.40 ± 8.87
Body weight (g)	388.60 ± 7.08	404.00 ± 5.71	369.30 ± 12.57	351.80 ± 7.74*
Weight gain percentage (%)	30.40 ± 3.18	23.42 ± 1.06	17.38 ± 2.49**	17.29 ± 5.41*
Average daily gain (g)	2.57 ± 0.25	2.09 ± 0.10	1.72 ± 0.20*	1.49 ± 0.17*
Average daily feed intake (g)	3.16 ± 0.05	3.27 ± 0.05	2.86 ± 0.05**	2.98 ± 0.08
Liver (g)	12.94 ± 0.45	12.98 ± 0.36	11.83 ± 0.74	10.66 ± 0.44*
Relative liver (%)	3.51 ± 0.07	3.30 ± 0.10	3.20 ± 0.21	2.95 ± 0.09*
Spleen (g)	0.77 ± 0.04	0.71 ± 0.03	0.76 ± 0.06	0.59 ± 0.04*
Relative Spleen (%)	0.21 ± 0.01	0.18 ± 0.01	0.20 ± 0.01	0.16 ± 0.01*
Kidney (g)	1.19 ± 0.04	1.27 ± 0.03	1.18 ± 0.07	1.00 ± 0.02*
Relative Kidney (%)	0.33 ± 0.01	0.32 ± 0.01	0.31 ± 0.01	0.29 ± 0.01*
Heart (g)	1.29 ± 0.05	1.40 ± 0.08	1.22 ± 0.12	1.16 ± 0.07
Relative Heart (%)	0.34 ± 0.01	0.36 ± 0.02	0.34 ± 0.04	0.33 ± 0.02
Lung (g)	2.33 ± 0.08	2.60 ± 0.12	2.40 ± 0.17	2.30 ± 0.10
Relative Lung (%)	0.61 ± 0.02	0.64 ± 0.03	0.69 ± 0.06	0.66 ± 0.03
Adrenal (g)	0.033 ± 0.002	0.034 ± 0.003	0.036 ± 0.003	0.038 ± 0.004
Relative Adrenal (%)	0.009 ± 0.001	0.009 ± 0.001	0.011 ± 0.001	0.011 ± 0.001

*The values shown are the mean ± SEM of 8 animals per group. Compared to control; *p < 0.05, **p < 0.01.*

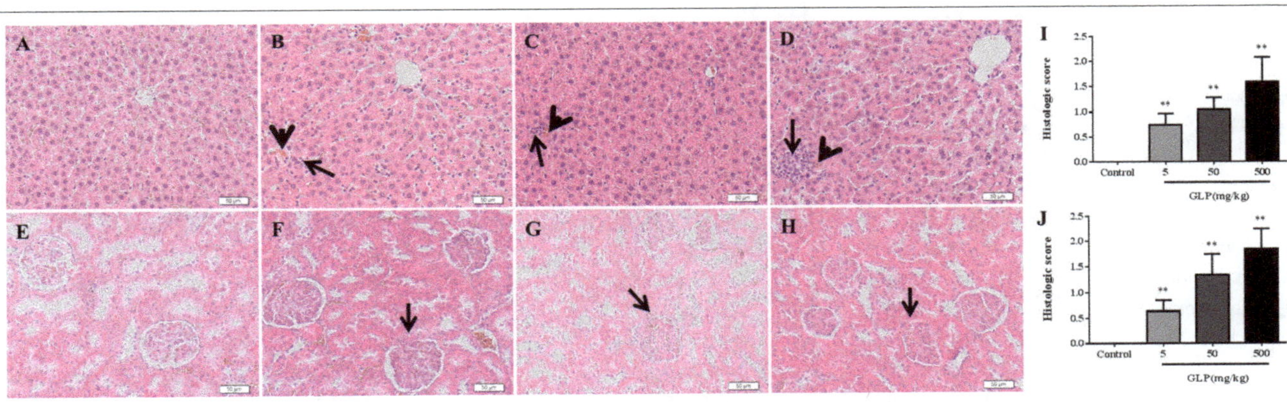

FIGURE 1 | Histopathological changes in the livers and kidneys of male rats following oral GLP administration through Hematoxylin and eosin staining. 200 × magnification. **(A)** Normal liver section. Hepatic lobules consisting of a central vein surrounded by radiating hepatocytes which were separated; **(B–D)** GLP (5, 50, and 500 mg/kg/day) treated presenting periportal expansion, structural disorder, monocyte infiltration (arrows), and congestion (arrowheads). **(E)** Normal kidney section. No signs of kidney damage were observed in the kidney of controls; **(F–H)** GLP (5, 50, and 500 mg/kg/day) treated presenting proximal and distal tubular necrosis and glomerular toxicity (arrows). **(I,J)** The hepatic and renal damages histologic score evaluating. Data shown are mean ± SEM of six liver sections in each group. Compared to control; $^{**}p < 0.01$.

exposure, SOD activity in the 500 mg/kg GLP-treated group showed significant decrease in the liver compared with the control ($p < 0.05$). However, the level of H_2O_2 in the 500 mg/kg GLP-treated group significantly increased compared with the control group ($p < 0.05$) (**Table 3**).

Next, the activity of antioxidant enzymes in the kidney was examined. As shown in **Table 3**, the MDA content in the 5 mg/kg GLP-treated group showed significant increase compared with the control group ($p < 0.01$). The SOD and GSH-PX activities were significantly decreased in the 500 mg/kg GLP-treated groups compared with the control group ($p < 0.05$). And the GSH activity also showed significant decrease in the 50 mg/kg GLP-treated groups compared with the control group ($p < 0.05$). However, there was no difference for the H_2O_2 and CAT activities between the control and treatment groups (**Table 3**).

Serum IL-1β and IL-6 Levels

The concentrations of inflammatory mediators IL-1β and IL-6 in serum were determined as shown in the **Figure 3**. The level of IL-1β has a significant increase in the 500 mg/kg GLP-treated group compared with the control rats ($p < 0.05$) (**Figures 3A,B**).

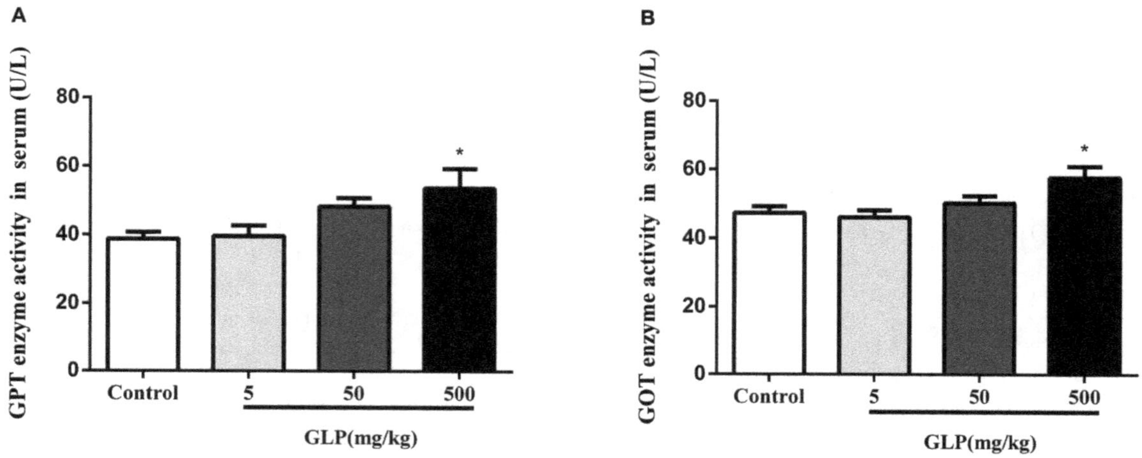

FIGURE 2 | Effect of GLP treatment on GPT **(A)** and GOT **(B)** enzyme activities in the serum. Data shown are mean ± SEM of eight animals in each group. Compared to control; $^{*}p < 0.05$.

TABLE 3 | Effects of GLP on antioxidant enzyme activities and lipid peroxidation levels in serum, liver, and kidney of rats.

	Control	GLP (mg/kg body weight)		
	0	5	50	500
SERUM				
SOD (U/mL)	13.29 ± 0.16	13.01 ± 0.58	12.89 ± 0.46	11.30 ± 0.28*
MDA (nmol/mL)	20.72 ± 2.16	22.06 ± 2.03	32.38 ± 2.00**	23.23 ± 1.99
H_2O_2 (nmol/mL)	113.50 ± 10.05	113.80 ± 8.87	117.50 ± 6.63	134.30 ± 7.45
CAT (U/mL)	28.33 ± 1.61	28.66 ± 2.22	30.51 ± 1.52	36.56 ± 1.60*
GSH (mg/L)	536.30 ± 22.76	431.90 ± 46.45	446.20 ± 52.51	423.40 ± 47.15
GSH-PX (U/L)	378.20 ± 37.47	400.80 ± 28.74	429.00 ± 37.64	453.00 ± 13.76
LIVER				
SOD (U/mgprot)	49.77 ± 2.06	50.30 ± 2.32	47.08 ± 1.49	41.53 ± 1.19*
MDA (nmol/mgprot)	1.93 ± 0.06	1.89 ± 0.08	1.86 ± 0.08	2.08 ± 0.07
H_2O_2 (nmol/mgprot)	5.10 ± 0.26	5.42 ± 0.27	5.90 ± 0.23	6.27 ± 0.14*
CAT (U/mgprot)	12.04 ± 0.68	13.01 ± 1.61	14.50 ± 1.22	14.48 ± 1.20
GSH (mg/gprot)	316.40 ± 27.98	342.20 ± 26.16	272.90 ± 25.01	357.80 ± 33.52
GSH-PX (U/mgprot)	64.09 ± 5.76	63.90 ± 7.62	56.43 ± 7.82	46.74 ± 4.39
KIDNEY				
SOD (U/mgprot)	97.67 ± 4.51	87.62 ± 6.51	75.10 ± 4.17*	73.06 ± 3.31*
MDA (nmol/mgprot)	1.87 ± 0.20	3.91 ± 0.25**	3.015 ± 0.49	3.026 ± 0.40
H_2O_2 (nmol/mgprot)	5.28 ± 0.34	6.03 ± 0.63	6.68 ± 0.46	5.58 ± 0.37
CAT (U/mgprot)	764.20 ± 38.35	873.70 ± 66.49	865.90 ± 83.28	819.60 ± 54.81
GSH (mg/gprot)	7.70 ± 1.85	4.31 ± 0.45	2.76 ± 1.06*	4.64 ± 0.75
GSH-PX (U/mgprot)	480.00 ± 19.96	421.80 ± 38.47	342.20 ± 40.60*	297.00 ± 36.08**

The values shown are the mean ± SEM of 8 animals per group. Compared to control; $^{*}p < 0.05$, $^{**}p < 0.01$.

Expression of mRNA Levels for Inflammation Related Genes in the Liver

We investigated the effects of GLP involved in the inflammatory response in the liver tissue (**Figure 4A**). Hepatic *IL-1α and IL-1β* mRNA expression were significantly increased after GLP exposure compared with the control group ($p < 0.05$); *IL-6, MAPK3, SIRT1, TNF-α, GPX2,* and *Caspase-3* mRNA expression were significantly increased in the 50 mg/kg and 500 mg/kg GLP-treated group compared with the control group ($p < 0.05$); *NF-κB* mRNA expression showed a significant increase in the 50 mg/kg GLP-treated group compared with the control group ($p < 0.05$); at the same time, we also observed a significant increase in *Keap1* mRNA expression in 5 mg/kg GLP-treated group compared with the control group ($p < 0.05$).

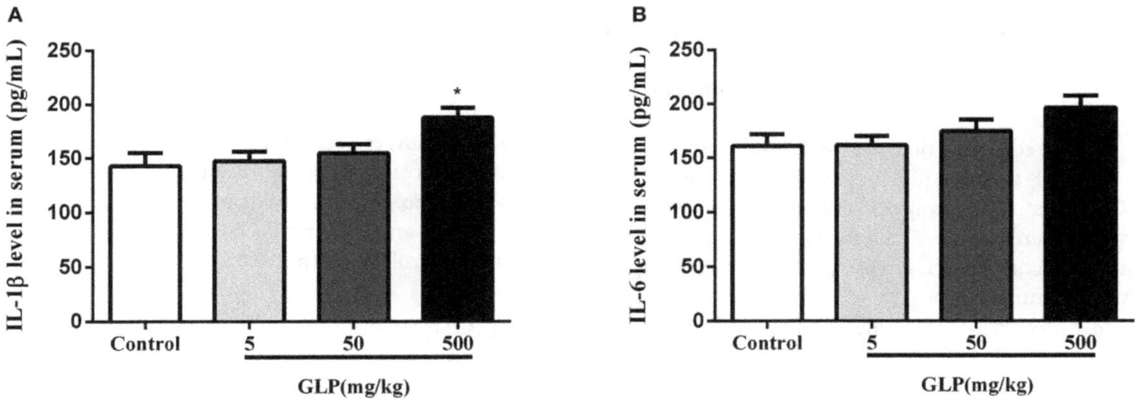

FIGURE 3 | The level of IL-1β **(A)** and IL-6 **(B)** in the serum was assayed by ELISA. Data shown are mean ± SEM of eight animals in each group. Compared to control; *$p < 0.05$.

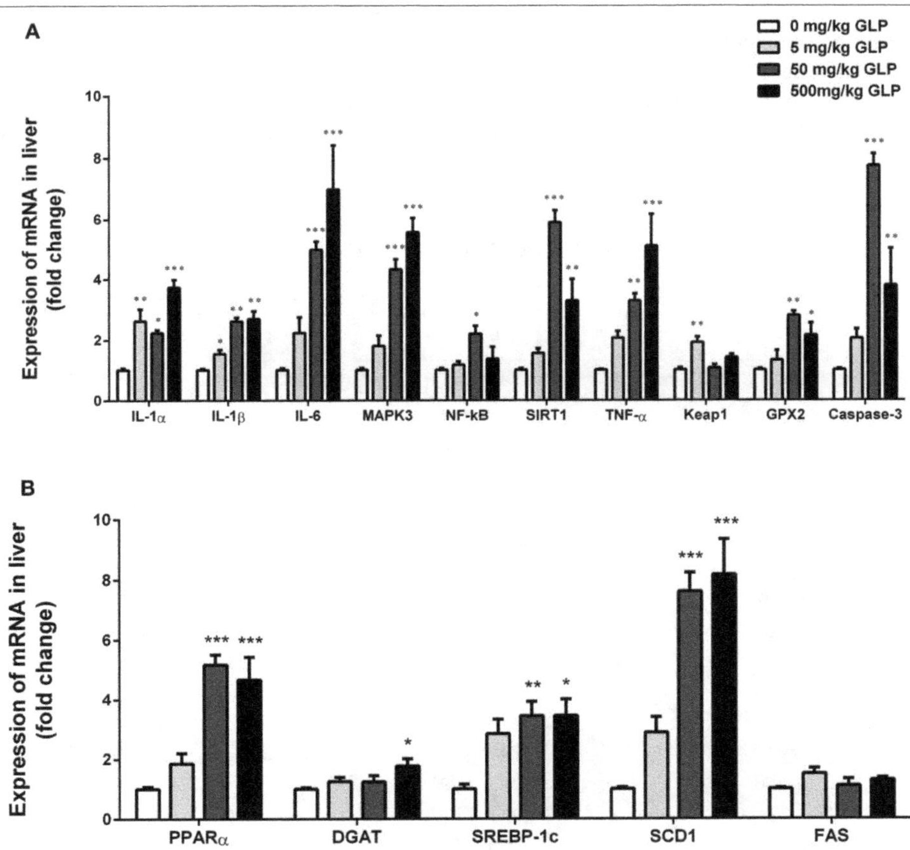

FIGURE 4 | Real-time RT-PCR analyses of IL-1α, IL-1β, IL-6, MAPK3, NF-kB, SIRT1, TNF-α, Keap1, GPX2, and Caspase-3 mRNA of liver **(A)**. Real-time RT-PCR analyses of PPARα, DGAT, SREBP1c, SCD1, and FAS mRNA of liver **(B)**. Data shown are mean ± SEM of eight animals in each group. Compared to control; *$p < 0.05$, **$p < 0.01$ and ***$p < 0.001$.

Expression of mRNA Levels for Lipid Metabolism Related Genes in the Liver

Compared with the control group, *PPARα*, *SREBP1c*, and *SCD1* mRNA expression were significantly increased in the 50 mg/kg and 500 mg/kg GLP treatment rats ($p < 0.05$); *DGAT* mRNA expression was significantly increased in the 500 mg/kg GLP-treated group compared with the control group ($p < 0.05$) (**Figure 4B**).

Concentrations of Ions in Liver, Kidney, Spleen, Heart, Lung, Brain, Muscle, and Fat

Concentrations of Al, Fe, Cu, Zn, and Mg in the liver, kidney, spleen, lung, heart, muscle, brain and fat were presented in **Tables 4, 5**.

In liver, compared with the control group, Al and Zn concentrations were significantly increased in 50 mg/kg and 500 mg/kg GLP treatment group ($p < 0.05$); Fe concentration was significantly increased in 5 mg/kg GLP treatment group ($p < 0.05$) and Mn concentration was significantly increased in 500 mg/kg GLP treatment group ($p < 0.05$); Mo concentration was significantly decreased in 5 mg/kg and 50 mg/kg GLP treatment group ($p < 0.05$) (**Table 4**).

In kidney, concentrations of Fe level was significantly increased in 50 mg/kg GLP treatment group compared with the control group ($p < 0.05$) (**Table 4**).

In spleen, Fe content showed significant increase in 50 mg/kg GLP treatment group compared with the control group ($p < 0.05$) (**Table 4**).

In lung, Al concentration was significantly decreased in 5 mg/kg and 50 mg/kg GLP treatment groups compared with the control group ($p < 0.05$); Fe concentration was significantly increased in 500 mg/kg GLP treatment group compared with the control group ($p < 0.05$) (**Table 5**).

In brain, Cu content was significantly increased in 500 mg/kg GLP treatment group compared with the control group ($p < 0.05$); Mg concentration significantly increased in 50 mg/kg and 500 mg/kg GLP treatment group compared with the control group ($p < 0.05$) (**Table 5**).

In muscle, Al concentration was significantly decreased in 500 mg/kg GLP treatment group ($p < 0.05$) (**Table 5**).

In fat tissue, concentrations of Cu was significantly increased in 50 mg/kg and 500 mg/kg GLP treatment groups compared with the control group ($p < 0.05$) (**Table 5**).

DISCUSSION

The present study demonstrated that GLP had an adverse effect on the histomorphology, inflammation, oxidative stress, lipid metabolism and ion concentration in adult male rats, and then discussed the relationship between them. This is the first report about the effects of GLP exposure on Al, Fe, Cu, Zn, and Mg content in main tissues of rats. Also we firstly revealed the connection between dysregulation of ion content and liver injury in rats exposed to GLP.

The results of our study showed that exposure to GLP for 35 days led to a significant reduction in body weight, body weight gain, average daily gain, and liver, spleen and kidney

TABLE 4 | The concentrations of Al, Fe, Cu, Zn, and Mg in the liver, kidney, spleen, and heart of rats.

	Control	GLP (mg/kg body weight)		
	0	5	50	500
LIVER				
Al (mg/kg)	1.75 ± 0.13	2.22 ± 0.14	2.88 ± 0.33*	3.14 ± 0.45*
Fe (mg/kg)	189.00 ± 12.56	244.0 ± 13.60*	218.10 ± 10.44	233.70 ± 13.64
Cu (mg/kg)	8.47 ± 0.13	8.14 ± 0.32	8.06 ± 0.15	8.64 ± 0.30
Zn (mg/kg)	63.45 ± 0.86	63.12 ± 3.46	72.24 ± 1.70*	73.46 ± 2.24*
Mg (mg/kg)	614.30 ± 12.87	579.60 ± 23.19	592.10 ± 11.77	608.90 ± 18.79
KIDNEY				
Al (mg/kg)	2.20 ± 0.37	2.52 ± 0.15	2.62 ± 0.33	2.53 ± 0.62
Fe (mg/kg)	150.80 ± 5.64	163.10 ± 7.22	216.70 ± 25.09*	151.00 ± 16.76
Cu (mg/kg)	11.15 ± 0.73	11.49 ± 0.34	11.45 ± 0.43	11.09 ± 0.52
Zn (mg/kg)	59.15 ± 3.53	58.93 ± 2.70	62.55 ± 1.61	56.06 ± 2.18
Mg (mg/kg)	593.90 ± 24.84	605.30 ± 27.81	669.20 ± 20.71	582.40 ± 15.86
SPLEEN				
Al (mg/kg)	10.27 ± 0.66	10.05 ± 1.09	9.37 ± 0.83	10.31 ± 0.68
Fe (mg/kg)	1162.00 ± 208.00	1704.00 ± 230.30	2049.00 ± 188.10*	1466.00 ± 98.26
Cu (mg/kg)	7.45 ± 0.35	7.15 ± 0.50	7.76 ± 0.35	7.16 ± 0.15
Zn (mg/kg)	117.10 ± 2.53	120.30 ± 11.39	111.60 ± 7.23	112.50 ± 4.94
Mg (mg/kg)	1185.00 ± 34.60	1182.00 ± 26.26	1240.00 ± 45.99	1159.00 ± 29.09
HEART				
Al (mg/kg)	7.07 ± 0.59	7.97 ± 0.37	7.43 ± 0.43	7.30 ± 1.04
Fe (mg/kg)	321.30 ± 11.96	367.70 ± 37.90	401.20 ± 27.08	313.20 ± 25.61
Cu (mg/kg)	20.58 ± 0.79	18.74 ± 0.27	18.63 ± 0.88	18.44 ± 0.47
Zn (mg/kg)	88.82 ± 5.52	79.85 ± 2.45	82.80 ± 5.42	78.39 ± 10.11
Mg (mg/kg)	1131.00 ± 24.37	1059.00 ± 40.66	1039.00 ± 56.45	987.80 ± 33.74

*The values shown are the mean ± SEM of 8 animals per group. Compared to control; *p < 0.05.*

TABLE 5 | The concentrations of Al, Fe, Cu, Zn, and Mg in the lung, brain, muscle and fat of rats.

	Control	GLP (mg/kg body weight)		
	0	5	50	500
LUNG				
Al (mg/kg)	26.55 ± 1.14	21.93 ± 1.05*	20.43 ± 0.71**	23.27 ± 1.52
Fe (mg/kg)	362.30 ± 31.16	446.00 ± 32.30	421.40 ± 35.80	647.30 ± 74.77**
Cu (mg/kg)	10.31 ± 0.27	10.13 ± 0.46	8.92 ± 0.40	9.94 ± 0.83
Zn (mg/kg)	211.00 ± 14.07	236.50 ± 14.07	187.10 ± 6.99	244.90 ± 20.62
Mg (mg/kg)	1133.00 ± 17.40	1114.00 ± 18.28	1045.00 ± 21.90	1016.00 ± 63.47
BRAIN				
Al (mg/kg)	4.74 ± 1.16	5.08 ± 0.73	5.38 ± 0.55	4.17 ± 0.24
Fe (mg/kg)	40.79 ± 0.59	50.21 ± 6.04	47.38 ± 2.20	53.01 ± 1.49
Cu (mg/kg)	4.08 ± 0.04	4.50 ± 0.06	5.35 ± 0.59	5.70 ± 0.24*
Zn (mg/kg)	35.59 ± 1.36	37.82 ± 1.08	51.28 ± 8.54	39.62 ± 1.71
Mg (mg/kg)	357.60 ± 8.83	357.90 ± 12.81	415.40 ± 3.05**	416.50 ± 6.58**
MUSCLE				
Al (mg/kg)	7.52 ± 0.55	7.54 ± 0.44	6.56 ± 0.54	5.48 ± 0.20*
Fe (mg/kg)	52.76 ± 2.45	57.89 ± 6.47	54.62 ± 4.48	72.62 ± 22.37
Cu (mg/kg)	3.68 ± 0.27	3.47 ± 0.24	3.51 ± 0.35	3.46 ± 0.15
Zn (mg/kg)	53.05 ± 4.89	53.28 ± 2.37	55.79 ± 3.83	58.50 ± 6.08
Mg (mg/kg)	1313.00 ± 14.13	1197.00 ± 26.59	1262.00 ± 33.24	1223.00 ± 55.23
FAT				
Al (mg/kg)	3.22 ± 0.29	2.37 ± 0.57	4.09 ± 0.40	3.23 ± 0.15
Fe (mg/kg)	11.16 ± 1.33	10.92 ± 4.01	16.44 ± 2.33	14.41 ± 1.82
Cu (mg/kg)	0.29 ± 0.05	0.35 ± 0.10	0.53 ± 0.03*	0.61 ± 0.04**
Zn (mg/kg)	5.65 ± 0.81	5.35 ± 0.53	6.36 ± 0.70	6.27 ± 1.02
Mg (mg/kg)	25.49 ± 1.25	25.99 ± 2.60	33.41 ± 1.96	33.57 ± 4.12

*The values shown are the mean ± SEM of 8 animals per group. Compared to control; *$p < 0.05$, **$p < 0.01$.*

coefficient. These results suggested that treated with GLP in male rats for 35 days could affect the growth performance of rats. In addition, our results also showed that exposure to GLP for 35 days caused significant hyperemia, cellular degeneration and necrosis accompanied inflammatory cell infiltration, renal tubular damage and glomerular filtration impairment in rats' hepatic and kidney cells, accompanied by significant increases in GPT and GOT levels. Transaminases are important enzymes and critical enzymes in the biological processes. GPT and GOT levels increased in serum can be a sign of liver damage and disruption of normal liver function (El-Demerdash et al., 2001; Celik and Suzek, 2008). Results showed that GLP caused damage in liver morphology and function.

Oxidative stress refers to the oxidation and anti-oxidation imbalance *in vivo* (Hou et al., 2013). Some studies reported that GLP is an organophosphate herbicide and can induce to oxidative stress and/or an impairment of the antioxidant defensive mechanisms (Larsen et al., 2012). Animals possess an antioxidant defense mechanism composed of enzymes including T-SOD and GPx, as well as non-enzymatic antioxidants including non-protein thiols, especially GSH. When the defenses of the organism are insufficient for neutralizing the ROS, oxidative damage can occur, and one of the most serious types of which is membrane lipid peroxidation (Ahmad et al., 2004). Liver is the major detoxification organ exposed to food or drinks contaminants (Gasnier et al., 2009). GLP-based herbicide has been demonstrated to damage carp or rat hepatocytes at low levels (Szarek et al., 2000; Malatesta et al., 2008).

MDA, the stable metabolite of lipid peroxidation (LPO) products, is a biomarker of LPO (Sun et al., 2001), and is presented as the total level of LPO products (Drewa et al., 2002). MDA can be produced by ozone, which reacts rapidly with cellular structures and generates hydrogen peroxide (Ajamieh et al., 2004). Hepatic SOD activity also can suggest the extent of liver damage (Li et al., 2013). CAT catalyzing the breakdown of H_2O_2 into O_2 and H_2O and catalyzing the oxidation of electron donors (Hou et al., 2013). In addition, GSH provide the major defense against oxidative stress induced cellular damage (Beuret et al., 2005; Ozden and Alpertunga, 2010). In the present study, our results showed that SOD activity significantly decreased in the serum, liver and kidney of the GLP-treated rats compared with the control group. MDA content showed significant increase in the serum and kidney of the GLP-treated rats. At the same time, CAT activity was also significantly increased in the serum of the GLP-treated rats compared with the control group. In addition, H_2O_2 increased in the liver tissue, suggesting *t* that rats were under the oxidant stress. Taken together, the data demonstrated that GLP could result in liver and kidney damage, the decreased SOD activity in the serum and tissue, and the increased MDA level in the serum, indicative of oxidative stress. On the other side, we have also tested the inflammatory Cytokines level in serum, our results showed that the level of IL-1β has a significant increase in the 500 mg/kg GLP-treated group compared with the control rats. Thus, we investigate whether the oxidative stress state of organism has a certain relationship with the inflammation related genes.

Inflammation, manifested as macrophage infiltration of adipose tissue, endoplasmic reticulum stress and oxidative stress (Trayhurn and Wood, 2004). In a few cases, steatosis causes apoptosis, necrosis, generation of oxidative stress and inflammation (Marchesini et al., 2008). Animal models of nonalcoholic fatty liver disease have also suggested a possible role of free fatty acids, not triglycerides, in the hepatocytes as factors promoting hepatocellular injury (Yamaguchi et al., 2007). GLP induced inflammation, which was found to be associated with induction of IL-33, which is known to induce TNF-α, IFN-γ, and IL-13 upon antigen challenge followed by activation and recruitment of inflammatory cells in the airways (Kumar et al., 2014). In this study, the mRNA expression of *IL-1α*, *IL-1β*, *IL-6*, *MAPK3*, *NF-κB*, *SIRT1*, *TNF-α*, *Keap1*, *GPX2* and *Caspase-3* were all increased in GLP treatment group compared with the liver tissue of control rats. Meanwhile, *PPARα*, *SREBP1c*, *DGAT*, and *SCD1* mRNA expressions were significantly increased in GLP treatment rats. It showed that GLP induced liver toxicity is mediated by inflammation, oxidative stress and lipid related pathways. In addition, in the present study, we only focus on changes in inflammatory markers and lipid metabolite levels in the liver, possible changes in kidneys will continue to be verified in future experiments.

Additionally, previous studies also indicated that GLP is bound to the soil constituent Fe, Al amorphous hydroxides and ferric oxides (Piccolo et al., 1994; Day et al., 1997). GLP negatively impact human health, and interference with cytochrome P450 (CYP) enzymes, which play many important roles in the body, meanwhile, GLP chelation of minerals, such as iron and cobalt (Samsel and Seneff, 2013). Al accumulation resulted in obvious damage to hepatic cells, including liver central venous hyperemia, lipid accumulation, and lymphocyte infiltration (Bogdanović et al., 2008; Türkez et al., 2010). Fe is an essential nutritional mineral for all life forms, both of Fe deficiency and excess in Fe also leads to oxidative DNA damage (Ames, 2001). Becaria reported that Al augmented oxidative stress injuries induced by Fe (Becaria et al., 2002). Zn has a relationship with many enzymes in the body (Powell, 2000; Ozturk et al., 2003; Ozdemir and Inanc, 2005). One study has shown that Zn deficiency increases lipid peroxidation in various rat tissues (Ozdemir and Inanc, 2005). Mg plays a pivotal role as an enzyme cofactor in biosynthesis of proteins and mineral administration. It is indispensable to osteogenesis and mineralization of bones (Rahnama and Marciniak, 2002). Subacute Mg deficiency can cause lymphopoietic neoplasms in young rats (Ilicin, 1971). Mg, Zn, and Cu are the cofactors of SOD. Fe and Cu overload could cause oxidative stress damage to rats' kidney and liver (Ozcelik et al., 2003; Bishu and Agarwal, 2006). This study results showed that the concentration of Al, Fe and Zn were significantly increased in GLP-treated rats' liver. Concentrations of Fe were also increased in the kidney, spleen, and lung tissue in GLP-treated rats. Al concentration was decreased in the muscle tissue of GLP-treated rats. In brain and fat tissue, Cu and Mg concentration were increased in GLP-treated rats. However, there showed no dose-dependent effect of GLP was found. Combined, these results suggested that GLP induced the ion-imbalance of Al, Fe, Mg, Cu, and Zn, which will make damage to hepatic cells and liver dysfunction, and the role of ion-imbalance in renal and other organs will continue to be verified in future experiments.

In summary, current study demonstrated that GLP causes obvious damage to rat liver, kidney and caused ion-imbalance in main tissue of rats, and the ion-imbalance is no dose-dependent effect of GLP was found. It may be due to the too large dose range we used in the study of the GLP. Ion imbalance-related oxidative stress may be involved in the mechanism of chronic liver injury caused by GLP. Simultaneously, GLP-induced ion imbalance and oxidative stress may also affect kidney damage. Therefore, the role of ion-imbalance in renal and other organs and its mechanism must be further confirmed by systematic experiments in the future.

AUTHOR CONTRIBUTIONS

JT, PH, YL, T-TW-S, and CL: Performed experiments and interpreted data; CL: Designed the study and provided funding; JT: Wrote the manuscript. All authors read and approved the final version of the manuscript.

ACKNOWLEDGMENTS

This work was supported by the National Key Research and Development Program of China (2016YFD0500505). National Nature Science Foundation of China (No. 31772648) and Graduate research and innovation projects of Jiangsu Province (KYLX15_0554).

REFERENCES

Aebi, H. (1984). Catalase *in vitro*. *Methods Enzymol.* 105, 121–126. doi: 10.1016/S0076-6879(84)05016-3

Ahmad, I., Pacheco, M., and Santos, M. (2004). Enzymatic and nonenzymatic antioxidants as an adaptation to phagocyte-induced damage in *Anguilla anguilla* L. following *in situ* harbor water exposure. *Ecotox. Environ. Saf.* 57, 290–302. doi: 10.1016/S0147-6513(03)00080-0

Ajamieh, H., Menéndez, S., Martínez-Sánchez, G., Candelario-Jalil, E., Re, L., Giuliani, A., et al. (2004). Effects of ozone oxidative preconditioning on nitric oxide generation and cellular redox balance in a rat model of hepatic ischaemia–reperfusion. *Liver Int.* 24, 55–62. doi: 10.1111/j.1478-3231.2004.00885.x

Ames, B. N. (2001). DNA damage from micronutrient deficiencies is likely to be a major cause of cancer. *Mutat. Res.* 475, 7–20. doi: 10.1016/S0027-5107(01)00070-7

Aust, S. D., Morehouse, L. A., and Thomas, C. E. (1985). Role of metals in oxygen radical reactions. *J. Free Radic. Biol. Med.* 1, 3–25. doi: 10.1016/0748-5514(85)90025-X

Ayoola, S. O. (2008). Toxicity of glyphosate herbicide on Nile tilapia (*Oreochromis niloticus*) juvenile. *Afr. J. Agr Res.* 3, 825–834.

Becaria, A., Campbell, A., and Bondy, S. (2002). Aluminum as a toxicant. *Toxicol. Ind. Health.* 18, 309–320. doi: 10.1191/0748233702th157oa

Bellaloui, N., Reddy, K. N., Zablotowicz, R. M., Abbas, H. K., and Abel, C. A. (2009). Effects of glyphosate application on seed iron and root ferric (III) reductase in soybean cultivars. *J. Agr. Food Chem.* 57, 9569–9574. doi: 10.1021/jf902175y

Benedetti, A. L., Vituri Cde, L., Trentin, A. G., Domingues, M. A., and Alvarez-Silva, M. (2004). The effects of sub-chronic exposure of Wistar rats to the herbicide Glyphosate-Biocarb. *Toxicol. Lett.* 153, 227–232. doi: 10.1016/j.toxlet.2004.04.008

Beuret, C. J., Zirulnik, F., and Giménez, M. S. (2005). Effect of the herbicide glyphosate on liver lipoperoxidation in pregnant rats and their fetuses. *Reprod. Toxicol.* 19, 501–504. doi: 10.1016/j.reprotox.2004.09.009

Bishu, K., and Agarwal, R. (2006). Acute injury with intravenous iron and concerns regarding long-term safety. *Clin. J. Am. Soc. Nephro.* 1, S19–S23. doi: 10.2215/CJN.01420406

Bogdanović, M., Janeva, A. B., and Bulat, P. (2008). Histopathological changes in rat liver after a single high dose of aluminium. *Arh. Hig. Rada Toksikol.* 59, 97–101. doi: 10.2478/10004-1254-59-2008-1859

Cattani, D., de Liz Oliveira Cavalli, V. L., Heinz Rieg, C. E., Domingues, J. T., Dal-Cim, T., Tasca, C. I., et al. (2014). Mechanisms underlying the neurotoxicity induced by glyphosate-based herbicide in immature rat hippocampus: involvement of glutamate excitotoxicity. *Toxicology* 320, 34–45. doi: 10.1016/j.tox.2014.03.001

Celik, I., and Suzek, H. (2008). The hematological effects of methyl parathion in rats. *J. Hazard. Mater.* 153, 1117–1121. doi: 10.1016/j.jhazmat.2007.09.067

Coutinho, C., Tanimoto, S., Galli, A., Gustavo, S., Takayama, M., Raquel, B., et al. (2005). Pesticides: action mechanism, degradation and toxicity. *Pesticidas* 15, 65–72.

Crisponi, G., Fanni, D., Gerosa, C., Nemolato, S., Nurchi, V. M., Crespo-Alonso, M., et al. (2013). The meaning of aluminium exposure on human health and aluminium-related diseases. *Biomol. Concepts* 4, 77–87. doi: 10.1515/bmc-2012-0045

Day, G., Hart, B., McKelvie, I., and Beckett, R. (1997). Influence of natural organic matter on the sorption of biocides onto goethite, II. Glyphosate. *Environ. Technol.* 18, 781–794. doi: 10.1080/09593331808616597

Draper, H. H., and Hadley, M. (1990). Malondialdehyde determination as index of lipid Peroxidation. *Methods Enzymol.* 186, 421–431. doi: 10.1016/0076-6879(90)86135-I

Drewa, G., Krzyzynska-Malinowska, E., Wozniak, A., Protas-Drozd, F., Mila-Kierzenkowska, C., Rozwodowska, M., et al. (2002). Activity of superoxide dismutase and catalase and the level of lipid peroxidation products reactive with TBA in patients with psoriasis. *Med. Sci. Monit.* 8, BR338–BR343.

Eker, S., Ozturk, L., Yazici, A., Erenoglu, B., Romheld, V., and Cakmak, I. (2006). Foliar-applied glyphosate substantially reduced uptake and transport of iron and manganese in sunfl ower (*Helianthus annuus* L.) plants. *J. Agric. Food Chem.* 54, 10019–10025. doi: 10.1021/jf0625196

El-Demerdash, F., Yousef, M., and Elagamy, E. (2001). Influence of paraquat, glyphosate, and cadmium on the activity of some serum enzymes and protein electrophoretic behavior (*in vitro*). *J. Environ. Sci. Health B* 36, 29–42. doi: 10.1081/PFC-100000914

El-Shenawy, N. S. (2009). Oxidative stress responses of rats exposed to Roundup and its active ingredient glyphosate. *Environ. Toxicol. Pharmacol.* 28, 379–385. doi: 10.1016/j.etap.2009.06.001

Elstner, E. F., and Heupel, A. (1976). Inhibition of nitrite formation from hydroxylammoniumchloride: a simple assay for superoxide dismutase. *Anal. Biochem.* 70, 616–620. doi: 10.1016/0003-2697(76)90488-7

Frisvold, G. B., Hurley, T. M., and Mitchell, P. D. (2010). Overview: herbicide resistant crops—diffusion, benefits, pricing and resistance management. *AgBioForum* 12, 244–248.

Gasnier, C., Dumont, C., Benachour, N., Clair, E., Chagnon, M.-C., and Séralini, G.-E. (2009). Glyphosate-based herbicides are toxic and endocrine disruptors in human cell lines. *Toxicology* 262, 184–191. doi: 10.1016/j.tox.2009.06.006

Geyikoglu, F., Turkez, H., Bakir, T. O., and Cicek, M. (2013). The genotoxic, hepatotoxic, nephrotoxic, haematotoxic and histopathological effects in rats after aluminium chronic intoxication. *Toxicol. Ind. Health* 29, 780–791. doi: 10.1177/0748233712440140

Hou, Y. J., Zhao, Y. Y., Xiong, B., Cui, X. S., Kim, N. H., Xu, Y. X., et al. (2013). Mycotoxin-containing diet causes oxidative stress in the mouse. *PLoS ONE* 8:e60374. doi: 10.1371/journal.pone.0060374

Ilicin, G. (1971). Serum copper and magnesium levels in leukaemia and malignant lymphoma. *Lancet* 2, 1036–1037. doi: 10.1016/S0140-6736(71)90 353-9

Ishak, K., Baptista, A., Bianchi, L., Callea, F., De Groote, J., Gudat, F., et al. (1995). Histological grading and staging of chronic hepatitis. *J. Hepatol.* 22, 696–699. doi: 10.1016/0168-8278(95)80226-6

Klopfleisch, R. (2013). Multiparametric and semiquantitative scoring systems for the evaluation of mouse model histopathology-a systematic review. *BMC Vet. Res.* 9:123. doi: 10.1186/1746-6148-9-123

Krewski, D., Yokel, R. A., Nieboer, E., Borchelt, D., Cohen, J., Harry, J., et al. (2007). Human health risk assessment for aluminium, aluminium oxide, and aluminium hydroxide. *J. Environ Sci. Health B* 10, 1–269. doi: 10.1080/10937400701597766

Kumar, S., Khodoun, M., Kettleson, E. M., McKnight, C., Reponen, T., Grinshpun, S. A., et al. (2014). Glyphosate-rich air samples induce IL-33, TSLP and generate IL-13 dependent airway inflammation. *Toxicology* 325, 42–51. doi: 10.1016/j.tox.2014.08.008

Kumar, V., and Gill, K. D. (2009). Aluminium neurotoxicity: neurobehavioural and oxidative aspects. *Arch. Toxicol.* 83, 965–978. doi: 10.1007/s00204-009-0455-6

Larini, L. (1999). In *Toxicologia dos Praguicidas*, ed Manole, 178–179.

Larsen, K., Najle, R., Lifschitz, A., and Virkel, G. (2012). Effects of sub-lethal exposure of rats to the herbicide glyphosate in drinking water: glutathione transferase enzyme activities, levels of reduced glutathione and lipid peroxidation in liver, kidneys and small intestine. *Environ. Toxicol. Pharmacol.* 34, 811–818. doi: 10.1016/j.etap.2012.09.005

Li, C.-M., Li, L., Bai, J.-Y., Wu, J., Huang, S., and Wang, G.-L. (2013). Correlation between heat shock protein 32 and chronic heat-induced liver injury in developing mice. *J. Therm. Biol.* 38, 513–519. doi: 10.1016/j.jtherbio.2013.08.006

Li, Y., Yang, L., Wang, W., Li, H., Lv, J., and Zou, X. (2011). Trace element concentrations in hair of healthy Chinese centenarians. *Sci. Total Environ.* 409, 1385–1390. doi: 10.1016/j.scitotenv.2011.01.017

Malatesta, M., Perdoni, F., Santin, G., Battistelli, S., Muller, S., and Biggiogera, M. (2008). Hepatoma tissue culture (HTC) cells as a model for investigating the effects of low concentrations of herbicide on cell structure and function. *Toxicol. In Vitro* 22, 1853–1860. doi: 10.1016/j.tiv.2008.09.006

Marchesini, G., Moscatiello, S., Di Domizio, S., and Forlani, G. (2008). Obesity-associated liver disease. *J. Clin Endocr. Metab.* 93, S74–S80. doi: 10.1210/jc.2008-1399

Modesto, K. A., and Martinez, C. B. (2010). Roundup® causes oxidative stress in liver and inhibits acetylcholinesterase in muscle and brain of the fish *Prochilodus lineatus*. *Chemosphere* 78, 294–299. doi: 10.1016/j.chemosphere.2009.10.047

Oteiza, P. I., Adonaylo, V. N., and Keen, C. L. (1999). Cadmium-induced testes oxidative damage in rats can be influenced by dietary zinc intake. *Toxicology* 137, 13–22. doi: 10.1016/S0300-483X(99)00067-0

Ozcelik, D., Ozaras, R., Gurel, Z., Uzun, H., and Aydin, S. (2003). Copper-mediated oxidative stress in rat liver. *Biol. Trace Elem. Res.* 96, 209–215. doi: 10.1385/BTER:96:1-3:209

Ozdemir, G., and Inanc, F. (2005). Zinc may protect remote ocular injury caused by intestinal ischemia reperfusion in rats. *Tohoku J. Exp. Med.* 206, 247–251. doi: 10.1620/tjem.206.247

Ozden, S., and Alpertunga, B. (2010). Effects of methiocarb on lipid peroxidation and glutathione level in rat tissues. *Drug Chem. Toxicol.* 33, 50–54. doi: 10.3109/01480540903130708

Ozturk, A., Baltaci, A. K., Mogulkoc, R., Oztekin, E., Sivrikaya, A., Kurtoglu, E., et al. (2003). Effects of zinc deficiency and supplementation on malondialdehyde and glutathione levels in blood and tissues of rats performing swimming exercise. *Biol. Trace Elem. Res.* 94, 157–166. doi: 10.1385/BTER:94:2:157

Piccolo, A., Celano, G., Arienzo, M., and Mirabella, A. (1994). Adsorption and desorption of glyphosate in some European soils. *J. Environ. Sci. Health B* 29, 1105–1115. doi: 10.1080/03601239409372918

Powell, S. R. (2000). The antioxidant properties of zinc. *J. Nutr.* 130 (Suppl. 5S), 1447S–1454S.

Rahnama, M., and Marciniak, A. (2002). Influence of estrogen deficiency on the level of magnesium in rat mandible and teeth. *Bull Vet. Inst. Pulawy* 46, 267–272.

Reitman, S., and Frankel, S. (1957). A colorimetric method for the determination of serum glutamic oxalacetic and glutamic pyruvic transaminases. *Am. J. Clin Pathol.* 28, 56–63. doi: 10.1093/ajcp/28.1.56

Samsel, A., and Seneff, S. (2013). Glyphosate, pathways to modern diseases II: celiac sprue and gluten intolerance. *Interdiscip. Toxicol.* 6, 159–184. doi: 10.2478/intox-2013-0026

Sedlak, J., and Lindsay, R. H. (1968). Estimation of total, protein-bound, and nonprotein sulfhydryl groups in tissue with Ellman's reagent. *Anal. Biochem.* 25, 192–205. doi: 10.1016/0003-2697(68)90092-4

Sun, F., Hamagawa, E., Tsutsui, C., Ono, Y., Ogiri, Y., and Kojo, S. (2001). Evaluation of oxidative stress during apoptosis and necrosis caused by carbon tetrachloride in rat liver. *Biochim. Biophys. Acta* 1535, 186–191. doi: 10.1016/S0925-4439(00)00098-3

Szarek, J., Siwicki, A., Andrzejewska, A., Terech-Majewska, E., and Banaszkiewicz, T. (2000). Effects of the herbicide Roundup^{TM} on the ultrastructural pattern of hepatocytes in carp (*Cyprinus carpio*). *Mar. Environ. Res.* 50, 263–266. doi: 10.1016/S0141-1136(00)00088-X

Temple, W. A., and Smith, N. A. (1992). Glyphosate herbicide poisoning experience in New Zealand. *New Z. Med. J.* 105, 173–174.

Trayhurn, P., and Wood, I. S. (2004). Adipokines: inflammation and the pleiotropic role of white adipose tissue. *Br. J. Nutr.* 92, 347–355. doi: 10.1079/BJN20041213

Türkez, H., Yousef, M. I., and Geyikoglu, F. (2010). Propolis prevents aluminium-induced genetic and hepatic damages in rat liver. *Food Chem. Toxicol.* 48, 2741–2746. doi: 10.1016/j.fct.2010.06.049

Williams, G. M., Kroes, R., and Munro, I. C. (2000). Safety evaluation and risk assessment of the herbicide Roundup and its active ingredient, glyphosate, for humans. *Regul. Toxicol. Phar.* 31, 117–165. doi: 10.1006/rtph.1999.1371

Yamaguchi, K., Yang, L., McCall, S., Huang, J., Yu, X. X., Pandey, S. K., et al. (2007). Inhibiting triglyceride synthesis improves hepatic steatosis but exacerbates liver damage and fibrosis in obese mice with nonalcoholic steatohepatitis. *Hepatology* 45, 1366–1374. doi: 10.1002/hep.21655

Zheng, Z., Schmidt-Ott, K. M., Chua, S., Foster, K. A., Frankel, R. Z., Pavlidis, P., et al. (2005). A Mendelian locus on chromosome 16 determines susceptibility to doxorubicin nephropathy in the mouse. *Proc. Natl. Acad. Sci. U.S.A.* 102, 2502–2507. doi: 10.1073/pnas.0409786102

8

Multi-Level Integration of Environmentally Perturbed Internal Phenotypes Reveals Key Points of Connectivity between Them

Nirupama Benis[1†], Soumya K. Kar[1†], Vitor A. P. Martins dos Santos[2,3], Mari A. Smits[4,5], Dirkjan Schokker[4†] and Maria Suarez-Diez[2†]*

[1] Host Microbe Interactomics, Wageningen University & Research, Wageningen, Netherlands, [2] Systems and Synthetic Biology, Department of Agrotechnology and Food Sciences, Wageningen University & Research, Wageningen, Netherlands, [3] Lifeglimmer GmbH, Berlin, Germany, [4] Wageningen Livestock Research, Wageningen University & Research, Wageningen, Netherlands, [5] Wageningen Bioveterinary Research, Wageningen University & Research, Wageningen, Netherlands

***Correspondence:**
Nirupama Benis
nirupama.benis@wur.nl

[†] These authors have contributed equally to this work.

The genotype and external phenotype of organisms are linked by so-called internal phenotypes which are influenced by environmental conditions. In this study, we used five existing -omics datasets representing five different layers of internal phenotypes, which were simultaneously measured in dietarily perturbed mice. We performed 10 pair-wise correlation analyses verified with a null model built from randomized data. Subsequently, the inferred networks were merged and literature mined for co-occurrences of identified linked nodes. Densely connected internal phenotypes emerged. Forty-five nodes have links with all other data-types and we denote them "connectivity hubs." In literature, we found proof of 6% of the 577 connections, suggesting a biological meaning for the observed correlations. The observed connectivities between metabolite and cytokines hubs showed higher numbers of literature hits as compared to the number of literature hits on the connectivities between the microbiota and gene expression internal phenotypes. We conclude that multi-level integrated networks may help to generate hypotheses and to design experiments aiming to further close the gap between genotype and phenotype. We describe and/or hypothesize on the biological relevance of four identified multi-level connectivity hubs.

Keywords: data integration, internal phenotype, transcriptomics, proteomics, metabolomics, microbiota, gastrointestinal tract, systems biology

INTRODUCTION

The information encoded in the genome (genotype) and the external quantitative traits or characteristics (phenotype) of an organism are linked to each other by several layers of so-called, intermediate (Leuchter et al., 2014; Fontanesi, 2016) or internal (Houle et al., 2010) phenotypes. Several of these internal phenotypic layers are shown in **Figure 1** that visualizes the conceptual relationship between the external phenotype (P), the genotype (G), the environment (E), and the G&E interactions. The epigenome is tightly associated with the genome and represents the programming of gene expression which is not dependent on the DNA code itself. The transcriptome layer represents direct effects of the environment on the gene expression of the

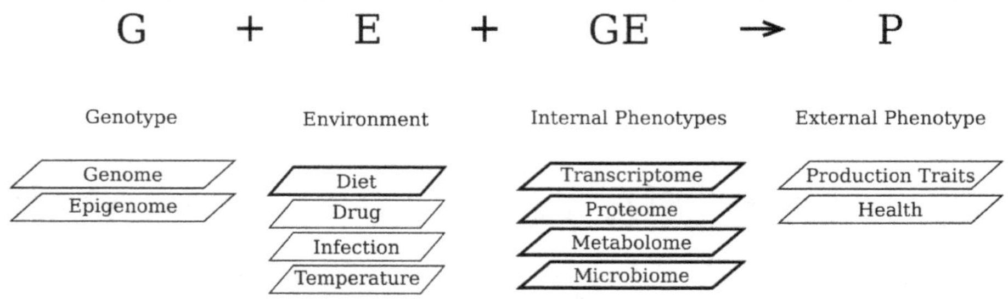

FIGURE 1 | Relationship between the external phenotype (P), the genotype (G), the environment (E), and the G&E interactions. The internal phenotypic layers and the environmental factor with a darker outline are included in the present study.

(epi-)genome. Translation of the transcriptome into proteins represents the next internal phenotype. The subsequent layer is represented by complex metabolite profiles. The organism-associated microbiota, especially those in the gut, can be regarded as a separate internal phenotypic layer, because it is not only dependent on the host genome but also heavily influenced by its environment, particularly by nutrition (Schwartz et al., 2012; Montiel-Castro et al., 2013). Although, for several traits the quantitative effects of the environment on the external phenotypes are known (Gentry et al., 2004; Cani et al., 2008; de Wit et al., 2011), the specific effects of the environment on the internal phenotypes are largely unknown. Furthermore, it is obvious to assume that the various layers of internal phenotypes are connected to each other and that their joint profiles ultimately determine the external phenotype (Leuchter et al., 2014; Fontanesi, 2016). Unfortunately, most of these assumptions are not based on solid evidence and at best represent oversimplifications of the dynamic nature of processes involved in determining external phenotypes. It, furthermore, partly explains the knowledge gap that exists between the genotype and the external phenotype.

Therefore, the objective of this study was to develop methodologies to identify components in the internal phenotypic layers that are connected to components in other internal phenotypic layers. To this end, we integrated multi-scale quantitative (–omics) data using a regression approach. The used data sets were derived from a single experiment with inbred mice which were exposed to five different dietary interventions as a means to perturb the different internal phenotypes. With a data-driven approach we were able to identify a large number of potential connections between the various intermediate phenotypes and for several we found proof of causal relationships in literature. We have used networks to represent the identified connections. The molecular components of each internal phenotype (such as genes, metabolites, cytokines, or bacterial groups) are represented as nodes in the network and the identified connections between each data type are represented as links or edges. The results of this study provide a basis to understand how various internal phenotypic layers are connected to each other. The identified connections may be crucial for the identification of causal relationships (Civelek and Lusis, 2014) between various biological scales and to uncover mechanisms involved in determining external phenotypes.

MATERIALS AND METHODS

Origin of Data

We used data from an experiment with 6-week old inbred mice that were fed for 4 weeks with six different semi-synthetic diets (Kar et al., submitted). In brief: thirty-six 21-day-old C57BL/6J mice (Harlan Laboratories, Horst, the Netherlands) were divided into 6 groups and housed in pairs with *ad libitum* access to diet and water. After adaptation for 1 week to a standard diet, the mice were fed semi-synthetic diets containing 300 g/kg (as fed basis) of one of the alternative protein sources for 28 days: soybean meal; casein; partially delactosed whey powder; spray dried plasma protein; wheat gluten meal and yellow meal worm. At the end of the experiment, mice were sacrificed to collect ileal tissue to acquire gene expression data, ileal digesta to study changes in microbiota, blood serum to profile cytokines and chemokines and blood and urine to profile amine metabolites. All procedures were approved by the Animal Experimentation Board at Wageningen University & Research Center (accession number 2012062.c) and carried out according to the guidelines of the European Council Directive 86/609/EEC dated November, 1986. Multi-omics data were obtained with regards to: whole genome gene expression profiles of ileal tissue as measured with Affymetrix GeneChip mouse gene 1.1 ST microarrays (Affymetrix, Santa Clara, CA, USA); community scale microbiota composition of ileal digesta by targeted-amplicon DNA sequencing of the bacterial 16S rDNA V3 region on an Illumina Mi-Seq sequencer; 23 serum cytokine and chemokine concentrations (pg/ml) using a Bio-Rad Mouse 23-plex kit (Bio-Rad, Hercules, CA, USA); and amine metabolic profiles of serum and urine using an ACQUITY UPLC system coupled online with a Xevo Tandem quadrupole mass spectrometer (Waters) operated using QuanLynx data acquisition software (version 4.1; Waters; Kar et al., in preparation). The data from the ileum reflects the local effects of the dietary interventions, the other three data assess the systemic effects.

Pre-processing and Selection of Data

An overview of the five types of data and their specifics are given in **Table 1**. Supplementary Figure 1 has an overview of all the analytical methods used in this study. Each dataset was pre-processed in a similar way using the R package limma (Smyth, 2005) to find the differentially significant data-points. The data

TABLE 1 | Pre-processing and specificities of each data-type.

Properties	Transcriptomics	Microbiota	Cytokine	Metabolomics serum	Metabolomics urine
Sampling	Ileum	Ileum	Serum	Serum	Urine
Before pre-processing	16,410 * 33	148 * 33	23 * 36	41 * 36	16 * 28
After pre-processing	52 * 33	22 * 33	13 * 36	26 * 36	16 * 28

Details of the site of sampling and data dimensions before and after pre-processing are indicated. The first number indicates the number of variables in the data and the second number denotes the number of samples.

is first log transformed and then this data is fitted to a linear model using the function lmFit (Phipson et al., 2016) which will give back information on the differences between the data-points in different samples and subsequently different comparisons of control vs. treatment. Then we used the function eBayes (Phipson et al., 2016) which applies an empirical Bayes method to compute p-values for a t-statistic under the assumption that only 1% of the data-points are differentially regulated among all the data-points in the samples. This p-value is then subjected to a Benjamini–Hochberg (Benjamini and Hochberg, 1995) multiple testing correction, also known as a False Discovery Rate (FDR).

This analysis was done by comparing the data of each dietary group against the data of the dietary group that received soy bean meal as protein source, which is the most common source of protein in animal diets. The FDR value of the data, is used to gauge significance and data-points that were significant in at least one of the five comparisons of the diets were included in the integration analysis. Except for the Cytokine and Metabolomics Serum (using the amine measurement), all the data-types had some samples thrown out due to quality control. Two types of metabolomics measurements were done on the sampled urine; Amine and Acyl-carnitine, the amine dataset did not have sufficient statistically significant data-points so was discarded. We only work with the Acyl-carnitine measurement in urine.

Data Integration, Network Generation, and Network Assessment

All significantly different data-points were used in the integration which was initially performed with two datasets at a time, so that from the 5 datasets 10 integrated networks were generated. The integration was performed using the function sPLS (sparse Partial Least Squares) in regression mode with ncomp = 5, from the R package mixOmics (Lê Cao et al., 2009; Dejean et al., 2011; González et al., 2012). The regression mode is used to model causal relationship between variables in both datasets by identifying combinations of variables between both datasets. Weight vectors used in the regression modeling are termed loading vectors. sPLS is used to perform simultaneous variable selection in the two datasets to be integrated and employs LASSO (Least Absolute Shrinkage and Selection Operator) penalization (Tibshirani, 2011) on the loading vectors. This approach requires one data set, $\boldsymbol{X}$ with n_x elements, to be designated the predictor and the other, $\boldsymbol{Y}$ with n_y elements, the response. As an output, the approach produces a matrix $Ma(\mathbf{X},\boldsymbol{Y})$ of size $n_x \times n_y$ representing the relevant correlations between both datasets, so that:

$$ma_{ij} = \begin{cases} 0, \; if \; Y_j \; independent \; of \; X_i \\ cor\left(X_i,\; Y_j\right), \; if \; Y_j \; dependent \; on \; X_i \end{cases}, \; with \; i \in \{1, \; \ldots, \; n_x\} \; and \; j \in \{1, \; \ldots, \; n_y\} \tag{1}$$

Where $cor\left(X_i,\; Y_j\right)$ is Pearson's correlation between elements i and j from datasets $\boldsymbol{X}$ and $\boldsymbol{Y}$, respectively. The correlation is computed across all available samples (here corresponding to dietary exposures).

Since it is not trivial to determine the predictor and response with biological data, we swapped the two types of data to compute $Mb(\boldsymbol{Y},\boldsymbol{X})$, a matrix of size $n_y \times n_x$ where the roles of $\boldsymbol{X}$ and $\boldsymbol{Y}$ have been interchanged. Both matrices, Ma and Mb where combined into a final matrix $M(\boldsymbol{X},\boldsymbol{Y})$ size $n_x \times n_y$ using

$$M(\mathbf{X},\mathbf{Y}) = Ma(\mathbf{X},\mathbf{Y}) + t(Mb(\mathbf{Y},\mathbf{X})) \tag{2}$$

where t represents matrix transposition. Thus, non-null elements of the matrix $M(\boldsymbol{X},\boldsymbol{Y})$ represent correlations between data types that have been deemed associated. This matrix can be seen as a weighted adjacency matrix representing a network where two nodes X_i and Y_j are connected via an edge if a non-null weight can be assigned to the edge. This weight is represented by the matrix value m_{ij}.

To further prune the network of (possibly) spurious interaction two additional thresholds ($th_l < 0$; and $th_h > 0$) were imposed to obtain an unweighted adjacency matrix $A(\boldsymbol{X}, \boldsymbol{Y})$of size $n_x \times n_y$

$$A_{ij} = \begin{cases} 1 \; if \; m_{ij} \geq th_h \; or \; m_{ij} \leq th_l \\ 0 \; if \; \left|m_{ij}\right| < \left|th_l\right| \; and \; m_{ij} < th_h \end{cases} \tag{3}$$

were |x| represents the absolute value. th_l and th_h where selected for each network so that only top 5% of the highest (positive) and lowest (negative) weights were kept for building the networks.

Networks represented by these adjacency matrix were transformed into the edge-list format, a two column table of the connected nodes in a network were each row represents an edge and visualized in Cytoscape (Shannon et al., 2003; Ono et al., 2015).

For each pair of integrated datasets a null model of the association networks was constructed using a strategy based on random permutations of measured values (Saccenti et al., 2015). Measured data-points were randomly permuted over samples before data integration to obtain randomized datasets that still retained the same value distribution for each variable. The randomized datasets were then used for data integration following the afore mentioned approach thereby generating randomized associations networks. The process was iterated $N_{it} = 1{,}000$ times for each pair of datasets; For each iteration, k, the values of the dynamic cut-offs (th_{lk} and th_{hk}) (5% of the highest and lowest correlation) were recorded. For the 10 pairwise combinations of datasets, the values obtained for th_l and th_h obtained using the unpermuted dataset, were compared with the distribution of values of th_{lk} and th_{hk} with $k = \{1,...,N_{it}\}$ to get networks from the random data to compare to the networks from the biological data.

Network Merging and Topological Analysis

The 10 networks arising from pair-wise data integration of the 5 data sets were merged in a combined network including all the nodes and edges of the 10 networks. This network is then restricted by only including nodes present in at least two of the separate networks. We used the igraph R package (Csardi and Nepusz, 2006) to further analyze the network, which was treated as non-directed, since no particular directionality was assigned to the edges. We obtained values for the following topological properties of the merged network (Barabasi and Oltvai, 2004; Csardi and Nepusz, 2006; Zhu et al., 2007): Degree: number of neighbors of a given node, that is the number of nodes connected to it. Clustering coefficient of a node is the ratio of the number of connections between the neighbors of a node and the total number of possible connections between said neighbors. Characteristic path length: median of the average distance between a node and all the rest. Network density: ratio between the total number of existing edges and the total number of possible edges (given the number of nodes in the network). Connected components maximal subgraphs in a network such that each node is connected to all the rest by means of network paths. For node level metrics, such as degree or clustering coefficient average values were computed over all nodes. Cytoscape was used for network visualization.

Literature Mining

To investigate the co-occurrence of the names of the connected nodes in the association network, we used the R package rentrez (Winter, 2016). This package searches for selected keywords in PubMed abstracts while making use of the MeSH (Medical Subject Headings) thesaurus to maximize results via the API from NCBI. The search was not restricted to a specific tissue type or organism. These results were examined, although not exhaustively, to find literature evidence of established relationships between nodes connected through identified edges; these were then considered as true positive search results.

The script used to generate all these results will be made available on request. All the above mentioned operations were performed using existing functions from R packages. The different steps involved are represented in Supplementary Figure 1.

RESULTS

Analysis of the Individual Datasets

A dietary intervention was performed on mice where the protein content was changed and multi-omics data were obtained with regard to: whole genome gene expression profiles of ileal tissue (Transcriptomics), community scale microbiota composition of ileal digesta (Microbiota), 24 different cytokine levels in blood serum (Cytokine), and protein-associated metabolic profiles of serum (Metabolomics Serum) and urine (Metabolomics Urine). These data were pre-processed and analyzed separately by fitting a linear model on the data-points and looking for differentially expressed readouts in each treatment vs. the control. Each dataset had its own p-value (corrected for multiple testing with the Benjamini–Hochberg method) threshold, ranging from 0.001 to 0.1 for difference between the tested and reference diets. The highest number of statistically significant entities was found in Transcriptomics. Furthermore, all the measured variables in Metabolomics Urine were found to be significantly different in at least one comparison.

Pairwise Data Association and Network Generation

We performed the integration by linking two data-types at a time and in such a way that after the pairwise analysis all the observed association data could be combined to build a multi-level interaction network. Therefore, each data-type was integrated with the other four types of data, resulting in 10 association networks. The topological characteristics of all these 10 networks are given in **Table 2** and **Figure 2**, and the network graphs are available in Supplementary Figure 2 as an image. Data Sheet 1 has the networks in a format that can be uploaded into Cytoscape in order to further explore the connectivities of these networks by simply clicking on these nodes. **Table 2** shows the positive and negative thresholds that were used separately for the association network. Connections between pairs of data points with correlation values between the threshold values, i.e., Low Threshold (negative threshold) and High Threshold (positive threshold) as indicated in **Table 2**, were discarded and the corresponding edges removed from the final network. There were two disconnected sub-graphs in five of the networks while the other five have only a single, fully connected graph. Supplementary Figure 3 shows the pattern of changes induced by the diet in three components of the network Microbiota & Transcriptomics.

The largest network, in terms of nodes, is the Microbiota & Transcriptomics network. This seems logical as it represents the most comprehensive datasets and spacial interactions between the two data-types are known to occur. Overall, networks involving Transcriptomics data had higher number of nodes than other networks. The smallest network with 18 nodes and 22 edges was the Metabolomics Urine & Cytokine network.

Technical Validation of Pairwise Integration Networks by Random Permutation

We performed the same method of integration on the five different data-types after randomly permuting the measured

TABLE 2 | The 10 individual correlation networks.

Network names (data A & data B)	Low threshold	High threshold	No. of nodes (A)	No. of nodes (B)	Connected components
Metabolomics Serum & Metabolomics Urine	−0.51	0.6	14	12	2
Metabolomics Serum & Microbiota	−0.38	0.3	21	14	1
Metabolomics Serum & Transcriptomics	−0.31	0.35	26	33	2
Metabolomics Serum & Cytokine	−0.33	0.5	18	13	2
Metabolomics Urine & Microbiota	−0.28	0.42	16	12	1
Metabolomics Urine & Transcriptomics	−0.55	0.54	14	29	1
Metabolomics Urine & Cytokine	−0.32	0.55	10	8	2
Microbiota & Transcriptomics	−0.28	0.27	19	48	1
Microbiota & Cytokine	−0.38	0.35	11	11	1
Transcriptomics & Cytokine	−0.27	0.34	31	13	2

Each row represents one of the 10 correlation networks. Low Threshold and High Threshold represent the thresholds used for the correlation values. The 3rd and 4th columns have the number of nodes in the network that belong to the first and second data, respectively. The last column displays the number of connected graphs in the network.

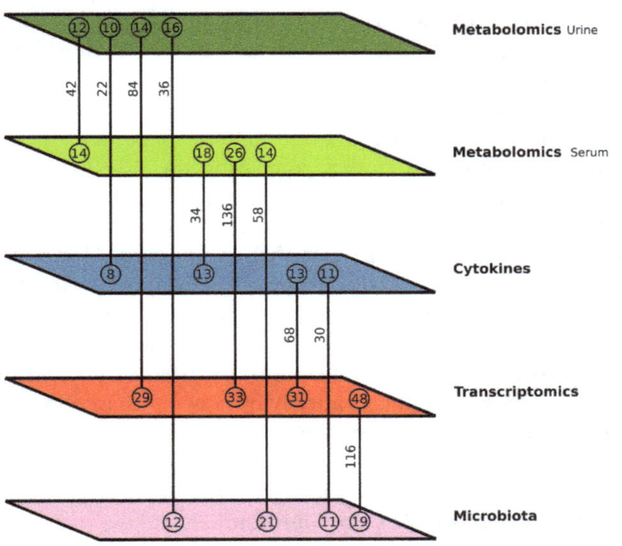

FIGURE 2 | Multilevel integration. This schematic image shows the number of connections between each internal phenotypic level with the other levels in a merged network. The colors of the parallelograms denote the internal phenotypic level to which the data-types belong. Green is Metabolomics (light green—Metabolite from Serum and dark green—Metabolite from Urine), blue is Cytokines, red is Transcriptomics, and pink is Microbiota. Each line connects two levels and the vertical number above the line indicates the number of edges in the correlation network between those two phenotypic levels. The number of connected nodes in each level is given in circles above and below the connecting lines.

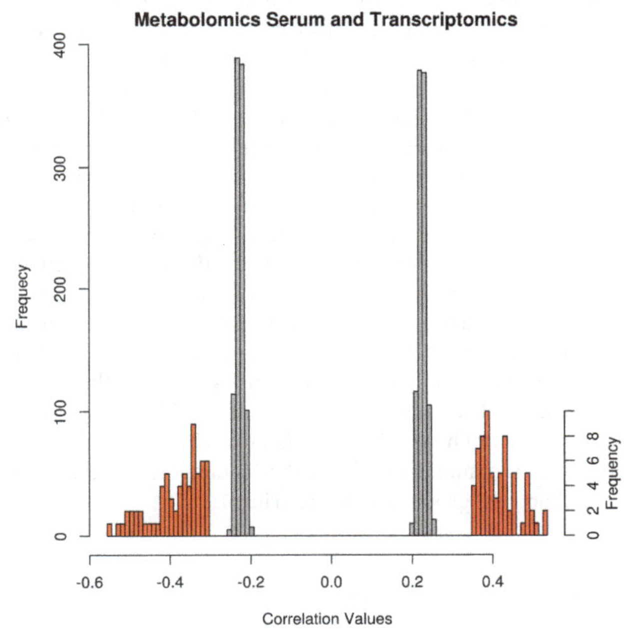

FIGURE 3 | Distribution of network correlations and random network cut-offs of the Metabolomics Urine and Transcriptomics networks. The x-axis depicts the range of correlation values and the y- axis shows its frequency. The gray bars denote the distribution of the thresholds of the 1,000 random correlation networks with frequency on the left y-axis. The red bars are distributions of the correlation values of the inferred network with frequency on the right y-axis.

data, this process was iterated a 1,000 times. In this way, the networks obtained from random permutations are considered a null model with no biological information, and used to assess the significance of the results obtained with the non-permuted data. **Figure 3** shows the spread of correlation values for the integration of Metabolomics Serum and Transcriptomics. The thresholds for network reconstruction were selected so that only the 5% highest and lowest correlations were kept. The separation between the values obtained for the integrated data and the randomly permutated datasets indicates the high significance of the edges in the integration networks. In this way, selection of the 5% highest and lowest correlations and significant limits the number of spurious correlations that could be due to chance alone while retaining maximum information in the networks.

Similar results were obtained for most of the integration networks (Supplementary Figure 3). In three of the networks, there is an overlap between the correlation values from the inferred network and the values arising from the randomly generated networks. The overlaps are in the networks Metabolomics Urine & Microbiota, Metabolomics Urine & Cytokine, and Transcriptomics & Cytokine network. The highest overlap appears in the first two and mostly affects edges with negative correlations.

Merged Network

All the 10 integration networks (Data Sheet 1) were merged and only nodes linked with nodes of at least two other data-types were kept (see **Table 3**). The gene expression data has the highest number of nodes in the merged network. However, nodes with the highest degree (number of connecting edges) arise from the microbiota data, with S24-7 having 57 neighbors and Bifidobacterium having 47 neighbors. The merged network encompasses 45 nodes that are connected to all the other types of data. For that reason we denote them "Connectivity hubs" and they are included in **Table 3** and Supplementary Table 1.

Functional Validation of Merged Network by Text Mining

A PubMed literature search for co-occurrence of linked nodes gave results for 6% of the links corresponding to 37 edges. We further investigated reported causality effects between the nodes in question. Most of the retrieved results are related to metabolites and cytokines measurements whereas a few results confirming causal relationships were found involving gene nodes. We were able to find literature confirmation pertaining to associations for six out of the 10 pair-wise connections between phenotypes, as summarized in **Table 4**. Supplementary Table 2 contains all the PubMed identifiers from the literature mining and Supplementary Table 3 has phrases from a maximum of three PubMed abstracts from the results. Among the nodes with literature results, four are from Microbiota, two from Transcriptomics, 15 from Metabolomics Serum, three from Metabolomics Urine, and six from Cytokines. The node with the highest number of hits in literature is Tnfa which co-occurs 8,563 times with nine metabolites from the Metabolomics Serum data and one bacterial group (Bifidobacterium).

TABLE 3 | Characteristics of the merged network.

Network statistics	
Total number of nodes	112 (45)
Total number of edges	577
Number of Metabolomics Urine nodes	15 (8)
Number of Metabolomics Serum nodes	24 (11)
Number of Cytokine nodes	13 (7)
Number of Transcriptomics nodes	43 (12)
Number of Microbiota nodes	17 (7)
Degree range	2–57
Average number of neighbors	10.35
Clustering coefficient	0.20
Characteristic path length	2.31
Network density	0.09
Connected components	1

Characteristics of the merged correlation network. The number of nodes from each data-type are given in rows three to seven. Between brackets the number of connectivity hubs is indicated.

Of the 30 data-points from all the types of data that have literature results, 15 are connectivity hubs. One such connectivity hub is Glutathione (GSH) which has 21 direct neighbors from four data-types as shown in **Figure 4**. This hub is especially interesting because six of the connected nodes (Carnitine, Tnfa, Il-1b, Il17c, Bifidobacterium, and Dapk2) have textual co-occurrences found by the text mining algorithm. The terms GSH and Tnfa were found 2,231 times in the abstracts of Pubmed indexed articles. Full text inspection shows that some of the connections are causal relationships as one of the connected nodes activates or inhibits the other.

DISCUSSION

In this study we developed and used a set of computational methods to identify components in internal phenotypic layers that are connected to components in other internal phenotypic layers of an organism. We successfully integrated multi-scale quantitative (-omics) data, derived from a single experiment with inbred mice and which were exposed to five different diets. Here the mice had been exposed to the dietary intervention for 4 weeks. Four weeks is a significant amount of time in the life of mice and previous studies comparing the development of mice and humans (specifically the immune system in Holladay and Smialowicz, 2000) indicate that the development of different systems is much faster in mice than in humans. Hence it is reasonable to assume that the mice have adapted to the new diet in 4 weeks. Since the data originated from an animal experiment that was not designed for the detection of genetically and/or dietarily induced differences in external phenotypes, we only focused on the connectivity between 5 intermediate phenotypic levels. Some studies have reported pairwise data integration of two (Lu et al., 2014; Rajasundaram et al., 2014; Benis et al., 2015) or three data sets (Adourian et al., 2008). But this is, to the best of our knowledge, the first time that an integration of such heterogeneous data-types from different tissues, arising from a single experiment, has been reported. The approach as described here could, in principle, be applied on any number and type of datasets, as long as they are from the same experiment, from samples at the same time-point and have comparable dimensions of differentially regulated data.

TABLE 4 | Overview of text mining results.

Data connections	PubMed Ids	Distinct edges
Cytokines & Metabolomics Serum	9,554	16
Metabolomics Serum & Metabolomics Urine	906	6
Microbiota & Metabolomics Serum	254	7
Microbiota & Cytokines	250	5
Transcriptomics & Microbiota	83	3
Metabolomics Serum & Transcriptomics	59	2

The first column shows the types of data that are connected by the edges that were found in the PubMed literature search.

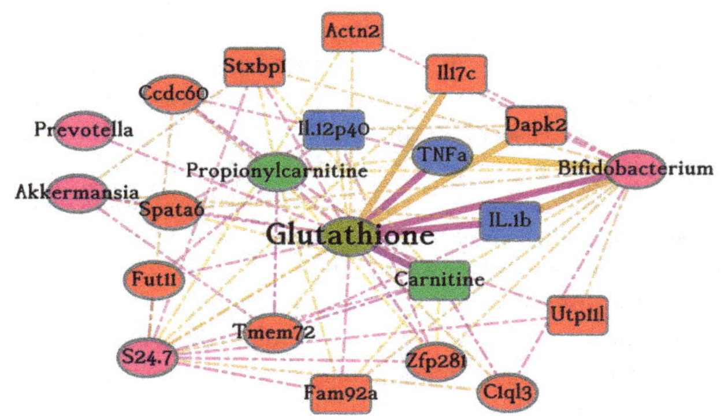

FIGURE 4 | Glutathione sub-network. This figure shows the 21 connections of the node Glutathione in the merged network. The different colors of nodes indicate the data-type of internal phenotypic level of that node, pink is Microbiota, red is Transcriptomics, blue is Cytokines, and green is Metabolites (light green—Metabolites from Serum and dark green—Metabolites from Urine). Oval nodes are connectivity hubs. Dotted lines show un-validated edges and continuous, thicker edges show connections also present in the results retrieved from scientific literature. Edge color, yellow and purple, indicates positive and negative correlations, respectively.

Internal Phenotypic Data and Pairwise Data Integration

Each used data-type represents a different internal phenotype and a different layer of the system that (co-) drives the manifestation of external phenotypes. We subjected each data-type to a separate analysis in order to correlate only those changes induced by the dietary intervention. Nodes with significantly different values could easily be identified in each of the sampled tissues and fluids (ileum, blood, and urine) thereby representing the local and systemic effects of the interventions and the need of a multi-scale approach.

In order to investigate connections between the five data-types we used sPLS, an integration method that can be applied to several types of data, two at a time. This method can also handle the dimensionality problem of biological datasets where the number of variables is usually higher than the number of samples. sPLS has been previously used for integration of microbiota with gene expression data (Benis et al., 2015; Steegenga et al., 2016), and measurements on cell wall polysaccharides of fibers with phenotypic characterizations of fibers in cotton balls (Rajasundaram et al., 2014).

We performed pairwise integration of the datasets, resulting in 10 networks with varying spreads of correlation values. Deciding on a threshold to distinguish genuine from spurious correlations is a major bottleneck for the definition of association networks. While a 0.8 threshold (absolute value) has been suggested for gene expression data (Schäfer and Strimmer, 2005), other authors suggested smaller values (0.6) in metabolomics data sets (Camacho et al., 2005). The correlation values greatly depend on the biological dataset under study and its dimensionality. There are several methods to choose a threshold based on the data: use assigned *p*-values as threshold; use network characteristics of the correlations; or use a percentage of the correlation distribution. When evaluated by Borate et al. (2009) they concluded that threshold selection methods based on network properties such as the clustering coefficient are best for gene co-expression networks. This would not work here because the generated networks always induce connections between data points of different type and as a result they have a zero clustering coefficient for every node. While integrating two types of metabolomics datasets with gene expression of the tissues in which they were measured Adourian et al. (2008) assigned *p*-values to the correlation values and then set a threshold. Selecting a threshold is further complicated by the possible appearance of spurious correlations due to a common response variable influencing the connecting nodes (A is correlated to B, A is correlated to C, therefore, B and C appear correlated). Regarding gene expression data, multiple methods (reviewed for example in Marbach et al., 2012) have been developed to minimize the number of falsely predicted associations. In this study, we used the top 5% of the correlation values because this dynamic threshold (separate for the positive and negative values) eliminates bias toward the size of the datasets. To further evaluate the impact of the correlation scores we have inspected the correlations between some linked nodes. Supplementary Figure 3 shows an extreme case in which transcript abundance of two genes negatively correlated with the abundance of a bacterial group. This might induce a spurious association between the genes. Spurious associations due to a common response variable influencing the connecting nodes are more likely to appear when both nodes are of the same type. Therefore, to further minimize the number of spurious associations we have focused on associations between different internal phenotypes.

We further validated the observed correlations by comparing them with a null model obtained by randomly permuting the data along the samples (Eguíluz et al., 2005; Saccenti et al., 2015). In the randomly permuted samples we expect all inferred associations to be spurious, as the permutation process destroys any possible correlation between the variables. In that case, even the correlations corresponding to the highest and lowest 5% of the population would be spurious. The values of the correlations deemed significant in the experimental data sets are found to be higher than these false positives. In two of the networks, Metabolomics Urine & Microbiota and Metabolomics Urine & Cytokine (the smallest network), the significance of the negative correlation values could not be established as we observed a considerable overlap between the negative correlation values of this network and the negative thresholds of the random networks. This calls for caution when biologically interpreting these networks. For five of the networks we observed a very clear separation of the random thresholds and the start of the correlation values in the network (Supplementary Figure 4). The other networks showed slight overlaps between the random threshold distribution and the network correlation distribution. This extra validation step reassured us that the observed correlations are rooted in biological phenomena. To our knowledge this technical validation step is not common in current studies of this type.

The edges of the inferred networks, indicate significant computationally-determined correlations between values of connected nodes. Our approach does not require a mechanistic model on how the associations are established and in each network these associations may be caused through entirely different mechanisms. In some cases the associations would be due to causal relationships between the connected nodes, such as increased expression levels of a cytokine gene linked to increased cytokine levels. However, in many cases, the associations could be indirect, mediated by elements that have not been measured in the experimental set up. In a formal mathematical model, they are considered hidden variables. Such would be the case of, for example, the changes in the metabolite levels of urine. These changes might have been caused by the colonic microbiota, in turn affected by the ileal microbiota. Since we only used the ileal microbiota data, we observe correlations between the ileal microbial populations and the urine metabolite levels which could be in reality, indirect relationships mediated by the colonic microbiota.

Network of Connected Internal Phenotypes

The pair-wise integration method allowed us to merge the 10 individual networks into a single network. Correlations within a dataset were deliberately excluded from this study because we only wanted to focus on connections between different internal phenotypes, where little work has been done. Thus, in the 10 networks, all detected connections are between two different data types and every node has a zero clustering coefficient. However, in the merged network, a non-zero clustering coefficient emerges as a result of nodes connecting to multiple data types (**Table 3**). This emphasizes the biological relevance of this method because the 10 networks were built without any information on cross-linking. Thus, we identified individual nodes that directly or indirectly participate in processes of the other four individual networks. Because they seem to connect different internal phenotypes, we denoted them "Connectivity Hubs." Starting the procedure as developed and applied here with networks with non-zero clustering coefficients (correlating within a dataset) would, however, not alter the connections between internal phenotypes.

Functional Validations of Phenotype Connections

Results of the text-mining were used to validate some of the identified links. This revealed insights into the mechanistic relationships between the variables predicted to be linked to each other. Thirty-seven of the 577 (6%) computational inferred links have already been described in literature as detected by our text-mining approach, which was not exhaustive because it focused only on text in journal abstracts. This indicates that our method identifies currently known biological interactions. The rest of the predicted links have not been discovered and investigated yet, have not been mentioned in abstracts, or do not exist in the biological system. Furthermore, by inspecting some of the retrieved abstracts and corresponding articles, we were even able to find causal relationships between some of the computational identified nodes where one of the nodes was used as an experimental perturbation and the other node was measured as a response parameter. Some examples are shown in Supplementary Table 3. Several indirect associations were also validated through reports on experiments where nodes, found to be connected in this study, were measured in response to another perturbation. During text-mining, in order to retrieve as many results as possible, search terms were matched against the MeSH thesaurus, irrespective of the organism, and all the synonyms were included in the search. The downside to this approach is the inclusion of several false textual associations. The most striking case is that of the identified association between Glutathione and Il17c. In the literature results, the reported association is between Glutathione and Il17a and not Il17c. Through the thesaurus, Il17c was mapped to Il17 and subsequently to Il17a thereby giving rise to that falsely identified association in literature.

In order to increase the precision and recall of text mining searches, and overcome problems associated to the use of a thesaurus, one needs to move from mining text, to mining the knowledge embedded in the text and the use of data hidden in public databases. Such an approach requires the use of knowledge management tools and representations that can be automatically accessed (Antezana et al., 2009). Semantic web technologies represent a new class of tools that include natural language processing, ontologies, machine learning algorithms and much more to facilitate integration knowledge from heterogeneous sources. The expansion of the use of semantic technologies in the life sciences domain will allow associating concepts such that inferences on causality, regulation, organism, or tissue can be made using high-throughput methods and automated reasoning.

Among the interactions retrieved from the automated literature search, a high prevalence of associations involving cytokines and/or metabolites was observed. In fact, such type of interactions represent 97% of the retrieved results. This probably highlights the extraordinary amount of work that has been done in these types of data in the past. On the opposite extreme, only 8% of the retrieved interactions involved associations between the expression of genes, reflecting the fact that most of the available gene expression data originates from genome-wide techniques. In such type of experiments, papers, especially abstracts, usually report on systems behaviors and pathways and less frequently on the individual behavior or role of individual genes and connected response nodes.

Validated Connectivity Hubs

Even though we only performed integrations of two datasets at a time, we find data-points (metabolites, cytokines, genes, or microbial groups) that correlate with different types of data. We identified 45 connectivity hubs in the merged network that seem to have associations with all four types of data. More than 30% of them are involved in links that were retrieved in literature. To further support the biological relevance of identified multi-level connectivities we discuss the implications of two of the 15 biologically validated connectivity hubs as examples. The two connectivity hubs were chosen because of the large amount of literature results for these hubs. The first hub, Tnfa has the highest number of literature results among all the nodes in the network and the other hub, Glutathione, has literature validations to the most number of data-types.

Tnfa is a connectivity hub in the merged network, with links to several neighbors belonging to the four other types of data. The position of this cytokine in our merged network shows that it plays a role in processes of the other internal phenotypes. The literature validated links are between Tnfa and two other types of data (Metabolomics Serum, Microbiota). Many of the validated links represent causal relationships. With regards to immune responses and as a drug target, Tnfa has been studied in great detail (Cicha and Urschel, 2015). The un-validated edges show that Tnfa could be a regulator of other internal phenotypes as well, than currently known.

The metabolite Glutathione (GSH) was measured in the serum and in the merged network is a connectivity hub proving that it is vital part of the system that connects several internal phenotypes. Among the 15 connectivity hubs with functionally validated links, GSH is the only one that has validated links to all other data-types based on our literature mining. These results support our claim of GSH being a connectivity hub, a biological component influencing several internal phenotypes. Several PubMed results for GSH are from *in-vivo* studies where GSH was administered to alleviate symptoms of a disease. Our literature results show that GSH has been studied in relation to all different types of data. Of the six validated links in our merged network, five represent proven causal relationships (see **Figure 4** and discussion of the functional validation). These neighboring nodes in the merged network are mostly related to immune and homeostatic mechanisms. GSH is a tripeptide, ubiquitously distributed in living cells and plays an important role in the intracellular defense mechanism against oxidative stress (Diaz-Vivancos et al., 2015; Couto et al., 2016). It is known that GSH metabolism is very important for the antioxidant and detoxifying action of the intestine. It is also essential for the maintenance of the luminal thiol-disulfide ratio involved in regulation mechanisms of the protein activity of epithelial cells (Iantomasi et al., 1997) which could be important since the intervention is changes in protein. Our results also demonstrate the manifold and central role of GSH when it comes to proteins, peptides and amino acids in nutrition. These observations indicate that the presented merged network represents, at least in part, associations of biological phenomena.

Potential Relevance of Selected Connectivity Hubs

There are 30 connectivity hubs in the merged network that do not co-occur with their connected nodes in our literature search. However, the prominence of these nodes in our merged network indicates that they could represent potential relevant interactions with components of the other internal phenotypes. In order to demonstrate how the results of this study may be used to hypothesize on functional relationships between different molecular components, we here describe the potential biological relevance of two highly linked connectivity hubs, Tmem72 and S24-7. Both hubs are not yet described in literature abstracts in conjunction with other data-types.

The high number of connectivity hubs in the Transcriptomics layer suggest that the expression of several intestinal genes is involved in many more interactions than currently known. None of the observed Transcriptomics connectivity hubs popped-up in our literature mining results. The most highly connected Transcriptomics node, Tmem72 (Transmembrane Protein 72), has only been studied in the kidney so far (Habuka et al., 2014) and not much information is available on it. But in the merged network this node has 27 links to other data-types (can be visualized in Data Sheet 1), mostly to metabolites from both the metabolomics datasets. Based on this, we hypothesize that Tmem72 is not specific to the kidney and that it has some sort of communication function in intestinal mucosa as well. The fact that Tmem72 is a transmembrane protein is supportive for this. Given its observed links with different microbiota, metabolites, and cytokines, it might be involved in diverse interactions with other internal phenotypes. Based on such an hypothesis, targeted experimental designs may be developed in order to investigate the hypothesized "communication" function of Tmem72 in intestinal mucosal tissue.

The most highly linked node of the merged network is the bacterial family classification, S24-7, suggesting an important role for this species in gut functionality. In some of the inferred individual association networks we already found it to be linked to a high number of nodes. Unfortunately, this node is not represented in literature abstracts together with the here observed neighbors. However, there is compelling literature that shows this microbial classification to be a significant part of the gut microbial community structure (Harris et al., 2014; Jakobsson et al., 2015). This family classification does not have a good functional definition, yet several studies show that it could be an important player in the functionality of the gut (Evans et al., 2014; Harris et al., 2014; Rooks et al., 2014). The latter claims are in line with the high number of neighbors that S24-7 has in our merged network. The current technical inability to cultivate S24-7 is most certainly due to the absence of knowledge on S24-7 interactions. However, a recent *in-silico* study (Ormerod et al., 2016) shows that S24-7 species have the ability to survive on different types of carbohydrate sources, similar to the genus Bifidobacteria. In the merged network, the connectivity hubs S24-7 and Bifidobacteria, share the highest number of neighbors (directly linked nodes). Among them are 16 genes, and neither S24-7 nor Bifidobacteria have literature results with any of these genes. An enrichment analysis on these shared network gene neighbors shows that they are involved in functions related to linoleic and linolenic acid metabolism (data not shown). It is known that these fatty acids are produced by Bifidobacteria (Teran et al., 2015) and that they are involved in the maintenance of the epidermal barrier function (Muñoz-Garcia et al., 2014). The observation that in our network these genes are shared between S24-7 and Bifidobacteria underscores the here hypothesized importance of S24-7 and indicates that these two bacterial groups are indeed closely related in function as hypothesized before (Ormerod et al., 2016).

From the results described in this paper, we conclude that we successfully developed methodologies to identify components in internal phenotypic layers that are connected to components in other internal phenotypic layers. By integrating multi-scale quantitative (-omics) data using a regression approach, we were able to provide provisional insight into potential ways internal phenotypic layers are connected to each other, including those between local and systemic layers. By a technical and functional validations, we underscored the relevance of our findings. Based on data generated by this type of integrated approaches, hypothesis driven and targeted research may be developed to identify causal relationships between various biological scales in order to diminish our knowledge gap between genotype and external phenotype. In addition, by expanding comparable approaches by incorporating data on genetic diversity and/or variation in external phenotypes, this knowledge gap may be even further closed down. The analysis pipeline that we developed is very general. Here we demonstrated this pipeline with datasets that address only one of the multiple environmental factors that might affect the internal phenotypes, namely the diet. However, the approach is very general and can be adapted to any type or number of data sets describing the impact of other perturbations.

AUTHOR CONTRIBUTIONS

NB performed the data analysis and prepared the manuscript. SK performed the animal experiment and contributed significantly to the biological interpretation of the results. VM contributed to the direction of the analysis and the manuscript. MS was involved in the animal experiment and helped with the direction and critical revision of the manuscript. DS was involved in the data analysis and biological interpretation. MS-D helped with the direction of the data analysis and the manuscript. All authors have read and approved of the final manuscript.

FUNDING

This work has been financially supported by the Systems Biology Investment Programme of Wageningen University, KB-17-003.02-022.

REFERENCES

Adourian, A., Jennings, E., Balasubramanian, R., Hines, W. M., Damian, D., Plasterer, T. N., et al. (2008). Correlation network analysis for data integration and biomarker selection. *Mol. Biosyst.* 4, 249–259. doi: 10.1039/b708489g

Antezana, E., Kuiper, M., and Mironov, V. (2009). Biological knowledge management: the emerging role of the Semantic Web technologies. *Brief. Bioinform.* 10, 392–407. doi: 10.1093/bib/bbp024

Barabasi, A.-L., and Oltvai, Z. N. (2004). Network biology: understanding the cell's functional organization. *Nat. Rev. Genet.* 5, 101–113. doi: 10.1038/nrg1272

Benis, N., Schokker, D., Suarez-Diez, M., Martins Dos Santos, V. A. P., Smidt, H., and Smits, M. A. (2015). Network analysis of temporal functionalities of the gut induced by perturbations in new-born piglets. *BMC Genomics* 16:556. doi: 10.1186/s12864-015-1733-8

Benjamini, Y., and Hochberg, Y. (1995). Controlling the false discovery rate: a practical and powerful approach to multiple testing. *J. R. Stat. Soc. Ser. B* 57, 289–300.

Borate, B. R., Chesler, E. J., Langston, M. A., Saxton, A. M., and Voy, B. H. (2009). Comparison of threshold selection methods for microarray gene co-expression matrices. *BMC Res. Notes* 2:240. doi: 10.1186/1756-0500-2-240

Camacho, D., De La Fuente, A., and Mendes, P. (2005). The origin of correlations in metabolomics data. *Metabolomics* 1, 53–63. doi: 10.1007/s11306-005-1107-3

Cani, P. D., Bibiloni, R., Knauf, C., Waget, A., Neyrinck, A. M., Delzenne, N. M., et al. (2008). Changes in gut microbiota control metabolic endotoxemia-induced inflammation in high-fat diet–induced obesity and diabetes in mice. *Diabetes* 57, 1470–1481. doi: 10.2337/db07-1403

Cicha, I., and Urschel, K. (2015). TNF-α in the cardiovascular system: from physiology to therapy. *Int. J. Interf. Cytokine Mediat. Res.* 7:9. doi: 10.2147/IJICMR.S64894

Civelek, M., and Lusis, A. J. (2014). Systems genetics approaches to understand complex traits. *Nat. Rev. Genet.* 15, 34–48. doi: 10.1038/nrg3575

Couto, N., Wood, J., and Barber, J. (2016). The role of glutathione reductase and related enzymes on cellular redox homeostasis network. *Free Radic. Biol. Med.* 95, 27–42. doi: 10.1016/j.freeradbiomed.2016.02.028

Csardi, G., and Nepusz, T. (2006). The igraph software package for complex network research. *InterJ. Complex Syst.* 1695, 1–9.

Dejean, S., Gonzalez, I., Lê, Cao, K.-A., and Monget, P. (2011). *mixOmics: Omics Data Integration Project*. R Package Version. 2–9.

de Wit, N. J. W., Boekschoten, M. V, Bachmair, E.-M., Hooiveld, G. J. E. J., de Groot, P. J., Rubio-Aliaga, I., et al. (2011). Dose-dependent effects of dietary fat on development of obesity in relation to intestinal differential gene expression in C57BL/6J mice. *PLoS ONE* 6:e19145. doi: 10.1371/journal.pone.0019145

Diaz-Vivancos, P., de Simone, A., Kiddle, G., and Foyer, C. H. (2015). Glutathione - linking cell proliferation to oxidative stress. *Free Radic. Biol. Med.* 89, 1154–1164. doi: 10.1016/j.freeradbiomed.2015.09.023

Eguíluz, V. M., Chialvo, D. R., Cecchi, G. A., Baliki, M., and Apkarian, A. V. (2005). Scale-free brain functional networks. *Phys. Rev. Lett.* 94:18102. doi: 10.1103/PhysRevLett.94.018102

Evans, C. C., LePard, K. J., Kwak, J. W., Stancukas, M. C., Laskowski, S., Dougherty, J., et al. (2014). Exercise prevents weight gain and alters the gut microbiota in a mouse model of high fat diet-induced obesity. *PLoS ONE* 9:e92193. doi: 10.1371/journal.pone.0092193

Fontanesi, L. (2016). Metabolomics and livestock genomics: Insights into a phenotyping frontier and its applications in animal breeding. *Anim. Front.* 6:11. doi: 10.2527/af.2016-0011

Gentry, J. G., McGlone, J. J., Miller, M. F., and Blanton, J. R. (2004). Environmental effects on pig performance, meat quality, and muscle characteristics1. *J. Anim. Sci.* 82, 209–217. doi: 10.2527/2004.821209x

González, I., Cao, K.-A. L., Davis, M. J., and Déjean, S. (2012). Visualising associations between paired "omics" data sets. *BioData Min.* 5:19. doi: 10.1186/1756-0381-5-19

Habuka, M., Fagerberg, L., Hallström, B. M., Kampf, C., Edlund, K., Sivertsson, Å., et al. (2014). The kidney transcriptome and proteome defined by transcriptomics and antibody-based profiling. *PLoS ONE* 9:e116125. doi: 10.1371/journal.pone.0116125

Harris, J. K., El Kasmi, K. C., Anderson, A. L., Devereaux, M. W., Fillon, S. A., Robertson, C. E., et al. (2014). Specific microbiome changes in a mouse model of parenteral nutrition associated liver injury and intestinal inflammation. *PLoS ONE* 9:e110396. doi: 10.1371/journal.pone.0110396

Holladay, S. D., and Smialowicz, R. J. (2000). Development of the murine and human immune system: differential effects of immunotoxicants depend on time of exposure. *Environ. Health Perspect.* 108(Suppl. 3), 463–473. doi: 10.1289/ehp.00108s3463

Houle, D., Govindaraju, D. R., and Omholt, S. (2010). Phenomics: the next challenge. *Nat. Rev. Genet.* 11, 855–866. doi: 10.1038/nrg2897

Iantomasi, T., Favilli, F., Marraccini, P., Magaldi, T., Bruni, P., and Vincenzini, M. T. (1997). Glutathione transport system in human small intestine epithelial cells. *Biochim. Biophys. Acta* 1330, 274–283. doi: 10.1016/S0005-2736(97)00097-7

Jakobsson, H. E., Rodríguez-Pi-eiro, A. M., Schütte, A., Ermund, A., Boysen, P., Bemark, M., et al. (2015). The composition of the gut microbiota shapes the colon mucus barrier. *EMBO Rep.* 16, 164–177. doi: 10.15252/embr.201439263

Lê Cao, K.-A., González, I., and Déjean, S. (2009). integrOmics: an R package to unravel relationships between two omics datasets. *Bioinformatics* 25, 2855–2856. doi: 10.1093/bioinformatics/btp515

Leuchter, A. F., Hunter, A. M., Krantz, D. E., and Cook, I. A. (2014). Intermediate phenotypes and biomarkers of treatment outcome in major depressive disorder. *Dialogues Clin. Neurosci.* 16, 525–537.

Lu, K., Abo, R. P., Schlieper, K. A., Graffam, M. E., Levine, S., Wishnok, J. S., et al. (2014). Arsenic exposure perturbs the gut microbiome and its metabolic profile in mice: an integrated metagenomics and metabolomics analysis. *Environ. Health Perspect.* 122, 284–291. doi: 10.1289/ehp.1307429

Marbach, D., Costello, J. C., Küffner, R., Vega, N. M., Prill, R. J., Camacho, D. M., et al. (2012). Wisdom of crowds for robust gene network inference. *Nat. Methods* 9, 796–804. doi: 10.1038/nmeth.2016

Montiel-Castro, A. J., González-Cervantes, R. M., Bravo-Ruiseco, G., and Pacheco-López, G. (2013). The microbiota-gut-brain axis: neurobehavioral correlates, health and sociality. *Front. Integr. Neurosci.* 7:70. doi: 10.3389/fnint.2013.00070

Muñoz-Garcia, A., Thomas, C. P., Keeney, D. S., Zheng, Y., and Brash, A. R. (2014). The importance of the lipoxygenase-hepoxilin pathway in the mammalian epidermal barrier. *Biochim. Biophys. Acta Mol. Cell Biol. Lipids* 1841, 401–408. doi: 10.1016/j.bbalip.2013.08.020

Ono, K., Muetze, T., Kolishovski, G., Shannon, P., and Demchak, B. (2015). CyREST: turbocharging cytoscape access for external tools via a RESTful API. 4:478. doi: 10.12688/f1000research.6767.1

Ormerod, K. L., Wood, D. L. A., Lachner, N., Gellatly, S. L., Daly, J. N., Parsons, J. D., et al. (2016). Genomic characterization of the uncultured Bacteroidales family S24-7 inhabiting the guts of homeothermic animals. *Microbiome* 4, 1–17. doi: 10.1186/s40168-016-0181-2

Phipson, B., Lee, S., Majewski, I. J., Alexander, W. S., and Smyth, G. K. (2016). Robust hyperparameter estimation protects against hypervariable genes and improves power to detect differential expression. *Ann. Appl. Stat.* 10, 946–963. doi: 10.1214/16-AOAS920

Rajasundaram, D., Runavot, J.-L., Guo, X., Willats, W. G. T., Meulewaeter, F., and Selbig, J. (2014). Understanding the relationship between cotton fiber properties and non-cellulosic cell wall polysaccharides. *PLoS ONE* 9:e112168. doi: 10.1371/journal.pone.0112168

Rooks, M. G., Veiga, P., Wardwell-Scott, L. H., Tickle, T., Segata, N., Michaud, M., et al. (2014). Gut microbiome composition and function in experimental colitis during active disease and treatment-induced remission. *ISME J.* 8, 1403–1417. doi: 10.1038/ismej.2014.3

Saccenti, E., Suarez-Diez, M., Luchinat, C., Santucci, C., and Tenori, L. (2015). Probabilistic networks of blood metabolites in healthy subjects as indicators of latent cardiovascular risk. *J. Proteome Res.* 14, 1101–1111. doi: 10.1021/pr501075r

Schäfer, J., and Strimmer, K. (2005). A shrinkage approach to large-scale covariance matrix estimation and implications for functional genomics. *Stat. Appl. Genet. Mol. Biol.* 4, 1175–1189. doi: 10.2202/1544-6115.1175

Schwartz, S., Friedberg, I., Ivanov, I. V, Davidson, L. A., Goldsby, J. S., Dahl, D. B., et al. (2012). A metagenomic study of diet-dependent interaction between gut microbiota and host in infants reveals differences in immune response. *Genome Biol.* 13, 1–16. doi: 10.1186/gb-2012-13-4-r32

Shannon, P., Markiel, A., Ozier, O., Baliga, N. S., Wang, J. T., Ramage, D., et al. (2003). Cytoscape: a software environment for integrated models of biomolecular interaction networks. *Genome Res.* 13, 2498–2504. doi: 10.1101/gr.1239303

Smyth, G. K. (2005). "limma: linear models for microarray data," in *Bioinformatics and Computational Biology Solutions Using R and Bioconductor SE - 23 Statistics for Biology and Health*, eds R. Gentleman, V. Carey, W. Huber, R. Irizarry, and S. Dudoit (New York, NY: Springer), 397–420.

Steegenga, W. T., Mischke, M., Lute, C., Boekschoten, M. V, Lendvai, A., Pruis, M. G. M., et al. (2016). Maternal exposure to a Western-style diet causes differences in intestinal microbiota composition and gene expression of suckling mouse pups. *Mol. Nutr. Food Res.* 61. doi: 10.1002/mnfr.201600141

Teran, V., Luna Pizarro, P., Zacarias, M. F., Vinderola, G., Medina, R., and Van Nieuwenhove, C. (2015). Production of conjugated dienoic and trienoic fatty acids by lactic acid bacteria and bifidobacteria. *J. Funct. Foods* 19, 417–425. doi: 10.1016/j.jff.2015.09.046

Tibshirani, R. (2011). Regression shrinkage and selection via the lasso: a retrospective. *J. R. Stat. Soc. Ser. B Stat. Methodol.* 73, 273–282. doi: 10.1111/j.1467-9868.2011.00771.x

Winter, D. (2016). *rentrez: Entrez in R.* Available online at: https://cran.r-project.org/web/packages/rentrez/rentrez.pdf

Zhu, X., Gerstein, M., and Snyder, M. (2007). Getting connected: analysis and principles of biological networks. *Genes Dev.* 21, 1010–1024. doi: 10.1101/gad.1528707

9

LiverSex Computational Model: Sexual Aspects in Hepatic Metabolism and Abnormalities

Tanja Cvitanović Tomaš [1], Žiga Urlep [1], Miha Moškon [2], Miha Mraz [2] and Damjana Rozman [1]*

[1] Faculty of Medicine, Centre for Functional Genomics and Bio-Chips, Institute of Biochemistry, University of Ljubljana, Ljubljana, Slovenia, [2] Faculty of Computer and Information Science, University of Ljubljana, Ljubljana, Slovenia

***Correspondence:**
Damjana Rozman
damjana.rozman@mf.uni-lj.si

The liver is to date the best example of a sexually dimorphic non-reproductive organ. Over 1,000 genes are differentially expressed between sexes indicating that female and male livers are two metabolically distinct organs. The spectrum of liver diseases is broad and is usually prevalent in one or the other sex, with different contributing genetic and environmental factors. It is thus difficult to predict individual's disease outcomes and treatment options. Systems approaches including mathematical modeling can aid importantly in understanding the multifactorial liver disease etiology leading toward tailored diagnostics, prognostics and therapy. The currently established computational models of hepatic metabolism that have proven to be essential for understanding of non-alcoholic fatty liver disease (NAFLD) and hepatocellular carcinoma (HCC) are limited to the description of gender-independent response or reflect solely the response of the males. Herein we present *LiverSex*, the first sex-based multi-tissue and multi-level liver metabolic computational model. The model was constructed based on *in silico* liver model *SteatoNet* and the object-oriented modeling. The crucial factor in adaptation of liver metabolism to the sex is the inclusion of estrogen and androgen receptor responses to respective hormones and the link to sex-differences in growth hormone release. The model was extensively validated on literature data and experimental data obtained from wild type C57BL/6 mice fed with regular chow and western diet. These experimental results show extensive sex-dependent changes and could not be reproduced *in silico* with the uniform model *SteatoNet*. *LiverSex* represents the first large-scale liver metabolic model, which allows a detailed insight into the sex-dependent complex liver pathologies, and how the genetic and environmental factors interact with the sex in disease appearance and progression. We used the model to identify the most important sex-dependent metabolic pathways, which are involved in accumulation of triglycerides representing initial steps of NAFLD. We identified PGC1A, PPARα, FXR, and LXR as regulatory factors that could become important in sex-dependent personalized treatment of NAFLD.

Keywords: sexual dimorphism, hepatic metabolism, systems medicine, large-scale metabolic model, NAFLD, liver

INTRODUCTION

The pharmacological and clinical discussions about the influence of gender on drug metabolism and disease susceptibility are raising, while on the other hand studies that would reveal the molecular basis of sex-based differences in humans are limited (Flórez-Vargas et al., 2016). Sexual dimorphism in animal kingdom has been known for centuries. Despite this, the majority of studies still focus on one sex and the results are discussed in a generalized manner. The choice of males as the dominant research model was justified by studies that showed females having higher biological variability associated with fluctuation of sex hormones during the reproductive cycle (McGregor et al., 2016).

Sexual dimorphism is a widespread phenomenon of somatic, physiologic, and behavioral differences between females and males (Söder, 2007; Urlep et al., 2017). Genes regulated by sex hormones differ in their tissue expression, which is particularly true for liver metabolism (Gustafsson et al., 1983). Transcriptome and proteome studies report that scope of described sexually dimorphic gene expression is significantly larger than previously recognized. Thousands of genes differ in expression between females and males not only in the liver (Laz et al., 2004; Yang et al., 2006; Waxman and Holloway, 2009) but also in adipose tissue and muscle, while brain expression seems to be less sexually dimorphic (Yang et al., 2006). In the context of the liver pathologies dissimilarities of sex hormones are listed among the main reasons for the differences in the prevalence of liver diseases. Hepatocellular carcinoma (HCC) is more frequent in males (Zheng et al., 2017), while females have increased risk of autoimmune liver diseases and exacerbated liver damage in alcoholic liver disease (Guy and Peters, 2013). In non-alcoholic fatty liver disease (NAFLD) the distinction is less clear with inconsistent reports of increased incidence in males and post-menopausal women, possibly due to increased tendency for visceral fat accumulation (Suzuki and Abdelmalek, 2009; Pan and Fallon, 2014).

A recent comprehensive review of NAFLD studies (Ballestri et al., 2017) identified age, sex, body construction, susceptibility to gaining weight, existence of metabolic syndrome and genetically determined characteristics as critical factors influencing NAFLD onset and/or progression. Studies show that the progression of NAFLD in males is independent of age (Kojima et al., 2003; Xu et al., 2013). This is in contrast to the correlation between age and NAFLD incidence in females, where NAFLD occurrence is decreased in premenopausal, but not in postmenopausal women (Hamaguchi et al., 2012; Florentino et al., 2013). Another study reported that women with NAFLD are approximately 10 years older than men (Carulli et al., 2006). Based on these studies, premenopausal women might be better protected from developing NAFLD compared to men and postmenopausal women. Estrogens might provide part of the explanation, as it has been reported that women with NAFLD have lower concentrations of serum estradiol than woman without NAFLD (Gutierrez-Grobe et al., 2010).

To describe the complex nature of liver metabolism and predict all possible consequences of genetic and metabolic insults computational approaches are applied (Petta et al., 2016; Hoehme et al., 2017; Lorente et al., 2017). Several large-scale metabolic models have been established to investigate liver metabolism (Holzhütter et al., 2012; Drasdo et al., 2014) and liver related diseases, such as NAFLD (Mardinoglu et al., 2014; Naik et al., 2014) and HCC (Agren et al., 2014). Large-scale metabolic models of liver metabolism and their clinical applications have recently been reviewed (Cvitanović et al., 2017). Among the most popular state-of-the-art computational approaches are genome-scale metabolic networks, where omics data are integrated to better understand the genotype-phenotype relationships (Lewis et al., 2012). Large-scale metabolic models, however, do not differentiate between genders and are mostly established and validated on the unified or male data. Gender-based differentiation has been performed only in smaller models, which do not account for the whole liver metabolism. Matthews et al. (2007) constructed a database and a model to predict reproductive toxicity in both genders, fetal dysmorphogenesis, functional toxicity, mortality, growth, and new-born behavioral toxicity of untested chemicals. A computational model of oxygenation and transport of solutes in the kidneys of spontaneously hypertensive female rats was used to investigate the sex differences in nitric oxide levels (Chen et al., 2017). Agren et al. (2014) established a liver metabolic model that indirectly accounted for gender-related differences. They reconstructed a personalized genome-scale metabolic model for each of the 27 patients with hepatocellular carcinoma. Ten of the 27 patients were females, which shows that personalized approaches can and should take gender into account. The major reason for the lack of human gender-based large-scale metabolic models might be an insufficient number of liver transcriptome-based studies that would account for both sexes (Zhang et al., 2012; Oshida et al., 2016).

Herein we present *LiverSex*, the first gender based multi-tissue and multi-level liver metabolic model. The construction of the model was performed with the extension and adaptation of the *SteatoNet* model (Naik et al., 2014), which was generated to investigate hepatic metabolism and liver related deregulations. *SteatoNet* as well as *LiverSex* feature two crucial characteristics: they account for (1) interactions between hepatic metabolic pathways and extra-hepatic tissues, and (2) regulations on transcriptional and post-translational levels. The experimentally observed sexual differences in liver gene expression were successfully reproduced *in silico* with *LiverSex*. Finally, the sensitivity analysis was applied to identify sex-dependent liver metabolic network deregulations that transform healthy liver to NAFLD.

MATERIALS AND METHODS

SteatoNet and Object Oriented Modeling

SteatoNet (*Steatosis Network*) (Naik et al., 2014) represents a dynamic semi-quantitative model based on a steady-state analysis of differential algebraic equations (DAEs). *SteatoNet* was established in object-oriented modeling language *Modelica*. It is based on the *Systems Bio*logy library *SysBio* (Belič et al., 2013), which was constructed to describe biological pathway entities. The *SysBio* library includes objects corresponding to the biological behavior of enzymes, metabolites, non-enzymatic regulatory proteins, mRNAs, flux sources, gene expression regulations, etc. Using object-oriented modeling approach models are easy to construct by linking the basic objects of *SysBio* library into a meaningful and hierarchical composition. Due to the steady-state normalization of the observed quantities most of the parameters describing the dynamics of the observed system are lumped when using *SysBio* library. This simplifies the model establishment, since only a small set of parameters needs to be evaluated. The main parameters governing the dynamical properties of the established models describe the metabolic flux distributions in each of the pathway branches. *SteatoNet* includes all major pathways of mammalian liver metabolism. Pathways that are included in the model were manually acquired from KEGG (Du et al., 2014) and REACTOME (Croft et al., 2011) databases and from the literature. *SteatoNet* additionally describes the transport of metabolites between liver, adipose tissue, pancreas, other extra-hepatic tissues, and macrophages *via* blood. The external sources of nutrients [influx of fatty acids and triglycerides (TG), glucose, cholesterol, and essential amino acids] have also been included into the model. Details of its structure have been extensively described before (Naik et al., 2014).

Data Availability

Freely accessible version of the *SteatoNet* and *LiverSex* along with the *SysBio* library can be downloaded from http://lrss.fri.uni-lj.si/bio/sysbio. The simulations can be executed with the open source Modelica simulation environment OpenModelica, which can be downloaded from https://openmodelica.org.

Construction of *LiverSex*

The hormonal regulation is simplified to a level that still ensures normal function. All included hormones are arranged into three groups: growth hormone, androgen, and estrogens. Androgen or estrogen groups represent any steroid hormones that regulate the development and maintenance of sex characteristics in vertebrates by binding to corresponding steroid hormone receptor (Sharma et al., 2017). Each group of hormones has its own source of flux. These sources display differences in hormonal regulation of liver between females and males. The growth hormone source acts as a daily oscillator in males or has a constant concentration in females (Norstedt and Palmiter, 1984; Waxman and O'connor, 2006). The female estradiol source mimics the monthly estrous cycle that cannot be found in males (Ciana et al., 2003; Shanle and Xu, 2010; Villa et al., 2012). In males, the androgen source is 10-fold higher than the estrogens source (Domonkos et al., 2017), while in females the androgen source is three-fold lower than the estrogen source (Simpson, 2003). Every hormone source is connected to its respective receptor. Each hormone receptor has an active and inactive form, which allows us to simulate different diseases connected with the perturbations of receptor functions. Active form of the receptors is in addition linked to *SteatoNet* according to the literature evidence (Heine et al., 2000; Barclay et al., 2011; Gårevik et al., 2012) and these connections than finally lead to the female and male *LiverSex* model. A more detailed description of sex-dependent hormonal regulation of liver metabolism is included in the Supplementary Data.

Validation of *LiverSex*

Expression profiling data (GEO database GSE78892) obtained from the hepatocyte specific *Cyp51* knockout mice (*Cyp51*$^{\text{flox/flox}}$; *Alb-Cre*) (Lorbek et al., 2013, 2015) are used for direct *LiverSex* validation. Female and male mice of mixed genetic background (129/Pas × C57BL/6J, close to 90% C57BL/6J) were included in the experiment and after the weaning period (age 3 weeks) put on a standard laboratory chow (Altromin) or isocaloric high-fat diet with 1.25% (w/w) of cholesterol (western diet) for another 16 weeks. For validation of *LiverSex* three objects defining the diet have been included in the model: sources of glucose, cholesterol, and triglycerides. Experimental conditions were simulated in the model by altering the nutrient (triglyceride and cholesterol) influx into the network, thus mimicking the experimental diets. Inconsistencies between biological observations and model simulations mainly occurred due to the missing components and regulatory connections in the model. A series of simulations was executed to identify the network components that caused erroneous behavior. Further in-depth literature searches were performed in the context of these components to identify the regulations that were absent in the network or were incorrectly depicted. The western diet was replicated *in silico* by increasing the influx of triglycerides (10-fold) and cholesterol (five-fold) (fold-changes were estimated from the strict composition of western diet and standard laboratory chow).

Sensitivity Analysis

Sensitivity analysis can provide valuable insight in the robustness of the computational model in dependence on the perturbations of model inputs, i.e., parameters values (Bentele et al., 2004). Moreover, sensitivity analysis can identify parameters with the greatest impact on the observed outputs. These parameters present potential targets for further experimental analysis (Zi, 2011). Sensitivity analysis has an important function in the analysis of computational models in systems biology and medicine (Ingalls, 2008). Metabolic Control Analysis (MCA) presents a sensitivity analysis method (Fell and Sauro, 1985) that was initially focused to the analysis of metabolic networks. The method was later adapted to the models of other biological networks such as cell signaling models, models of genetic networks, and models of other biological processes (Westerhoff et al., 1984; Heinrich and Schuster, 1996). MCA assesses the sensitivity of the model output with respect to the selected input with evaluation of control coefficients. Here, metabolic fluxes through the observed metabolic reactions or concentration of metabolites can be used as model outputs while model parameters can be used as model inputs. The MCA of the distribution of the metabolic fluxes in each of the pathway branches can be performed with the following equation:

$$C_f^X = \frac{d(X)}{df} = \frac{X^* - X}{f^* - f} \times \frac{f}{X}. \tag{1}$$

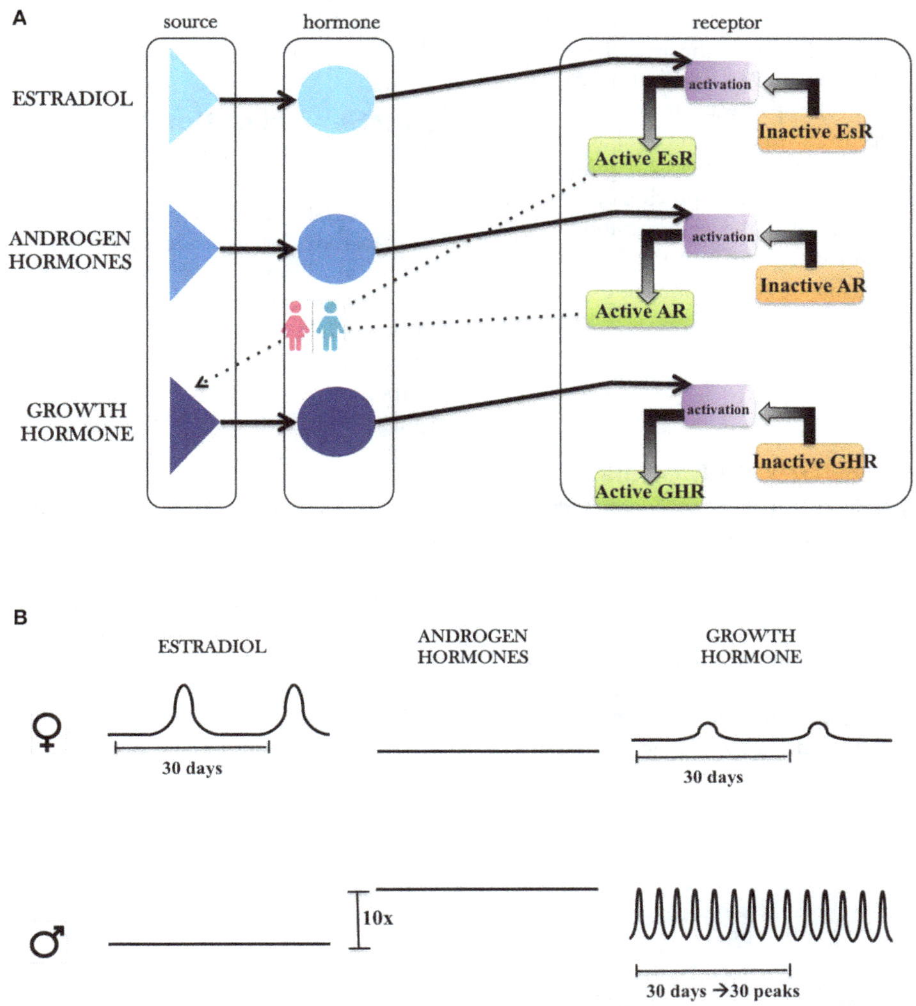

FIGURE 1 | Modeling hormonal regulation with *SysBio* library. **(A)** Graphical presentation of hormonal object in *SysBio* library. Each hormone group contains its own source, the hormone and corresponding receptor, which is further connected with hepatocyte based on literature evidence. **(B)** Differences between hormone sources based on the literature evidence. FEMALES: Estrogen concentrations are three-fold higher than androgens, and estrogens have one peak, which is consistent with the monthly oestrous cycle. Because of the estrogen receptor feedback regulation on growth hormone, we can observe the influence of estrous cycle on growth hormone. MALES: Androgen concentrations are 10-fold higher than concentrations of estrogens. Growth hormone concentrations show daily oscillations with ~24-h period.

where C_f^X represents the concentration control coefficient of parameter f with regard to X. X^* and X describe the concentration of the observed metabolite, which presents a variable under study at nominal (f) and perturbed flux distribution value (f^*). The ratio between f and X is normalized to achieve the relative value of sensitivity coefficient.

According to our previous experimental data and the literature data the NAFLD pathogenesis can be associated with *de novo* lipogenesis (Lorbek et al., 2013, 2015; Green et al., 2015; Sanders and Griffin, 2016; Softic et al., 2016). Our analyses of NAFLD progression were thus based on the observation of triglyceride accumulation. The variations in their accumulation were observed in dependence on the distribution of metabolic fluxes at pathway branch points, which can be described as model inputs. The concentration control coefficient from the Equation (1) was thus defined as a partial derivate of the alterations in triglyceride concentration with respect to the small changes in the distribution of fluxes at pathway branch points:

$$C_f^{TG} = \frac{d(TG)}{df} = \frac{TG^* - TG}{f^* - f} \times \frac{f}{TG}, \tag{2}$$

where TG^* and TG are triglyceride concentrations with flux distribution parameter values of f^* and f, respectively. The described method was used to identify the branch points with the largest sensitivities in each of the models. Moreover, the obtained values were used to identify branch points and their corresponding metabolic pathways, which have the largest gender-dependent influence on NAFLD progression.

To evaluate the sensitivity of hepatic triglyceride concentration in dependence on the metabolic flux distribution of *LiverSex*, the triglyceride influx into the model was raised by 10-fold to imitate high fat diet. The distribution parameter for each branch point in the pathway model was varied incrementally by 5% up to a maximum of 30%. Further investigation was focused on the analysis of gender-based influences of regulatory factors on the previously identified metabolic pathways. We calculated the concentration control coefficient of regulatory factors, i.e., C_f^R, using Equation (1), where $\boldsymbol{X}$ is replaced with regulator $\boldsymbol{R}$ from the list of molecular regulators (see Supplementary Table 2). Analyses were performed for each of the molecular regulators.

RESULTS

Construction of *LiverSex* by Modeling Hormonal Regulation With *SysBio* Library

LiverSex is composed of mathematical expressions of relationships between sex hormones and growth hormone, their corresponding receptors in hepatocytes and is based on literature evidence. An object named *hormonal regulation* is inserted into the blood section of the model. This object is connected with corresponding pathways in the hepatocyte. As explained in detail in the Materials and Methods section, it includes androgens, estrogens, and growth hormone (**Figure 1**). Each group of hormones has an effect on its corresponding receptor. The behavior of hormones is determined by gender, which results in two gender-specific models.

LiverSex Validation With Experimental Data

Three objects describing the diet have been included in *LiverSex*: glucose source, cholesterol source, and triglyceride source. Experimental conditions were mimicked in the model by altering the substrate (triglyceride and cholesterol) influx into the network in dependence on the experimental diets investigated (standard laboratory diet and western diet).

The set of 45 genes that were differentially expressed between females and males in mice fed with altromin and western diets (Lorbek et al., 2013, 2015) was screened for genes that are regulated inversely in females and males: either upregulated in males and downregulated in females or *vice versa*. Three inversely expressed genes were obtained (**Figure 2A**). The 1-AcylGlycerol-3-Phosphate O-AcylTransferase gene *Agpat* which is involved in lipid and glucose metabolism, and Protein Kinase AMP-Activated catalytic subunit Alpha gene *Prkaa* were downregulated in males and upregulated in females, while the Insulin Receptor Substrate gene *Irs*, which is involved in insulin signaling pathway, was upregulated in males and downregulated in females. While the simulation results obtained by the *SteatoNet* could only be attributed to males (**Figure 2B**), *LiverSex* correctly described the data from both genders (**Figures 2C,D**).

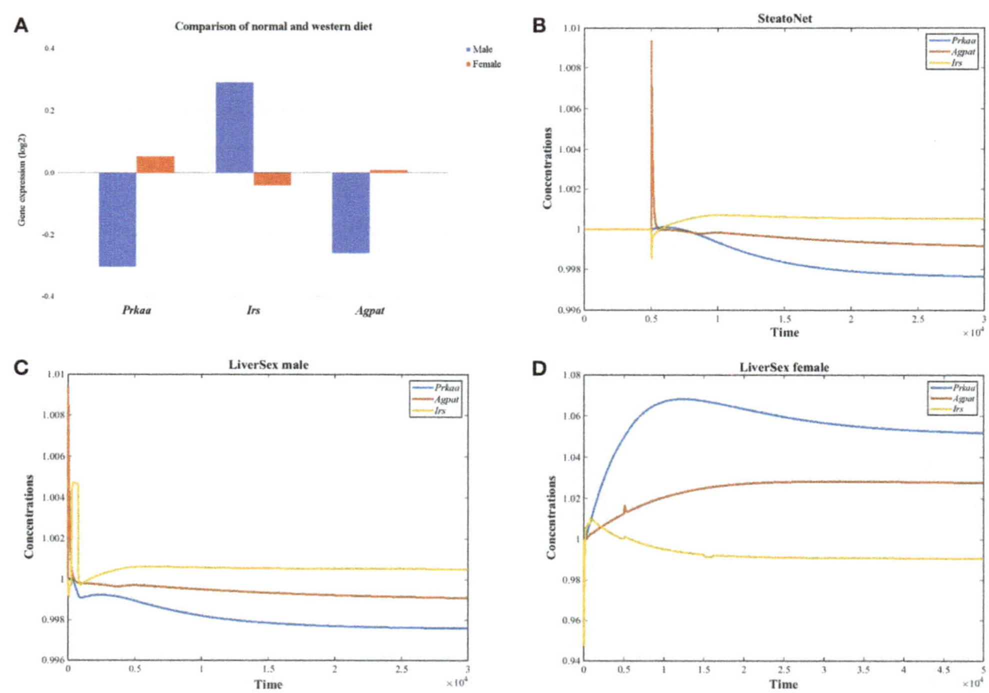

FIGURE 2 | *LiverSex* validation with experimental data. **(A)** Graph represents gender based gene expression data obtained with the experiment (mice fed with standard laboratory diet and western diet). For these genes, we looked up the log2 fold change values and *p*-values for the comparison of both diets in wild-type female and male mice. **(B)** *SteatoNet* simulation results represent only the male gender. **(C)** *LiverSex* simulation results represent the male gene expression response on the high fat diet. **(D)** The female *LiverSex* response to the high fat diet.

LiverSex Prediction of Signaling Pathways That Trigger NAFLD

With sensitivity analysis we were able to identify metabolic reactions with the largest gender dependent influence on hepatic triglyceride accumulation, which is considered as the initial stage of NAFLD. **Table 1** shows concentration control coefficients with respect to hepatic triglyceride accumulation listed in direction from the maximal to the minimal differences in sensitivity values for males and females. Only the first 20 parameters are listed in **Table 1** (see Supplementary Material for the full list of parameters—Supplementary Table 1). If we classify the metabolic reaction with $C_f^{TG} > 1$ as highly sensitive with respect to hepatic triglyceride accumulation, only 3 reactions can be regarded as highly sensitive: transformation of monoacylglycerol to glycerol (*k159*), transport of triglycerides from liver to adipose triglyceride lipid droplets (*k177*), and transformation of acetoacetate to β-hydroxybutyrate (*k152*). Transformation of monoacylglycerol to glycerol and transport of hepatic triglycerides to adipose triglyceride lipid droplets are highly sensitive metabolic pathways in both genders, but metabolic reaction from acetoacetate to β-hydroxybutyrate, which is a part of the body ketone metabolism, shows a higher tendency for female hepatic triglyceride accumulation only.

TABLE 1 | Concentration control coefficients C_f^{TG} with respect to hepatic triglyceride accumulation in *LiverSex* for males in females.

C_f^{TG} for males		C_f^{TG} for females	
Parameter	**Sensitivity**	**Parameter**	**Sensitivity**
k159	88.19979	k159	109.4524
k177	2.179425	k177	2.373645
k500	0.609015	k152	1.469995
k180	0.248614	k500	0.661528
k179	0.082083	k180	0.114715
k142	0.06897	k163	0.052388
k163	0.061144	k142	0.046768
k1051	0.053941	k179	0.044451
k154	0.053466	k800	0.030237
k152	0.051326	k102	0.017683
k155	0.043668	k154	0.01731
k169	0.042516	k176	0.015594
k800	0.039541	k169	0.015429
k150	0.03319	k144	0.01494
k170	0.030855	k155	0.014034
k187	0.026241	k1051	0.012309
k166	0.025481	k187	0.011062
k165	0.025479	k150	0.010651
k164	0.025467	k170	0.010537
k144	0.025462	k105	0.009198

k102, *Hepatic glucose → Glucose-6P;* ***k105,*** *Hepatic glucose → Blood glucose;* ***k142,*** *Fructose-1,6BP → DHAP;* ***k144,*** *mito AcetylCoA + Oxaloacetate → Citrate;* ***k150,*** *Acetoacetate → blood Acetoacetate;* ***k152,*** *Acetoacetate → β-hydroxybutyrate;* ***k154,*** *blood β-hydroxybutyrate → adipose β-hydroxybutyrate;* ***k155,*** *blood → Acetoacetate adipose Acetoacetate;* ***k159,*** *MAG → Glycerol;* ***k163,*** *[Cholesterol source + (LDL cholesterol → Cholesterol) + (A 2 HDL → Cholesterol) + (HMGCoA → Cholesterol)] → Cholesterol utilization;* ***k164,*** *blood → Cholesterol macrophage Cholesterol;* ***k165,*** *blood → Cholesterol adipose Cholesterol;* ***k166,*** *blood Cholesterol → tissue Cholesterol;* ***k169,*** *adipose Fatty → acids Unsaturated FattyAcylCoA;* ***k170,*** *adipose Fatty → acids Saturated FattyAcylCoA;* ***k172,*** *UnsaturatedFattyAcylCoA adipocyte → FattyAcylCoA Glycerol3P to LPA adipocyte;* ***k173,*** *DAG → TG;* ***k177,*** *TG → adipose TG lipid droplet;* ***k179,*** *blood Fatty → acids tissue Fatty acids;* ***k180,*** *Chylomicron → Chylomicron remnants;* ***k187,*** *Oxoglutarate + Ammonia → Glutamate;* ***k172,*** *FattyAcylCoA + Glycerol2P → LPA;* ***k500,*** *TG → VLDL;* ***k800,*** *(TG → DAG) + (PA → DAG) + (MAG DAG);* ***k1051,*** *Blood → glucoseAdipose glucose;* ***k1071****-Hepatic glucoseBlood → glucose.*

The concentration control coefficients reflect the impact of perturbations on metabolite concentration. In our case, these coefficients measure the relative steady-state change in triglyceride accumulation in response to the relative change in fluxes at metabolic branch points. Data obtained with sensitivity analysis are sorted by descending absolute difference of sensitivity values between male and female. It is interesting that the first few pathways show a predominant effect in females (**Figure 3**). The terminal degradation of triglycerides by conversion of monoacylglycerol to glycerol (k159) seems to be the most powerful flux in the network in both sexes. However, upon perturbation with the diet, triglyceride accumulation is affected more in females. Hepatic glycerol utilization is a metabolic pathway, which is preferentially connected with carbohydrate metabolism in men and lipid metabolism in women (Rodríguez et al., 2015). Females display a higher sensitivity to ketone body metabolism (*k152*), transport of triglycerides (*k177*), and VLDL transport (*k500*), which carries triglycerides from the liver, possibly to avoid the development of fatty liver, taking them to the peripheral tissues for storage in adipose or for use in skeletal muscle.

Regulatory Factors Involved in Sex-Dependent Differences in NAFLD Progression

Pathway branch points with the most significant absolute difference of C_f^{TG} between sexes were further investigated to identify regulatory factors, which are sensitive to alterations in flux distribution at these branches. By calculating C_f^R with respect to various regulatory factors in the *LiverSex*, we obtained results presented in **Table 2** and Supplementary Table 2. **Figure 4** illustrates the regulatory factors with high sensitivity to alterations in flux distributions within the respective metabolic pathways. PGC1A (Peroxisome proliferator-activated receptor gamma coactivator 1-alpha, known also as PPARGC1A), which induces mitochondrial biogenesis, PPARα (Peroxisome Proliferator Activated Receptor alpha), the major regulator of lipid metabolism, FXR (Farnesoid X Receptor), a regulator of bile acid synthesis and excretion, LXR (Liver X Receptor), involved in lipid and cholesterol metabolism, and ADIPO (adiponectin), which is involved in glucose regulation and fatty acid oxidation, display global sensitivity to alterations in metabolic flux distribution at the majority of the high sensitivity pathway branches, indicating the broad role of these transcription factors.

DISCUSSION

Object oriented modeling can be successfully employed to support hierarchical structuring, reuse and evolution of more complex models, independently of the application domain.

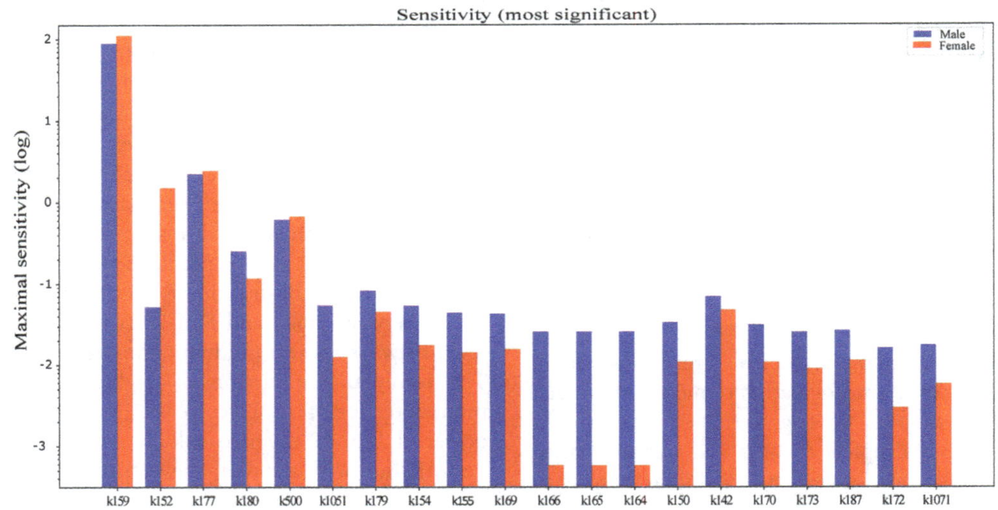

FIGURE 3 | Difference between gender dependent concentration control coefficients C_f^{TG} with respect to hepatic triglyceride accumulation in *LiverSex*. Data are obtained with sensitivity analysis and sorted by descending absolute difference of sensitivity values in males and females. Data are presented in the logarithmic scale. ***k159***, MAG → Glycerol; ***k152***, Acetoacetate → β-hydroxybutyrate; ***k177***, TG → adipose TG lipid droplet; ***k180***, Chylomicron → Chylomicron remnants; ***k500***, TG → VLDL; ***k1051***, Blood glucose → Adipose glucose; ***k179***, blood Fatty acids → tissue Fatty acids; ***k154***, blood β-hydroxybutyrate → adipose β-hydroxybutyrate; ***k155***, blood Acetoacetate adipose Acetoacetate; ***k169***, adipose Fatty acids → Unsaturated FattyAcylCoA; ***k166***, blood Cholesterol → tissue Cholesterol; ***k165***, blood Cholesterol → adipose Cholesterol; ***k164***, blood Cholesterol → macrophage Cholesterol; ***k150***, Acetoacetate → blood Acetoacetate; ***k142***, Fructose-1,6BP → DHAP; ***k170***, adipose Fatty → acids Saturated FattyAcylCoA; ***k173***, DAG → TG; ***k187***, Oxoglutarate + Ammonia → Glutamate; ***k172***, FattyAcylCoA + Glycerol2P LPA; ***k1071***, Hepatic glucose → Blood glucose.

This also holds true for the *LiverSex,* where *SteatoNet* is reused for adaptation to gender specific data. An object with hormonal regulation is added to the *SysBio* library and after that positioned into *SteatoNet* and connected to the liver based on literature data. These models are constructed manually, i.e., by connecting the *SysBio* objects that correspond to the biological entities within the observed network. We are, however, currently working on the automation of this construction process. The *LiverSex* model by itself has certain limitations, which mainly originate from the derivation of the *SysBio* library, which is used for model construction. In order to reduce the space of unknown parameters, the *SysBio* library objects presume the normalized steady-state of the system. Obtained results thus do not correspond to the actual concentrations of observed metabolites due to the normalization of their concentrations (Naik et al., 2014). The *LiverSex* was, however, successful in replicating the results that correspond to different mice strains as well as human data found in the literature.

The mechanism responsible for NAFLD progression in humans is not yet fully understood. Furthermore, sex differences have a big impact on the prevalence of NAFLD. Based on the current data, premenopausal women are better protected from developing NAFLD compared to men and postmenopausal women (Ballestri et al., 2017). In this study, we tried to expose the sexual differences in NAFLD based on hepatic triglyceride accumulation. After performing sensitivity analyses, metabolic differences between sexes in NAFLD were identified (see **Figure 4**). Sensitivity analyses pinpointed to metabolic pathways, in which the same perturbations cause the largest differences in hepatic triglyceride accumulation. According to the literature data all metabolic pathways with a high sensitivity for hepatic triglyceride accumulation as reported by *LiverSex* are involved in the earliest stage of NAFLD pathogenesis (Cohen et al., 2011). One of the initial steps of NAFLD is hepatic steatosis, which is characterized by the deposition of triglycerides as lipid droplets (Reingold et al., 2005) and according to the results of the sensitivity analyses of *LiverSex*, this metabolic step is more sensitive in females.

Microsomal triglyceride transfers protein (MTTP) facilitates triglyceride, cholesteryl ester, and phospholipid transport between phospholipid surfaces (*k500*). A defect in lipid export from the liver may also contribute to the pathogenesis of steatosis (Fabbrini et al., 2008). MTTP is necessary for the assembly and secretion of VLDL from hepatocytes (Jamil et al., 1995). It is responsible for lipoprotein assembly by transferring triglycerides, to nascent apolipoproteins B. The *LiverSex* demonstrates that transferring triglycerides by MTTP, which is involved in NAFLD progression, is more sensitive in females. It was previously reported that MTTP expression is sex-dependent and that female GH secretory pattern has a significant influence on its expression (Améen and Oscarsson, 2003).

Hormone sensitive lipase (HSL) converts monoacylglycerides to free fatty acids and glycerol (MGLL or MAGL) (*k159*) and this step regulates the quantity of fatty acids, which are used as signaling molecules and have been shown to promote cancer cell migration, invasion and tumor growth (Nomura et al., 2010). MAGL is a crucial lipolytic enzyme and an important regulator of tumor progression. It can promote hepatocellular carcinoma

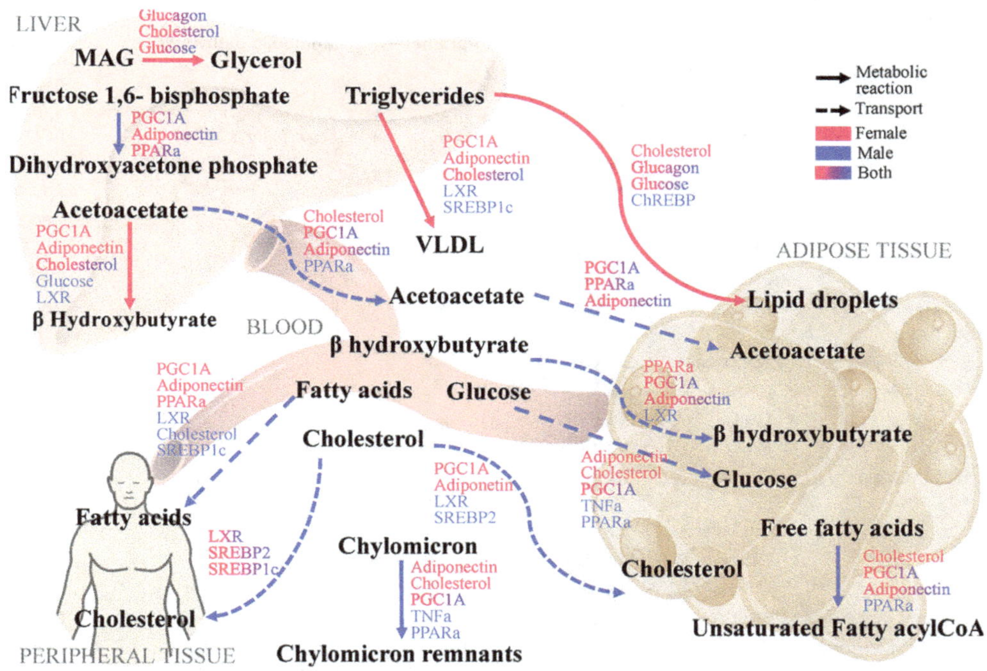

FIGURE 4 | *LiverSex* identified pathways and regulatory factors with largest difference between genders and with respect to hepatic triglyceride accumulation as the first step of NAFLD. The displayed pathways that show the largest differences between genders and determine the change in hepatic triglyceride accumulation highlight branch-points with high dynamic sensitivity. Regulatory factors that are affected by modifications in flux distribution are categorized at the corresponding reaction to which they are sensitive. MAG, Monoacylglycerol; PGC1A, Peroxisome Proliferator-Activated Receptor Gamma Coactivator 1 alpha; PPARa, Peroxisome Proliferator-Activated Receptor alpha; FXR, Farnesoid X Receptor; LXR, Liver X Receptor; ChREBP, Carbohydrate Response Element-Binding Protein; SREBP-1c, Sterol Regulatory Element-Binding Protein-1c; SREBP-2, Sterol Regulatory Element-Binding Protein-2; VLDL, Very-Low Density Lipoprotein; TNFa, Tumor Necrosis Factor alpha.

progression and was recently suggested as a potential therapeutic target and as a biomarker for prognosis in patients with HCC (Zhu et al., 2016). Expression of HSL is decreased in NAFLD compared with normal liver (Kohjima et al., 2007), which was also observed in our simulation results. There is currently no literature data describing the sex-specific differences in the expression of liver HSL. However, differences were reported previously in skeletal muscles, where women were found to have a higher intramuscular triacylglycerol during exercise than men, and also higher mRNA levels of HSL in the muscle. Yet, as HSL activity during prolonged exercise is higher in men it is likely that the enzyme-substrate interactions differ between the sexes (Roepstorff et al., 2006). In addition, our results show that women have a higher susceptibility to changes in lipolysis. show that women have a higher susceptibility to changes in lipolysis.

Removal of FA from the liver occurs by secretion as VLDL (*k500*) and by FA oxidation (*k152*) (Hodson and Frayn, 2011). Some studies suggest women have enhanced production and clearance of VLDL compared to men (Wang et al., 2011). Few studies have investigated sex-specific differences in FA oxidation and found out that after a prolonged overnight fasting, women metabolize FA toward 3-hydroxybutyrate (3OHB) to a greater extent than men (Halkes et al., 2003; Marinou et al., 2011). Other studies (Koutsari et al., 2011; Marinou et al., 2011) indicate that women exhibit a higher non-oxidative FFA disposal (i.e., esterification and storage as triglycerides) and, after an overnight fast, they are prone to partition fatty acids toward ketone body production rather than VLDL. These differences were also reflected by our *LiverSex* model.

Partition of fatty acids to ketone body production, VLDL synthesis and fatty acids oxidation, together with deposition of triglycerides as lipid droplets are considered as parts of NAFLD pathology, which were all found to be more sensitive in females in response to a high-fat diet challenge. The ability to partition fatty acids into different pathways might be one of the possible protective mechanisms in females leading to delayed NAFLD progression compared to males. However, further research is needed to confirm this hypothesis.

There are few metabolic pathways for which regulators do not show sexual dimorphism, such as transformation of monoacylglycerides to glycerol, fructose-1,6 bisphosphate to dihidroxyacetone phosphate and transport of cholesterol from blood to peripheral tissues. However, transport of fatty acids from blood to peripheral tissues and cholesterol from blood to the adipose tissue are pathways, in which regulatory factors differ substantially between genders. The activity of regulatory factors such as PGC1A, PPARα, FXR, and LXR is highly related to gender (see **Figure 4**).

Several studies have focused on the analysis of mice with liver-specific knockouts crucial for growth hormone signaling

TABLE 2 | Regulatory factors with high concentration control coefficients to alterations in flux distribution at presented branch points.

Parameter	Metabolic pathway	Regulatory factors	
		Female	**Male**
k159	MAG→ Glycerol	Glucagon	Glucagon
		Cholesterol	Cholesterol
		Glucose	Glucose
		ChREBP	ChREBP
		SREBP2	SREBP2
k152	Acetoacetate→ BHydroxybutyrate	PGC1A	Cholesterol
		Adiponectin	Glucose
		Cholesterol	LXR
		PPARα	ChREBP
		FXR	PGC1A
k177	TG→ Adipose TG lipid droplet	Glucagon	Glucagon
		Cholesterol	Glucose
		Glucose	ChREBP
		ChREBP	Cholesterol
		SREBP2	SREBP2
k180	Chylomicron→ Chylomicron remnants	PGC1A	PGC1A
		Adiponectin	TNFa
		Cholesterol	PPARα
		PPARα	LXR
		FXR	Adiponectin
k500	Triglycerides→ VLDL	PGC1A	LXR
		Adiponectin	Cholesterol
		Cholesterol	SREBP1c
		PPARα	SREBP2
		FXR	PGC1A
k1051	Blood glucose→ Adipose glucose	PGC1A	PGC1A
		Adiponectin	TNFa
		Cholesterol	PPARα
		PPARα	Adiponectin
		FXR	Glucocorticoid
k179	Blood Fatty acids→ Tissue Fatty acids	PGC1A	LXR
		Adiponectin	Cholesterol
		PPARα	SREBP1c
		FXR	PGC1A
		TNFa	Adiponectin
k154	Blood BHydroxybutyrate→ Adipose BHydroxybutyrate	PGC1A	Adiponectin
		Adiponectin	PGC1A
		PPARα	LXR
		FXR	PPARα
		TNFA	FXR
k155	Blood Acetoacetate→ Adipose Acetoacetate	PGC1A	Adiponectin
		Adiponectin	PGC1A
		PPARα	PPARα
		FXR	LXR
		TNFA	FXR

(Continued)

TABLE 2 | Continued

Parameter	Metabolic pathway	Regulatory factors	
		Female	**Male**
k169	Adipo Fatty acids→ Unsaturated FattyAcylCoA	PGC1A	PGC1A
		Adiponectin	PPARα
		Cholesterol	Adiponectin
		PPARα	TNFA
		FXR	FXR
k166	Blood Cholesterol→ Tissue Cholesterol	Cholesterol	Cholesterol
		LXR	LXR
		SREBP2	SREBP2
		SREBP1c	SREBP1c
		ChREBP	Glucose
k165	Blood Cholesterol→ Adipose Cholesterol	PGC1A	Cholesterol
		Adiponectin	LXR
		Cholesterol	SREBP2
		PPARα	SREBP1c
		FXR	Glucose
k164	Blood Cholesterol→ Macrophage Cholesterol	Cholesterol	Cholesterol
		LXR	LXR
		SREBP2	SREBP2
		SREBP1c	SREBP1c
		ChREBP	Glucose
k150	Acetoacetate→ Blood Acetoacetate	PGC1A	Adiponectin
		Adiponectin	PGC1A
		Cholesterol	PPARα
		PPARα	LXR
		FXR	FXR
k142	Fructose-1,6BP→ DHAP	PGC1A	PGC1A
		Adiponectin	Adiponectin
		PPARα	PPARα
		FXR	TNFa
		TNFa	FXR

proteins indicating an important role of growth hormone in hepatic triglyceride secretion (Cui et al., 2007; Fan et al., 2009; Barclay et al., 2011; Sos et al., 2011). *Pgc1a* has been proposed as one of the transcriptional targets responsible for steatosis (Cui et al., 2007; Fan et al., 2009; Barclay et al., 2011; Sos et al., 2011) and based on our observations women are more susceptible for this. Skeletal muscle-specific PGC-1a overexpression increased glucose uptake, glycogen and lipid droplets quantity (Mormeneo et al., 2012), raising the possibility that PGC1A could also promote triglyceride accumulation into adipose lipid droplets as predicted by our model.

PPARα is known to be highly expressed in the liver and exhibits a sex-dimorphic nature. In the liver, PPARα promotes fatty acid oxidation, which makes it a possible drug target for treating hypertriglyceridemia (Rando and Wahli, 2011). In PPARα-null mice, gross hepatic abnormalities, disclosed to the steatotic liver and hepatomegaly, were found in males, but not females (Costet et al., 1998). *LiverSex* revealed a higher capacity of females to secrete triglycerides *via* VLDL compared to males, which was also the presumed cause for the increased steatosis resistance in female PPARα-null mice (Lindén et al., 2001).

Literature search did not reveal any sex-dependent FXR and LXR correlation to liver. FXR modulates hepatic inflammation, thus, FXR sex-dimorphic function in that context is less clear (Rando and Wahli, 2011). Indication that many of the FXR, PPARα, LXRα overlapping binding sites are functional (Boergesen et al., 2012) might present the reason for sex-dimorphic behavior of these nuclear receptors. Higher FXR sensitivity to the triglycerides accumulation in females could be correlated with higher binding of Retinoic X Receptor (RXRα), which is obligate heterodimerization partner of FXR to female hepatic chromatin for the essential lipid processing genes (Kosters et al., 2013). In addition, these sex-specific binding patterns and differences in ligand responsiveness may be the reasons for sex-specific distinctive effects of drugs. LXRs act as liver lipid sensors and regulate the metabolism of cholesterol and fatty acids (Schultz et al., 2000). LXR indirectly regulates *Srebp1c*, which is directly acting on *Pnpla3* (Huang et al., 2010). It has been previously reported that LXR is not the subject of regulation by either dietary cholesterol or sex (Lorbek et al., 2013; Feillet et al., 2016), but *LiverSex* reported higher sensitivity of LXR in males in the initial steps of NAFLD.

Several nuclear receptors together with their molecular cascades are promising pharmacological targets for NAFLD treatment (Serviddio et al., 2013). Based on the results obtained by *LiverSex*, PGC1A, PPARα, FXR, and LXR could provide novel pharmacological targets for sex-based therapy in the future. Although the various studies emphasize the importance of regulators in modulating hepatic lipid homeostasis, data regarding the sex-dependent effects on the development of steatosis is still missing, emphasizing the need for further studies.

Our results suggest that one of the major hepatic characteristics is its sexually dimorphic nature. Sex steroids and growth hormone play a crucial role in fine-tuning the sex-dependent metabolic pathways in the liver. Further studies of sexually dimorphic genes and pathways as well as differences in their expression, are required for better insights into the complex functions of the liver and the relation to disease progression in both sexes. *LiverSex* and its future extensions in the context of personalized models may help with finding preventive approaches for NAFLD as well as other liver related sex-specific diseases.

AUTHOR CONTRIBUTIONS

TC: Wrote the manuscript and conducted the computational part of the study; TC and ŽU: Conducted the experimental work and analyzed the data; MMo: Devised and supervised the computational part of the study; DR, MMo, and MMr: Provided critical feedback and helped shape the research, analysis, and manuscript.

FUNDING

Supported by the resources of FP7 CASyM (Coordinating Action Systems Medicine Europe, grant no. 305033) and by Slovenian Research Agency grants P1-0390, P2-0359, and the infrastructure grant ELIXIR.

REFERENCES

Agren, R., Mardinoglu, A., Asplund, A., Kampf, C., Uhlen, M., and Nielsen, J. (2014). Identification of anticancer drugs for hepatocellular carcinoma through personalized genome-scale metabolic modeling. *Mol. Syst. Biol.* 10:721. doi: 10.1002/msb.145122

Améen, C., and Oscarsson, J. (2003). Sex difference in hepatic microsomal triglyceride transfer protein expression is determined by the growth hormone secretory pattern in the rat. *Endocrinology* 144, 3914–3921. doi: 10.1210/en.2003-0518

Ballestri, S., Nascimbeni, F., Baldelli, E., Marrazzo, A., Romagnoli, D., and Lonardo, A. (2017). NAFLD as a sexual dimorphic disease: role of gender and reproductive status in the development and progression of nonalcoholic fatty liver disease and inherent cardiovascular risk. *Adv. Ther.* 34, 1291–1326. doi: 10.1007/s12325-017-0556-1

Barclay, J. L., Nelson, C. N., Ishikawa, M., Murray, L. A., Kerr, L. M., McPhee, T. R., et al. (2011). GH-dependent STAT5 signaling plays an important role in hepatic lipid metabolism. *Endocrinology* 152, 181–192. doi: 10.1210/en.2010-0537

Belič, A., Ačimovič, J., Naik, A., and Golićnik, M. (2013). Analysis of the steady-state relations and control-algorithm characterisation in a mathematical model of cholesterol biosynthesis. *Simul. Model. Pract. Theor.* 33, 18–27. doi: 10.1016/j.simpat.2011.12.010

Bentele, M., Lavrik, I., Ulrich, M., Stösser, S., Heermann, D., Kalthoff, H., et al. (2004). Mathematical modeling reveals threshold mechanism in CD95-induced apoptosis. *J. Cell. Biol.* 166, 839–851. doi: 10.1083/jcb.200404158

Boergesen, M., Pedersen, T. Å., Gross, B., van Heeringen, S. J., Hagenbeek, D., Bindesbøll, C., et al. (2012). Genome-wide profiling of liver X receptor, retinoid X receptor, and peroxisome proliferator-activated receptor α in mouse liver reveals extensive sharing of binding sites. *Mol. Cell. Biol.* 32, 852-867. doi: 10.1128/MCB.06175-11

Carulli, L., Lonardo, A., Lombardini, S., Marchesini, G., and Loria, P. (2006). Gender, fatty liver and GGT. *Hepatology* 44, 278–279. doi: 10.1002/hep.21218

Chen, Y., Sullivan, J. C., Edwards, A., and Layton, A. T. (2017). Sex-specific computational models of the spontaneously hypertensive rat kidneys: factors affecting nitric oxide bioavailability. *Am. J. Physiol. Renal.* 313, 174–183. doi: 10.1152/ajprenal.00482.2016

Ciana, P., Raviscioni, M., Mussi, P., Vegeto, E., Que, I., Parker, M. G., et al. (2003). *In vivo* imaging of transcriptionally active estrogen receptors. *Nat. Med.* 9, 82–86. doi: 10.1038/nm809

Cohen, J. C., Horton, J. D., and Hobbs, H. H. (2011). Human fatty liver disease: old questions and new insights. *Science* 332, 1519–1523. doi: 10.1126/science.1204265

Costet, P., Legendre, C., Moré, J., Edgar, A., Galtier, P., and Pineau, T. (1998). Peroxisome proliferator-activated receptor α-isoform deficiency leads to progressive dyslipidemia with sexually dimorphic obesity and steatosis. *J. Biol. Chem.* 273, 29577–29585. doi: 10.1074/jbc.273.45.29577

Croft, D., O'Kelly, G., Wu, G., Haw, R., Gillespie, M., Matthews, L., et al. (2011). Reactome: a database of reactions, pathways and biological processes. *Nucleic Acids Res.* 39(Database issue), D691–D697. doi: 10.1093/nar/gkq1018

Cui, Y., Hosui, A., Sun, R., Shen, K., Gavrilova, O., Chen, W., et al. (2007). Loss of signal transducer and activator of transcription 5 leads to hepatosteatosis and impaired liver regeneration. *Hepatology* 46, 504–513. doi: 10.1002/hep.21713

Cvitanović, T., Reichert, M. C., Moškon, M., Mraz, M., Lammert, F., and Rozman,

D. (2017). Large-scale computational models of liver metabolism: how far from the clinics? *Hepatology* 66, 1323–1334. doi: 10.1002/hep.29268

Domonkos, E., Borbelyova, V., Csongova, M., Bosy, M., Kacmarova, M., Ostatnikova, D., et al. (2017). Sex differences and sex hormones in anxiety-like behavior of aging rats. *Horm. Behav.* 93, 159–165. doi: 10.1016/j.yhbeh.2017.05.019

Drasdo, D., Bode, J., Dahmen, U., Dirsch, O., Dooley, S., Gebhardt, R., et al. (2014). The virtual liver: state of the art and future perspectives. *Arch. Toxicol.* 88, 2071–2075. doi: 10.1007/s00204-014-1384-6

Du, J., Yuan, Z., Ma, Z., Song, J., Xie, X., and Chen, Y. (2014). KEGG-PATH: kyoto encyclopedia of genes and genomes-based pathway analysis using a path analysis model. *Mol. Biosyst.* 10, 2441–2447. doi: 10.1039/C4MB00287C

Fabbrini, E., Mohammed, B. S., Magkos, F., Korenblat, K. M., Patterson, B. W., and Klein, S. (2008). Alterations in adipose tissue and hepatic lipid kinetics in obese men and women with nonalcoholic fatty liver disease. *Gastroenterology* 134, 424–431. doi: 10.1053/j.gastro.2007.11.038

Fan, Y., Menon, R. K., Cohen, P., Hwang, D., Clemens, T., DiGirolamo, D. J., et al. (2009). Liver-specific deletion of the growth hormone receptor reveals essential role of growth hormone signaling in hepatic lipid metabolism. *J. Biol. Chem.* 284, 19937–19944. doi: 10.1074/jbc.M109.014308

Feillet, C., Guérin, S., Lonchampt, M., Dacquet, C., Gustafsson, J. Å., Delaunay, F., et al. (2016). Sexual dimorphism in circadian physiology is altered in LXRα deficient mice. *PLoS ONE* 11:e0150665. doi: 10.1371/journal.pone.0150665

Fell, D. A., and Sauro, H. M. (1985). Metabolic control and its analysis. *FEBS J.* 148, 555–561.

Florentino, G. S., Cotrim, H. P., Vilar, C. P., Florentino, A. V., Guimarães, G. M., and Barreto, V. S. (2013). Nonalcoholic fatty liver disease in menopausal women. *Arq. Gastroenterol.* 50, 180–185. doi: 10.1590/S0004-28032013000200032

Flórez-Vargas, O., Brass, A., Karystianis, G., Bramhall, M., Stevens, R., Cruickshank, S., et al. (2016). Bias in the reporting of sex and age in biomedical research on mouse models. *Elife* 5:e13615. doi: 10.7554/eLife.13615

Gårevik, N., Skogastierna, C., Rane, A., and Ekström, L. (2012). Single dose testosterone increases total cholesterol levels and induces the expression of HMG CoA Reductase. *Subst. Abuse Treat. Prev. Policy* 7:12. doi: 10.1186/1747-597X-7-12

Green, C. J., Pramfalk, C., Morten, K. J., and Hodson, L. (2015). From whole body to cellular models of hepatic triglyceride metabolism: man has got to know his limitations. *Am. J. Physiol. Endocrinol. Metab.* 308, E1–E20. doi: 10.1152/ajpendo.00192.2014

Gustafsson, J. A., Mode, A., Norstedt, G., and Skett, P. (1983). Sex steroid induced changes in hepatic enzymes. *Annu. Rev. Physiol.* 45, 51–60. doi: 10.1146/annurev.ph.45.030183.000411

Gutierrez-Grobe, Y., Ponciano-Rodríguez, G., Ramos, M. H., Uribe, M., and Méndez-Sánchez, N. (2010). Prevalence of non alcoholic fatty liver disease in premenopausal, postmenopausal and polycystic ovary syndrome women. The role of estrogens. *Ann. Hepatol.* 9, 402–409.

Guy, J., and Peters, M. G. (2013). Liver disease in women: the influence of gender on epidemiology, natural history, and patient outcomes. *Gastroenterol. Hepatol.* 9, 633–639.

Halkes, C., Van Dijk, H., Verseyden, C., de Jaegere, P. T., Plokker, H., Meijssen, S., et al. (2003). Gender differences in postprandial ketone bodies in normolipidemic subjects and in untreated patients with familial combined hyperlipidemia. *Arterioscl. Thromb. Vasc.* 23, 1875–1880. doi: 10.1161/01.ATV.0000092326.00725.ED

Hamaguchi, M., Kojima, T., Ohbora, A., Takeda, N., Fukui, M., and Kato, T. (2012). Aging is a risk factor of nonalcoholic fatty liver disease in premenopausal women. *World J. Gastroenterol.* 18:237. doi: 10.3748/wjg.v18.i3.237

Heine, P., Taylor, J., Iwamoto, G., Lubahn, D., and Cooke, P. (2000). Increased adipose tissue in male and female estrogen receptor-α knockout mice. *Proc. Natl. Acad. Sci. U.S.A.* 97, 12729–12734. doi: 10.1073/pnas.97.23.12729

Heinrich, R., and Schuster, S. (1996). *The Regulation of Cellular Systems*. New York, NY: Springer Science & Business Media. doi: 10.1007/978-1-4613-1161-4

Hodson, L., and Frayn, K. N. (2011). Hepatic fatty acid partitioning. *Curr. Opin. Lipidol.* 22, 216–224. doi: 10.1097/MOL.0b013e3283462e16

Hoehme, S., Friebel, A., Hammad, S., Drasdo, D., and Hengstler, J. G. (2017). Creation of three-dimensional liver tissue models from experimental images for systems medicine. *Methods Mol. Biol.* 1506, 319–362. doi: 10.1007/978-1-4939-6506-922

Holzhütter, H. G., Drasdo, D., Preusser, T., Lippert, J., and Henney, A. M. (2012). The virtual liver: a multidisciplinary, multilevel challenge for systems biology. *Wires Syst. Biol. Med.* 4, 221–235. doi: 10.1002/wsbm.1158

Huang, Y., He, S., Li, J. Z., Seo, Y.-K., Osborne, T. F., Cohen, J. C., et al. (2010). A feed-forward loop amplifies nutritional regulation of PNPLA3. *Proc. Natl. Acad. Sci. U.S.A.* 107, 7892–7897. doi: 10.1073/pnas.1003585107

Ingalls, B. (2008). Sensitivity analysis: from model parameters to system behaviour. *Essays Biochem.* 45, 177–194. doi: 10.1042/bse0450177

Jamil, H., Dickson, J. K., Chu, C. H., Lago, M. W., Rinehart, J. K., Biller, S. A., et al. (1995). Microsomal triglyceride transfer protein specificity of lipid binding and transport. *J. Biol. Chem.* 270, 6549–6554. doi: 10.1074/jbc.270.12.6549

Kohjima, M., Enjoji, M., Higuchi, N., Kato, M., Kotoh, K., Yoshimoto, T., et al. (2007). Re-evaluation of fatty acid metabolism-related gene expression in nonalcoholic fatty liver disease. *Int. J. Mol. Med.* 20, 351–358. doi: 10.3892/ijmm.20.3.351

Kojima, S. I., Watanabe, N., Numata, M., Ogawa, T., and Matsuzaki, S. (2003). Increase in the prevalence of fatty liver in Japan over the past 12 years: analysis of clinical background. *J. Gastroenterol.* 38, 954–961. doi: 10.1007/s00535-003-1178-8

Kosters, A., Sun, D., Wu, H., Tian, F., Felix, J. C., Li, W., et al. (2013). Sexually dimorphic genome- wide binding of retinoid X receptor alpha (RXRα) determines male-female differences in the expression of hepatic lipid processing genes in mice. *PLoS One* 8:e71538. doi: 10.1371/journal.pone.0071538

Koutsari, C., Basu, R., Rizza, R. A., Nair, K. S., Khosla, S., and Jensen, M. D. (2011). Nonoxidative free fatty acid disposal is greater in young women than men. *J. Clin. Endocrinol. Metab.* 96, 541–547. doi: 10.1210/jc.2010-1651

Laz, E. V., Wiwi, C. A., and Waxman, D. J. (2004). Sexual dimorphism of rat liver nuclear proteins: regulatory role of growth hormone. *Mol. Cell. Proteomics* 3, 1170–1180. doi: 10.1074/mcp.M400102-MCP200

Lewis, N. E., Nagarajan, H., and Palsson, B. O. (2012). Constraining the metabolic genotype-phenotype relationship using a phylogeny of *in silico* methods. *Nat. Rev. Microbiol.* 10:291. doi: 10.1038/nrmicro2737

Lindén, D., Alsterholm, M., Wennbo, H., and Oscarsson, J. (2001). PPARα deficiency increases secretion and serum levels of apolipoprotein B-containing lipoproteins. *J. Lipid Res.* 42, 1831–1840.

Lorbek, G., Perše, M., Horvat, S., Björkhem, I., and Rozman, D. (2013). Sex differences in the hepatic cholesterol sensing mechanisms in mice. *Molecules* 18, 11067–11085. doi: 10.3390/molecules180911067

Lorbek, G., Perše, M., Jeruc, J., Juvan, P., Gutierrez-Mariscal, F. M., Lewinska, M., et al. (2015). Lessons from hepatocyte-specific Cyp51 knockout mice: impaired cholesterol synthesis leads to oval cell-driven liver injury. *Sci. Rep.* 5:8777. doi: 10.1038/srep08777

Lorente, D., Martínez-Martínez, F., Rupérez, M., Lago, M., Martínez-Sober, M., Escandell-Montero, P., et al. (2017). A framework for modelling the biomechanical behaviour of the human liver during breathing in real time using machine learning. *Expert Syst. Appl.* 71, 342–357. doi: 10.1016/j.eswa.2016.11.037

Mardinoglu, A., Agren, R., Kampf, C., Asplund, A., Uhlen, M., and Nielsen, J. (2014). Genome-scale metabolic modelling of hepatocytes reveals serine deficiency in patients with non-alcoholic fatty liver disease. *Nat. Commun.* 5:3083. doi: 10.1038/ncomms4083

Marinou, K., Adiels, M., Hodson, L., Frayn, K. N., Karpe, F., and Fielding, B. A. (2011). Young women partition fatty acids towards ketone body production rather than VLDL-TAG synthesis, compared with young men. *Br. J. Nutr.* 105, 857–865. doi: 10.1017/S0007114510004472

Matthews, E. J., Kruhlak, N. L., Daniel Benz, R., and Contrera, J. F. (2007). A comprehensive model for reproductive and developmental toxicity hazard identification: I development of a weight of evidence QSAR database. *Regul. Toxicol. Pharmacol.* 47, 115–135. doi: 10.1016/j.yrtph.2006.11.002

McGregor, A. J., Hasnain, M., Sandberg, K., Morrison, M. F., Berlin, M., and Trott, J. (2016). How to study the impact of sex and gender in medical research: a review of resources. *Biol. Sex. Differ.* 7:46. doi: 10.1186/s13293-016-0099-1

Mormeneo, E., Jimenez-Mallebrera, C., Palomer, X., De Nigris, V., Vázquez-Carrera, M., Orozco, A., et al. (2012). PGC-1α induces mitochondrial and myokine transcriptional programs and lipid droplet and glycogen accumulation in cultured human skeletal muscle cells. *PLoS ONE* 7:e29985. doi: 10.1371/journal.pone.0029985

Naik, A., Rozman, D., and Belic, A. (2014). SteatoNet: the first integrated human metabolic model with multi-layered regulation to investigate liver-associated pathologies. *PLoS Comput. Biol.* 10:e1003993. doi: 10.1371/journal.pcbi.1003993

Nomura, D. K., Long, J. Z., Niessen, S., Hoover, H. S., Ng, S. W., and Cravatt, B. F. (2010). Monoacylglycerol lipase regulates a fatty acid network that promotes cancer pathogenesis. *Cell* 140, 49–61. doi: 10.1016/j.cell.2009.11.027

Norstedt, G., and Palmiter, R. (1984). Secretory rhythm of growth hormone regulates sexual differentiation of mouse liver. *Cell* 36, 805–812. doi: 10.1016/0092-8674(84)90030-8

Oshida, K., Waxman, D. J., and Corton, J. C. (2016). Correction: chemical and hormonal effects on STAT5b- dependent sexual dimorphism of the liver transcriptome. *PLoS ONE* 11:e0161519. doi: 10.1371/journal.pone.0161519

Pan, J. J., and Fallon, M. B. (2014). Gender and racial differences in nonalcoholic fatty liver disease. *World J. Hepatol.* 6:274. doi: 10.4254/wjh.v6.i5.274

Petta, S., Valenti, L., Bugianesi, E., Targher, G., Bellentani, S., and Bonino, F. (2016). A "systems medicine" approach to the study of non-alcoholic fatty liver disease. *Digest. Liver Dis.* 48, 333–342. doi: 10.1016/j.dld.2015.10.027

Rando, G., and Wahli, W. (2011). Sex differences in nuclear receptor-regulated liver metabolic pathways. *Biochim. Biophys. Acta* 1812, 964–973. doi: 10.1016/j.bbadis.2010.12.023

Reingold, J. S., McGavock, J. M., Kaka, S., Tillery, T., Victor, R. G., and Szczepaniak, L. S. (2005). Determination of triglyceride in the human myocardium by magnetic resonance spectroscopy: reproducibility and sensitivity of the method. *Am. J. Physiol. Endocrinol. Metab.* 289, E935–E939. doi: 10.1152/ajpendo.00095.2005

Rodríguez, A., Marinelli, R. A., Tesse, A., Frühbeck, G., and Calamita, G. (2015). Sexual dimorphism of adipose and hepatic aquaglyceroporins in health and metabolic disorders. *Front. Endocrinol.* 6:171. doi: 10.3389/fendo.2015.00171

Roepstorff, C., Donsmark, M., Thiele, M., Vistisen, B., Stewart, G., Vissing, K., et al. (2006). Sex differences in hormone-sensitive lipase expression, activity, and phosphorylation in skeletal muscle at rest and during exercise. *Am. J. Physiol. Endocrinol. Metab.* 291, E1106–E1114. doi: 10.1152/ajpendo.00097.2006

Sanders, F. W., and Griffin, J. L. (2016). *De novo* lipogenesis in the liver in health and disease: more than just a shunting yard for glucose. *Biol. Rev.* 91, 452–468. doi: 10.1111/brv.12178

Schultz, J. R., Tu, H., Luk, A., Repa, J. J., Medina, J. C., Li, L., et al. (2000). Role of LXRs in control of lipogenesis. *Gene. Dev.* 14, 2831–2838.

Serviddio, G., Bellanti, F., and Vendemiale, G. (2013). Free radical biology for medicine: learning from nonalcoholic fatty liver disease. *Free Radic. Biol. Med.* 65, 952–968. doi: 10.1016/j.freeradbiomed.2013.08.174

Shanle, E. K., and Xu, W. (2010). Endocrine disrupting chemicals targeting estrogen receptor signaling: identification and mechanisms of action. *Chem. Res. Toxicol.* 24, 6–19. doi: 10.1021/tx100231n

Sharma, G., Mauvais-Jarvis, F., and Prossnitz, E. R. (2017). Roles of G protein-coupled estrogen receptor GPER in metabolic regulation. *J. Steroid Biochem. Mol. Biol.* 176, 31–37. doi: 10.1016/j.jsbmb.2017.02.012

Simpson, E. (2003). Sources of estrogen and their importance. *J. Steroid Biochem. Mol. Biol.* 86, 225–230. doi: 10.1016/S0960-0760(03)00360-1

Söder, O. (2007). Sexual dimorphism of gonadal development. *Best Pract. Res. Clin. Endocrinol. Metab.* 21, 381–391. doi: 10.1016/j.beem.2007.05.002

Softic, S., Cohen, D. E., and Kahn, C. R. (2016). Role of dietary fructose and hepatic *de novo* lipogenesis in fatty liver disease. *Dig. Dis. Sci.* 61, 1282–1293. doi: 10.1007/s10620-016-4054-0

Sos, B. C., Harris, C., Nordstrom, S. M., Tran, J. L., Balázs, M., Caplazi, P., et al. (2011). Abrogation of growth hormone secretion rescues fatty liver in mice with hepatocyte-specific deletion of JAK2. *J. Clin. Invest.* 121, 1412–1423. doi: 10.1172/JCI42894

Suzuki, A., and Abdelmalek, M. F. (2009). Nonalcoholic fatty liver disease in women. *Womens Health* 5, 1–13. doi: 10.2217/17455057.5.2.191

Urlep, Ž., Lorbek, G., Perše, M., Jeruc, J., Juvan, P., Matz-Soja, M., et al. (2017). Disrupting hepatocyte Cyp51 from cholesterol synthesis leads to progressive liver Injury in the developing mouse and decreases RORC signalling. *Sci. Rep.* 7:40775. doi: 10.1038/srep40775

Villa, A., Della Torre, S., Stell, A., Cook, J., Brown, M., and Maggi, A. (2012). Tetradian oscillation of estrogen receptor α is necessary to prevent liver lipid deposition. *Proc. Natl. Acad. Sci. U.S.A.* 109, 11806–11811. doi: 10.1073/pnas.1205797109

Wang, X., Magkos, F., and Mittendorfer, B. (2011). Sex differences in lipid and lipoprotein metabolism: it's not just about sex hormones. *J. Clin. Endocrinol. Metab.* 96, 885–893. doi: 10.1210/jc.2010-2061

Waxman, D. J., and Holloway, M. G. (2009). Sex differences in the expression of hepatic drug metabolizing enzymes. *Mol. Pharmacol.* 76, 215–228. doi: 10.1124/mol.109.056705

Waxman, D. J., and O'connor, C. (2006). Growth hormone regulation of sex-dependent liver gene expression. *Mol. Endocrinol.* 20, 2613–2629. doi: 10.1210/me.2006-0007

Westerhoff, H. V., Groen, A. K., and Wanders, R. J. (1984). Modern theories of metabolic control and their applications. *Biosci. Rep.* 4, 1–22. doi: 10.1007/BF01120819

Xu, C., Yu, C., Ma, H., Xu, L., Miao, M., and Li, Y. (2013). Prevalence and risk factors for the development of nonalcoholic fatty liver disease in a nonobese Chinese population: the Zhejiang Zhenhai Study. *Am. J. Gastroenterol.* 108, 1299–1304. doi: 10.1038/ajg.2013.104

Yang, X., Schadt, E. E., Wang, S., Wang, H., Arnold, A. P., Ingram-Drake, L., et al. (2006). Tissue-specific expression and regulation of sexually dimorphic genes in mice. *Genome Res.* 16, 995–1004. doi: 10.1101/gr.5217506

Zhang, Y., Laz, E. V., and Waxman, D. J. (2012). Dynamic, sex-differential STAT5 and BCL6 binding to sex-biased, growth hormone-regulated genes in adult mouse liver. *Mol. Cell Biol.* 32, 880–896. doi: 10.1128/MCB.06312-11

Zheng, B., Zhu, Y. J., Wang, H. Y., and Chen, L. (2017). Gender disparity in hepatocellular carcinoma (HCC): multiple underlying mechanisms. *Sci. China Life Sci.* 60, 575–584. doi: 10.1007/s11427-016-9043-9

Zhu, W., Zhao, Y., Zhou, J., Wang, X., Pan, Q., Zhang, N., et al. (2016). Monoacylglycerol lipase promotes progression of hepatocellular carcinoma via NF-κB-mediated epithelial-mesenchymal transition. *J. Hematol. Oncol.* 9:127. doi: 10.1186/s13045-016-0361-3

Zi, Z. (2011). Sensitivity analysis approaches applied to systems biology models. *IET Syst. Biol.* 5, 336–346. doi: 10.1049/iet-syb.2011.0015

10

Network Modeling of Liver Metabolism to Predict Plasma Metabolite Changes During Short-Term Fasting in the Laboratory Rat

Kalyan C. Vinnakota[1,2], Venkat R. Pannala[1,2], Martha L. Wall[3], Mohsin Rahim[3], Shanea K. Estes[4], Irina Trenary[3], Tracy P. O'Brien[4], Richard L. Printz[4], Jaques Reifman[2], Masakazu Shiota[4], Jamey D. Young[3,4]* and Anders Wallqvist[2]**

[1] Henry M. Jackson Foundation for the Advancement of Military Medicine, Inc., Bethesda, MD, United States, [2] Department of Defense Biotechnology High Performance Computing Software Applications Institute, Telemedicine and Advanced Technology Research Center, United States Army Medical Research and Materiel Command, Fort Detrick, MD, United States, [3] Department of Chemical and Biomolecular Engineering, Vanderbilt University School of Engineering, Nashville, TN, United States, [4] Department of Molecular Physiology and Biophysics, Vanderbilt University School of Medicine, Nashville, TN, United States

***Correspondence:**
Kalyan C. Vinnakota
kvinnakota@bhsai.org
Jamey D. Young
j.d.young@vanderbilt.edu
Anders Wallqvist
sven.a.wallqvist.civ@mail.mil

The liver—a central metabolic organ that integrates whole-body metabolism to maintain glucose and fatty-acid regulation, and detoxify ammonia—is susceptible to injuries induced by drugs and toxic substances. Although plasma metabolite profiles are increasingly investigated for their potential to detect liver injury earlier than current clinical markers, their utility may be compromised because such profiles are affected by the nutritional state and the physiological state of the animal, and by contributions from extrahepatic sources. To tease apart the contributions of liver and non-liver sources to alterations in plasma metabolite profiles, here we sought to computationally isolate the plasma metabolite changes originating in the liver during short-term fasting. We used a constraint-based metabolic modeling approach to integrate central carbon fluxes measured in our study, and physiological flux boundary conditions gathered from the literature, into a genome-scale model of rat liver metabolism. We then measured plasma metabolite profiles in rats fasted for 5–7 or 10–13 h to test our model predictions. Our computational model accounted for two-thirds of the observed directions of change (an increase or decrease) in plasma metabolites, indicating their origin in the liver. Specifically, our work suggests that changes in plasma lipid metabolites, which are reliably predicted by our liver metabolism model, are key features of short-term fasting. Our approach provides a mechanistic model for identifying plasma metabolite changes originating in the liver.

Keywords: metabolic network, rat, liver, plasma, metabolomics, fasting, central carbon flux, gluconeogenesis

INTRODUCTION

The liver is the primary organ responsible for metabolizing drugs and toxicants, a process collectively known as xenobiotic metabolism. This function makes the liver highly susceptible to injury and potential failure (Zimmerman, 1999). Current clinical markers of liver cell damage, such as the enzymes alanine amino transferase (ALT) and aspartate amino transferase (AST), which appear one to several days following exposure to a toxicant, are often limited in sensitivity and specificity to detect the pathology or injury (Zimmerman, 1999). Metabolite profiles, as measured in the plasma and urine of laboratory animal models of liver injury, are actively being investigated for their potential to detect liver damage earlier than current clinical markers and thereby facilitate timely intervention (Kamp et al., 2012; Mattes et al., 2014; Beger et al., 2015; Iruzubieta et al., 2015; Chang et al., 2017; Jarak et al., 2017). Additionally, they are being analyzed to identify canonical metabolic pathways (i.e., not including xenobiotic metabolism), such as lipid, amino acid, and oxidative stress pathways, which are perturbed during a drug- or toxicant-induced liver injury. However, plasma metabolite profiles and canonical metabolic pathways are also affected by the nutritional and physiological state of an animal, which could confound the identification of liver injury-induced changes in the plasma metabolite profile (Mellert et al., 2011; Mu et al., 2015). Importantly, the plasma metabolite profile consists of contributions from all other organs in the body, each of which is determined by the physiological state of the organ. It is important, therefore, to identify the contributions of liver metabolism to the plasma metabolite profile, and the metabolic pathways contributing to the observed changes under physiological and pathophysiological perturbations.

Genome-scale computational modeling of organ metabolism constitutes an important approach toward obtaining mechanistic insights into organ metabolism and canonical metabolic pathways under various conditions (Blais et al., 2017). Here, we subjected rats to short-term fasting in vehicle control groups of a larger study involving three different toxicants, and applied a genome-scale rat metabolic network to assess liver contributions to plasma metabolite profiles and to identify the responsible metabolic pathways. The short-term fasting conditions studied here were dominated by hormonally regulated changes in liver glycogen breakdown without significant transcriptomic changes of liver enzymes, which created a challenge in applying a genome-scale network modeling approach to describe liver function. We made our modeling analysis represent the liver mainly by constraining the model with the measured metabolic fluxes in this study and fluxes reported in the literature under similar conditions. Specifically, we measured the evolution of key metabolic fluxes in the liver, the liver transcriptome, and plasma metabolite profiles in three *in vivo* studies during which the rats underwent short-term food deprivation for up to 13 h. We used a recently published algorithm to integrate the measurements with a rat metabolic network model, and predicted the direction of change in extracellular metabolite concentrations resulting from a perturbation of metabolic fluxes in the network (Blais et al., 2017; Pannala et al., 2018). By comparing model predictions of the directions of metabolite changes with measured plasma metabolite profiles, we assessed the contributions of the liver to those changes.

MATERIALS AND METHODS

Animals and Study Groups

Male Sprague-Dawley rats at 10 weeks of age were purchased from Charles River Laboratories (Wilmington, MA, United States). The rats were fed with Formulab Diet 5001 (Purina LabDiet; Purina Miles, Richmond, IN, United States) and given water *ad libitum* in an environmentally controlled room with a 12:12-h light-dark cycle at 23°C. All experiments were conducted in accordance with the Guide for the Care and Use of laboratory Animals of the United States Department of Agriculture, using protocols approved by the Vanderbilt University Institutional Animal Care and Use Committee, and by the United States Army Medical Research and Materiel Command Animal Care and Use Review Office.

Three types of measurements, plasma metabolite profiles, liver gene expression, and stable isotope tracer-based metabolic flux profiles, were made at one or two time points in three experimental studies. The three studies described here were the vehicle control groups of a larger study involving three different toxicants. The vehicle for each toxicant was different due to their differing physical and chemical properties. The time points also varied slightly because of the differences in their toxicity in the larger study. **Table 1** summarizes the number of animals for each measurement in each study.

Catheter Implantation for Infusions and Sampling

Catheter implantation surgery was performed 7 days before each experiment, as previously described (Shiota, 2012). Rats were anesthetized with isoflurane, after which one of two procedures was performed depending on the type of measurement to be collected during the experiment. To measure changes in gene expression and plasma metabolite profiles, the right external jugular vein was cannulated with a sterile silicone catheter [0.51 mm inner diameter (ID) and 0.94 mm outer diameter (OD)]. Alternatively, to measure metabolic flux, both the carotid artery and the right external jugular vein were cannulated with sterile silicone catheters (0.51 mm ID and 0.94 mm OD). The free ends of the implanted catheters were passed subcutaneously to the back of the neck, where they were fixed. Finally, each

TABLE 1 | Number of animals used for each measurement per time point in Studies 1–3.

Measurement	Study 1		Study 2		Study 3	
	5 h	10 h	5 h	10 h	7 h	13 h
Metabolic flux	–	9	–	8	–	8
Plasma metabolite profiles	8	8	8	8	9	9
Liver gene expression	8	8	8	8	8	8

implanted catheter was occluded with a metal plug after a flush with heparinized saline solution (200 U heparin/ml). The rats were housed individually after the surgery.

Procedures for Measuring Changes in Gene Expression and Plasma Metabolite Profiles

Two time points were selected for sampling tissue and blood after vehicle administration in each of the three studies analyzed in the present paper: they were 5 h and 10 h for Studies 1 and 2, and 7 h and 13 h for Study 3. The administered vehicles and their dosages were polyethylene glycol at 6 ml/kg, corn oil at 2 ml/kg, and saline at 2 ml/kg in Studies 1, 2, and 3, respectively. Following blood collection, animals were given vehicle by oral gavage at 7 a.m. and moved to a new housing cage, where they were given access to water *ad libitum* but not food. Then, at 12 p.m. (5 h group) or 5 p.m. (10 h group), after blood collection, animals in Studies 1 and 2 were anesthetized by intravenous injection of sodium pentobarbital through the jugular vein catheter and immediately subjected to laparotomy. The same procedures were performed at 2 p.m. (7 h group) or 8 p.m. (13 h group) in Study 3. After laparotomy, the liver was dissected and frozen using Wollenberger tongs precooled in liquid nitrogen. The collected plasma and liver samples were stored at −80°C until use for further analyses.

Methods for Measuring Metabolite Flux

In vivo Procedures in the Rat

At 7 a.m. on the day of the study, rats in all three studies were administered vehicle (50% polyethylene glycol or 6 ml/kg of either saline or corn oil) by oral gavage. Then, after food and water were removed, they were anesthetized with isoflurane at 12:50 p.m. (Studies 1 and 2) or 3:50 p.m. (Study 3). Subsequently, a 200-μl arterial blood sample was collected through the carotid artery catheter to determine the natural isotopic abundance of circulating glucose, after which a bolus of [$^2H_2$]water (99.9%) was delivered subcutaneously to enrich total body water to 4.5%. A [6,6-$^2H_2$]glucose prime (80 $mg \cdot kg^{-1}$) was dissolved in the bolus. Post-awakening, at 1 p.m. or 4 p.m. (i.e., 6 or 9 h after dosing), rats were connected to sampling and infusion lines and placed in bedded containers without food or water. Following the bolus, [6,6-$^2H_2$]glucose was administered as a continuous infusion (0.8 $mg \cdot kg^{-1} \cdot min^{-1}$) into the systemic circulation through the jugular vein catheter for the duration of the study. Sodium [$^{13}C_3$]propionate (99%) was delivered as a primed (110 $mg \cdot kg^{-1}$), continuous (5.5 $mg \cdot kg^{-1} \cdot min^{-1}$) infusion starting 120 min after delivery of the [$^2H_2$] water bolus. All infusates were prepared in a 4.5% [$^2H_2$] water-saline solution unless otherwise specified. Stable isotopes were obtained from Cambridge Isotope Laboratories (Tewksbury, MA, United States). Blood glucose was monitored (AccuCheck; Roche Diagnostics, Indianapolis, IN, United States) and donor erythrocytes were infused to maintain hematocrit throughout the study. Three blood samples (300 μl each) were collected over a 20-min period following 100 min of [$^{13}C_3$]propionate infusion. Arterial blood samples were centrifuged in EDTA-coated tubes for plasma isolation, and the three 100-μl plasma samples were stored at −20°C prior to glucose derivatization and gas chromatography-mass spectrometry (GC-MS) analysis. Rats were rapidly euthanized through the carotid artery catheter immediately after the final steady-state sample was collected.

Preparation of Glucose Derivatives

Plasma samples were divided into three aliquots and derivatized separately to obtain di-*O*-isopropylidene propionate, aldonitrile pentapropionate, and methyloxime pentapropionate derivatives of glucose. For di-*O*-isopropylidene propionate preparation, proteins were precipitated from 20 μl of plasma using 300 μl of cold acetone, and the protein-free supernatant was evaporated to dryness in screw-cap culture tubes. Derivatization proceeded as described previously (Antoniewicz et al., 2011) to produce glucose 1,2,5,6-di-isopropylidene propionate. For aldonitrile and methyloxime derivatization, proteins were precipitated from 10 μl of plasma using 300 μl of cold acetone and the protein-free supernatants were evaporated to dryness in microcentrifuge tubes. Derivatizations then proceeded as described previously (Antoniewicz et al., 2011) to produce glucose aldonitrile pentapropionate and glucose methyloxime pentapropionate. All derivatives were evaporated to dryness, dissolved in 100 μl of ethyl acetate, and transferred to GC injection vials with 250 μl glass inserts for GC-MS analysis.

GC-MS Analysis

GC-MS analysis was performed using an Agilent 7890A gas chromatography system with an HP-5 ms (30 m × 0.25 mm × 0.25 μm, Agilent J&W Scientific; Agilent Technologies Inc., Santa Clara, CA, United States) capillary column interfaced with an Agilent 5975C mass spectrometer. Samples were injected into a 270°C injection port in splitless mode. Helium flow was maintained at 0.88 $ml \cdot min^{-1}$. For analysis of di-*O*-isopropylidene and aldonitrile derivatives, the column temperature was held at 80°C for 1 min, ramped at 20°C $\cdot min^{-1}$ to 280°C and held for 4 min, then ramped at 40°C $\cdot min^{-1}$ to 325°C. For methyloxime derivatives, the same oven program was used except the ramp to 280°C was 10°C $\cdot min^{-1}$. After a 5 min solvent delay, the MS collected data in scan mode from m/z 300 to 320 for di-*O*-isopropylidene derivatives, m/z 100 to 500 for aldonitrile derivatives, and m/z 144 to 260 for methyloxime derivatives. Each derivative peak was integrated using a custom MATLAB®(Mathworks Inc., Natick, MA, United States) function (Antoniewicz et al., 2007) to obtain mass isotopomer distributions (MIDs) for six specific ion ranges: aldonitrile – m/z 173–177, 259–265, 284–288, 370–374; methyloxime – m/z 145–149; di-*O*-isopropylidene – m/z 301–308. To assess uncertainty, root mean square error was calculated by comparing the baseline MID of unlabeled glucose samples to the theoretical MID computed from the known abundances of naturally occurring isotopes.

$^2H/^{13}C$ Metabolic Flux Analysis (MFA)

A detailed description of the *in vivo* metabolic flux analysis methodology employed in these studies has been previously provided (Hasenour et al., 2015). Briefly, a reaction network was constructed using the INCA software package (Young, 2014). The reaction network defined the carbon and hydrogen transitions for biochemical reactions linking hepatic glucose production and associated intermediary metabolism reactions. Flux through each reaction was estimated relative to citrate synthase (fixed at 100) by minimizing the sum of squared residuals between simulated and experimentally determined MIDs of the six fragment ions previously described. Flux estimation was repeated at least 25 times from random initial values. Goodness-of-fit was assessed by a chi-square test, and 95% confidence intervals were computed by evaluating the sensitivity of the sum-of-squared residuals to variations in flux values (Antoniewicz et al., 2006). The average sum of squares of residuals (SSR) of each experimental group fell within the 95% confidence interval of the corresponding chi-square distribution with D degrees of freedom: Study 1 ($D = 22$): SSR = 29.65 ± 7.05; Study 2 ($D = 23$): SSR = 28.77 ± 2.83; Study 3 ($D = 26$): SSR = 22.69 ± 1.83. Relative fluxes were converted to absolute values using the known [6,6-$^2H_2$]glucose infusion rate and rat weights. Flux estimates for the steady-state samples were averaged to obtain a representative set of values for each rat.

Metabolomic Analysis

Sample Preparation and Ultrahigh Performance Liquid Chromatography/Mass Spectrometry (UHPLC/MS)

Sample preparation was carried out at Metabolon, Inc. in a manner similar to a previous study (Hatano et al., 2016). Briefly, individual samples were subjected to methanol extraction and then split into aliquots for analysis by UHPLC/MS. The global biochemical profiling analysis comprised four unique arms: reverse phase chromatography positive ionization methods optimized for hydrophilic compounds (LC/MS Pos Polar) and hydrophobic compounds (LC/MS Pos Lipid); reverse phase chromatography with negative ionization conditions (LC/MS Neg), and a hydrophilic interaction liquid chromatography (HILIC) method coupled to negative ionization (LC/MS Polar) (Evans et al., 2014). All of the methods alternated between full scan MS and data-dependent MS^n scans. The scan range varied slightly between methods but generally covered 70–1,000 m/z.

Metabolites were identified by automated comparison of the ion features in the experimental samples to a reference library of chemical standard entries that included retention time, molecular weight (m/z), preferred adducts, and in-source fragments as well as associated MS spectra, and curated by visual inspection for quality control using software developed at Metabolon. Identification of known chemical entities was based on comparison to metabolomic library entries of purified standards (Dehaven et al., 2010).

Statistical Analysis of Metabolomic Data

We performed statistical analysis to identify metabolites that changed significantly with the duration of fasting. The raw data consisted of MS counts for each metabolite detected in a given plasma sample. We imputed any missing values with the minimum observed value for each metabolite. We then computed distributions of fold-change values for each metabolite and pooled them across the three studies to resolve changes during short-term fasting above experimental and biological noise. From these pooled distributions, we calculated 99% confidence intervals for the mean fold-change values of each metabolite using the percentile approach (Efron and Hastie, 2016). Briefly, for each metabolite at each of the two points in a study, we constructed $n \times 10^5$ instances of MS count data by random sampling with replacement, where n is the number of animals. Then, for each metabolite in the given study, we calculated $n \times 10^5$ fold-change values from the synthetic data sets generated in the previous step. We pooled these fold-change values across studies for a given metabolite, and calculated 10^5 sample means, which constitute the bootstrapped distribution of the mean fold-change. To obtain the 99% confidence interval of the mean fold value for each metabolite, we identified a percentile-based confidence interval from the bootstrapped distribution of the mean fold-change value, which excluded values above the highest 0.5th percentile and those below the lowest 0.5th percentile. A metabolite was determined to have significantly increased or decreased if both bounds of the 99% confidence interval of its mean fold-change value were above or below the value 1. All statistical analyses were performed in MATLAB®R2017b (Mathworks Inc., Natick, MA, United States). We have provided MATLAB code for this analysis in the **Supplementary Material.**

RNA Sequencing and Data Analysis

RNA Isolation and Sequencing

Total RNA was isolated from the liver, using TRIzol Reagent (Thermo Fisher Scientific, Waltham, MA, United States) and the direct-zol RNA Mini Prep kit (Zymo Research, Irvine, CA, United States). The isolated RNA samples were then submitted to the Vanderbilt University Medical Center VANTAGE Core (Nashville, TN, United States) for RNA quality determination and sequencing. Total RNA quality was assessed using a 2100 Bioanalyzer (Agilent, Santa Clara, CA, United States). At least 200 ng of DNase-treated total RNA with high RNA integrity was used to generate poly-A-enriched mRNA libraries, using KAPA Stranded mRNA sample kits with indexed adaptors (Roche, Indianapolis, IN, United States). Library quality was assessed using the 2100 Bioanalyzer (Agilent), and libraries were quantitated using KAPA library Quantification kits (Roche). In Study 1, pooled libraries were subjected to 75-bp single-end sequencing according to the manufacturer's protocol (Illumina HiSeq 3000, San Diego, CA, United States). In contrast, in Studies 2 and 3, the respective pooled libraries were subjected to 150-bp paired-end sequencing on Illumina NovaSeq 6000 and 75-bp paired-end sequencing on Illumina HiSeq 3000 according to the manufacturer's protocol. Bcl2fastq2 Conversion Software (Illumina) was used to generate de-multiplexed Fastq files.

Analysis of RNA-Seq Data

Analysis of RNA-seq data consists of two stages: (1) determination of transcript abundance and (2) determination of differentially expressed genes. We determined transcript abundance from Fastq files, consisting of raw sequence reads, using a recently published software tool Kallisto (Bray et al., 2016). Using Kallisto, we first generated a reference transcriptome index from cDNA files based on genome assembly Rnor6.0 for rat, published on ENSEMBL Release 92 (Zerbino et al., 2018). We then determined transcript abundance using Kallisto, which is based on pseudoalignment of raw sequence reads to the reference transcriptome index. We used appropriate Kallisto settings for processing single-end sequence reads from Study 1, and paired-end sequence reads from Studies 2 and 3. Using these transcription data, expressed in units of transcripts per million (TPM), we used the analytical tool Sleuth (Pimentel et al., 2017) to investigate differential expression of genes between two time points in each. Within Sleuth, we applied a likelihood ratio test to identify statistically significant gene expression changes and a Wald test to compute the effect sizes (logarithms of the fold-changes), between the two time points in each study, for each test. From these results, we obtained effect sizes for the genes that were identified by the likelihood ratio test to have changed significantly. Finally, we designated the genes with absolute effect sizes in the top 10th percentile as biologically significant, conditional upon statistical significance.

Curation of Rat Metabolic Network *iRno* and Assignment of Physiological Flux Bounds

We first updated a recently published functional rat genome-scale network reconstruction *iRno*, which contains 2,325 genes and 5,620 metabolites in 8,336 reactions and eight compartments connected by Gene-Protein-Reaction rules, and is capable of simulating 327 liver-specific metabolic functions (Blais et al., 2017). The updates to *iRno* included additional reactions or modification of existing reactions based on experimental evidence (**Supplementary Table S1**). For instance, we removed a reaction (S)-lactate:ferricytochrome-c 2-oxidoreductase, which was determined to be non-existent in mammalian systems. Additionally, we added 90 transport and 105 exchange reactions to *iRno* to improve its coverage of exchangeable metabolites that were detected in plasma metabolite profiles in the present study. The updated *iRno* contains 2,325 genes and 5,709 metabolites including 3,201 unique metabolites in 8,534 reactions including 595 exchange reactions in eight compartments. **Supplementary Table S1** provides the updated *iRno*.

The liver operates in a gluconeogenic mode during the short-term fasting trajectory in the present study. In this state, the liver takes up amino acids, lactate, and glycerol to produce glucose and urea. The liver also takes up non-esterified fatty acids to produce ketone bodies. We constrained the uptake rates of amino acids, fatty acids, lactate, and glycerol, using values reported in the literature from *in vivo* measurements in rats undergoing short-term fasting (**Supplementary Table S2**).

Application of Transcriptionally Inferred Metabolic Biomarker Response (TIMBR) Algorithm

Transcriptionally inferred metabolic biomarker response (TIMBR) is a recently published method developed for predicting changes in extracellular metabolites due to gene expression changes under defined physiological operating conditions by integrating those changes into genome-scale network reconstructions (see Blais et al., 2017 for details). In the present study, we applied TIMBR to predict metabolite changes during a 5–6-h window of short-term fasting, where gene expression changes have little influence on metabolic state (Ikeda et al., 2014), in contrast to the changes in the central carbon metabolism fluxes. TIMBR calculates the global network demand required for producing a metabolite (X_{met}) by minimizing the weighted sum of fluxes across all reactions for each condition and metabolite, while satisfying the steady-state mass balance and a defined optimal fraction of maximum network production flux capability (ν_{opt}) to produce a metabolite as shown below:

$$\begin{aligned} X_{met} &= \min \sum |v| \\ s.t.:\ & v_X \geq v_{opt};\ v_{lb} < v < v_{ub};\ S \cdot v = 0 \end{aligned} \tag{1}$$

where ν is a vector of reaction fluxes and S is the stoichiometric matrix. We included boundary conditions for uptake and secretion rates into the algorithm by fixing the respective lower (ν_{lb}) and upper bounds (ν_{ub}) of the metabolite exchange reactions (ν_{ex}), as shown in Eq. (2). Similarly, we integrated measurements from ^{13}C-labeled tracer studies for some of the central carbon metabolism fluxes into the TIMBR algorithm by constraining the lower and upper bounds of the respective reactions in the model (ν_{mfa}) (Eq. 3).

$$v_{lb} < v_{ex} < v_{ub} \tag{2}$$

$$v_{lb} < v_{mfa} < v_{ub} \tag{3}$$

Using this method, we determined the relative production scores for all metabolites (X_{raw}) from 5 to 7 h (X_{5-7}) and 10 to 13 h (X_{10-13}) time points (Eq. 4), and then calculated the TIMBR production scores (X_s) as the z-transformed scores across all exchangeable metabolites (Eq. 5).

$$X_{raw} = \frac{X_{5-7} - X_{10-13}}{X_{5-7} + X_{10-13}} \tag{4}$$

$$X_s = \frac{X_{raw} - \mu}{\sigma} \tag{5}$$

Figure 1 shows the workflow for the application of the TIMBR algorithm (adapted from Pannala et al., 2018). We performed the model computations in MATLAB R2017b using the linear programming solver provided in the GNU Linear Programming Kit. We refer the reader to the original publication for detailed descriptions of the TIMBR algorithm and the corresponding computer codes (Blais et al., 2017).

RESULTS AND DISCUSSION

Liver Glucose Production and Glycogenolysis Fluxes Decrease With Fasting Duration

During fasting, the liver produces glucose by synthesizing it from glycerol, lactate, and amino acids, as well as by breaking down glycogen. **Figure 2** shows a schematic of the

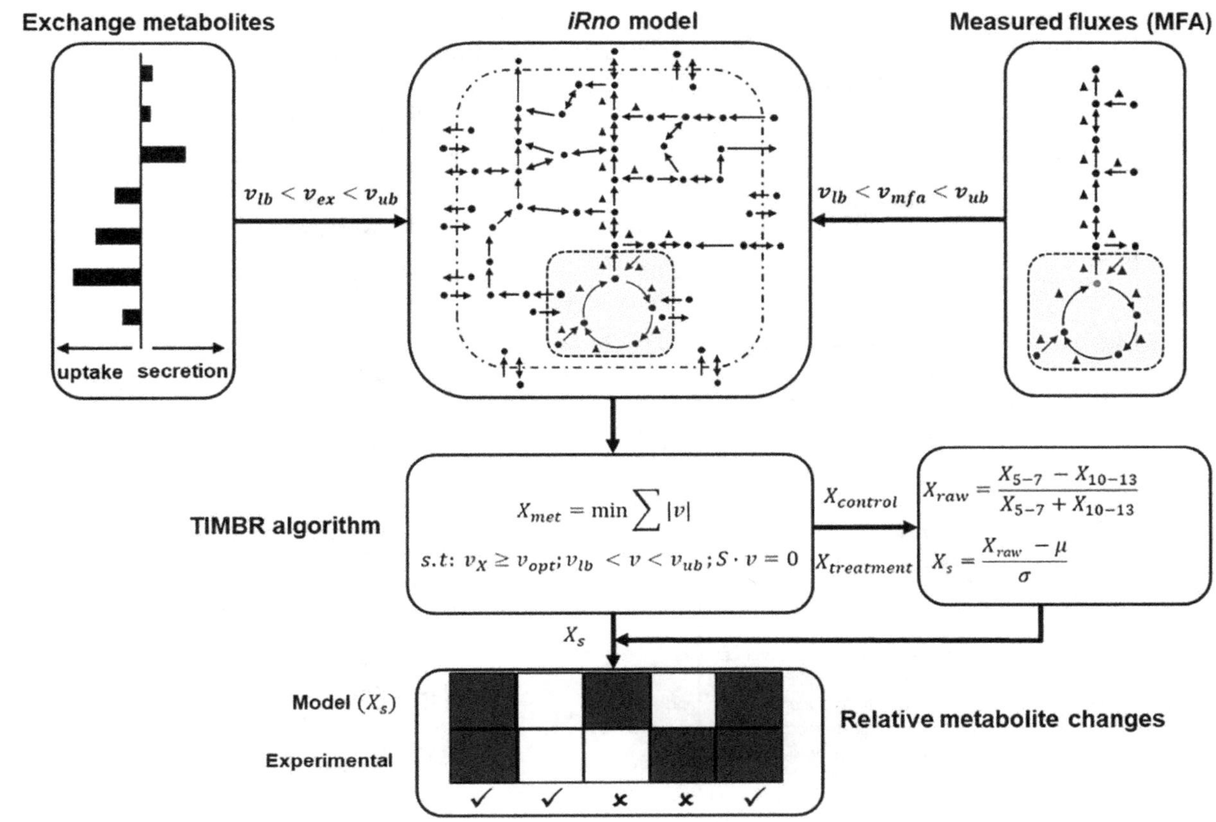

FIGURE 1 | Schematic (adapted from Pannala et al., 2018) illustrates how we integrated physiological flux bounds for exchangeable metabolites (v_{ex}), measured central carbon fluxes (v_{mfa}) with the rat metabolic network model *iRno* to compute global network demand (X_{met}) using TIMBR, by minimizing the sum of the absolute value of flux across all reactions at the earlier (X_{5-7}) and later (X_{10-13}) time points. We then calculated a z-transformed TIMBR score (X_s) from the raw metabolite production score (X_{raw}) for each metabolite, whose positive or negative sign indicated its predicted tendency to increase or decrease in plasma. The TIMBR scores were compared with the measured fold-change values of significantly changed metabolites in the plasma to assess the contributions of liver metabolism to those changes.

liver glucose production pathways, which include reactions of glycogenolysis, gluconeogenesis, and the tricarboxylic acid cycle. The aforementioned fluxes are collectively termed central carbon fluxes. The flux values through individual reactions at 10 and 13 h of fasting (**Figure 3**, Studies 1–3) were measured by stable isotope tracer studies, and those at 5–7 h of fasting (**Figure 3**, Est. 5–7 h) were compiled from the literature under conditions similar to our studies. In all studies considered for flux values at 5–7 h, food was withdrawn at the beginning of the light cycle. To reduce the influence of potential confounding factors, we first obtained absolute flux of liver glucose production from Rossetti et al.'s (1993) study conducted in 322 g male Sprague-Dawley rats [standard error (*SE*) = 7 g, *n* = 35] fed standard chow under conscious unrestrained conditions. The fractional contribution of glycogen to liver glucose production (48%) at 5–7 h was reported to be invariant to rat strain, body weight, state of anesthesia, and measurement technique (Rossetti et al., 1993; Neese et al., 1995; Peroni et al., 1997; Sena et al., 2007; Jin et al., 2013). The remaining 52% of glucose output came from glycerol, and lactate and amino acids (Rossetti et al., 1993; Neese et al., 1995; Peroni et al., 1997; Sena et al., 2007; Jin et al., 2013). The reported range of glycerol contribution was 15–19% and that of lactate and amino acids was 37–41% (Peroni et al., 1997; Sena et al., 2007; Jin et al., 2013) in various rat strains and a wide range of body weights. We selected fractional contributions of glycerol and lactate from the study of Jin et al. (2013) where they used 324 g male Sprague-Dawley rats (*SE* = 4 g, *n* = 9). **Table 2** shows the fractional contributions of various precursors to liver glucose output at 5–7 h and **Figure 3** shows the absolute flux values.

Overall glucose output progressively decreased by 30% from 5 to 7 h until 13 h of fasting. Much of this reduction was due to a decrease in the flux of glycogenolysis, whose fractional contribution to glucose output decreased from 48% at 5 h to 2.3% at 13 h of fasting (**Table 2**). Thus, the contributions of the remaining precursors—glycerol, lactate, and amino acids—to glucose output remained nearly constant as absolute values but increased as fractions of glucose output. As a result, the absolute fluxes through the reactions downstream of glycogen breakdown (PYGL in **Figure 2**), beginning with glucose-6-phosphate isomerase (GPI in **Figure 2**) and ending in the tricarboxylic acid cycle at succinate dehydrogenase (SDH in **Figure 2**), were nearly

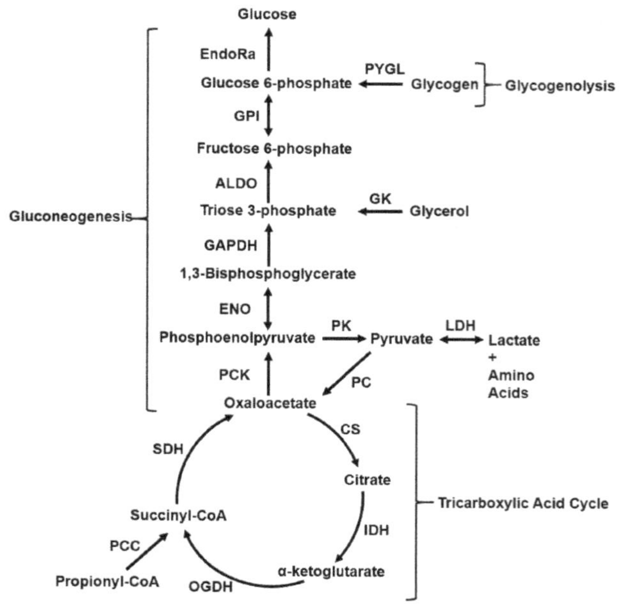

FIGURE 2 | Figure (adapted from Pannala et al., 2018) depicts liver central carbon metabolism pathways that produce glucose by breaking down glycogen (glycogenolysis) and by gluconeogenesis from glycerol, lactate, and amino acids during fasting. Unidirectional arrows indicate reactions that operate far from thermodynamic equilibrium and are practically irreversible. Bidirectional arrows indicate reactions that operate closer to thermodynamic equilibrium and are reversible under physiological conditions. ALDO, aldolase; CS, citrate synthase; EndoRa, endogenous liver glucose production; ENO, enolase; GAPDH, glyceraldehyde phosphate dehydrogenase; GK, glycerol kinase; GPI, glucose-6-phosphate isomerase; IDH, isocitrate dehydrogenase; LDH, lactate dehydrogenase; OGDH, oxoglutarate dehydrogenase; PC, pyruvate carboxylase; PCC, propionyl-CoA carboxylase; PCK, phos-phosphoenolpyruvate carboxykinase; PK, pyruvate kinase; PYGL, glycogen phosphorylase; SDH, succinate dehydrogenase.

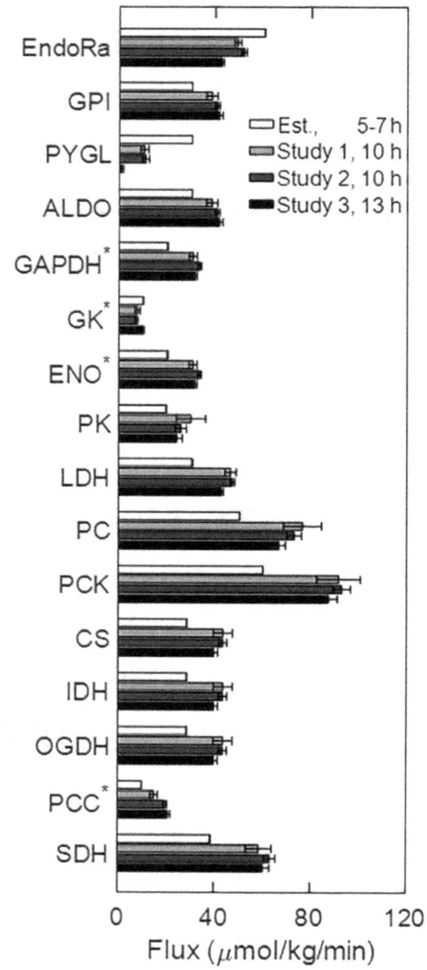

FIGURE 3 | Central carbon metabolic pathway fluxes through the reactions illustrated in **Figure 2**, measured in Studies 1–3 (10 and 13 h time points), and estimated from the literature at 5–7 h time interval. Bars represent mean flux values, and the error bars represent the SE of the means. The numbers of biological replicates in Studies 1–3 were 9, 8, and 8, respectively. Fluxes labeled by an asterisk (GAPDH, GK, ENO, and PCC) were expressed in hexose units, i.e., divided by a factor of two from their actual values. Abbreviated reaction names on the *y*-axis follow their definitions in the legend for **Figure 2**.

equal in magnitude at 10 and 13 h of fasting but higher than the values at 5–7 h of fasting (**Figure 3**).

The major conclusions from the central carbon flux data (**Figure 3**) were that glycogenolysis and overall glucose output decline with fasting duration. A key observation was that the glycogenolysis flux was almost completely depleted after 13 h of fasting. The flux analysis assumption that liver metabolism operated in a pseudo-steady state at 5–7 h and 10–13 h is consistent with numerous observations reported in the literature (McGarry et al., 1973; Rossetti et al., 1993). The 5–7-h time interval represented the end of an early post-absorptive period—where glycogen breakdown contributed to half of the liver glucose output—which was followed by a steep decline in glycogenolysis and a steep increase in ketogenesis plateauing at the 10–13-h time interval. Although the absolute flux of gluconeogenesis from glycerol was nearly equal at all time points, the flux of gluconeogenesis from lactate and amino acids was higher at the 10–13-h time interval, which indicated the coupling of liver metabolism to extra-hepatic sources of precursors for gluconeogenesis after longer fasting durations. Finally, a key approximation in the central carbon flux analysis was that the liver provided all of the glucose output. Although the kidney is also known to contribute to overall gluconeogenesis, its contribution is important only at fasting durations beyond 24 h (Mithieux et al., 2006). Together with previous evidence, our data suggest the presence of distinct metabolic states after 5–7 h and 10–13 h of fasting.

Metabolite Changes Observed During Short-Term Fasting

Plasma metabolites changed after short-term fasting (**Table 3**). Given the similarity in liver central carbon fluxes, we treated the 5-h (Studies 1 and 2) and 7-h (Study 3) fasting durations as early time points, and the 10-h (Studies 1 and 2) and 13-h (Study 3)

TABLE 2 | Fractional contributions of metabolic precursors glycogen, glycerol, and lactate and amino acids to liver glucose production at varying durations of fasting.

Metabolic precursor	Percent contribution to liver glucose output		
	5–7 h	10 h	13 h
Glycogen	48[a]	20[b]	2.3[b]
Glycerol	15[a]	16[b]	23.4[b]
Lactate and amino acids (lactate)	37[a] (33[a])	64[b] (51[c])	74.3[b] (59[c])

The fractional contribution of lactate alone to liver glucose production is shown in parentheses adjacent to that of lactate and amino acids in total. [a]*(Rossetti et al., 1993; Jin et al., 2013).* [b]*This study.* [c]*(Lopez et al., 1998).*

TABLE 3 | Observed changes in metabolites between early (5–7 h) and late (10–13 h) time intervals, experimentally measured in the plasma, and in the subset that is represented in the rat metabolic network model as exchangeable between the hepatocyte and plasma.

	Elevated	Depressed	
Metabolite set	Total	($p < 0.01$)	($p < 0.01$)
Experimentally measured in plasma	824	121	72
Model represented and exchangeable with plasma	216	33	6

durations as later time points for determining metabolite fold-change values and their statistical significance. Of the 884 metabolites observed across the three studies, 198 changed significantly ($p < 0.01$). Of these, 39 metabolites were represented in the rat metabolic network model (*iRno*) as exchangeable between liver cells and the extracellular space or plasma. We compared our model predictions for the direction of change with fasting to those for the 39 metabolites, 33 of which showed an increase and 6 of which showed a decrease.

We also compared the significant changes in plasma metabolites observed in the present study to those reported in the literature on short-term fasting in the rat (McGarry et al., 1973; Ho, 1976; Brass and Hoppel, 1978; Palou et al., 1981; Kotal et al., 1996; Ikeda et al., 2014). In terms of major metabolite pathways, most of the changes reported in the literature were in agreement with those found in our study (**Table 4**). Important changes indicative of fasting were a reduction in glucose and phospholipids, and an elevation of ketone bodies, fatty acyl carnitines, corticosterone, and choline. Furthermore, key liver-specific metabolite changes observed here and in the literature were the elevation of primary and secondary bile acids, and the elevation of bile pigments bilirubin and biliverdin. **Supplementary Table S3** provides detailed lists of those metabolites and the entire summary of statistical analysis of all metabolites.

Reports on large-scale data on plasma metabolite changes during a short-term fast, the number of biological replicates required to resolve them, and their sensitivity to the type of vehicle administered, do not exist in the literature. The number of metabolites measured in Studies 1, 2, and 3 were 569, 645, and 633, respectively, where the vehicle administered to the rats was different for each study. The metabolite fold-change values needed to be pooled across the three studies to resolve metabolite changes above experimental and biological noise during short-term fasting. The sum total of unique metabolites measured in the plasma in all three studies was 824 (**Table 3**), of which 420 were common to all three studies, 183 were common to exactly any two studies, and 221 were observed in exactly any one study. We calculated bootstrapped 99% confidence intervals of the fold-change values of the 420 common metabolites and confirmed that the vehicle was not a significant factor influencing metabolite changes (see **Supplementary Table S3**).

Among the 193 significantly changed metabolites (**Table 3**), 104 (54%) were measured in all three studies, 44 (23%) in exactly any two studies, and 45 (23%) in exactly any one study. Similarly, among the 631 unchanged metabolites, 316 (50%) were measured in all three studies, 139 (22%) in exactly any two

TABLE 4 | Concordance of observed changes in plasma metabolite data with reported changes in the literature due to short-term fasting.

Pathway	Number of metabolites reported in this study (and in the literature)			Fraction in agreement with this study	Reference
	Elevated	Unchanged	Depressed		
Amino acid	3 (6)	18 (13)	1 (3)	0.6	Palou et al., 1981
Carbohydrate	0	0	1 (1)	1.0	McGarry et al., 1973; Palou et al., 1981
Hemoglobin and porphyrin metabolism	3 (3)	0	0	1.0	Kotal et al., 1996
Lipid/carnitine	0 (0)	0	1 (0)	1.0	Brass and Hoppel, 1978
Lipid/corticosteroids	1 (1)	0	0 (0)	1.0	Dauchy et al., 2010; Ikeda et al., 2014
Lipid/diacylglycerol	1 (0)	0	7 (8)	0.9	Ikeda et al., 2014
Lipid/acyl carnitine	23 (23)	0	0	1.0	Brass and Hoppel, 1978
Lipid/ketone bodies	2 (2)	0	0	1.0	McGarry et al., 1973; Palou et al., 1981
Lipid/phosphatidylcholine	0	0	11 (11)	1.0	Ikeda et al., 2014
Lipid/phosphatidylinositol	0	0	5 (5)	1.0	Ikeda et al., 2014
Lipid/choline	1 (1)	0	0	1.0	Ikeda et al., 2014
Lipid/bile acids	9 (9)	0	0	1.0	Ho, 1976
Lipid/sterol	0	0	1 (1)	1.0	Ikeda et al., 2014

studies, and 176 (27%) in exactly any one study. Taken together, there was no study-wise representation bias in the proportion of metabolites among the changed and unchanged groups, nor was there any differential effect of the vehicle on metabolite changes between studies, ensuring that pooling of metabolite fold-change data across studies was not confounded by known experimental differences between studies.

Of the 216 metabolites represented in *iRno* as exchangeable metabolites, 163 (76%) were measured in all three studies, which indicated the overall reliability of the data on exchangeable metabolites. Similarly, among the 39 significantly changed metabolites, 35 (90%) were measured in all three studies, which indicated the reliability of the metabolite data against which our model predictions were compared. Of the remaining four, *N*-carbamoylaspartate was measured in Study 3, acetylcarnitine in Study 1, inosine in Studies 1 and 2, and isocitrate in Studies 1 and 3.

Metabolite pathway annotations showed that lipids, amino acids, and cofactors and vitamins account for 49%, 23%, and 4% of the 824 metabolites, respectively, which indicated that lipid metabolites constituted the single largest category. Among the 193 metabolites that changed significantly, lipid metabolites again constituted the single largest group at 58%. The fraction of significantly changed lipid metabolites among all lipid metabolites was also highest at 28%, when compared to changes in other major pathways (19% or less). These results underscore the significance of lipids during short-term fasting.

Metabolic Gene Expression Did Not Change Significantly During Short-Term Fasting

Gene expression changes in the liver during short-term fasting in all three studies (**Table 5**) revealed that the transcripts from each study mapped to a similar total number of genes (about 14,000), of which 2,258 were mapped to 2,240 in *iRno*. Out of the 2,325 genes in *iRno,* which were annotated with NCBI gene identifiers, 2,240 had 2,258 ENSEMBL gene identifiers that were used to annotate our transcriptomic data, with several genes mapping to than one ENSEMBL identifier. Based on the criteria of a false discovery rate of less than 0.1 and a biological effect size cutoff of 0.6 (corresponding to the 90th percentile), we found no statistically and biologically significant change in the expression of metabolic genes mapping to *iRno* in Studies 1 and 3 except for 100 genes in Study 2. Therefore, we did not use any differential gene expression-based weights in our implementation of the TIMBR algorithm to predict plasma metabolite changes. **Supplementary Table S4** shows the results of the gene expression analysis.

TABLE 5 | Summary of gene expression changes with fasting.

Study	Number of genes		
	Total	Mapped to *iRno* (total)	Mapped to *iRno* ($q < 0.1$)
1	14,115	2,240	0
2	14,581	2,240	100
3	14,419	2,240	0

Liver Metabolism Accounts for 64% of Plasma Metabolite Changes

We integrated liver central carbon flux data, as well as known physiological flux bounds for metabolite exchange fluxes at early (after 5–7 h of fasting) and late (after 10–13 h of fasting) time points, with *iRno* using the TIMBR algorithm. We then used the TIMBR algorithm to compute a TIMBR score, whose positive or negative sign indicated the tendency of a metabolite to increase or decrease in the plasma, respectively, owing to changes in the liver metabolic network demand induced by fasting. The TIMBR predictions agreed overall with the metabolite changes observed here; TIMBR scores accurately predicted five out of six depressed, and 20 out of 33 elevated metabolites (**Table 6**). A summary of the 39 metabolites, their observed $\log_2$(fold-change) values, and corresponding TIMBR scores (**Figure 4**) revealed an overall accuracy of 64% for predicting any changes, and accuracies of 61% and 83% for predicting elevated and depressed metabolites, respectively. The probability that 64% or higher prediction accuracy could be achieved by chance was calculated to be 0.054, using the exact binomial test. Therefore, our network model of liver metabolism could account for 64% of plasma metabolite changes (increase or decrease) that were represented in the model, during short-term fasting.

The results in **Figure 4**, organized by metabolite pathways, revealed three major pathways represented in our data set: amino acids (8 metabolites), cofactors and vitamins (7 metabolites), and lipids (18 metabolites). The model accuracy in predicting metabolite changes for these three major pathways was 75% for amino acids, 42% for cofactors and vitamins, and 78% for lipids, providing estimates of both the reliability of the network model and the hepatic origin of metabolite changes in the pathways. In particular, the model achieved 100% accuracy in predicting the elevation of five primary and secondary bile acids (under lipids in **Figure 4**), and two bile pigments (under cofactors and vitamins), which are specific to the liver.

Computational Model Assumptions, Limitations, and Interpretation of Predictions

The rat metabolic network model, *iRno*, currently the most comprehensive genome-scale model of rat metabolism, instantiated with physiological flux bounds pertinent to the

TABLE 6 | Concordance of TIMBR predictions with observed directions of change in metabolite data.

Direction of change	Number of metabolites measured	Concordant model predictions
Elevated	33	20
Depressed	6	5
All	39	25

Metabolite	Data	TIMBR	Group
dimethylglycine	0.32	0.98	Amino Acid
glycine	0.19	-0.89	Amino Acid
cysteine	1.39	-0.87	Amino Acid
5-methylthioadenosine (MTA)	0.29	0.72	Amino Acid
serotonin	1.65	0.79	Amino Acid
3-(4-hydroxyphenyl)lactate	-0.32	-0.30	Amino Acid
tyrosine	-0.30	-0.88	Amino Acid
arginine	-0.14	-0.88	Amino Acid
mannose	0.18	-0.44	Carbohydrate
oxalate (ethanedioate)	0.26	-0.71	Cofactors and Vitamins
threonate	0.61	-0.47	Cofactors and Vitamins
bilirubin (Z,Z)	0.38	1.64	Cofactors and Vitamins
biliverdin	0.59	1.58	Cofactors and Vitamins
quinolinate	0.67	0.82	Cofactors and Vitamins
dihydrobiopterin	0.66	-0.06	Cofactors and Vitamins
pyridoxate	0.57	-0.77	Cofactors and Vitamins
isocitrate	1.83	-0.11	TCA cycle
carnitine	-0.16	0.98	Lipid
deoxycarnitine	0.31	0.94	Lipid
corticosterone	0.84	1.43	Lipid
acetylcarnitine	0.81	1.02	Lipid
16-hydroxypalmitate	0.34	2.35	Lipid
choline	0.35	1.40	Lipid
arachidonate (20:4n6)	0.26	-0.90	Lipid
eicosapentaenoate (EPA; 20:5n3)	0.80	-0.89	Lipid
mead acid (20:3n9)	0.69	2.87	Lipid
tauro-beta-muricholate	1.41	1.39	Lipid
taurochenodeoxycholate	0.80	1.35	Lipid
taurocholate	1.20	1.36	Lipid
deoxycholate	2.50	1.36	Lipid
glycodeoxycholate	3.37	1.43	Lipid
taurodeoxycholate	1.77	1.65	Lipid
taurohyodeoxycholic acid	1.28	1.73	Lipid
stearoyl sphingomyelin (d18:1/18:0)	0.38	-2.13	Lipid
cholesterol	-0.25	-0.84	Lipid
inosine	1.59	-0.17	Nucleotide
cytidine	0.57	-0.41	Nucleotide
N-carbamoylaspartate	-0.64	-0.66	Nucleotide
phenylacetylglycine	0.86	0.21	Peptide

FIGURE 4 | Binary heat map of TIMBR scores of significantly changed exchangeable metabolites in plasma represented in *iRno* compared with measured fold-change values, grouped by major biochemical pathways: amino acid, carbohydrate, cofactors, and vitamins, TCA cycle, lipid, nucleotide, and peptide. The values in the left-hand side column (data) are measured $\log_2$(fold change) values of metabolites, grouped as depressed (black background), or elevated (white background) metabolites. The values in the right-hand side column are the computed TIMBR scores whose negative (black background) or positive (white background) sign indicates a predicted tendency of the metabolite to be depressed or elevated in plasma.

liver, was tested for satisfying defined liver-specific metabolic functionalities (Blais et al., 2017). The implicit assumption in our model was that overall liver metabolism could be represented by a single network with a representative set of physiological boundary conditions. This assumption seemed to contradict the known metabolic differences in hepatocytes between perivenous and periportal regions in the liver (Thurman et al., 1986). Despite not representing those different kinds of hepatocytes in our model, the overall satisfaction of liver metabolic tasks attested to a sufficient representation of liver metabolic functions originating in both regions. Additionally, the physiological flux bounds and central carbon fluxes employed to constrain the model did not include any metabolic heterogeneity. Finally, a key assumption in analyzing the model was that the network maintained a steady state, which was reasonable given the known metabolic flux conditions at 5–7 h and 10–13 h.

A limitation of our modeling analysis was the restricted coverage of metabolites exchanged between the plasma and liver cells. Additional curation of *iRno*, which included addition of exchange fluxes to improve network coverage of plasma metabolites, was limited by the paucity of literature evidence on the exchangeability of those metabolites. Consequently, the fraction of lipid metabolites among the 216 exchangeable metabolites (37%) was lower than that of the overall data set (49%). However, the fraction of lipid metabolites among the 39 significantly changing metabolites was higher at 46%, which is consistent with the trend in lipid metabolite fractions observed in the overall data set. Therefore, metabolite changes mapped to the network model are not biased by their limited coverage.

The measured changes in the circulating metabolites in plasma reflected the fasting response of the whole body. Our modeling effort sought to investigate plasma metabolite changes that can be associated with changes in liver metabolism under short-term fasting conditions where the primary observation was a decrease in the hormonally regulated flux of liver glycogenolysis and no significant transcriptomic changes of liver enzymes (Lin and Accili, 2011). Our metabolic network analysis was made liver specific and relevant to liver metabolism by the flux constraints.

We used the *in vivo* central carbon fluxes derived from our tracer-infusion studies under short-term fasting conditions coupled with literature data from several studies during short-term fasting that sets the overall metabolite uptake and secretion fluxes of the liver (Lopez et al., 1998; Jin et al., 2013). This analysis assumed that the bulk of the glucose production flux captured by the *in vivo* metabolic flux analysis was of hepatic origin under these conditions (Hasenour et al., 2015). Thus, even though the measured metabolite changes were reflective of the overall systemic response, our computational analysis estimated those changes that were in concordance with a hepatic origin. To assess the impact of liver transcriptomic changes, we repeated our implementation of the TIMBR method using all of the transcriptomic changes regardless of their statistical significance and found that the predicted directions of metabolite changes were unaltered from those shown in **Figure 4** (see **Supplementary Figures S1–S3**).

Finally, the estimated model accuracy in predicting bile acids and bile pigments (100%, p = 0.004, subset of lipids), lipids (78%, p = 0.03), and amino acids (75%, p = 0.29) demonstrated the capability of the model to describe liver metabolic functions, and provided estimates of contributions of liver metabolism that agreed with metabolite changes observed in those pathways. In particular, lipid metabolite changes emerged as indicators of changes in liver metabolism, which were characterized both experimentally and computationally with sufficient statistical significance.

CONCLUSION

Liver glycogenolysis became vanishingly small over the course of a short-term fast of 13 h, which resulted in a decline in the overall liver glucose output from 5 h until 13 h. Metabolites in plasma during this period showed changes known to be associated with short-term fasting, whereas liver gene expression did not change significantly. Finally, our computational analysis showed that two-thirds of the metabolite changes in plasma between 5–7 h and 10–13 h of fasting could be explained by central carbon flux changes in the liver without significant changes in gene expression.

AUTHOR CONTRIBUTIONS

KV conceived the short-term fasting analysis, analyzed RNA-seq and metabolomics data, computed model predictions, and wrote the manuscript. VP curated the rat metabolic network model. MW and MR performed metabolic flux calculations based on isotope labeling measurements. SE performed all of the animal studies, including catheterization surgeries. IT processed plasma samples for metabolic flux analysis. TO collected and analyzed all of the blood samples. RP contributed to RNA extraction from tissue and purifications. JR helped to conceive and supervise the study, and helped to edit the manuscript. MS conceived the study, supervised and carried out the experiments on rats to generate the raw data, and helped to write the manuscript. JY conceived the study, supervised the metabolic flux analysis, and helped to write the manuscript. AW conceived and supervised the study, and helped to edit and write the final manuscript.

FUNDING

This study was supported by the United States Army Medical Research and Materiel Command, Fort Detrick, MD, United States, as part of the United States Army's Network Science Initiative and under Contract No. W81XWH-14-C-0058 (to JY). Vanderbilt University Medical Center's Vanderbilt Technologies for Advanced Genomics (VANTAGE Core) was supported in part by CTSA grant (5UL1 RR024975-03), the Vanderbilt Ingram Cancer Center (P30 CA68485), the Vanderbilt Vision Center (P30 EY08126), and NIH/NCRR (G20 RR030956).

ACKNOWLEDGMENTS

The authors gratefully acknowledge the assistance of Drs. Shivendra Tewari, Francisco Vital-Lopez, and Srinivas Laxminarayan for helpful discussions at various stages of this study. The authors also gratefully acknowledge Dr. Tatsuya Oyama contributions in editing the manuscript. The Vanderbilt University Medical Center's VANTAGE Core provided the genome-wide RNA sequencing data; Metabolon Inc. provided the global metabolic profiling data and some technical assistance for this work. The opinions and assertions contained herein are the private views of the authors and are not to be construed as official or as reflecting the views of the United States Army, the United States Department of Defense, or the Henry M. Jackson Foundation for the Advancement of Military Medicine, Inc. This paper has been approved for public release with unlimited distribution.

SUPPLEMENTARY MATERIAL

FIGURE S1 | Binary heat map of TIMBR scores of significantly changed exchangeable metabolites in plasma represented in *iRno* compared with measured fold-change values, computed using both liver physiological flux changes and gene expression changes in Study 1 and grouped by major biochemical pathways: amino acid, carbohydrate, cofactors, and vitamins, TCA cycle, lipid, nucleotide, and peptide. The values in the left-hand side column (data) are measured $\log_2$ (fold change) values of metabolites, grouped as depressed (black background), or elevated (white background) metabolites. The values in the right-hand side column are the computed TIMBR scores whose negative (black background) or positive (white background) sign indicates a predicted tendency of the metabolite to be depressed or elevated in plasma.

FIGURE S2 | Binary heat map of TIMBR scores of significantly changed exchangeable metabolites in plasma represented in *iRno* compared with measured fold-change values, computed using both liver physiological flux changes and gene expression changes in Study 2 and grouped by major biochemical pathways: amino acid, carbohydrate, cofactors, and vitamins, TCA cycle, lipid, nucleotide, and peptide. The values in the left-hand side column (data) are measured $\log_2$ (fold change) values of metabolites, grouped as depressed (black background), or elevated (white background) metabolites. The values in the right-hand side column are the computed TIMBR scores whose negative (black background) or positive (white background) sign indicates a predicted tendency of the metabolite to be depressed or elevated in plasma.

FIGURE S3 | Binary heat map of TIMBR scores of significantly changed exchangeable metabolites in plasma represented in *iRno* compared with measured fold-change values, computed using both liver physiological flux changes and gene expression changes in Study 3 and grouped by major biochemical pathways: amino acid, carbohydrate, cofactors, and vitamins, TCA cycle, lipid, nucleotide, and peptide. The values in the left-hand side column (data) are measured $\log_2$ (fold change) values of metabolites, grouped as depressed (black background), or elevated (white background) metabolites. The values in the right-hand side column are the computed TIMBR scores whose negative (black background) or positive (white background) sign indicates a predicted tendency of the metabolite to be depressed or elevated in plasma.

TABLE S1 | Rat genome-scale metabolic network reconstruction *iRno*, with modifications.

TABLE S2 | Flux constraints for *iRno* during short-term fasting obtained from the literature.

TABLE S3 | Metabolomic imputed data from Studies 1–3, and the summary of statistical analysis of metabolite changes during short-term fasting in all three studies.

TABLE S4 | Results of RNA-seq data analysis, using the Wald and the likelihood ratio tests, to assess gene expression changes during short-term fasting in Studies 1–3.

DATA SHEET S1 | Rat genome-scale metabolic network reconstruction *iRno* in SBML format.

DATA SHEET S2 | Computer code to analyze metabolomics data.

DATA SHEET S3 | Computer code to reproduce TIMBR analysis results in **Figure 1** and **Supplementary Figures S1–S3**.

REFERENCES

Antoniewicz, M. R., Kelleher, J. K., and Stephanopoulos, G. (2006). Determination of confidence intervals of metabolic fluxes estimated from stable isotope measurements. *Metab. Eng.* 8, 324–337. doi: 10.1016/j.ymben.2006.01.004

Antoniewicz, M. R., Kelleher, J. K., and Stephanopoulos, G. (2007). Accurate assessment of amino acid mass isotopomer distributions for metabolic flux analysis. *Anal. Chem.* 79, 7554–7559. doi: 10.1021/ac0708893

Antoniewicz, M. R., Kelleher, J. K., and Stephanopoulos, G. (2011). Measuring deuterium enrichment of glucose hydrogen atoms by gas chromatography/mass spectrometry. *Anal. Chem.* 83, 3211–3216. doi: 10.1021/ac200012p

Beger, R. D., Bhattacharyya, S., Yang, X., Gill, P. S., Schnackenberg, L. K., Sun, J., et al. (2015). Translational biomarkers of acetaminophen-induced acute liver injury. *Arch. Toxicol.* 89, 1497–1522. doi: 10.1007/s00204-015-1519-4

Blais, E. M., Rawls, K. D., Dougherty, B. V., Li, Z. I., Kolling, G. L., Ye, P., et al. (2017). Reconciled rat and human metabolic networks for comparative toxicogenomics and biomarker predictions. *Nat. Commun.* 8:14250. doi: 10.1038/ncomms14250

Brass, E. P., and Hoppel, C. L. (1978). Carnitine metabolism in the fasting rat. *J. Biol. Chem.* 253, 2688–2693.

Bray, N. L., Pimentel, H., Melsted, P., and Pachter, L. (2016). Near-optimal probabilistic RNA-seq quantification. *Nat. Biotechnol.* 34, 525–527. doi: 10.1038/nbt.3519

Chang, H., Meng, H. Y., Liu, S. M., Wang, Y., Yang, X. X., Lu, F., et al. (2017). Identification of key metabolic changes during liver fibrosis progression in rats using a urine and serum metabolomics approach. *Sci. Rep.* 7:11433. doi: 10.1038/s41598-017-11759-z

Dauchy, R. T., Dauchy, E. M., Tirrell, R. P., Hill, C. R., Davidson, L. K., Greene, M. W., et al. (2010). Dark-phase light contamination disrupts circadian rhythms in plasma measures of endocrine physiology and metabolism in rats. *Comp. Med.* 60, 348–356.

Dehaven, C. D., Evans, A. M., Dai, H., and Lawton, K. A. (2010). Organization of GC/MS and LC/MS metabolomics data into chemical libraries. *J. Cheminform.* 2:9. doi: 10.1186/1758-2946-2-9

Efron, B., and Hastie, T. (2016). *Computer Age Statistical Inference: Algorithms, Evidence, and Data Science*. New York, NY: Cambridge University Press. doi: 10.1017/CBO9781316576533

Evans, A. M., Bridgewater, B. R., Liu, Q., Mitchell, M. W., Robinson, R. J., Dai, H., et al. (2014). High resolution mass spectrometry improves data quantity and quality as compared to unit mass resolution mass spectrometry in high-throughput profiling metabolomics. *Metabolomics* 4:132. doi: 10.4172/2153-0769.1000132

Hasenour, C. M., Wall, M. L., Ridley, D. E., Hughey, C. C., James, F. D., Wasserman, D. H., et al. (2015). Mass spectrometry-based microassay of (2)H and (13)C plasma glucose labeling to quantify liver metabolic fluxes *in vivo*. *Am. J. Physiol. Endocrinol. Metab.* 309, E191–E203. doi: 10.1152/ajpendo.00003.2015

Hatano, T., Saiki, S., Okuzumi, A., Mohney, R. P., and Hattori, N. (2016). Identification of novel biomarkers for parkinson's disease by metabolomic technologies. *J. Neurol. Neurosurg. Psychiatry* 87, 295–301. doi: 10.1136/jnnp-2014-309676

Ho, K. J. (1976). Circadian distribution of bile acids in the enterohepatic circulatory system in rats. *Am. J. Physiol.* 230, 1331–1335. doi: 10.1152/ajplegacy.1976.230.5.1331

Ikeda, I., Metoki, K., Yamahira, T., Kato, M., Inoue, N., Nagao, K., et al. (2014). Impact of fasting time on hepatic lipid metabolism in nutritional animal studies. *Biosci. Biotechnol. Biochem.* 78, 1584–1591. doi: 10.1080/09168451.2014.923297

Iruzubieta, P., Arias-Loste, M. T., Barbier-Torres, L., Martinez-Chantar, M. L., and Crespo, J. (2015). The need for biomarkers in diagnosis and prognosis of drug-induced liver disease: does metabolomics have any role? *Biomed. Res. Int.* 2015:386186. doi: 10.1155/2015/386186

Jarak, I., Carrola, J., Barros, A. S., Gil, A. M., Pereira, M. L., Corvo, M. L., et al. (2017). From the cover: metabolism modulation in different organs by silver nanoparticles: an NMR metabolomics study of a mouse model. *Toxicol. Sci.* 159, 422–435. doi: 10.1093/toxsci/kfx142

Jin, E. S., Beddow, S. A., Malloy, C. R., and Samuel, V. T. (2013). Hepatic glucose production pathways after three days of a high-fat diet. *Metabolism* 62, 152–162. doi: 10.1016/j.metabol.2012.07.012

Kamp, H., Strauss, V., Wiemer, J., Leibold, E., Walk, T., Mellert, W., et al. (2012). Reproducibility and robustness of metabolome analysis in rat plasma of 28-day repeated dose toxicity studies. *Toxicol. Lett.* 215, 143–149. doi: 10.1016/j.toxlet.2012.09.015

Kotal, P., Vitek, L., and Fevery, J. (1996). Fasting-related hyperbilirubinemia in rats: the effect of decreased intestinal motility. *Gastroenterology* 111, 217–223. doi: 10.1053/gast.1996.v111.pm8698202

Lin, H. V., and Accili, D. (2011). Hormonal regulation of hepatic glucose production in health and disease. *Cell Metab.* 14, 9–19. doi: 10.1016/j.cmet.2011.06.003

Lopez, H. W., Moundras, C., Morand, C., Demigne, C., and Remesy, C. (1998). Opposite fluxes of glutamine and alanine in the splanchnic area are an efficient mechanism for nitrogen sparing in rats. *J. Nutr.* 128, 1487–1494. doi: 10.1093/jn/128.9.1487

Mattes, W., Davis, K., Fabian, E., Greenhaw, J., Herold, M., Looser, R., et al. (2014). Detection of hepatotoxicity potential with metabolite profiling (metabolomics) of rat plasma. *Toxicol. Lett.* 230, 467–478. doi: 10.1016/j.toxlet.2014.07.021

McGarry, J. D., Meier, J. M., and Foster, D. W. (1973). The effects of starvation and refeeding on carbohydrate and lipid metabolism *in vivo* and in the perfused rat liver. The relationship between fatty acid oxidation and esterification in the regulation of ketogenesis. *J. Biol. Chem.* 248, 270–278.

Mellert, W., Kapp, M., Strauss, V., Wiemer, J., Kamp, H., Walk, T., et al. (2011). Nutritional impact on the plasma metabolome of rats. *Toxicol. Lett.* 207, 173–181. doi: 10.1016/j.toxlet.2011.08.013

Mithieux, G., Gautier-Stein, A., Rajas, F., and Zitoun, C. (2006). Contribution of intestine and kidney to glucose fluxes in different nutritional states in rat. *Comp. Biochem. Physiol. B Biochem. Mol. Biol.* 143, 195–200. doi: 10.1016/j.cbpb.2005.11.007

Mu, C., Yang, Y., Luo, Z., and Zhu, W. (2015). Metabolomic analysis reveals distinct profiles in the plasma and urine of rats fed a high-protein diet. *Amino Acids* 47, 1225–1238. doi: 10.1007/s00726-015-1949-6

Neese, R. A., Schwarz, J. M., Faix, D., Turner, S., Letscher, A., Vu, D., et al. (1995).

Gluconeogenesis and intrahepatic triose phosphate flux in response to fasting or substrate loads. Application of the mass isotopomer distribution analysis technique with testing of assumptions and potential problems. *J. Biol. Chem.* 270, 14452–14466. doi: 10.1074/jbc.270.24.14452

Palou, A., Remesar, X., Arola, L., Herrera, E., and Alemany, M. (1981). Metabolic effects of short term food deprivation in the rat. *Horm. Metab. Res.* 13, 326–330. doi: 10.1055/s-2007-1019258

Pannala, V. R., Wall, M. L., Estes, S. K., Trenary, I., O'Brien, T. P., Printz, R. L., et al. (2018). Metabolic network-based predictions of toxicant-induced metabolite changes in the laboratory rat. *Sci. Rep.* 8:11678. doi: 10.1038/s41598-018-30149-7

Peroni, O., Large, V., Diraison, F., and Beylot, M. (1997). Glucose production and gluconeogenesis in postabsorptive and starved normal and streptozotocin-diabetic rats. *Metabolism* 46, 1358–1363. doi: 10.1016/S0026-0495(97)90244-4

Pimentel, H., Bray, N. L., Puente, S., Melsted, P., and Pachter, L. (2017). Differential analysis of RNA-seq incorporating quantification uncertainty. *Nat. Methods* 14, 687–690. doi: 10.1038/nmeth.4324

Rossetti, L., Giaccari, A., Barzilai, N., Howard, K., Sebel, G., and Hu, M. (1993). Mechanism by which hyperglycemia inhibits hepatic glucose production in conscious rats. Implications for the pathophysiology of fasting hyperglycemia in diabetes. *J. Clin. Invest.* 92, 1126–1134. doi: 10.1172/JCI116681

Sena, C. M., Barosa, C., Nunes, E., Seica, R., and Jones, J. G. (2007). Sources of endogenous glucose production in the goto-kakizaki diabetic rat. *Diabetes Metab.* 33, 296–302. doi: 10.1016/j.diabet.2007.03.002

Shiota, M. (2012). Measurement of glucose homeostasis *in vivo*: combination of tracers and clamp techniques. *Methods Mol. Biol.* 933, 229–253. doi: 10.1007/978-1-62703-068-7_15

Thurman, R. G., Kauffman, F. C., and Jungermann, K. (1986). *Regulation of Hepatic Metabolism: Intra- and Intercellular Compartmentation*. New York, NY: Plenum Press. doi: 10.1007/978-1-4684-5041-5

Young, J. D. (2014). INCA: a computational platform for isotopically non-stationary metabolic flux analysis. *Bioinformatics* 30, 1333–1335. doi: 10.1093/bioinformatics/btu015

Zerbino, D. R., Achuthan, P., Akanni, W., Amode, M. R., Barrell, D., Bhai, J., et al. (2018). Ensembl 2018. *Nucleic Acids Res.* 46, D754–D761. doi: 10.1093/nar/gkx1098

Zimmerman, H. J. (1999). *Hepatotoxicity: The Adverse Effects of Drugs and Other Chemicals on the Liver*. Philadelphia, PA: Lippincott Williams & Wilkins.

11

Understanding the Representative Gut Microbiota Dysbiosis in Metformin-Treated Type 2 Diabetes Patients Using Genome-Scale Metabolic Modeling

Dorines Rosario[1†], Rui Benfeitas[1†], Gholamreza Bidkhori[1], Cheng Zhang[1], Mathias Uhlen[1], Saeed Shoaie[2,3] and Adil Mardinoglu[1,4*]*

[1] Science for Life Laboratory, Royal Institute of Technology, Stockholm, Sweden, [2] Centre for Host-Microbiome Interactions, Dental Institute, King's College London, London, United Kingdom, [3] Centre for Translational Microbiome Research, Department of Microbiology, Tumor and Cell Biology, Karolinska Institute, Stockholm, Sweden, [4] Department of Biology and Biological Engineering, Chalmers University of Technology, Gothenburg, Sweden

***Correspondence:**
Saeed Shoaie
saeed.shoaie@kcl.ac.uk
Adil Mardinoglu
adilm@scilifelab.se

[†] These authors have contributed equally to this work.

Dysbiosis in the gut microbiome composition may be promoted by therapeutic drugs such as metformin, the world's most prescribed antidiabetic drug. Under metformin treatment, disturbances of the intestinal microbes lead to increased abundance of *Escherichia* spp., *Akkermansia muciniphila, Subdoligranulum variabile* and decreased abundance of *Intestinibacter bartlettii*. This alteration may potentially lead to adverse effects on the host metabolism, with the depletion of butyrate producer genus. However, an increased production of butyrate and propionate was verified in metformin-treated Type 2 diabetes (T2D) patients. The mechanisms underlying these nutritional alterations and their relation with gut microbiota dysbiosis remain unclear. Here, we used Genome-scale Metabolic Models of the representative gut bacteria *Escherichia* spp., *I. bartlettii, A. muciniphila,* and *S. variabile* to elucidate their bacterial metabolism and its effect on intestinal nutrient pool, including macronutrients (e.g., amino acids and short chain fatty acids), minerals and chemical elements (e.g., iron and oxygen). We applied flux balance analysis (FBA) coupled with synthetic lethality analysis interactions to identify combinations of reactions and extracellular nutrients whose absence prevents growth. Our analyses suggest that *Escherichia* sp. is the bacteria least vulnerable to nutrient availability. We have also examined bacterial contribution to extracellular nutrients including short chain fatty acids, amino acids, and gasses. For instance, *Escherichia* sp. and *S. variabile* may contribute to the production of important short chain fatty acids (e.g., acetate and butyrate, respectively) involved in the host physiology under aerobic and anaerobic conditions. We have also identified pathway susceptibility to nutrient availability and reaction changes among the four bacteria using both FBA and flux variability analysis. For instance, lipopolysaccharide synthesis, nucleotide sugar metabolism, and amino acid metabolism are pathways susceptible to changes in *Escherichia* sp. and *A. muciniphila*. Our observations highlight important commensal and competing behavior, and their association with cellular metabolism for prevalent gut microbes. The results of our analysis have potential important implications for development of new therapeutic approaches in T2D patients through the development of prebiotics, probiotics, or postbiotics.

Keywords: gut microbiota, dysbiosis, host–microbiome interactions, genome-scale metabolic models, systems biology

INTRODUCTION

Dysbiosis in the gut bacterial community and concomitant metabolic changes have an impact on human health (Qin et al., 2012; Tremaroli and Bäckhed, 2012; Karlsson et al., 2013; Forslund et al., 2015; Mardinoglu et al., 2016; Magnusdottir et al., 2017). Gut microbiome could affect host metabolism (Brillat-Savarin, 1826; Tremaroli and Bäckhed, 2012; Shoaie et al., 2013, 2015; Magnusdottir et al., 2017) through degrading non-enzymatically digestible foods, and synthesis of amino acids and short chain fatty acids (SCFAs). Dysbiosis may have detrimental effects on host metabolism such as alterations in abundance of nutrients crucial for homeostasis including butyrate (Forslund et al., 2015; Mardinoglu et al., 2016; Wu et al., 2017). Perturbations of intestinal microbiota are recognized as a risk factor for type 2 diabetes (T2D), a complex chronic disorder associated with genetic and environmental risk factors such as age, diet, and lifestyle (Karlsson et al., 2013; Forslund et al., 2015; Shoaie et al., 2015; Mardinoglu et al., 2016; Magnusdottir et al., 2017). Recently, compositional shifts in representative gut microbes were identified in T2D patients undergoing metformin treatment, the most prescribed antidiabetic drug. These patients display increased abundance of *Escherichia* sp., *Akkermansia muciniphila* (*A. muciniphila*), and *Subdoligranulum variabile* (*S. variabile*) (Forslund et al., 2015; Mardinoglu et al., 2016; Wu et al., 2017), and lower of *Intestinibacter bartlettii* (Forslund et al., 2015; Wu et al., 2017), as well as increased levels of the SCFAs butyrate and propionate. Thus, despite potentially detrimental effects of gut microbiota dysbiosis, metformin-treated patients display beneficial alterations in gut SCFA abundances (Forslund et al., 2015; Mardinoglu et al., 2016). However, the relationship between the metabolism of representative gut bacteria such as *Escherichia* sp., *A. muciniphila*, *S. variabile* and *I. bartlettii*, and compounds in the intestinal lumen such as SCFAs or amino acids is unclear.

Clarifying complex metabolic responses and relationships between gut microbes and host metabolism requires an analysis of large and highly intertwined reaction networks. GEnome-scale Metabolic models (GEMs) allow for the analysis of such complex networks and have successfully been applied to clarify the mechanisms underlying insulin resistance (Varemo et al., 2015; Zhang and Hua, 2016; Mardinoglu et al., 2018; Turanli et al., 2018) and to identify important nutritional interactions between gut microbes and the host (Shoaie et al., 2013; Ji and Nielsen, 2015; Mardinoglu et al., 2015; Zhang and Hua, 2016). Synthetic lethality analysis (Pratapa et al., 2015) is an approach commonly used in constraint-based modeling to clarify biological phenomena (Mardinoglu and Nielsen, 2012; Mardinoglu et al., 2016; Magnusdottir et al., 2017). It is used to identify vital interconnected metabolic processes underlying a phenotype of interest (Qin et al., 2012; Shoaie et al., 2013; Magnusdottir et al., 2017) and has been extensively applied in health and disease (O'Neil et al., 2017). While synthetic lethality analysis traditionally seeks to identify genes that are individually essential, this approach may assist in identifying whether the simultaneous knock-out of two genes of interest leads to cell lethality, but their individual knock-out maintains cell viability, i.e., synthetic lethality interactions (Kaelin, 2005).

Through reconstruction and analysis of GEMs, we sought to understand the contribution of the four bacteria in the physiology of T2D patients undergoing metformin treatment. We used AGORA GEM reconstructions of *Escherichia* sp., *A. muciniphila*, *S. variabile*, and *I. bartlettii* to analyze relationships between the bacterial metabolism and the extracellular environment, as well as predicting the survivability of the bacteria against nutritional alterations (Magnusdottir et al., 2017). Here, we employed the concept of synthetic lethality analysis to identify sets of individual and pairs of reactions that, when not present, abolished growth. Additionally, we implemented nutritional interactions analysis to understanding how the presence or absence of gut nutrients influences bacterial growth by focusing on nutrient transport reactions (i.e., exchange reactions). Moreover, we assessed the influence of available nutrients and synthetic lethal reactions on cellular metabolic pathways to clarify which metabolic pathways were mostly dependent on nutritional alterations and under survivability threat, respectively. Lastly, interactions between the gut microbiota and the environment (host intestine) were evaluated through a novel approach based on the production and consumption of substrates of interest under maximal growth and minimal media conditions of each organism. Our observations highlight important association between cellular metabolism of these four prevalent gut microbes and point important implications for development of new therapeutic approaches in T2D patients.

MATERIALS AND METHODS

Genome Scale Metabolic Model Retrieval, Curation, and Modeling

AGORA (Assembly of Gut Organisms through Reconstruction and Analysis) model reconstructions (Magnusdottir et al., 2017) were downloaded in SBML format from Virtual Metabolic Human (VMH) database[1] for *Escherichia* sp. 4_1_40B, and

[1] https://vmh.uni.lu/#microbes/search

I. bartlettii (*Clostridium bartlettii* DSM 16795) on the 27th of January 2017, for *A. muciniphila* ATCC BAA-835 and *S. variabile* DSM 15176 on the 2nd April 2018. Details regarding microorganism AGORA reconstructions are accessible in **Supplementary Table S1**. The models were manually curated to ensure biological functionality. The computations were performed on resources provided by the Swedish National Infrastructure for Computing (SNIC) through Uppsala Multidisciplinary Center for Advanced Computational Science (UPPMAX).

The RAVEN (Reconstruction, Analysis and Visualization of Metabolic Networks) Toolbox (Agren et al., 2013) was used to define and set parameters for simulations and perform analyses of the originated predictions. Unless otherwise stated, all flux balance analyses (FBAs) considered biomass production as objective function. For flux variability analysis (FVA), minimum and maximum flux ranges were calculated for each reaction for the optimized value of the objective function through the COBRA (Constraint-Based Reconstruction and Analysis) Toolbox (Schellenberger et al., 2012).

Synthetic Lethality Analysis

Lethality analysis was performed by adapting the Fast-SL algorithm (Pratapa et al., 2015) from the COBRA Toolbox (Schellenberger et al., 2012) to RAVEN Toolbox (Agren et al., 2013). Fast-SL-derived single and double lethal reactions predictions (**Supplementary Table S2**) were further validated by constraining methods, setting lower and upper bounds to zero, with biomass maximization defined as objective function. Single lethal reactions were determined and treated as essential reactions for cell growth. Double lethal reactions were considered as those pairs of reactions that induce no growth when blocked simultaneously but not individually. Exchange reactions were determined using default RAVEN functions, and only those involving nutrient exchange with the extracellular space are reported (i.e., *outside reactions*, and not *inside reactions* which include DNA replication, RNA transcription, protein biosynthesis and biomass, and are treated as intracellular reactions). This permits the identification of essential exchange reactions, which are the nutrients required to be uptaken from the environment by the organism in order to guarantee cell survival.

Metabolic Pathway Sensitivity to Essential Reactions and Nutrient Changes

The built-in subsystems of the model were used for defining the pathways (**Supplementary Table S5**) and unclassified pathways were ignored. We applied modeling-constraints (lower and upper bounds set to zero and objective function defined as biomass maximization) going through each of the single and double lethal reactions (essential reactions) and non-essential exchange reactions. Pathway sensitivity to changes was determined based on the proportion of reactions that presented absolute flux changes above 0.01 mmol/gDW/h relative to the respective flux in the reference model where no constraints were set on lower/upper bounds. This value was conservatively considered based on the observation that FBA-based approaches often use 0.001 mmol/gDW/h as threshold for identifying reactions that have fluxes (Hyotylainen et al., 2016).

Additionally, these results were compared with those from FVA in response to the inhibition of single and paired synthetic lethal (essential) and non-essential exchange reactions, and compared to a reference output without applied constraints on lethal neither exchange reactions. Only solutions on flux variation that achieve $\geq$90% of the reference solution were considered. Using the minimum and maximum fluxes determined for each reaction, we computed the mean and ranges for all reactions in each subsystem.

Extracellular Nutrient Uptake and Alternative Aerobic and Anaerobic *Escherichia* sp. Growth

We have employed a novel approach which allowed us to identify which are the minimal sufficient nutrients that when combined are capable of providing cellular growth when uptaken by the organism. In order to identify which nutrients are on the first line promoting cellular growth under environmental limited conditions, the target reactions of this approach were non-essential exchange reactions. No constraint was applied for single essential exchange reactions to ensure that growth inhibition was not due to the block of required essential nutrients. Cellular intake through non-essential exchange reactions was blocked with lower bounds set to zero. Based on FBA methods, non-essential exchange reactions were blocked one-by-one, two-by-two, and three-by-three. Future work should test how this approach compares with existing methods for determining minimum growth conditions (e.g., Imielinski et al., 2006; Eker et al., 2013). This was performed for all organisms under anaerobiosis, and also for *Escherichia* sp. under aerobiosis. A biomass flux threshold of 10^{-5} was defined as minimum to consider cell growth.

Maximal Growth-Coupled Extracellular Nutrient Production and Consumption

We developed a novel approach to assess the contribution of each bacteria for nutrient production and consumption under the maximum growth rate permitted under minimum media conditions. Specifically, we determined the maximal rate of secretion or intake of each metabolite when the organism is at its highest growth yield by individually setting each metabolite of interest as objective function at a time, therefore maximizing its production or consumption. Maximum organism growth was determined based on FBA under minimal media for each organism (**Supplementary Table S7**). Thus, the predicted maximal growth (0.6387, 0.2268, 0.2599, 0.2460 mmol/gDW/h, respectively for *Escherichia* sp., *I. bartlettii, A. muciniphila,* and *S. variabile*) was used as lower bound constraint for biomass together with minimal media conditions and under anaerobic conditions (with oxygen exchange constrained to zero in both models).

RESULTS

In Silico Identification of Different Growth Requirements in Representative Gut Bacteria

To assess growth requirements of *Escherichia* sp., *I. bartlettii, A. muciniphila* and *S. variabile,* we retrieved AGORA (Magnusdottir et al., 2017) models for these organisms (**Supplementary Table S1**). These models comprise the entire known metabolic reaction networks of these organisms, and contain 1757, 1095, 1125, and 1057 reactions, and 1267, 730, 592, and 1313 genes, respectively. Using the FAST-SL algorithm (Pratapa et al., 2015) based on FBAs) with biomass as objective function, we performed synthetic lethality interaction analysis (**Figure 1**) on these four organisms. Through this approach, we revealed the influence of an inhibited (i.e., without flux) reaction on the metabolic network. This allowed for the identification of single essential reactions (**Figure 1A**), and those combinations of reaction pairs that become lethal when blocked simultaneously but not individually (**Figure 1B**). In total, this represents between 559,153 to 1,544,403 different conditions (including single and double reaction combinations) tested.

Additionally, this approach allowed for understanding the consequences of unavailability of environmental compounds (e.g., amino acids or oxygen) on cell growth by inhibiting transport reactions with the extracellular environment (i.e., exchange reactions). *Escherichia* sp., *I. bartlettii, A. muciniphila,* and *S. variabile* respectively displayed 211, 153, 142, and 130 exchange reactions. *I. bartlettii* was the bacteria with higher proportion of exchange reactions, while *S. variabile* was the organism with higher proportion of single lethal reactions. *Escherichia* sp. was the bacteria with lower proportion of essential exchange reactions (**Figure 1A** and **Supplementary Table S2**). These four organisms commonly shared 46 single lethal reactions. *A. muciniphila* presented 182 organism specific single lethal reactions and 45 additional single lethal reactions shared with *Escherichia* sp. Among all exchange reactions, 10 single-lethal were shared by these four organisms: environmental exchange of calcium, chloride, carbon dioxide, copper, potassium, magnesium, manganese, sulfate, zinc, and ferrous (Fe^{2+}) iron (**Figure 1C**). *Escherichia* sp. did not present organism-specific essential exchange reactions, whereas *I. bartlettii, S. variabile,* and *A. muciniphila* respectively had 1, 2, and 6 single-lethal exchange reactions found only in these organisms. Both *A. muciniphila* and *S. variabile* presented shared single-lethal exchange reactions with *I. bartlettii,* where exchange of ferric iron (Fe^{3+}) was essential in the three organisms. Exchange of vitamin B5 and tryptophan were essential exchange reactions found in *I. bartlettii* and *S. variabile,* whereas exchange of hydrogen phosphate is commonly essential in *I. bartlettii* and *A. muciniphila.*

When considering all possible pairs of combinations, *A. muciniphila* presented the highest proportion of double lethal reaction pairs and pairs that include at least 1 exchange reaction. *I. bartlettii* was the organism with higher number of organism-specific lethal reaction pairs with $\geq$1 exchange reaction, followed by *A. muciniphila* (**Figure 1B**). There were no lethal reaction pairs ($\geq$1 exchange reactions) exclusively shared by the two organisms. However, ornithine exchange comprised 7 and 4 organism-specific double lethal reactions in *I. bartlettii* and *A. muciniphila,* respectively. Among those combinations found together with ornithine exchange, the urea cycle was the only common pathway between the two bacteria, where arginine and proline metabolism are specific for *A. muciniphila,* and alanine and aspartate metabolism, pyrimidine synthesis, citric acid cycle are specific for *I. bartlettii.*

Intracellular reactions involving $NADP^+$/NADPH became lethal when combined with riboflavin or diaminoheptanedioate exchange in *I. bartlettii*. In turn, intracellular reactions involving $NADP^+$/NADPH together with environmental exchange of vitamin B_5, the fatty acid laurate or thymidine were synthetic lethal reaction pairs in *Escherichia* sp., but not in *I. bartlettii. Escherichia* sp. displayed the lowest proportion of double lethal reactions, as well as the lowest proportion of double lethal reactions with $\geq$1 exchange reactions, and the lowest number of organism-specific lethal reaction pairs with $\geq$1 exchange reactions. Among these pairs with $\geq$1 exchange reaction which involved fatty acids, *Escherichia* sp. and *A. muciniphila* respectively displayed 20 of 21 shared reaction pairs involving laurate exchange and an intracellular reaction associated with fatty acid synthesis or oxidation. Simultaneous inhibition of acetate exchange and acetate kinase or phosphotransacetylase reactions were lethal in *A. muciniphila.*

Several double lethal pairs involving nicotinate exchange were present in *S. variabile* (three pairs) and *I. bartlettii* (four pairs). Lethal pairs involving nicotinamide mononucleotide (NMN) exchange were also found for *S. variabile* (three pairs) and *Escherichia* sp. (two pairs), where one pair involves nicotinate-nucleotide adenylyltransferase in both organisms. Reactions involved in hypoxanthine exchange and purine synthesis were found in 10 double lethal pairs exclusive of *S. variabile.*

The inhibition of L-lysine exchange simultaneously with diaminopimelate decarboxylase reaction was the only lethal pair found in the four organisms. Reaction pairs including exchange of arginine, alanine, asparagine, aspartate, isoleucine, lysine, tyrosine, valine, thymidine, or thiamine (vitamin B1) were synthetic lethal in one or more organisms. *S. variabile, A. muciniphila, Escherichia* sp., and *I. bartlettii* respectively had 4, 2, 1 and 1 double lethal pairs involving 2 exchange reactions. Simultaneous inhibition of NMN exchange and nicotinate, or L-tyrosine coupled with glycyl-L-tyrosine, or phosphate paired with glycerol 3-phosphate and uracil paired with succinate became lethal in *S. variabile.* In *A. muciniphila* inhibiting the exchange of L-asparagine together with glycyl-L-asparagine or thiamin led to lethality. Notably, simultaneous blocking of exchange of oxygen with ferric iron (Fe^{3+}) or nicotinate, respectively prevented growth in *Escherichia* sp. and *I. bartlettii.* While *I. bartlettii* is an obligate anaerobe (**Supplementary Table S1**), the observation that O_2 exchange is present in this model could indicate that the model failed to describe its aerotolerance. However, the two following points indicate that the model predictions are robust to O_2 availability. First, the Spearman correlation between model fluxes in presence vs. absence of O_2 was very high (Spearman's

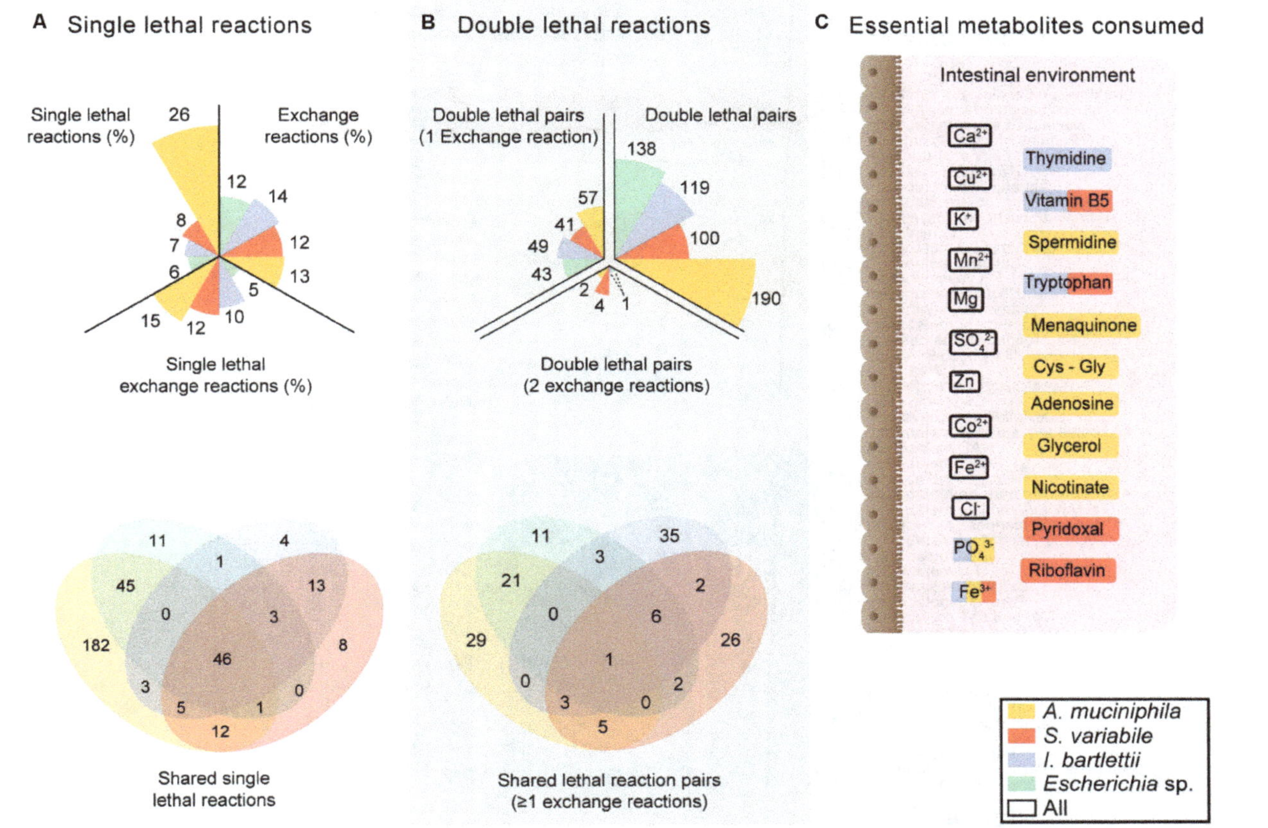

FIGURE 1 | Specific growth requirements suggest lower vulnerability of *Escherichia* sp. to environmental nutritional deficiencies. **(A)** Proportions of single lethal reaction sets for the entire metabolic network and for exchange reactions in the four organisms, and number of exclusive and shared single lethal reactions (**Supplementary Table S2**) **(B)** Number of double lethal reaction pairs. **(C)** Essential metabolites consumed by the four organisms. Multiple colored metabolites are consumed by several bacteria according to the legend.

$\rho > 0.82$, $P < 10^{-70}$ considering all 304 non-null fluxes of both models). Second, the reactions catalyzed by antioxidants against reactive oxygen species (hydrogen peroxide reductase) showed activity in a model encompassing oxygen exchange, but not in its absence (**Supplementary Table S3**). We finally, removed oxygen exchange from the *I. bartlettii* model and repeated the lethality analysis for the entire reaction network. The comparison of synthetic lethality analysis under aerobic versus anaerobic conditions changes the number of single lethal reactions from 80 to 85, and from 124 to 171 lethal pairs (**Supplementary Table S4**), respectively. However, only one additional single lethal exchange reaction (methionine exchange) was identified in the *I. bartlettii* model. These observations reinforce the confidence in the predictions of the model in terms of environmental dependency or synthetic lethal reactions.

Identification of Sensitive Pathways to Inhibition of Lethal and Non-essential Exchange Reactions

We investigated which pathways were mostly altered by single and double synthetic lethal reactions (i.e., essential reactions) and non-essential exchange reactions. *Escherichia* sp. displays 73 metabolic pathways, *I. bartlettii* displays 66, *A. muciniphila* has 68 and *S. variabile* displays 63, of which 54 are commonly present in the four organisms (**Supplementary Table S5**). Considering the entire metabolic network and sets of single, paired essential reactions, and non-essential exchange reactions individually and coupled in pairs, we computed the proportion of reactions that are altered in each pathway in comparison with each bacteria's reference model, i.e., the model with no reaction blocking. To do so, we used FBA to identify flux distribution between pathways while maximizing for bacterial growth, i.e., "pathway sensitivity" to reaction blocking. Additionally and to complement this methodology, we employed FVA (**Supplementary Table S6**). We observed (**Figures 2, 3**) that several pathways show significant alterations in >50% of their reactions. For instance, cholesterol (and squalene) synthesis but not other reactions involved in cholesterol metabolism, were highly perturbed by essential reactions and partly by environmental exchange reactions in *Escherichia* sp. In turn, cholesterol metabolism was highly perturbed by essential and environmental exchange reactions under the same constraints in *A. muciniphila* but not in *I. bartlettii* and *S. variabile*.

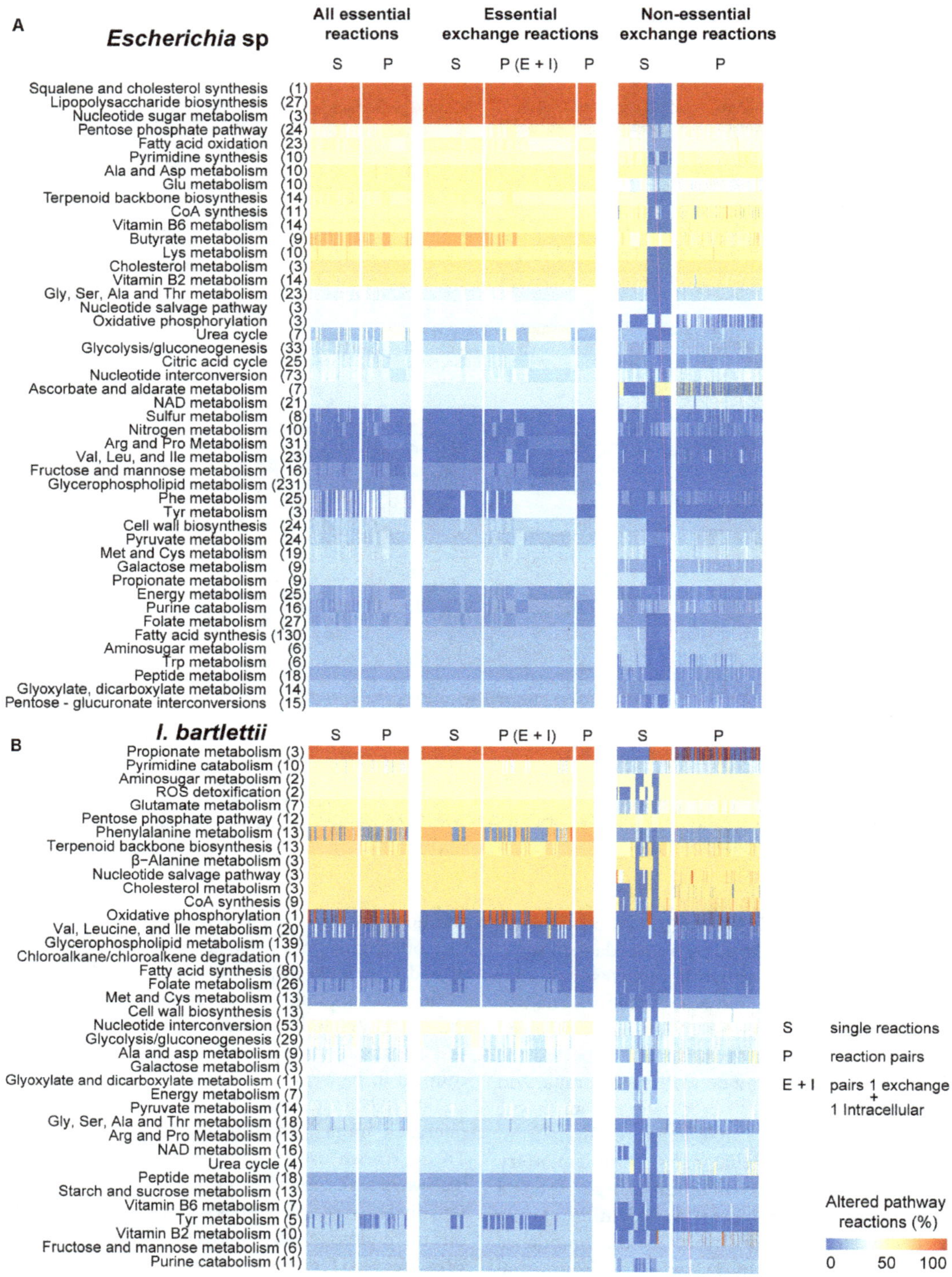

FIGURE 2 | Pathways of *Escherichia* sp. and *Intestinibacter bartlettii* show distinct vulnerability to environmental nutritional changes. Synthetic lethality analysis was performed in *Escherichia* sp. **(A)** and *I. bartlettii* **(B)** for blocking of single reactions or pairs of reactions belonging to the entire metabolic network ("All essential reactions"), for exchange reactions, or for non-essential exchange reactions and then we determined the fraction of pathway reactions altered (>1% change with respect to the reference model). For reaction pairs, we also considered pairs comprising 1 exchange reaction and 1 intracellular reaction. Columns have different number of blocked reactions, and only one pair of essential exchange reactions was found in each organism (see text). Columns leading to no pathway changes are not shown; for non-essential exchange reactions, only those in the top 30% inducing most pathway changes are shown. Amino acids are abbreviated by their common three-letter names. Total number of reactions in each pathway are presented in brackets. Due to the large number of possible combinations, only those pairs of non-essential exchange reactions that resulted in high pathway changes are shown (sum over all pathways >4).

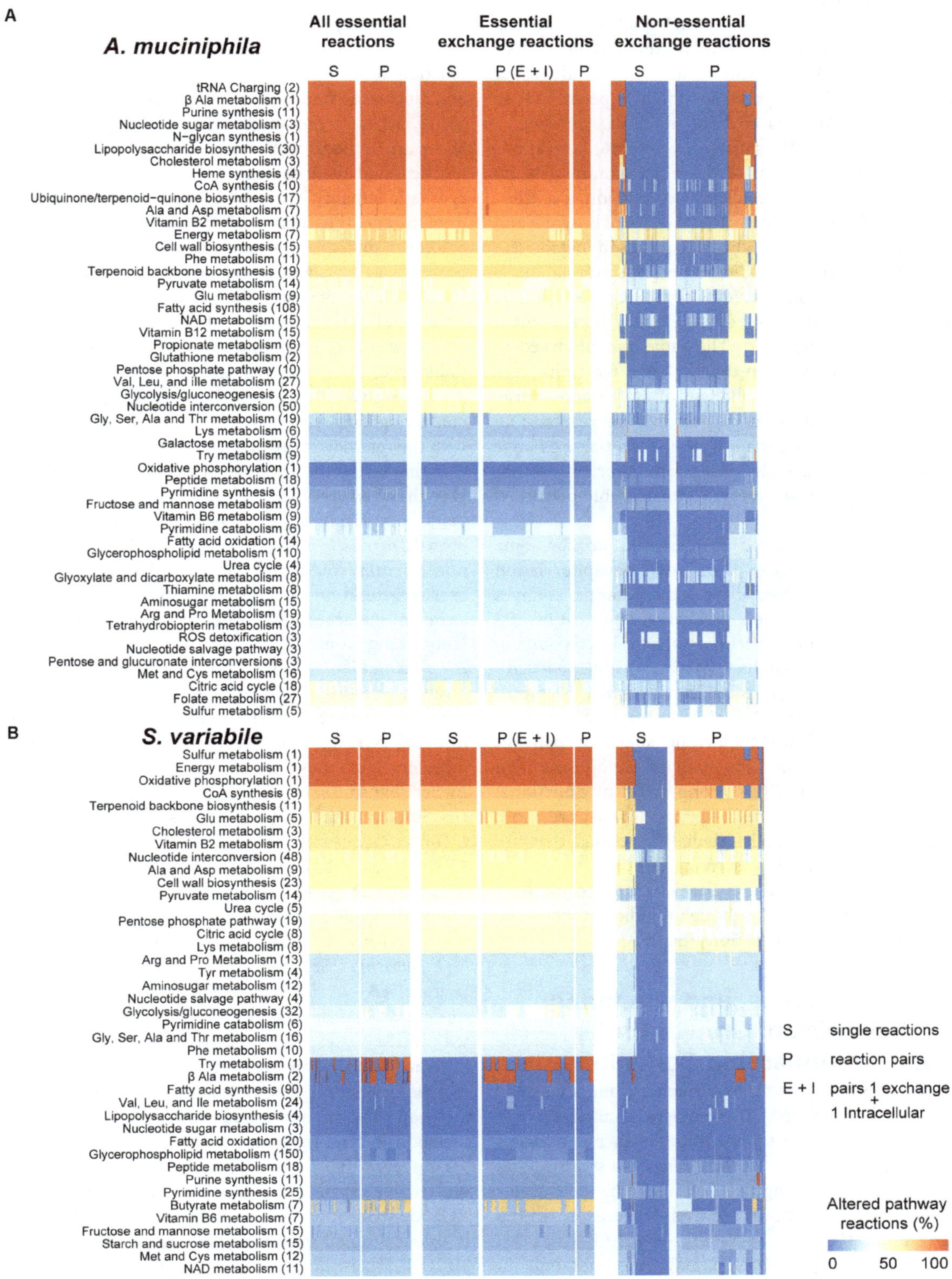

FIGURE 3 | Pathway susceptibility to environmental changes in *Akkermansia muciniphila* and *Subdoligranulum variabile*. Synthetic lethality analysis was performed in *A. muciniphila* **(A)** and *S. variabile* **(B)** similarly to **Figure 2**. Amino acids are abbreviated by their common three-letter names. Total number of reactions in each pathway are presented in brackets. Due to the large number of possible combinations, only those pairs of non-essential exchange reactions that resulted in high pathway changes are shown (sum over all pathways >4).

Akkermansia muciniphila showed the most significant cellular pathway alterations in response to essential reactions including N-glycan synthesis, exclusive to this bacteria (**Figure 3A**). Lipopolysaccharide (LPS) biosynthesis and nucleotide sugar metabolism were metabolic pathways highly perturbed in *A. muciniphila* and *Escherichia* sp., but not in *S. variabile. I. bartlettii* showed (**Figure 2B**) substantial (>50%) alterations in metabolism of propionate, phenylalanine, alanine but no change in chloroalkane and chloroalkene degradation, a species-exclusive metabolic pathway. In turn, metabolism of butyrate and vitamin B2 showed substantial (>50%) alterations in metabolism in *Escherichia* sp. (**Figure 2A**). Oxidative phosphorylation, a metabolic pathway found in the four organisms, was highly perturbed in *S. variabile* when any of its lethal or non-essential exchange reactions were inhibited. The same was observed in *I. bartlettii,* however mainly when double lethal reactions were blocked simultaneously. The metabolism of sulfur and energy were equally highly perturbed in *S. variabile* in response to inhibition of any of its essential or non-essential exchange reactions, while sulfur metabolism was poorly affected in other species and energy metabolism was only considerably perturbed in *A. muciniphila.*

While some of the pronounced changes exhibited by some pathways reflect their small size (e.g., oxidative phosphorylation with $\leq$3 reactions), other pathways showed substantial changes though they comprise more reactions. This is the case of LPS biosynthesis (27 reactions in *Escherichia* sp. and 30 reactions in *A. muciniphila*), butyrate metabolism (9 reactions in *I. bartlettii* and *Escherichia* sp.), or phenylalanine metabolism (25 and 10 reactions in *Escherichia* sp. and *S. variabile*). Importantly, these trends were also observed when blocking single or pairs of essential exchange reactions, and for many of the non-essential exchange reactions, indicating the strong effect of nutritional availability in these pathways. Metabolic pathways were more sensitive to inhibition of essential (lethal) reactions that are intracellular and environmentally exchanged, comparatively to non-essential exchange reactions in the four organisms. FVA showed qualitatively similar results, though it indicates that more pathways were sensitive to perturbations than FBA.

Tyrosine, Phenylalanine, and Vitamin B6 Permit *Escherich*ia sp. Growth Under Aerobic but Not Anaerobic Conditions

Bacteria present different growth requirements, and thus may present selective advantages and disadvantages. Among the four bacteria tested here, all are strict anaerobes with exception to *Escherichia* sp., a facultative aerobe. In *Escherichia* sp., blocking of oxygen and iron exchange together induces lethality (but not individually, since production of ferric iron depends on oxygen through the reaction $4H^{+} + O_2 + 4Fe^{2+} \rightarrow 2H_2O + 4Fe^{3+}$). We questioned if pathway utilization may differ not only in response to nutrients but also in response to oxygen availability (**Figure 4A**, top). Such differential nutritional responses may present an added selective advantage over anaerobic bacteria.

We investigated pathway response to oxygen availability in *Escherichia* sp., and determined the minimum growth requirements for the four organisms. We developed an approach complementary to those used above for assessing pathway sensitivity (**Figure 4A**, bottom). Briefly, from the entire metabolic reaction network, we selected those involving exchange reactions and blocked all non-essential single exchange reactions identified above, whereas the single-lethal exchange reactions identified above are unblocked. All non-lethal exchange reactions are firstly blocked, and then unblocked one by one, two by two, etc. The synthetic lethality approach employed above optimized for cell growth, and thus allowed for identification of those exchange reactions that most penalize cell growth and whose blocking prevents cell growth using otherwise unconstrained models. In turn, the approach used here optimizes flux distribution in a tightly constrained model and permits identifying those combinations of exchange reactions that, when simultaneously unblocked, promote cell growth. This additionally permits identifying those pathways showing the greatest changes while conferring the greatest increments to cell growth by comparison with the reference fully unconstrained model.

None of the four gut bacteria under study displayed cellular growth when unblocking any single exchange reaction. Only pairs comprising either oxygen or iron exchange resulted in growth for *Escherichia* sp. when combinations of two-by-two non-essential reactions were allowed. In combinations of three exchange reactions, oxygen and iron exchange is always present as one of the necessary reactions for growth (results not shown). Unblocking combinations of two non-essential reactions in *A. muciniphila* and *S. variabile* provided significant cellular growth. Notably, employing this approach yielded no growth in *I. bartlettii* using combinations of 1, 2, and even 3 unblocked non-essential exchange reactions (results not shown), suggesting that more nutrients must be available in order to permit growth. The *Escherichia* sp. model shows growth with as few as 12 exchange reactions (of which 10 are single-essential), whereas the model for *I. bartlettii* does not grow with 18 exchange reactions (including 15 single-essential). Additionally, *A. muciniphila* shows growth with only 23 exchange reactions (which includes 21 single-essential), while *S. variabile* shows growth with only 14 exchange reactions (of which 12 single-essential).

Escherichia sp. displays substantial pathway changes (**Figure 4B**) in LPS, squalene and cholesterol biosynthesis, nucleotide sugar metabolism (>90% pathway reactions with >1% fluxes under all assessed conditions), purine and butyrate metabolism (>74% reactions altered), as well as metabolism of histidine, tryptophan, valine, leucine, isoleucine, aspartate, alanine, and lysine (>70%). Glutathione and nitrogen metabolism tend to be mostly unchanged (<2%). Additionally, we observed that *Escherichia* sp. responds differently depending on oxygen availability. As expected from aerobic growth, ROS detoxification is significantly active when O_2 exchange is unconstrained versus no changes when Fe^{3+} is unblocked but O_2 exchange is blocked (respectively, >33 vs. 0%, compare **Figure 4B**, left with right). Slight increased fluxes are also identified under aerobic conditions in energy metabolism (mean pathway reaction changes >21% aerobic vs. 16% anaerobic), pentose phosphate pathway (57 vs. 50%), starch and sucrose metabolism (14 vs. 3%), and metabolism of

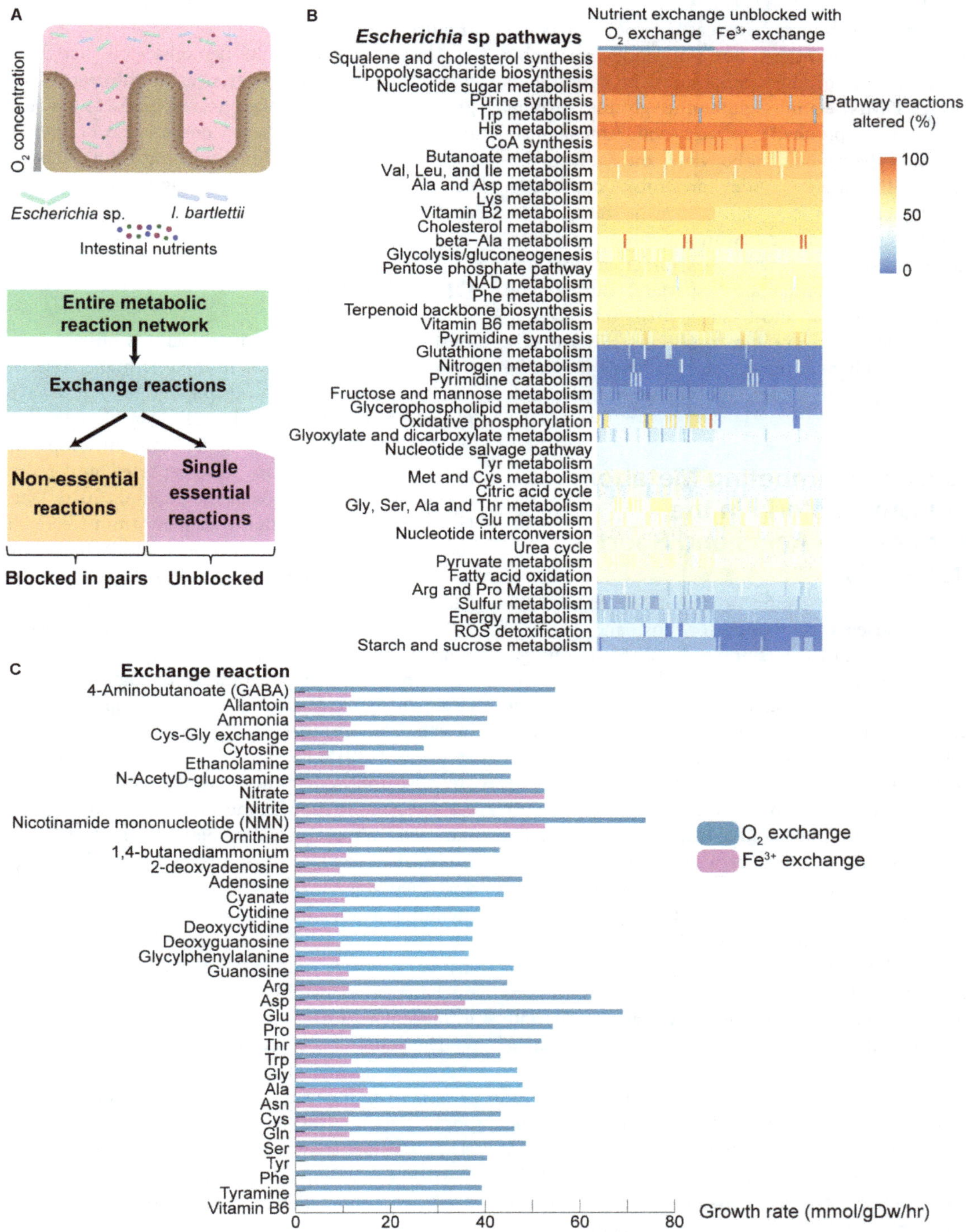

FIGURE 4 | Effect of availability of environmental nutrients on pathway responses and growth rates in *Escherichia* sp. under aerobic and anaerobic growth. **(A)** Due to their aerotolerance, the facultative *Escherichia* sp. may respond differently to environmental nutrients under aerobic versus anaerobic growth, which may provide a selective advantage with respect to the obligate anaerobe *I. bartlettii*. We employed a novel *in silico* approach where all single essential reactions are kept unblocked, and the non-essential exchange reactions (in **Figure 2**) are unblocked one-by-one and two-by-two. This approach may thus assist in identifying those combinations that confer the highest increments on cell growth, as well as determining which pathways most support this response. **(B)** *Escherichia* sp. pathway reactions that are altered (% from total) as response to availability of specific nutrients, together with oxygen or iron exchange (only pairs that either included oxygen or iron exchange resulted in growth). No growth is observed when unblocking single reactions for *Escherichia* sp., or in *I. bartlettii* for single, pairs, or triplets of reactions (results not show). Reactions were considered altered when their flux were altered >1% against the reference model. **(C)** Growth rates for *Escherichia* sp. achieved by unblocking exchange reactions together with O_2 exchange (i.e., aerobic conditions) or iron exchange (i.e., anaerobic conditions).

vitamins B6 (64 vs. 57%) and B2 (71 vs. 64%). Oxidative phosphorylation shows substantial increases (>66%) in some entries under aerobic conditions, but not under anaerobic conditions, when exchange of some compounds and amino acids is unblocked (e.g., NMN, alanine, glutamine, glycine, proline, serine, threonine, and tryptophan). In turn, sulfur metabolism (18 vs. 25%) and glyoxylate/dicarboxylate metabolism (29 vs. 35%) are slightly altered under anaerobic conditions. Practically all nutrients confer highest growth rates under aerobic than anaerobic conditions, with exception to nitrate exchange that elicits similar growth rates under aerobic and anaerobic growth. NMN, glutamate, aspartate, nitrate, and nitrite exchange confer the most substantial increases to growth under aerobic and anaerobic conditions (**Figure 4C**). Interestingly, tyrosine, phenylalanine, tyramine, and vitamin B6 uptake allow for cell growth under aerobic but not anaerobic conditions.

Commensal and Competing Metabolic Behavior of Gut Bacteria in the Utilization of Amino Acids and Short Chain Fatty Acids

We also determined how amino acids, short chain fatty acids, and other nutrients important for host and bacterial metabolism (Shoaie et al., 2013; Forslund et al., 2015; Mardinoglu et al., 2016) were produced or used by the four bacteria. To this extent, we aimed to determine for each metabolite its maximum growth-coupled uptake/secretion fluxes under maximal growth and minimal media conditions in anaerobiosis (**Supplementary Table S7**, see section "Materials and Methods"), since the human intestinal environment is predominantly anaerobic (Tremaroli and Bäckhed, 2012; Donaldson et al., 2015). We observed that the four organisms may contribute for the production of extracellular acetate, whereas all but *S. variabile* produced propionate. Predictions have shown butyrate production by *S. variabile.* In turn, *I. bartlettii* produced isobutyrate (**Figure 5A** and **Supplementary Table S8**), while both *Escherichia* sp. and *I. bartlettii* revealed to compete for ribose, deoxyribose and cysteinylglycine, as well as for aspartate and phosphate, which were both products of *S. variabile* (**Figure 5B**).

Potential commensal behavior may occur, since some of these compounds may be produced by *A. muciniphila* and *S. variabile* (e.g., threonine and glycine), while consumed by *Escherichia* sp. and *I. bartlettii.* Phenylalanine produced by the three other bacteria may be consumed by *I. bartlettii,* which in turn is predicted to secrete phenylacetate. Proline and glutamine were produced by *A. muciniphila, I. bartlettii* and *S. variabile* and consumed by *Escherichia* sp. Finally, *Escherichia* sp. was involved in the production of the gasses hydrogen and, together with *A. muciniphila,* both may produce hydrogen sulfide; whereas *I. bartlettii* produced methanethiol (**Figure 5C**). Because *Escherichia* sp. is a facultative aerobe we repeated these analyses under aerobic conditions, and observed some differences in comparison with the results under anaerobiosis, specifically in the secretion of amino acids (e.g., proline, glutamate, and threonine) and nucleobases (**Figure 5B**).

Altogether, our results demonstrated that the four bacteria displayed substantial differences in substrate requirements for growth, as well as metabolic responses to nutritional changes in the environment. As a consequence of their metabolisms, these four organisms differently contributed and competed for nutrients in the gut, which among those were short chain fatty acids, amino acids, and gasses.

DISCUSSION

Dysbiosis is one of the main features observed in metformin-treated T2D patients, where there is higher relative abundance of *Escherichia* spp., *A. muciniphila, S. variabile* but lower of *I. bartlettii* (Forslund et al., 2015; Mardinoglu et al., 2016; Wu et al., 2017). Moreover, larger concentrations of the SCFAs propionate and butyrate were reported under drug treatment (Forslund et al., 2015; Mardinoglu et al., 2016; Wu et al., 2017). However, the observation that metformin-treated T2D patients show a depletion in Firmicutes bacteria including *I. bartlettii* (Forslund et al., 2015; Wu et al., 2017), and that Firmicutes and Clostridia are major sources of butyrate (Tremaroli and Bäckhed, 2012; Shoaie et al., 2013, 2015), raises questions about the possible sources of SCFAs. Systems biology approaches have consistently been applied to clarify complex biological processes (Benfeitas et al., 2017; Lee et al., 2017, 2018; Uhlen et al., 2017) including in the relationship between host and gut microbiota (Shoaie et al., 2013, 2015; Forslund et al., 2015; Mardinoglu et al., 2015). Here, we used systems biology methodologies including genome-scale metabolic models and flux balance optimization to clarify the metabolic relationships between the prevalent gut bacteria *Escherichia* sp., *A. muciniphila, S. variabile,* and *I. bartlettii* and their contributions for extracellular pool of compounds including SCFAs and amino acids. Based on synthetic lethality, we also examined the influence of uptake reactions, which involve substrate exchange with the extracellular space, not only on bacterial growth rates but also on flux distribution across intracellular pathways.

The cumulative evidence presented here suggests that the shifts in microbiota diversity reported under metformin treatment and their resulting increase in butyrate and propionate pool (Forslund et al., 2015; Mardinoglu et al., 2016; Wu et al., 2017) may be due to an increased abundance of *S. variabile,* a butyrate-producing anaerobe (Louis and Flint, 2009). *A. muciniphila* may produce aminobutyrate, while *I. bartlettii* produces isobutyrate, a branched chain fatty acid that has been associated with increased risk of colon cancer (Shoaie et al., 2015). In turn, while the enzyme-coding genes involved in butyrate production are present in *Escherichia* sp., this compound is not produced by the wild-type bacterium but may be engineered to do so (Baek et al., 2013). It remains to test if other butyrate-producing bacteria (Forslund et al., 2015) show similar trends. Moreover, our modeling simulations indicate that *I. bartlettii, A. muciniphila,* and *Escherichia* sp. may contribute for the extracellular pool of propionate, of which *A. muciniphila*

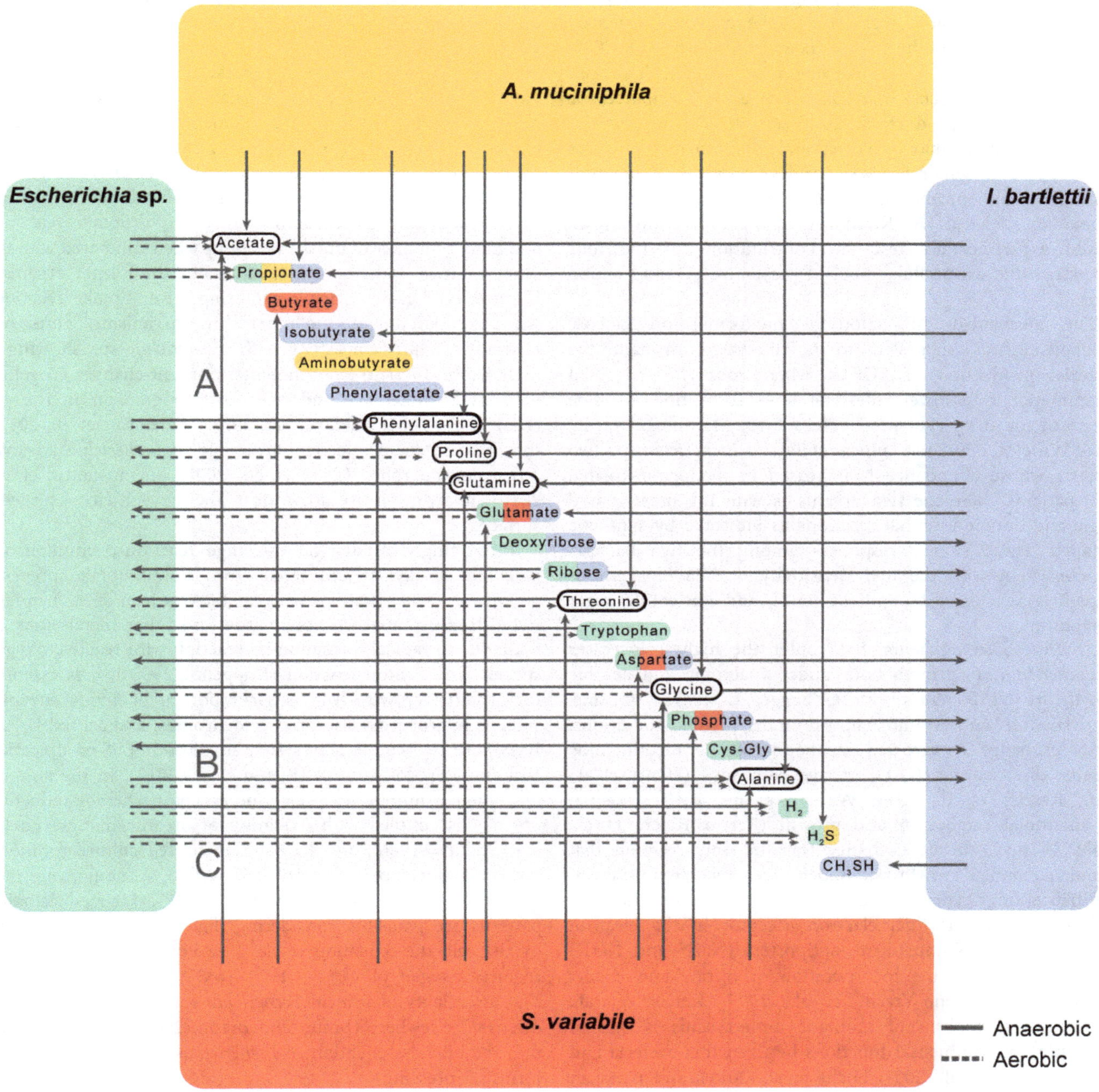

FIGURE 5 | Contribution and competition of the four bacteria for extracellular substrates including short chain fatty acids **(A)**, amino acids and nucleobases **(B)**, and gases **(C)**. Metabolic models for all organisms considered biomass maximization under minimal media anaerobic or aerobic conditions (respectively, solid and dashed arrows, see section "Materials and Methods" and **Supplementary Tables S7**, **S8**). Cys–Gly indicates Cysteinylglycine. Glutamine, deoxyribose, aspartate, and Cys–Gly show no flux under aerobic growth. Metabolite colors indicate the bacteria that influence its extracellular levels. For all bacteria we considered minimal medium conditions (see section "Materials and Methods") with exception to *A. muciniphila*, which additionally requires mucin to grow (de la Cuesta-Zuluaga et al., 2017).

had previously been observed to produce propionate (Derrien et al., 2004). These observations were associated with the major changing pathways in the four organisms. Propionate metabolism was the pathway displaying the highest responses to alterations in nutrient uptake in *I. bartlettii*, together with metabolism of phenylalanine. In turn, butyrate metabolism in *S. variabile* was perturbed depending on the inhibited reactions.

Bloating and intestinal discomfort are reported side-effects of metformin medication (Forslund et al., 2015), and gasses produced by gut microbiota enhance these adverse side effects

(Lewis and Cochrane, 2007; Jahng et al., 2012; Forslund et al., 2015). Colonic transit may be beneficially influenced by the production of hydrogen (Lewis and Cochrane, 2007; Jahng et al., 2012). Our observations show that hydrogen was produced by *Escherichia* sp., which also contributed for hydrogen sulfide production together with *A. muciniphila*. Hydrogen sulfide may have several beneficial effects for both host and gut microbes, displaying anti-inflammatory properties, and promoting smooth muscle relaxation and antioxidant defense (Al Khodor et al., 2017). Future work should experimentally test the contributions of the four bacteria to the extracellular pool of gasses, SCFAs, and amino acids.

The mechanism of action of metformin on glucose metabolism was suggested to be mediated through the bacterial production of SCFAs, where local LPS-triggered inflammation and lower intestinal lipid absorption are side effects of the drug (Forslund et al., 2015; Mardinoglu et al., 2016; Wu et al., 2017). *A. muciniphila* and *Escherichia* sp., two bacteria whose abundance is increased in metformin-treated T2D patients, were the two organisms with the most shared single and double essential reactions as indicated by synthetic lethality. These similar responses among the two bacteria are consistent with the high sensitivity of LPS biosynthesis (a pathway exclusive of both bacteria), and nucleotide sugar metabolism.

Among those nutrients that confer the highest increases to *Escherichia* sp. growth both under anaerobic and aerobic growth are NMN and nitrate exchange, as well as tyrosine, phenylalanine, and tyramine uptake under aerobic conditions. NMN exchange is involved in the coenzyme nicotinamide adenine dinucleotide (NAD) salvage pathway I (Henry et al., 2010; Keseler et al., 2013; Wattam et al., 2017) essential for microbial catabolism and growth (Berríos-Rivera et al., 2002). In turn, nitrate exchange was the only reaction that stimulated similar growth rate under alternative circumstances. Denitrification occurs as part of anaerobic respiration by replacing oxygen as final electron acceptor in the electron transport chain. Nitrate:nitrite antiporters (NarU and NarK) are responsible for the incorporation of nitrate and export of nitrogen (Moreno-Vivian et al., 1999; Keseler et al., 2013). The catabolism of aromatic amino acids is one of the important commensal functions between this bacteria and the host (Díaz et al., 2001; Fuchs et al., 2011), and plays an important role in microbial-mediated food digestion in the intestine (Donaldson et al., 2015; Shoaie et al., 2015). Our observations further suggest that potential commensal behavior may be displayed by *Escherichia* sp. and *I. bartlettii* under anaerobic growth, where on one hand the former produces phenylalanine required by the latter, and on the other hand *I. bartlettii* produces proline, glutamine, and glutamate that are uptaken by *Escherichia* sp. Moreover, phenylalanine, tryptophan, and threonine are essential amino acids which must be ingested by the host for nutritional availability, and which are part of the set minimal sufficient sources promoting cellular growth of *Escherichia* sp. Complementarily, arginine, cysteine, glutamine, glycine, proline, and tyrosine are conditionally non-essential amino acids as well as contributing as first line of sufficient sources for *Escherichia* sp. growth.

The dysbiosis induced by metformin treatment of T2D patients promotes nutritional imbalances (Forslund et al., 2015; Mardinoglu et al., 2016) that may impose fitness disadvantages for specific bacterial taxa. The alterations in relative abundance of *Escherichia* sp. was consistent with our observed growth organism requirements. *Escherichia* sp. is a facultative aerobe and displays a slightly lower number of *essential* uptake reactions and higher number of uptake reactions when compared with the other bacteria under study. Additionally, the former organism is capable of growing while requiring fewer uptake reactions when compared with the other three organisms. Thus, our observations are consistent with *Escherichia* sp. showing a higher robustness to environmental nutrient changes. Together with its aerotolerance and steep oxygen gradient in the gut (Díaz et al., 2001; Bueno et al., 2012; Donaldson et al., 2015), this may confer a selective advantage to *Escherichia* sp. over other gut microbes (Díaz et al., 2001; Magnusdottir et al., 2017), allowing it to grow near the oxygen-rich epithelial surface.

Interestingly, among all exchange reactions, simultaneous blocking of oxygen and ferric iron (Fe^{3+}) uptake prevents growth of *Escherichia* sp, whereas ferrous iron (Fe^{2+}) uptake is by itself essential. Although iron and other metals may be toxic due to radical formation by reaction with reactive oxygen species [i.e., Fenton reaction (Koppenol, 1993)], it is essential for bacterial growth. Iron is a component of hemic enzymes such as hydroperoxidases and cytochromes, and sensed by the BasS-BasR two-component system involved in LPS modification and anoxic redox control (Bueno et al., 2012). In the absence of oxygen, iron may act as electron acceptor whereby reduction of Fe^{3+} is coupled with oxidation of organic matter (Lovley and Phillips, 1986), and its addition to cell culture promotes growth under anoxia (Bueno et al., 2012). Although one may question whether the observed O_2/Fe^{3+}-associated lethality patterns are plausible considering that Fe^{2+} iron is uptaken by the cell, the oxidation of Fe^{2+} to Fe^{3+} by bacterioferritin requires oxygen ($4Fe^{2+} + 4H^+ + O_2 \rightarrow 4Fe^{3+} + 2H_2O$). The essentiality of iron in *Escherichia* sp. has been extensively discussed elsewhere (Braun and Braun, 2002), and is encoded into the biomass equation of *Escherichia* sp. where both redox forms are present.

Overall, our *in silico* observations suggest commensal and competing behavior in the production of extracellular compounds including short chain fatty acids and amino acids, among which the metabolism of *Escherichia* sp., *A. muciniphila*, *S. variabile,* and *I. bartlettii* may explain the observed features in metformin-treated type 2 diabetes patients. These observations remain to be experimentally tested, though the above observations indicate good agreement with previously known features of these organisms; multiple studies have shown that growth predictions by FBA and gene essentiality prediction are in good agreement with experimental observations (Edwards et al., 2001; Feist et al., 2007). Microbiota modulation approaches based on probiotics, prebiotics, and postbiotics are considered as potential therapies in type 2 diabetes patients. Thus, identification of intestinal bacteria playing a beneficial role or promoting adverse effects on glucose and fatty acids metabolism, will allow the identification of potential microbial targets to improve host metabolism.

AUTHOR CONTRIBUTIONS

AM conceived and supervised the study. DR, RB, GB, and CZ designed the experiments. DR performed the experiments. SS assisted in model acquisition and refining of the model. DR and RB analyzed the data and wrote the manuscript. All authors have revised and contributed to the final manuscript.

FUNDING

This work was funded by Knut and Alice Wallenberg Foundation and King's College London.

SUPPLEMENTARY MATERIAL

TABLE S1 | Organism and AGORA reconstruction details.

TABLE S2 | Single and double essential reactions in *Escherichia* sp. and *Intestinibacter bartlettii*.

TABLE S3 | Flux changes in reactive oxygen species (ROS) reactions of *I. bartlettii* under aerobic and anaerobic conditions.

TABLE S4 | Influence of oxygen exchange reaction on Synthetic Lethality Analysis of *I. bartlettii*.

TABLE S5 | Organism exclusive and shared cellular metabolic pathways.

TABLE S6 | Flux variability analysis for the four bacteria.

TABLE S7 | Short chain fatty acids and metabolite consumption (negative flux) and production (positive flux) under maximal growth and minimal media constraints.

TABLE S8 | Minimal media constraints applied on *Escherichia* sp. and *I. bartlettii* models.

REFERENCES

Agren, R., Liu, L., Shoaie, S., Vongsangnak, W., Nookaew, I., and Nielsen, J. (2013). The RAVEN toolbox and its use for generating a genome-scale metabolic model for *Penicillium chrysogenum*. *PLoS Comput. Biol.* 9:e1002980. doi: 10.1371/journal.pcbi.1002980

Al Khodor, S., Reichert, B., and Shatat, I. F. (2017). The microbiome and blood pressure: can microbes regulate our blood pressure? *Front. Pediatr.* 5:138. doi: 10.3389/fped.2017.00138

Baek, J. M., Mazumdar, S., Lee, S. W., Jung, M. Y., Lim, J. H., Seo, S. W., et al. (2013). Butyrate production in engineered *Escherichia coli* with synthetic scaffolds. *Biotechnol. Bioeng.* 110, 2790–2794. doi: 10.1002/bit.24925

Benfeitas, R., Uhlen, M., Nielsen, J., and Mardinoglu, A. (2017). New challenges to study heterogeneity in cancer redox metabolism. *Front. Cell Develop. Biol.* 5:65. doi: 10.3389/fcell.2017.00065

Berríos-Rivera, S. J., Bennett, G. N., and San, K.-Y. (2002). The effect of increasing NADH availability on the redistribution of metabolic fluxes in *Escherichia coli* chemostat cultures. *Metab. Eng.* 4, 230–237. doi: 10.1006/mben.2002.0228

Braun, V., and Braun, M. (2002). Iron transport and signaling in *Escherichia coli*. *FEBS Lett.* 529, 78–85.

Brillat-Savarin, A. (1826). You are what you eat. *Physiol. Gout* 32, 243–245. doi: 10.1002/cind.786-16.x

Bueno, E., Mesa, S., Bedmar, E. J., Richardson, D. J., and Delgado, M. J. (2012). Bacterial adaptation of respiration from oxic to microoxic and anoxic conditions: redox control. *Antioxid. Redox Signal.* 16, 819–852. doi: 10.1089/ars.2011.4051

de la Cuesta-Zuluaga, J., Mueller, N. T., Corrales-Agudelo, V., Velasquez-Mejia, E. P., Carmona, J. A., Abad, J. M., et al. (2017). Metformin is associated with higher relative abundance of mucin-degrading *Akkermansia muciniphila* and several short-chain fatty acid-producing microbiota in the gut. *Diabetes Care* 40, 54–62. doi: 10.2337/dc16-1324

Derrien, M., Vaughan, E. E., Plugge, C. M., and De Vos, W. M. (2004). *Akkermansia muciniphila* gen. nov., sp. nov., a human intestinal mucin-degrading bacterium. *Int. J. Syst. Evol. Microbiol.* 54, 1469–1476. doi: 10.1099/ijs.0.02873-0

Díaz, E., Ferrández, A., Prieto, M. A., and García, J. L. (2001). Biodegradation of aromatic compounds by *Escherichia coli*. *Microbiol. Mol. Biol. Rev.* 65, 523–569. doi: 10.1128/MMBR.65.4.523

Donaldson, G. P., Lee, S. M., and Mazmanian, S. K. (2015). Gut biogeography of the bacterial microbiota. *Nat. Rev. Microbiol.* 14, 20–32. doi: 10.1038/nrmicro3552

Edwards, J. S., Ibarra, R. U., and Palsson, B. O. (2001). *In silico* predictions of *Escherichia coli* metabolic capabilities are consistent with experimental data. *Nat. Biotechnol.* 19, 125–130. doi: 10.1038/84379

Eker, S., Krummenacker, M., Shearer, A. G., Tiwari, A., Keseler, I. M., Talcott, C., et al. (2013). Computing minimal nutrient sets from metabolic networks via linear constraint solving. *BMC Bioinformatics* 14:114. doi: 10.1186/1471-2105-14-114

Feist, A. M., Henry, C. S., Reed, J. L., Krummenacker, M., Joyce, A. R., Karp, P. D., et al. (2007). A genome-scale metabolic reconstruction for *Escherichia coli* K-12 MG1655 that accounts for 1260 ORFs and thermodynamic information. *Mol. Syst. Biol.* 3:121. doi: 10.1038/msb4100155

Forslund, K., Hildebrand, F., Nielsen, T., Falony, G., Le Chatelier, E., Sunagawa, S., et al. (2015). Disentangling type 2 diabetes and metformin treatment signatures in the human gut microbiota. *Nature* 528, 262–266. doi: 10.1038/nature15766

Fuchs, G., Boll, M., and Heider, J. (2011). Microbial degradation of aromatic compounds — from one strategy to four. *Nat. Rev. Microbiol.* 9, 803–816. doi: 10.1038/nrmicro2652

Henry, C. S., Dejongh, M., Best, A. A., Frybarger, P. M., Linsay, B., and Stevens, R. L. (2010). High-throughput generation, optimization and analysis of genome-scale metabolic models. *Nat. Biotechnol.* 28, 977–982. doi: 10.1038/nbt.1672

Hyotylainen, T., Jerby, L., Petaja, E. M., Mattila, I., Jantti, S., Auvinen, P., et al. (2016). Genome-scale study reveals reduced metabolic adaptability in patients with non-alcoholic fatty liver disease. *Nat. Commun.* 7:8994. doi: 10.1038/ncomms9994

Imielinski, M., Belta, C., Rubin, H., and Halasz, A. (2006). Systematic analysis of conservation relations in *Escherichia coli* genome-scale metabolic network reveals novel growth media. *Biophys. J.* 90, 2659–2672. doi: 10.1529/biophysj.105.069278

Jahng, J., Jung, I. S., Choi, E. J., Conklin, J. L., and Park, H. (2012). The effects of methane and hydrogen gases produced by enteric bacteria on ileal motility and colonic transit time. *Neurogastroenterol. Motil.* 24, 185–191. doi: 10.1111/j.1365-2982.2011.01819.x

Ji, B., and Nielsen, J. (2015). From next-generation sequencing to systematic modeling of the gut microbiome. *Front. Genet.* 6:219. doi: 10.3389/fgene.2015.00219

Kaelin, W. G. Jr. (2005). The concept of synthetic lethality in the context of anticancer therapy. *Nat. Rev. Cancer* 5, 689–698. doi: 10.1038/nrc1691

Karlsson, F. H., Tremaroli, V., Nookaew, I., Bergstrom, G., Behre, C. J., Fagerberg, B., et al. (2013). Gut metagenome in European women with normal, impaired and diabetic glucose control. *Nature* 498, 99–103. doi: 10.1038/nature12198

Keseler, I. M., Mackie, A., Peralta-Gil, M., Santos-Zavaleta, A., Gama-Castro, S., Bonavides-Martínez, C., et al. (2013). EcoCyc: fusing model organism databases with systems biology. *Nucleic Acids Res.* 41, 605–612. doi: 10.1093/nar/gks1027

Koppenol, W. H. (1993). The centennial of the Fenton reaction. *Free Radic. Biol. Med.* 15, 645–651.

Lee, S., Zhang, C., Arif, M., Liu, Z., Benfeitas, R., Bidkhori, G., et al. (2018). TCSBN: a database of tissue and cancer specific biological networks. *Nucleic Acids Res.* 46, D595–D600. doi: 10.1093/nar/gkx994

Lee, S., Zhang, C., Liu, Z., Klevstig, M., Mukhopadhyay, B., Bergentall, M., et al. (2017). Network analyses identify liver-specific targets for treating liver diseases. *Mol. Syst. Biol.* 13:938. doi: 10.15252/msb.20177703

Lewis, S., and Cochrane, S. (2007). Alteration of sulfate and hydrogen metabolism in the human colon by changing intestinal transit rate. *Am. J. Gastroenterol.* 102, 624–633. doi: 10.1111/j.1572-0241.2006.01020.x

Louis, P., and Flint, H. J. (2009). Diversity, metabolism and microbial ecology of butyrate-producing bacteria from the human large intestine. *FEMS Microbiol. Lett.* 294, 1–8. doi: 10.1111/j.1574-6968.2009.01514.x

Lovley, D. R., and Phillips, E. J. (1986). Organic matter mineralization with reduction of ferric iron in anaerobic sediments. *Appl. Environ. Microbiol.* 51, 683–689.

Magnusdottir, S., Heinken, A., Kutt, L., Ravcheev, D. A., Bauer, E., Noronha, A., et al. (2017). Generation of genome-scale metabolic reconstructions for 773 members of the human gut microbiota. *Nat. Biotechnol.* 35, 81–89. doi: 10.1038/nbt.3703

Mardinoglu, A., Boren, J., and Smith, U. (2016). Confounding effects of metformin on the human gut microbiome in type 2 diabetes. *Cell Metab.* 23, 10–12. doi: 10.1016/j.cmet.2015.12.012

Mardinoglu, A., Boren, J., Smith, U., Uhlen, M., and Nielsen, J. (2018). Systems biology in hepatology: approaches and applications. *Nat. Rev. Gastroenterol. Hepatol.* 15, 365–377. doi: 10.1038/s41575-018-0007-8

Mardinoglu, A., and Nielsen, J. (2012). Systems medicine and metabolic modelling. *J. Intern. Med.* 271, 142–154. doi: 10.1111/j.1365-2796.2011.02493.x

Mardinoglu, A., Shoaie, S., Bergentall, M., Ghaffari, P., Zhang, C., Larsson, E., et al. (2015). The gut microbiota modulates host amino acid and glutathione metabolism in mice. *Mol. Syst. Biol.* 11:834. doi: 10.15252/msb.20156487

Moreno-Vivian, C., Cabello, P., Martinez-Luque, M., Blasco, R., and Castillo, F. (1999). Prokaryotic nitrate reduction: molecular properties and functional distinction among bacterial nitrate reductases. *J. Bacteriol.* 181, 6573–6584.

O'Neil, N. J., Bailey, M. L., and Hieter, P. (2017). Synthetic lethality and cancer. *Nat. Rev. Genet.* 18, 613–623. doi: 10.1038/nrg.2017.47

Pratapa, A., Balachandran, S., and Raman, K. (2015). Fast-SL: an efficient algorithm to identify synthetic lethal sets in metabolic networks. *Bioinformatics* 31, 3299–3305. doi: 10.1093/bioinformatics/btv352

Qin, J., Li, Y., Cai, Z., Li, S., Zhu, J., Zhang, F., et al. (2012). A metagenome-wide association study of gut microbiota in type 2 diabetes. *Nature* 490, 55–60. doi: 10.1038/nature11450

Schellenberger, J., Thiele, I., and Orth, J. D. (2012). Quantitative prediction of cellular metabolism with constraint-based models. *Nat. Prot.* 6, 1290–1307. doi: 10.1038/nprot.2011.308

Shoaie, S., Ghaffari, P., Kovatcheva-Datchary, P., Mardinoglu, A., Sen, P., Pujos-Guillot, E., et al. (2015). Quantifying diet-induced metabolic changes of the human gut microbiome. *Cell Metab.* 22, 320–331. doi: 10.1016/j.cmet.2015.07.001

Shoaie, S., Karlsson, F., Mardinoglu, A., Nookaew, I., Bordel, S., and Nielsen, J. (2013). Understanding the interactions between bacteria in the human gut through metabolic modeling. *Sci. Rep.* 3:2532. doi: 10.1038/srep02532

Tremaroli, V., and Bäckhed, F. (2012). Functional interactions between the gut microbiota and host metabolism. *Nature* 489, 242–249. doi: 10.1038/nature11552

Turanli, B., Grøötli, M., Borén, J., Nielsen, J., Uhlen, M., Arga, K. Y., et al. (2018). Drug repositioning for effective prostate cancer treatment. *Front. Physiol.* 9:500. doi: 10.3389/fphys.2018.00500

Uhlen, M., Zhang, C., Lee, S., Sjostedt, E., Fagerberg, L., Bidkhori, G., et al. (2017). A pathology atlas of the human cancer transcriptome. *Science* 357:eaan2507. doi: 10.1126/science.aan2507

Varemo, L., Scheele, C., Broholm, C., Mardinoglu, A., Kampf, C., Asplund, A., et al. (2015). Proteome- and transcriptome-driven reconstruction of the human myocyte metabolic network and its use for identification of markers for diabetes. *Cell Rep.* 11, 921–933. doi: 10.1016/j.celrep.2015.04.010

Wattam, A. R., Davis, J. J., Assaf, R., Boisvert, S., Brettin, T., Bun, C., et al. (2017). Improvements to PATRIC, the all-bacterial bioinformatics database and analysis resource center. *Nucleic Acids Res.* 45, D535–D542. doi: 10.1093/nar/gkw1017

Wu, H., Esteve, E., Tremaroli, V., Khan, M. T., Caesar, R., Mannerås-Holm, L., et al. (2017). Metformin alters the gut microbiome of individuals with treatment-naive type 2 diabetes, contributing to the therapeutic effects of the drug. *Nat. Med.* 23, 850–858. doi: 10.1038/nm.4345

Zhang, C., and Hua, Q. (2016). Applications of genome-scale metabolic models in biotechnology and systems medicine. *Front. Physiol.* 6:413. doi: 10.3389/fphys.2015.00413

12

Analysis of Genes Involved in Ulcerative Colitis Activity and Tumorigenesis Through Systematic Mining of Gene Co-expression Networks

Wanting Shi[1,2†], Rongjun Zou[3†], Minglei Yang[4†], Lei Mai[1], Jiangnan Ren[2], Jialing Wen[5,6], Zhaoshi Liu[1,2] and Renxu Lai[1,2]*

[1] Department of Gastroenterology, Fifth Affiliated Hospital, Sun Yat-sen University, Zhuhai, China, [2] Digestive Endoscopy Center, Fifth Affiliated Hospital, Sun Yat-sen University, Zhuhai, China, [3] Department of Cardiovascular Surgery, Sun Yat-sen Memorial Hospital, Sun Yat-sen University, Guangzhou, China, [4] Department of Genetics, Zhongshan School of Medicine, Sun Yat-sen University, Guangzhou, China, [5] Guangdong Institute of Gastroenterology, Guangdong, China, [6] Guangdong Provincial Key Laboratory of Colorectal and Pelvic Floor Diseases, The Sixth Affiliated Hospital, Sun Yat-sen University, Guangzhou, China

***Correspondence:**
Renxu Lai
lairenxu@mail.sysu.edu.cn*

† These authors have contributed equally to this work

Ulcerative colitis (UC) is an idiopathic, chronic inflammatory disorder of the colon, characterized by continuous mucosal inflammation. Recently, some studies have considered it as part of an inflammatory bowel disease-based global network. Herein, with the aim of identifying the underlying potential genetic mechanisms involved in the development of UC, multiple algorithms for weighted correlation network analysis (WGCNA), principal component analysis (PCA), and linear models for microarray data algorithm (LIMMA) were used to identify the hub genes. The map of platelet activation, ligand-receptor interaction, calcium signaling pathway, and cAMP signaling pathway showed significant links with UC development, and the hub genes *CCR7*, *CXCL10*, *CXCL9*, *IDO1*, *MMP9*, and *VCAM1*, which are associated with immune dysregulation and tumorigenesis in biological function, were found by multiple powerful bioinformatics methods. Analysis of The Cancer Genome Atlas (TCGA) also showed that the low expression of *CCR7*, *CXCL10*, *CXCL9*, and *MMP9* may be correlated with a poor prognosis of overall survival (OS) in colorectal cancer (CRC) patients (all $p < 0.05$), while no significance detected in both of *IDO1* and *VCAM1*. In addition, low expression of *CCR7*, *CXCL10*, *CXCL9*, *MMP9*, and *IDO1* may be associated with a poor prognosis in recurrence free survival (RFS) time (all $p < 0.05$), but no significant difference was identified in *VCAM1*. Moreover, the *NFKB1*, *FLI1*, and *STAT1* with the highest enrichment score were detected as the master regulators of hub genes. In summary, these results indicated the central role of the hub genes of *CCR7*, *CXCL10*, *CXCL9*, *IDO1*, *VCAM1*, and *MMP9*, in response to UC progression, as well as the development of UC to CRC, thus shedding light on the molecular mechanisms involved and assisting with drug target validation.

Keywords: ulcerative colitis, colorectal cancer, pathway enrichment, molecular mechanism, bioinformatics analysis

INTRODUCTION

Ulcerative colitis (UC) is a global, progressive and complex disease, the incidence of which is still growing, according to large-scale epidemiological statistics studies (Ng et al., 2018). Epidemiological reports shows that the highest annual incidence of UC was 24.3 per 100,000 person-years in Europe, 6.3 per 100,000 person-years in Asia and the Middle East, and 19.2 per 100,000 person-years in North America; and adjusted prevalences have exceeded 0.3% in many countries, especially in Europe and North America (Molodecky et al., 2012; Ng et al., 2018). A further concern is that the incidence of UC and the widespread use of therapeutic agents are associated with an increased risk of cancer (Biancone et al., 2015). Regarding the pathogenesis of UC, most of the emerging evidence supports the concept of an "inflammatory bowel disease (IBD) interactome," that is, UC is considered as part of a global disease network, with a complex interplay between host genetics, immunity, and environmental factors (Dabritz and Menheniott, 2014). According to this model, gene–environment interactions have pivotal roles in UC progression and mediate UC-related comorbidities and complications, including colitis-associated cancer (Dabritz and Menheniott, 2014). In the past two decades, novel genotyping and sequencing technologies, including RNA expression profiling, DNA methylation profiling, single-cell DNA analysis, chromatin immunoprecipitation sequencing, and RNA sequencing, have launched the era of genetic diseases; so far, 242 susceptibility loci and over 50 hub genes have been discovered in relation to IBD and various phenotypes (Mirkov et al., 2017). Moon et al. performed deep resequencing of UC-associated genes, showing that genetic variants of rs10035653 in *C5orf55*, rs41417449 in *BTNL2*, rs3117099 in *HCG23*, rs7192 in *HLA-DRA*, rs3744246 in *ORMDL3*, and rs713669 in *IL17REL* were significant (Moon et al., 2018). Hong et al. (2018) performed a *trans*-ethnic meta-analysis based on Asian IBD patients and subsequently identified three novel susceptibility loci at *MYO10-BASP1*, *PPP2R3C/KIAA0391/PSMA6/NFKB1A*, and *LRRK1*; as well as four previously known loci at *NCF4*, *TSPAN32*, *CIITA*, and *VANGL2*. Similarly, Peters et al. (2017) presented a predictive model of immune-related genes and further analyzed the functional and regulatory annotations based on genome-wide association studies. Consequently, a driver set including *DOCK2*, *GPSM3*, *AIF1*, *NCKAP1L*, and *DOK3* was selected, representing a high predictive efficiency in the integrated circuits of genetics, molecular, and clinical traits of IBD (Peters et al., 2017). The candidate biomarkers identification of UC activity and tumorigenesis in prior studies were presented in **Table 1**.

TABLE 1 | The candidate biomarkers identification of ulcerative colitis activity and tumorigenesis in prior studies.

Terms	Investigator	Candidate biomarker
UC activity	Moon et al., 2018	C5orf55, BTNL2, HCG23, and HLA-DRA, et al.
	Hong et al., 2018	MYO10-BASP1, PPP2R3C, KIAA0391, and PSMA6, et al.
	Wu et al., 2014	VCAM1, IL6, IL18, ICAM1, and TNFα
	McNamee et al., 2015	CCR7
	Ciorba et al., 2010	IDO1, STAT1, TLR9, and CD11
UC-associated cancer	Zhang et al., 2017	TNFα, IL1β, IFNγ, IL6, IL17a, IL23a, IL4, and IL12a
	Liu et al., 2014	IL1β, IL6, TNFα, NFκB, and STAT3
	Shukla et al., 2016	CXCL9, CXCL10, CCL5, IL1α, IL6, and TNFα
	Pujada et al., 2017	MMP9 and S100A8
	Thaker et al., 2013	IDO1 and IFNγ
	Xu et al., 2018	CCR7, CCL19 and CD31

In summary, these novels genotyping and sequencing technologies and validated hub gene or susceptibility loci not only confer new regulators of pathophysiology, but also open a new horizon to find drug targets and redefine the disease's regulatory framework. However, these genetic variants combined only explain one in four cases of UC (Uhlig and Muise, 2017). The results also suggest that: (1) The genetic variants considered as personal pathogenic components cannot be isolated in the gene-environment network; (2) These hub genes show better statistical significance while loss of the functional and regulatory annotations or may play an important part in protein-protein interaction (PPI) networks without statistical power; (3) some of the hub gene information may have been missed, owing to low abundance or small fold change (FC); and (4) disease-based co-expression network analysis may further improve the mining efficiency beyond classical methods (Uhlig and Muise, 2017). Based on the above notes, we may apply linear models for microarray data power differential expression analyses (LIMMA), weighted correlation network analysis (WGCNA), and principal component analysis (PCA) to explore the hub gene regulatory network, using high-throughput gene expression arrays in UC, to further elucidate the molecular mechanisms of gene–environment interactions.

MATERIALS AND METHODS

Materials

Raw expression microarray array (CEL data) from the GSE13367, GSE38713, GSE16879, GSE48958, GSE75214, GSE4183, GSE37283, and GSE31106 datasets were downloaded from Gene Expression Omnibus[1] (Barrett et al., 2013). Probe annotations and platform information were generated by matching with the GPL6244 (HuGene-1_0-st) Affymetrix Human Gene 1.0 ST Array (Affymetrix, Santa Clara, CA, United States).

In this study, we analyzed the patients with colitis exclusively, no other IBD cases included. Here, GSE48958 and GSE75214 are matching with the GPL6244 (HuGene-1_0-st) Affymetrix Human Gene 1.0 ST Array, while GSE13367, GSE38713, GSE16879, GSE37283, and GSE4183 are pairing with the GPL570 (HG-U133_Plus_2) Affymetrix Human Genome U133 Plus 2.0 Array and the GSE31106 is in line with GPL1261 (Mouse430_2) Affymetrix Mouse Genome 430 2.0 Array. Total RNA extracted from mucosal biopsies was used to analyze mRNA expression via Affymetrix arrays, and corresponding grouping

[1] http://ncbi.nlm.nih.gov/geo/

information from each sample was subsequently pooled for further correlation analysis. Statistical analysis was performed with the R (version 3.3.2).

Data Processing

To remove bias and variability (resulting from heterogeneity and latent variables) from the high-throughput data for the different microarrays, the "ComBat" function in the SVA package was used to directly adjust the batch effects and latent variables (Leek et al., 2012). Subsequently, all of the microarray raw data analyzed using bioinformatics methods, including background correction, quantile normalization, and probe summarization of the expression values (Irizarry et al., 2003; Ritchie et al., 2015). Some advanced algorithms were used, including: (1) robust multi-array average for background-adjusted, normalized, and log-transformed probe expression values; (2) k-nearest-neighbor for displacing missing values of probes; (3) the *t*-test in the "LIMMA" package to identify differentially expressed genes (DEGs) in mucosal biopsy specimens from the comparative analysis among normal, UC, adenoma, and colorectal cancer (CRC) for GSE4183; and (4) the Benjamini–Hochberg method to adjust *p*-values and thus calculate the false discovery rate and FC (Irizarry et al., 2003; Ritchie et al., 2015). Gene expression values with $|\log_2 FC| > 1.5$ and adjusted p-value < 0.05 were used to define DEGs. The co-annotated genes (a total of 16,653 genes) between GPL570 and GPL6244 platform were selected for further co-expression network analysis. The analysis strategy is presented in **Figure 1**.

Weighted Co-expression Network Construction and Module Detection

The advantages of co-expression network analysis include the ability to integrate external information and avoid information loss in the case of low-abundance or small-FC genes. Systems-level insight gives WGCNA an edge over other approaches (Langfelder and Horvath, 2008). Therefore, we carried out a systems-level analysis based on WGCNA. The analysis involved the following processes: (1) identifying the appropriate sample basing on the flash-Clust method; (2) selecting a "soft" threshold using the scale-free topology criterion; (3) identifying co-expression modules by employed the dynamic hybrid cut method; (4) relating the co-expression modules to sample traits based on the gene significance (GS) measures, which are defined as the statistical significance of the difference between the gene profile and the sample trait; and (5) accessing the interactions and connectivity of eigengenes among different co-expression modules by the topological overlap matrix method (Langfelder and Horvath, 2008).

PPI Networks and Functional Enrichment Analysis

We accessed gene biological knowledge, protein functional associations, and PPIs with respect to genetic function, using a web-based analytic tool. The analysis flowchart as flowing that: (1) the gene ontology (GO) functions enrichment was extracted from the DAVID database[2] (Huang et al., 2007) for annotation, visualization, and integrated discovery bioinformatics resources; GO terms for which $p < 0.05$ were considered to be significantly enriched in the gene modules of interest; and (2) the network of Kyoto Encyclopedia of Genes and Genomes (KEGG) pathway was identified form Metascape database[3] (Zhou et al., 2019), and $p < 0.05$ and enrichment score > 1.0 was set as the cut-off criteria; (3) after carried out for the genes enriched in KEGG pathway of immunity, inflammation and tumorigenesis for the interesting gene modules, we subsequently constructed the PPI biological networks based on the STRING online database (V10.5[4]) with the nodes association confidence score > 0.4 (Szklarczyk et al., 2017). In addition, the Cytoscape software (V3.5.1[5]) was used to visualize and evaluate interactions and identifying the hub gene in functional networks (Szklarczyk et al., 2017). The top 10 highest-degree nodes were defined as functional hub genes in the PPI network.

Identification of Candidate Biomarkers Involving in UC-Associated Carcinogenesis

Additionally, raw data of GSE4183 was used to analysis the co-DEGs involved in UC, adenoma, and CRC. Here, we overlapped the co-DEGs and the PPI network's functional hub genes, which constructed by WGCNA key modules and identified as important parts in response to the pathway of UC immunity-inflammation and tumorigenesis, to detect the UC-associated carcinogenesis in hub genes. Additionally, the suitable dataset of GSE37283, including the expression profiling of UC with neoplasia, UC and normal mucosa samples, was used to validate the UC-associated carcinogenesis biomarkers; as well as the mouse dataset of GSE31106 involved in the multistep process of "inflammation-dysplasia-cancer." The human and mouse genes were matched by Gene database[6] (Brown et al., 2015).

The Cancer Genome Atlas (TCGA) colon adenocarcinoma normalized gene expression value (fragments per kilobase of exon model per million reads mapped, FPKM) were downloaded from the "TCGA biolinks" package (Colaprico et al., 2016). Subsequently, the FPKM data transformed into transcripts per kilobase million (TPM; Li et al., 2010), a comparable data type, which used to apply the survival analysis. The sample and corresponding clinical features were included in further survival and DEGs analysis.

Investigating the Functional Role and Transcription Factor of Hub Genes

Importantly, the DAVID[7] and Metascape database were used to explore the GO terms and KEGG pathway enrichment analysis of candidate targets, respectively. The enrichment cut-off criteria

[2]http://david.abcc.ncifcrf.gov/
[3]http://metascape.org/
[4]http://string-db.org/
[5]http://cytoscape.org/
[6]https://www.ncbi.nlm.nih.gov/gene/
[7]http://david.abcc.ncifcrf.gov/

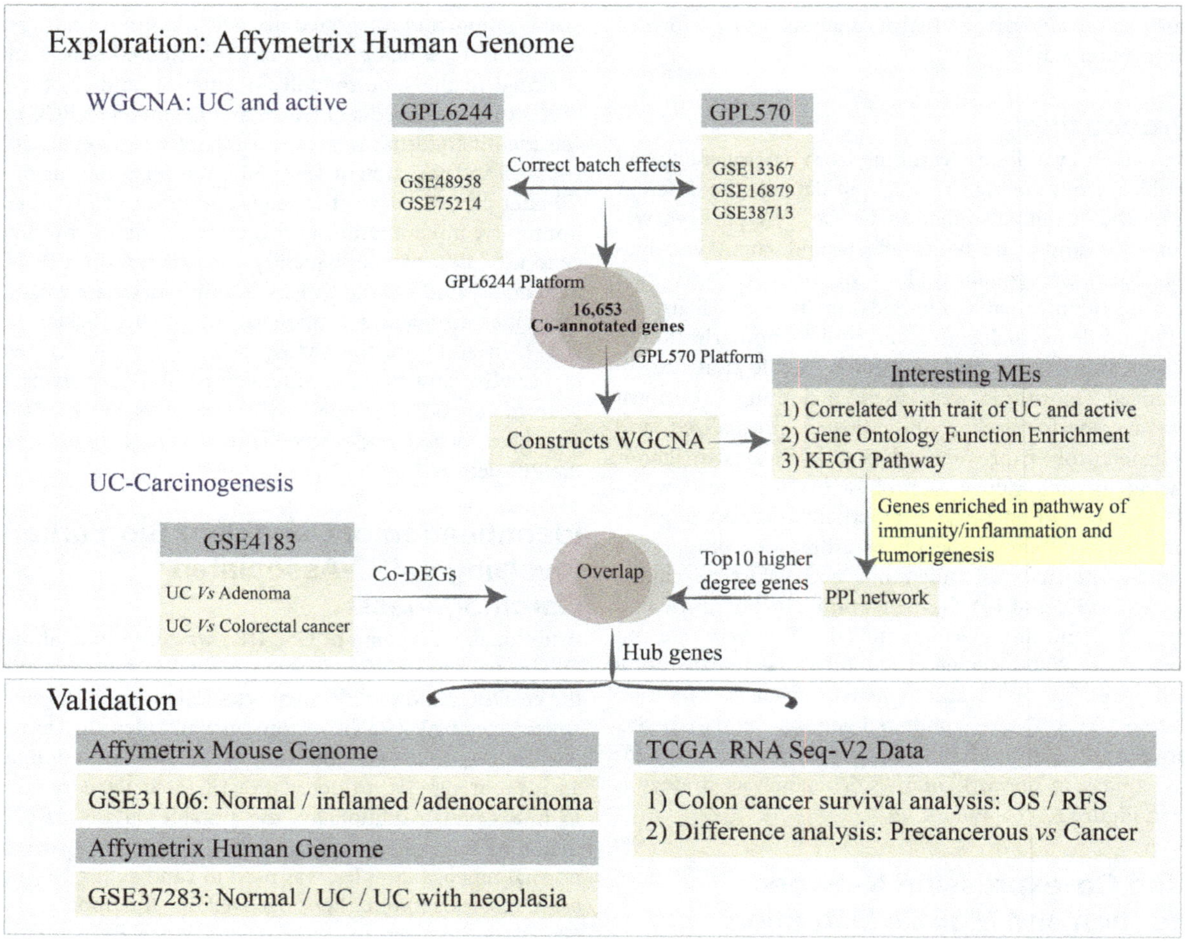

FIGURE 1 | Strategy used for the integrative gene microarray bioinformatics analyses.

keep the same with the chapter and Section "PPI Networks and Functional Enrichment Analysis." Subsequently, to identify the transcription factor (TF) of the hub genes, the plug in iRegulon for Cytoscape software was applied, with the parameters were set to: (1) minimum identity between orthologous genes = 0.05; (2) maximum FDR for motif similarity = 0.001; and (3) normalized enrichment score (NES) $\geq$ 3.0 (Janky et al., 2014). Here, the top three regulators with the highest NES value were detected to construct the regulatory network involved in UC-associated carcinogenesis process.

RESULTS

Data Processing

The normal and UC mucosa without additional treatment from GPL6244 (GSE48958 and GSE75214) and GPL570 (GSE13367, GSE38713, and GSE16879) platform were selected in their entirety for further analysis, including the 58 normal, 55 UC inactive and 170 UC active samples (**Supplementary Table S1**). After merging the co-annotated genes, 16,653 genes were retained in further analysis (**Figure 2A** and **Supplementary Table S1**). The PCA of co-annotated genes in response to pre- and post-correct the batch effects were showing in **Figure 2B**, which presenting a significant distinction between control, UC inactive and UC active samples.

Construction of Co-expression Network and Gene Modules

After sample cluster analysis, the 283 samples with 16,653 gene variables were divided into 13 clusters (MEblack, MEblue, MEbrown, MEgreen, MEgreenyellow, MEgrey, MEmagenta, MEpink, MEpurple, MEred, MEtan, MEturquoise, and MEyellow; **Figure 2C**), and no samples removed in this process (**Supplementary Figure S1A**).

Following the WGCNA: (1) when the critical parameter of the power value was 12, the scale independence was up to 0.8 and had a higher mean connectivity (**Supplementary Figure S1B**); (2) two key modules and the relationship with the clinical traits were detected (Colitis: MEbrown Pearson coefficient = 0.94, p = 7E-134, MEgreen Pearson coefficient = 0.75, p = 2E-51; UC

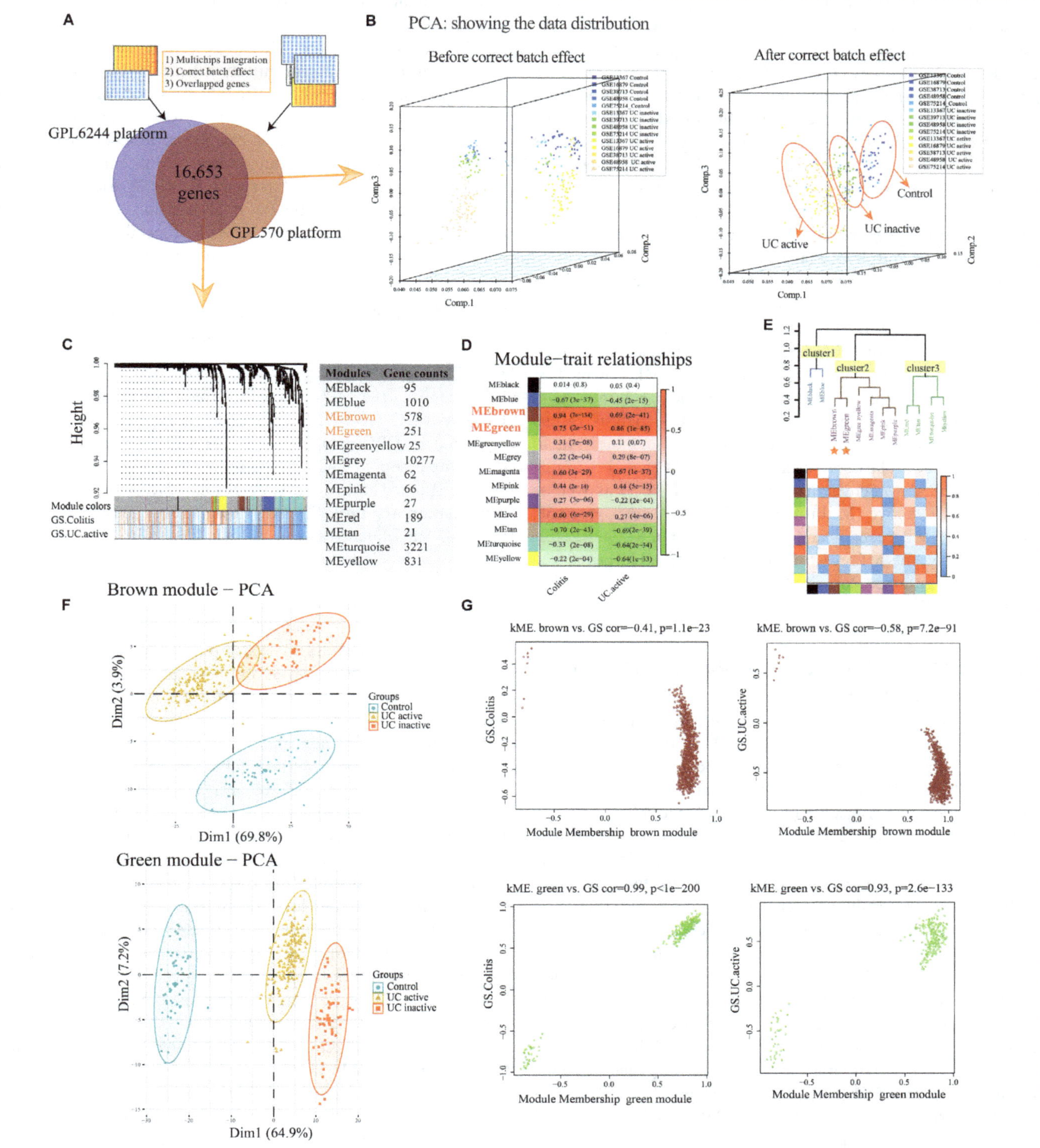

FIGURE 2 | Co-expression modules construction and identify interesting modules of ulcerative colitis and activity. **(A)** Venn diagram showing the overlap of the co-annotated genes in GPL6244 and GPL570 platform. **(B)** The principal component analysis (PCA) for co-annotated genes among the various microarrays in response to pre- and post-adjusting of the batch effects of the status of ulcerative colitis activity. **(C)** Construction of co-expression modules based on a dynamic branch-cutting method. **(D)** The relationship between the co-expression modules and clinical traits. Red represents a positive correlation, and the green represents a negative correlation. **(E)** The connectivity of eigengenes. Red represents a positive correlation, and blue represents a negative correlation. **(F)** The PCA for interesting module genes in response to the status of ulcerative colitis activity. **(G)** The gene significance (GS) and module membership (MM) analysis of interesting modules in response to ulcerative colitis and activity.

active: MEbrown Pearson coefficient = 0.69, p = 2E-41; MEgreen Pearson coefficient = 0.86, p = 1E-85; **Figure 2D**); (3) the result of interaction analysis among co-expression modules suggested a high degree of independence among different module genes, such that the heatmap showed no significant interaction among module genes (**Supplementary Figure S1C**); and (4) The connectivity of eigengenes in different modules allowed us to identify three clusters identified, and the eigengenes of different modules within the same cluster showed significant connectivity, whereas there was no difference among different clusters' modules (**Figure 2E**). The interesting module gene list was presented in **Supplementary Table S2**.

Additionally, in related to UC activity, two-dimensional PCA results also showing satisfactory connectivity and distinguish ability of MEgreen and MEbrown module genes in response to UC and activity (**Figure 2F**; MEgreen: first principal component: 64.9%, second principal component: 7.2%; MEbrown: first principal component: 69.8%, second principal component: 23.9%). And, as shown in **Figure 2G**, the GS analysis results showing a tight correlation between the gene and the trait of colitis (MEbrown: Pearson coefficient = −0.41, p = 1.1E-23; MEgreen: Pearson coefficient = 0.99, p < 1E-200), as well as the trait of UC active (MEbrown: Pearson coefficient = −0.58, p = 7.2E-91; MEgreen: Pearson coefficient = 0.93, p = 2.6E-133). Similarly, the MEbrown and MEgreen module genes also presented a significant contribution to the module membership (MM; **Figure 2G**).

Functional Enrichment Analysis and PPI Networks Construction

The MEgreen and MEbrown modules were assessed for further functional enrichment, consisting of GO term enrichment analysis of module genes of interest. Regarding GO terms enrichment, the MEgreen module was mainly enriched in GO: 0007041~lysosomal transport (5 genes enriched; p = 1.11E-05), GO: 0098609~cell-cell adhesion (13 genes enriched; p = 1.68E-04), and GO: 0043254~regulation of protein complex assembly (4 genes enriched; p = 6.43E-04). Genes in the MEbrown module were predominantly enriched in GO: 0071805~ion transmembrane transport (21 genes enriched; p = 3.98E-11), GO: 0042391~regulation of membrane potential (13 genes enriched; p = 4.80E-07), and GO: 0034765~regulation of ion transmembrane transport (18 genes enriched; p = 3.95E-09). These results are illustrated in **Figure 3A**. Regarding the KEGG pathway enrichment, the MEgreen module genes were significantly enriched in viral carcinogenesis (15 genes enriched; enrichment score = 5.01; p = 3.51E-05), proteoglycans in cancer (10 genes enriched; enrichment score = 3.97; p = 1.01E-03), and platelet activation (8 genes enriched; enrichment score = 4.91; p = 1.46E-03). However, genes in the MEbrown module were significantly enriched in ligand-receptor interaction (22 genes enriched; enrichment score = 3.55; p = 3.41E-07), calcium signaling pathway (13 genes enriched; enrichment score = 3.21; p = 1.72E-03), and adenosine 3′, 5′-cyclic monophosphate (cAMP) signaling pathway (12 genes enriched; enrichment score = 2.72; p = 2.36E-03).

Additionally, the **Figure 3B** illustrating a part of the visible pathway that tightly correlated with cancer from the KEGG pathway network (**Table 2**). These cancer-correlated pathways were related to immunity-inflammation response and tumorigenesis. These results also illustrated in **Table 2.** After submitting the genes enriched in cancer-correlated pathways to the STRING database, 50 and 48 PPI nodes were obtained for the MEbrown and MEgreen modules, respectively, with a confidence threshold greater than 0.4. After analyzed by Cytoscape software as an undirected method, the top 10 highest connectivity nodes of each PPI network were considered to be central agents. The PPI network of interesting modules was presented in **Figure 3B.**

Identification of Candidate Biomarkers Involving in UC-Associated Carcinogenesis

What's more, 184 DEGs were obtained in the comparison of UC and CRC (160 DEGs down-regulated and 24 DEGs up-regulated in CRC samples), and 344 DEGs were identified in the comparison of UC and adenoma in GSE4183 (332 DEGs down-regulated and 12 DEGs up-regulated in adenoma samples) (**Supplementary Table S3**). After overlapped, 106 co-DEGs were selected. Subsequently, we've further identified the same genes between co-DEGs and central agents of each PPI network, which have been selected as UC-related tumorigenesis genes. And 6 (*CXCL10*, *VCAM1*, *CXCL9*, *MMP9*, *IDO1*, and *CCR7*) out of the 106 co-DEGs remained after selection (**Figure 2B** and **Supplementary Table S5**). We also found a statistical difference in the gene expression levels of these genes between healthy individuals and UC patients (**Figure 4A** and **Supplementary Table S4**), as well as the expression levels between healthy individuals, UC, adenoma, and CRC patients of GSE4183 dataset (**Figure 4B** and **Supplementary Table S5**).

After validated by GSE37283 and GSE31106 datasets, the six hub gene expression levels in phases of UC were significantly increased in compared with the normal sample in both of the human and mouse's colonic mucosa (all the p < 0.05; **Supplementary Table S6**). Additionally, in comparison with UC mucosa, the expression level of six hub genes was decreased in phases of adenocarcinoma in human's colonic mucosa (all the p < 0.05; **Figures 4C,D**). Additionally, in comparison with normal samples, the expression level of *CCR7*, *CXCL10*, *IDO1*, and *MMP9* were increased in phases of adenocarcinoma's tissue, while the expression level of *CXCL9* and *VCAM1* were decreased. These results are shown in **Figure 4** and **Supplementary Table S6**.

To extend our findings, the gene expression levels in CRC and para-cancerous tissues were compared based on TCGA database. Consequently, the gene differential expression level with regrading to hub genes was constructed; and all of the hub genes shown a significant difference in expression level between cancer and para-cancer tissues (all the p < 0.05; **Figure 5A**). Importantly, the Kaplan–Meier survival curves indicated that a higher expression level of *CXCL10* (hazard ratio = 0.63; p = 0.035), *CXCL9* (hazard ratio = 0.63; p = 0.037), *MMP9* (Hazard Ratio = 0.61; p = 0.023), and *CCR7* (Hazard Ratio = 0.59;

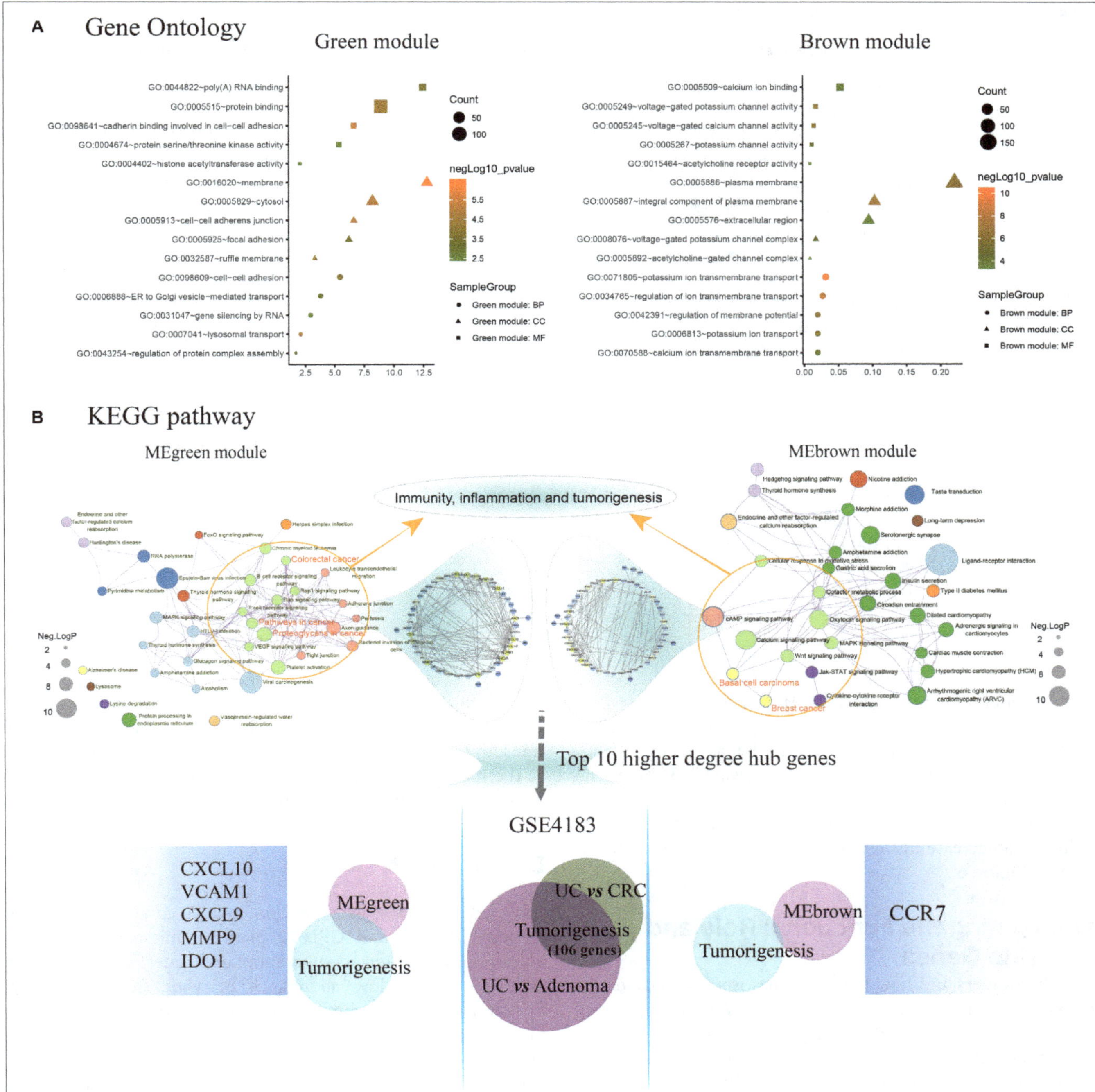

FIGURE 3 | Identification of key pathways and hub genes in the progression of ulcerative colitis activity and tumorigenesis. **(A)** Gene ontology (GO) terms enrichment analyzing was performed using the Database for Annotation, Visualization, and Integration Discovery (DAVID) database. The sizes of the dots represent the counts of enriched module genes, and the dot color represents the negative Log_{10} (p-value). **(B)** Kyoto Encyclopedia of Genes and Genomes (KEGG) pathway enrichment was constructed by Metascape database. The sizes of the dots represent the negative Log_{10} (p-value). Subsequently, the genes enriched in the pathway of immunity, inflammation, and tumorigenesis were selected to construct the protein-protein interaction (PPI) network basing on the STRING database for modules with a threshold value >0.4, respectively. And the Venn diagram showing the overlap of the top 10 functional hub genes in the MEgreen and MEbrown PPI networks, and tumorigenesis genes detected in GSE4183. The font sizes represent the degree of gene interaction in the PPI network.

$p = 0.013$) were significantly associated with the poor prognosis for CRC patients; although the difference in overall survival (OS) between high and low expression of *IDO1* (Hazard Ratio = 0.78; $p = 0.27$) and *VCAM1* (Hazard Ratio = 0.74; $p = 0.215$) were not significant. Additionally, there was a clear tendency for lower expression of *CXCL10* (Hazard Ratio = 0.38; $p < 0.001$), *CXCL9*

TABLE 2 | Identifying the cancer-correlated terms form the KEGG pathway network of the interesting modules.

MEmodule	KEGG term	*p* Value	Enriched genes
MEgreen	Platelet activation	0.001	AKT2, RHOA, ITGB1, MMP9, PRKACA, et al.
	Proteoglycans in cancer	0.001	AKT2, RHOA, ITGB1, MDM2, PRKACA, et al.
	B cell receptor signaling pathway	0.005	AKT2, PPP3R1, RAC1, IKBKG
	Chronic myeloid leukemia	0.005	AKT2, MDM2, PTPN11, IKBKG
	Pathways in cancer	0.006	AKT2, RHOA, DAPK3, ITGB1, MDM2, et al.
	Bacterial invasion of epithelial cells	0.007	RHOA, RAC1, CXCL10, CXCL9, CXCL11, et al.
	Ras signaling pathway	0.008	AKT2, RHOA, PRKACA, PTPN11, RAC1, et al.
	T cell receptor signaling pathway	0.019	AKT2, RHOA, PPP3R1, IKBKG, CCL19
	Rap1 signaling pathway	0.019	AKT2, RHOA, ITGB1, RAC1, TLN1, et al.
	VEGF signaling pathway	0.021	AKT2, PPP3R1, RAC1, VCAM1, PTPN11
	Colorectal cancer	0.022	AKT2, RHOA, RAC1, CD19, CD274
	Leukocyte transendothelial migration	0.027	RHOA, ITGB1, PTPN11, RAC1
	Adherens junction	0.035	RHOA, PTPN1, RAC1, TNFSF13B, IDO1, et al.
	Pertussis	0.041	RHOA, CFL1, ITGB1, GZMB
Mebrown	Calcium signaling pathway	0.000	ATP2B3, AVPR1B, CCKAR, CACNA1B, CAMK2B, et al.
	cAMP signaling pathway	0.002	ATP2B3, HCN2, CAMK2B, CNGA4, DRD2, et al.
	Oxytocin signaling pathway	0.002	CAMK2B, KCNJ5, OXT, PRKACG, PRKCG, et al.
	MAPK signaling pathway	0.013	CACNA1B, FGF6, MAPT, PRKACG, PRKCG, et al.
	Wnt signaling pathway	0.015	CAMK2B, PRKACG, PRKCG, CCR7, SFRP5, et al.
	Jak-STAT signaling pathway	0.024	CNTFR, EPO, GFAP, GH2, IFNA2, et al.
	Cofactor metabolic process	0.026	CAMK2B, DCT, PRKACG, PRKCG, WNT7B, et al.
	Basal cell carcinoma	0.034	GLI1, WNT7B, WNT8A, CCR7, APC2, et al.
	Cytokine-cytokine receptor interaction	0.041	AMHR2, CNTFR, EPO, GH2, IFNA2, et al.
	Breast cancer	0.043	FGF6, PGR, WNT7B, WNT8A, FGF23, et al.

(Hazard Ratio = 0.11; p = 0.004), *MMP9* (Hazard Ratio = 0.59; p = 0.046), *IDO1* (Hazard Ratio = 0.53; p = 0.012) and *CCR7* (Hazard Ratio = 0.61; p = 0.051) to be associated with a better prognosis in the recurrence free survival (RFS) time. This suggests that, to some extent, the effect of *CXCL10*, *CXCL9*, *MMP9*, *IDO1*, and *CCR7* overexpression on early survival time resulted in a decrease in the survival rate. And these results are shown in **Figure 6**.

Investigating the Functional Role and TF of Hub Genes

To further understand how the hub genes were correlated with UC-associated carcinogenesis, we applied DAVID and Metascape online database to explore the biological function. The results of GO term enrichment indicated that the GO:0032496~response to lipopolysaccharide (Enriched genes: *CCR7*, *CXCL9*, *IDO1*, *CXCL10*; p = 1.87E-06), GO:0030816~regulation of cAMP metabolic process (Enriched genes: *CXCL9*, *CXCL10*; p = 1.25E-03), and GO:0006954~inflammatory/immune response (Enriched genes: *CCR7*, *CXCL9*, *CXCL10*; p = 2.11E-03) were mainly enriched, while pathway of Ecb04668: TNF signaling pathway (Enriched genes: *CXCL10*, *VCAM1*, *MMP9*; p = 1.36E-03), Ecb04062: Chemokine signaling pathway (enriched genes: *CCR7*, *CXCL9*, *CXCL10*; p = 3.76E-03), and Ecb04060: Cytokine-cytokine receptor interaction (enriched genes: *CCR7*, *CXCL9*, *CXCL10*; p = 4.64E-03) (**Figure 5B**).

Finally, we predicted TFs and found that nuclear factor NF-kappa-B1 (*NFKB1*) (NES = 14.21, target genes = 5, motifs = 30), friend leukemia integration 1 TF (*FLI1*) (NES = 7.57, target genes = 3, motifs = 5), and signal transducer and activator of transcription 1 (*STAT1*) (NES = 7.71, target genes = 3, motifs = 2) as the master regulators of the hub genes are involved in UC-associated carcinogenesis (**Figure 5C**).

DISCUSSION

After adjusting the batch effects, 16,653 co-annotated genes among GPL6244 and GPL570 platform microarray datasets. Subsequently, we included co-annotated genes, some of which were present in low abundance or with small FC, in a further analysis, in which combination with WGCNA could integrate external traits and avoid information loss at a system level. According to the results, both MEbrown and MEgreen appeared to be moderately effective in revealing the UC-based global network. Biologically, following the functional enrichment analysis, the pathways of viral carcinogenesis, proteoglycans in cancer, platelet activation, ligand-receptor interaction, calcium signaling pathway, and cAMP signaling pathway were identified as being significantly associated with UC active. And cancer with highly correlated pathway and enriched genes were selected to construct the PPI network. The most critical genes were *CXCL10*, *VCAM1*, *CXCL9*, *MMP9*, *IDO1*, and *CCR7*, indicating that genetic variability influences susceptibility to the disease global network, and subsequently revealing potential regulatory roles in UC-associated carcinogenesis. Furthermore, these hub genes majorly enriched in tumor necrosis factor (TNF) signaling

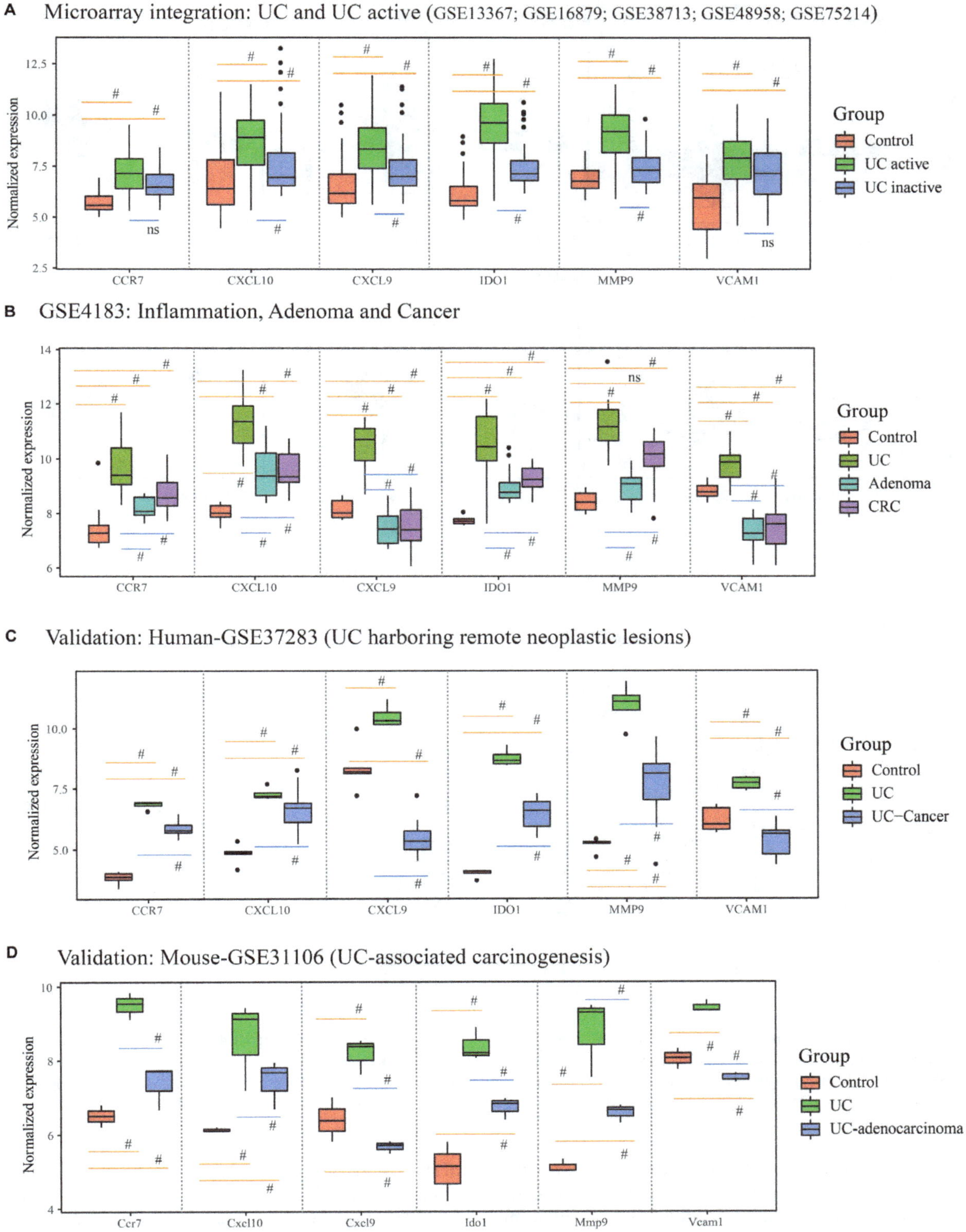

FIGURE 4 | The gene expression analysis and validation in response to the ulcerative colitis activity and tumorigenesis of hub genes. **(A)** The hub gene's expression in response to ulcerative colitis and activity in integrative microarray datasets. **(B)** The hub gene's expression detection of GSE4183 involved in inflammation, adenoma and colonic cancer. **(C,D)** The validation in the progression of UC-associated carcinogenesis for six candidate genes in human and mouse microarray datasets. #Represent $p < 0.05$ among the multi-comparison between normal, UC, and adenocarcinoma mucosa.

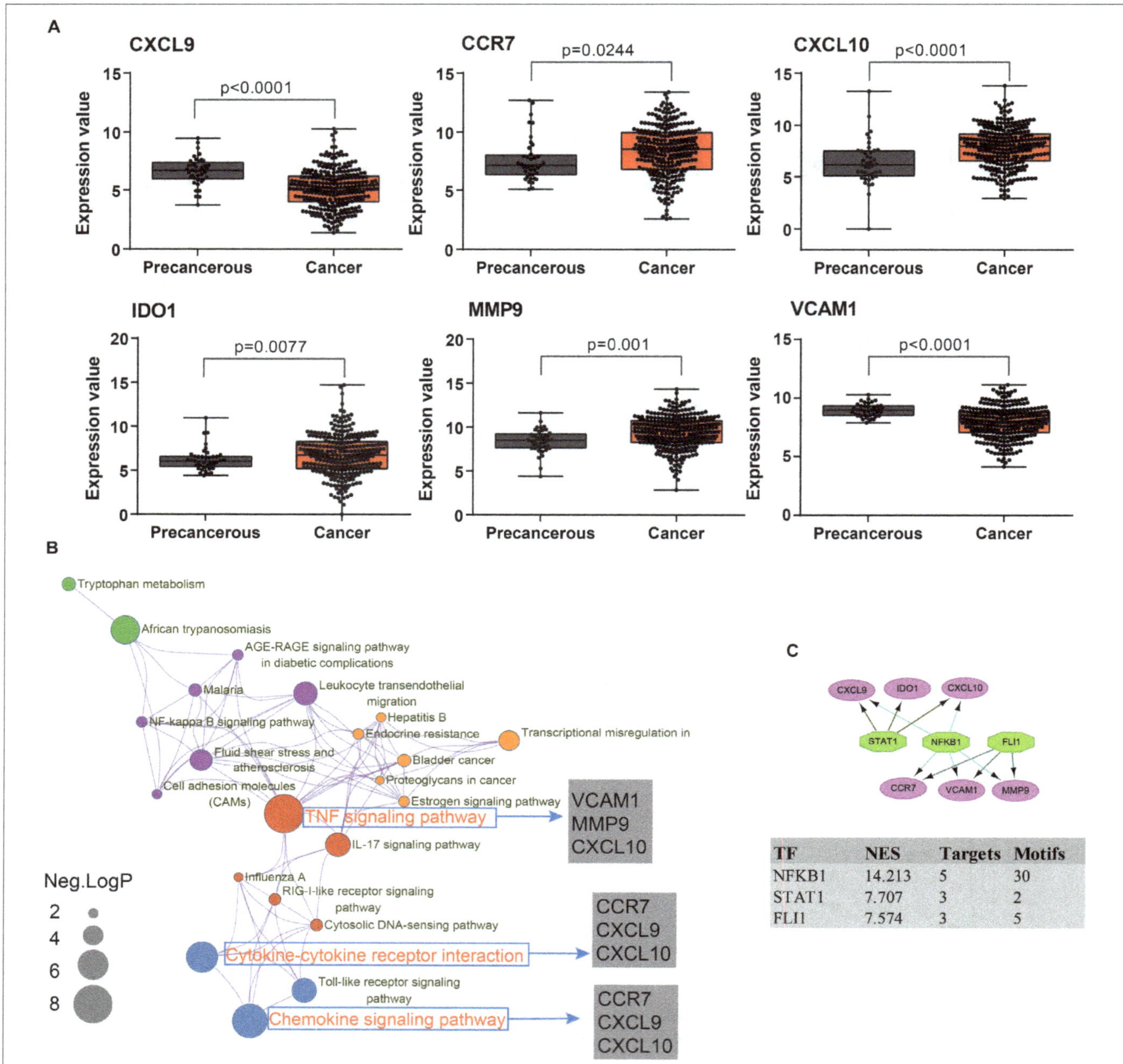

TF	NES	Targets	Motifs
NFKB1	14.213	5	30
STAT1	7.707	3	2
FLI1	7.574	3	5

FIGURE 5 | The molecular mechanism and transcription factors investigation for candidate biomarkers involved in ulcerative colitis activity and tumorigenesis. **(A)** The hub gene's expression levels analysis among cancer and para-cancerous tissues. **(B)** The KEGG pathway enrichment analysis of detected hub genes based on Metascape database. The sizes of the dots represent the negative Log_{10} (*p*-value). **(C)** The regulatory network results, based on the iRegulon plugin, showing that the top three regulators of *NFKB1*, *STAT1*, and *FLI1* in a set of six hub genes, were selected with the highest normalized enrichment score (NES).

pathway, chemokine signaling pathway, and cytokine-cytokine receptor interaction; and potentially regulated by *NFKB1*, *FLI1*, and *STAT1* in TFs network analysis. Furthermore, a significant association of *CCR7*, *CXCL10*, *CXCL9*, *IDO1*, and *MMP9* with UC-correlated CRC development was identified by integrating gene expression and survival analysis.

Emerging evidence has revealed the central role of gene-environment interaction in UC-based disease networks. Extrinsic and intrinsic environmental factors may cause chronic or acute inflammation in UC patients. Wang et al. found that calcium signaling pathway contributes to the development of colonic dysmotility in UC and intestinal inflammation, may be related with the calcium-transporting ATPase dysregulation in epithelial cells (Wang et al., 2016). And, additionally, the evidence for the interdependence of platelet abnormalities in UC model and patients, suggesting

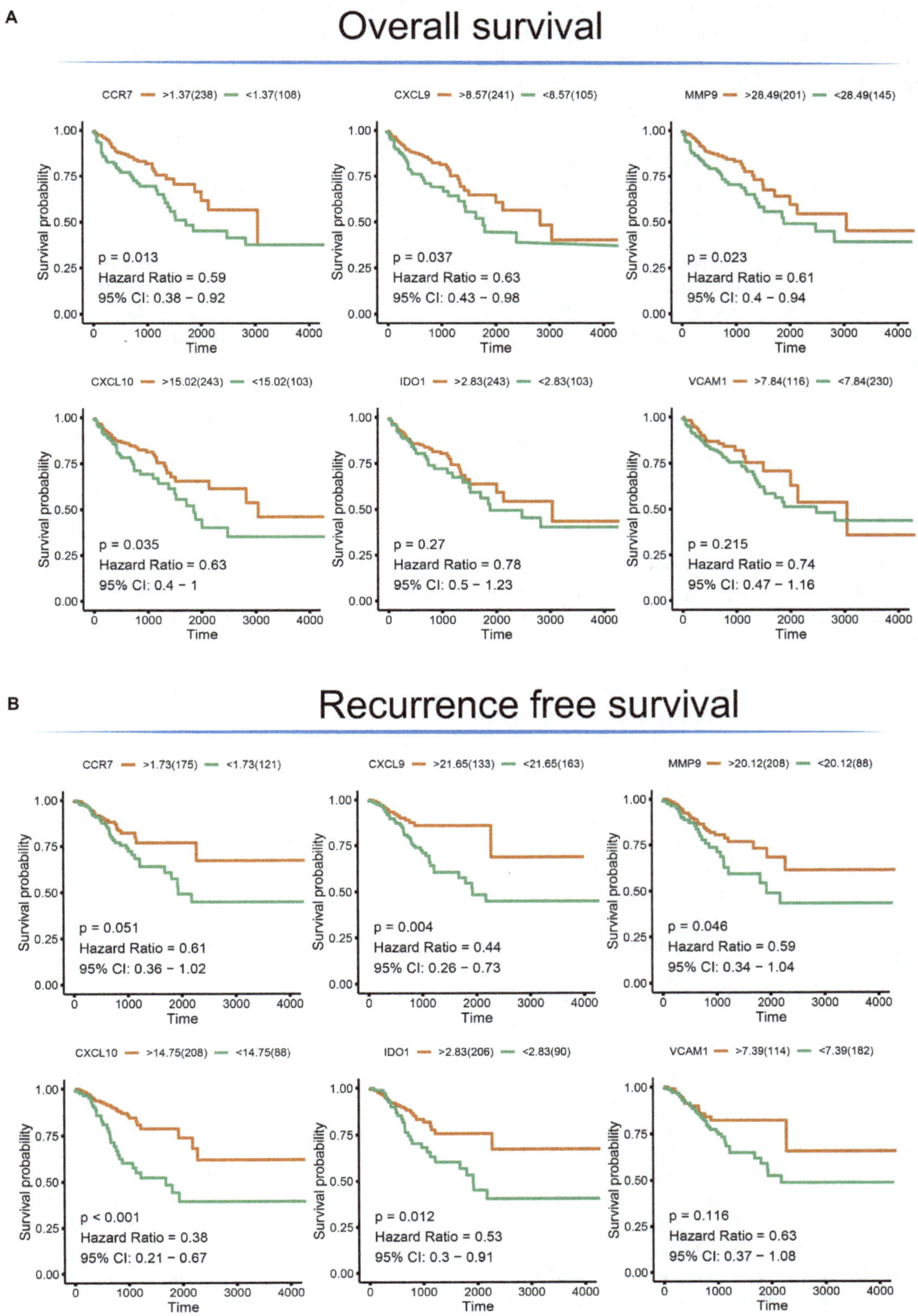

FIGURE 6 | The Kaplan–Meier survival analysis for the hub genes. **(A)** Overall survival analysis illustrating the significant difference between higher expression level and lower expression level of *CXCL10*, *CXCL9*, *MMP9*, and *CCR7* gene with respect to patient survival time; no difference was observed for the *VCAM1* and *IDO1* gene. **(B)** Significant differences were detected for the *CXCL10*, *CXCL9*, *MMP9*, *IDO1*, and *CCR7* in recurrence free survival time; no difference was observed for the *VCAM1* gene.

that the pathological state of changes in platelet parameters and their activation, may be linked to the inflammatory response and enhanced platelet-leukocyte, and aggregate formation associated with colitis (Senchenkova et al., 2015; Gawronska et al., 2017). Proteoglycans have been found to be critical in the regulation of stem cell through inducing precise and coordinated modulation of key growth factors, resulting in selective mitogen-activated protein kinases (MAPK) and/or another intracellular signaling, demonstrating an aberrant expression of ligand-receptor interaction on immune cells in IBD patients (Elshal et al., 2016; Gawronska et al., 2017). Li et al. demonstrated the multiple proinflammatory signaling pathways and candidate biomarkers, including *STAT1*, *STAT6*, and cAMP signaling pathway, in the exacerbation of UC (Li et al., 2012). Boothello et al. (2019) revealed that proteoglycans mediate cancer stem cells induced CRC xenograft's growth in a dose-dependent fashion. Moreover, syndecan-2, a type of proteoglycan, up-regulates MMP-7 expression in colon cancer cells via PKCγ-mediated activation of FAK/ERK signaling (Jang et al., 2017). Therefore, the pathway of the calcium signaling pathway, ligand-receptor interaction, platelet activation, cAMP signaling pathway and the none-cancer pathway involved, may provide insight into the immunological and inflammatory response, and the hypothesis of phospholipid-related barrier defects in the intestinal mucosa offers an opportunity to further understand UC-based pathogenesis.

The association between UC-related chronic inflammation and colon cancer has long been recognized (**Table 1**). According to a systemic review reported by Tatiya-Aphiradee, the pathway immuno-inflammatory response was closely linked to the regulation and maintenance of UC pathogenesis, that directly mediated by dynamic and complex communication between immune cells and cytokines (Tatiya-Aphiradee et al., 2018). Biologically, the dysregulation of antigen recognition, neutrophil chemotaxis, commensal microflora, and epithelial barrier defects may provide insight into the immunological and inflammatory response, it might offer an opportunity to further understand UC-based pathogenesis (Hindryckx et al., 2016). Gene expression profiling by Zhang's group shown the pathways includes PI3K-Akt signaling, cytokine-cytokine receptor interaction and ECM-receptor interaction was significantly associated with the process of colitis-associated carcinogenesis (Zhang et al., 2017). Several potential biomarkers of TNF signaling pathway, including *TNF-α*, *IL-6*, *IL-1*, *TGF-β*, and *IL-10*, have been confirmed to be involved in the process of malignant transformation of cells and carcinogenesis (Zhang et al., 2017). The pathway of cytokine-cytokine receptor interaction may also be closely linked to UC-related inflammation and tumorigenesis. Fang et al. (2015) compared IBD microarray datasets and found an important role for cytokine-cytokine receptor pathway dysregulation in both pediatric and mouse models of colitis. In sum, during the procession of intestinal inflammation and carcinogenesis, a variety of immunological and inflammatory signaling events, including the TNF signaling pathway, chemokine signaling pathway, and cytokine-cytokine receptor interaction, are activated and involved in a complex biological process.

Among the candidate biomarkers, the current understanding of the function of *CXCL10* and *CXCL9* may recruit the leukocytes to inflammation sites. However, a novel report from Shukla's group demonstrated that both *CXCL10* and *CXCL9* may promote colonic tumorigenesis via promotes the cytokine-mediated mucosal injury and inflammation response (Shukla et al., 2016). Additionally, *IDO1* were over-expressed in inflamed and adenoma of the colon, also functioned in promotes colitis-associated tumorigenesis independent of T-cell immune surveillance (Thaker et al., 2013). *MMP9* could maintain the microbiota and colonic epithelium mucosal barrier, also correlated with tissue remodeling and carcinogenesis via activates the EGFR signaling pathway (Pujada et al., 2017). The adhesion molecules VCAM-1 and ICAM-1, associated with macrophage infiltration, are directly associated with cell transmigration in inflamed colonic tissue (Wu et al., 2014). In addition, Bernhard et al. revealed that VCAM1 was correlated with different subsets of three immune cells and with high densities of T-cell subpopulations within specific tumor regions in CRC, thus the expression of adhesion molecules also associated with survival prognosis (Mlecnik et al., 2010). What's more, the lymphoid chemokine receptor CCR7 was re-expressed by activated T cells, allowing them to flow from the tissue to the lymph nodes through afferent lymphatics. McNamee's data showed a critical role for CCR7 in orchestrating immune cell traffic (McNamee et al., 2015). The role of chemokines in tumor angiogenesis was achieved in a CCR7-dependent manner through inhibiting Met/ERK/Elk-1/HIF-1α/VEGF-A pathway in CRC (Xu et al., 2018).

Finally, the TFs analysis results shown that *NFKB1*, *FLI1*, and *STAT1* were significantly predicted in hub gene's regulatory network, correlated with UC-correlated tumorigenesis. Here, *STAT1*, the first member of signal transducer and activator of transcription (STAT) family, has been involved in cancer suppression, including CRC (Zamanian-Azodi and Rezaei-Tavirani, 2019). Schwiebs et al. (2019) found that *STAT1* has involved in the process of tumor immune microenvironment during the crosstalk of "inflammation-to-tumor." NF-kappa-B1 (*NF-κB1*) signaling is a prominent and widely studied inflammatory signaling cascade in the field of immunology (Eden et al., 2017). Increased transcription of NF-κB is associated with inflammation and angiogenesis. Burkitt proposed that *NF-κB1* differentially regulate susceptibility to colitis-associated adenoma development (Burkitt et al., 2015). *FLI1*, a member of the family of ETS TFs, contains a highly conserved domain that recognizes ETS core consensus sites (GGAA/T; Hollenhorst et al., 2011; Tang et al., 2015). EWS-FLI1 regulates multiple target genes through binding to typical ETS core consensus sites or GGAA microsatellites, then participates in the carcinogenic process (Lessnick and Ladanyi, 2012; Tang et al., 2015). Azuara et al. (2018) have defined *FLI1* as a DNA methylation signature that can be distinguished in the early detection of CRC associated with IBD.

In summary, we found that the pathways of platelet activation, ligand-receptor interaction, calcium signaling pathway, and cAMP signaling pathway may play an important role in UC development via multiple physiological and pathophysiological processes, revealing a potentially attractive therapeutic target for UC-based disease networks. The overlapping results for *CXCL10*, *VCAM1*, *CXCL9*, *MMP9*, *IDO1*, and *CCR7* were obtained, which are considered to be hub biomarkers involved in UC-correlated tumorigenesis. Following the expression validation, survival analysis, and functional analysis, our results indicated that the novel biomarkers of *CXCL10*, *VCAM1*, *CXCL9*, *MMP9*, *IDO1*, and *CCR7* has powerful statistical efficiency and biological function. These genes are also linked to immune dysregulation and inflammation response, and thus provide new insights into the pathogenetic mechanisms of UC development and tumorigenic processes. Finally, our results also subsequently identified that the master regulators of *NFKB1*, *FLI1*, and *STAT1* have significantly associated with UC activity and carcinogenesis via target the candidate biomarkers.

AUTHOR CONTRIBUTIONS

WS, RZ, and MY took the responsibility for all aspects of the reliability and freedom from bias of the data presented and their discussed interpretation, and drafting the article. LM, JR, ZL, and JW took the responsibility for statistical analyses and interpretation of data. RL took the responsibility for full-text evaluation and guidance, and final approval of the version to be submitted.

FUNDING

This work was supported by National Key Clinical Discipline-National Natural Science Foundation of China (Grant No. 81372142), National Basic Research Program of China (Grant No. 2015CB554001), and Zhuhai science and technology project (Grant No. 20171009E030062).

REFERENCES

Azuara, D., Ausso, S., Rodriguez-Moranta, F., Guardiola, J., Sanjuan, X., Lobaton, T., et al. (2018). New methylation biomarker panel for early diagnosis of dysplasia or cancer in high-risk inflammatory bowel disease patients. *Inflamm. Bowel. Dis.* 24, 2555–2564. doi: 10.1093/ibd/izy255

Barrett, T., Wilhite, S. E., Ledoux, P., Evangelista, C., Kim, I. F., Tomashevsky, M., et al. (2013). NCBI GEO: archive for functional genomics data sets–update. *Nucleic Acids Res.* 41, D991–D995. doi: 10.1093/nar/gks1193

Biancone, L., Onali, S., Petruzziello, C., Calabrese, E., and Pallone, F. (2015). Cancer and immunomodulators in inflammatory bowel diseases. *Inflamm. Bowel. Dis.* 21, 674–698. doi: 10.1097/mib.0000000000000243

Boothello, R. S., Patel, N. J., Sharon, C., Abdelfadiel, E. I., Morla, S., Brophy, D. F., et al. (2019). A unique nonsaccharide mimetic of heparin hexasaccharide inhibits colon cancer stem cells via p38 MAP kinase activation. *Mol. Cancer Ther.* 18, 51–61. doi: 10.1158/1535-7163.Mct-18-0104

Brown, G. R., Hem, V., Katz, K. S., Ovetsky, M., Wallin, C., Ermolaeva, O., et al. (2015). Gene: a gene-centered information resource at NCBI. *Nucleic Acids Res.* 43, D36–D42. doi: 10.1093/nar/gku1055

Burkitt, M. D., Hanedi, A. F., Duckworth, C. A., Williams, J. M., Tang, J. M., O'Reilly, L. A., et al. (2015). NF-kappaB1, NF-kappaB2 and c-Rel differentially regulate susceptibility to colitis-associated adenoma development in C57BL/6 mice. *J. Pathol.* 236, 326–336. doi: 10.1002/path.4527

Ciorba, M. A., Bettonville, E. E., McDonald, K. G., Metz, R., Prendergast, G. C., Newberry, R. D., et al. (2010). Induction of IDO-1 by immunostimulatory DNA limits severity of experimental colitis. *J. Immunol.* 184, 3907–3916. doi: 10.4049/jimmunol.0900291

Colaprico, A., Silva, T. C., Olsen, C., Garofano, L., Cava, C., Garolini, D., et al. (2016). TCGAbiolinks: an R/Bioconductor package for integrative analysis of TCGA data. *Nucleic Acids Res.* 44:e71. doi: 10.1093/nar/gkv1507

Dabritz, J., and Menheniott, T. R. (2014). Linking immunity, epigenetics, and cancer in inflammatory bowel disease. *Inflamm. Bowel. Dis.* 20, 1638–1654. doi: 10.1097/mib.0000000000000063

Eden, K., Rothschild, D. E., McDaniel, D. K., Heid, B., and Allen, I. C. (2017). Noncanonical NF-kappaB signaling and the essential kinase NIK modulate crucial features associated with eosinophilic esophagitis pathogenesis. *Dis. Model. Mech.* 10, 1517–1527. doi: 10.1242/dmm.030767

Elshal, M. F., Aldahlawi, A. M., Saadah, O. I., and McCoy, J. P. (2016). Expression of CD200R1 and its ligand CD200 on T-helper lymphocytes of pediatric patients with ulcerative colitis and Crohn's disease. *Clin. Lab.* 62, 1521–1529. doi: 10.7754/Clin.Lab.2016.151231

Fang, K., Grisham, M. B., and Kevil, C. G. (2015). Application of comparative transcriptional genomics to identify molecular targets for pediatric IBD. *Front. Immunol.* 6:165. doi: 10.3389/fimmu.2015.00165

Gawronska, B., Matowicka-Karna, J., Kralisz, M., and Kemona, H. (2017). Markers of inflammation and influence of nitric oxide on platelet activation in the course of ulcerative colitis. *Oncotarget* 8, 68108–68114. doi: 10.18632/oncotarget.19202

Hindryckx, P., Jairath, V., and D'Haens, G. (2016). Acute severe ulcerative colitis: from pathophysiology to clinical management. *Nat. Rev. Gastroenterol. Hepatol.* 13, 654–664. doi: 10.1038/nrgastro.2016.116

Hollenhorst, P. C., McIntosh, L. P., and Graves, B. J. (2011). Genomic and biochemical insights into the specificity of ETS transcription factors. *Annu. Rev. Biochem.* 80, 437–471. doi: 10.1146/annurev.biochem.79.081507.103945

Hong, M., Ye, B. D., Yang, S. K., Jung, S., Lee, H. S., Kim, B. M., et al. (2018). Immunochip meta-analysis of inflammatory bowel disease identifies three novel loci and four novel associations in previously reported loci. *J. Crohns Colitis* 12, 730–741. doi: 10.1093/ecco-jcc/jjy002

Huang, D. W., Sherman, B. T., Tan, Q., Kir, J., Liu, D., Bryant, D., et al. (2007). DAVID bioinformatics resources: expanded annotation database and novel algorithms to better extract biology from large gene lists. *Nucleic Acids Res.* 35, W169–W175. doi: 10.1093/nar/gkm415

Irizarry, R. A., Hobbs, B., Collin, F., Beazer-Barclay, Y. D., Antonellis, K. J., Scherf, U., et al. (2003). Exploration, normalization, and summaries of high density oligonucleotide array probe level data. *Biostatistics* 4, 249–264. doi: 10.1093/biostatistics/4.2.249

Jang, B., Jung, H., Choi, S., Lee, Y. H., Lee, S. T., and Oh, E. S. (2017). Syndecan-2 cytoplasmic domain up-regulates matrix metalloproteinase-7 expression via the protein kinase Cgamma-mediated FAK/ERK signaling pathway in colon cancer. *J. Biol. Chem.* 292, 16321–16332. doi: 10.1074/jbc.M117.793752

Janky, R., Verfaillie, A., Imrichova, H., Van de Sande, B., Standaert, L., Christiaens, V., et al. (2014). iRegulon: from a gene list to a gene regulatory network using large motif and track collections. *PLoS Comput. Biol.* 10:e1003731. doi: 10.1371/journal.pcbi.1003731

Langfelder, P., and Horvath, S. (2008). WGCNA: an R package for weighted correlation network analysis. *BMC Bioinformatics* 9:559. doi: 10.1186/1471-2105-9-559

Leek, J. T., Johnson, W. E., Parker, H. S., Jaffe, A. E., and Storey, J. D. (2012). The sva package for removing batch effects and other unwanted variation in high-throughput experiments. *Bioinformatics* 28, 882–883. doi: 10.1093/bioinformatics/bts034

Lessnick, S. L., and Ladanyi, M. (2012). Molecular pathogenesis of ewing sarcoma: new therapeutic and transcriptional targets. *Annu. Rev. Pathol.* 7, 145–159. doi: 10.1146/annurev-pathol-011110-130237

Li, B., Ruotti, V., Stewart, R. M., Thomson, J. A., and Dewey, C. N. (2010). RNA-Seq gene expression estimation with read mapping uncertainty. *Bioinformatics* 26, 493–500. doi: 10.1093/bioinformatics/btp692

Li, Y., Deuring, J., Peppelenbosch, M. P., Kuipers, E. J., de Haar, C., and van der Woude, C. J. (2012). STAT1, STAT6 and adenosine 3',5'-cyclic monophosphate (cAMP) signaling drive SOCS3 expression in inactive ulcerative colitis. *Mol. Med.* 18, 1412–1419. doi: 10.2119/molmed.2012.00277

Liu, Y., Fang, X., Yuan, J., Sun, Z., Li, C., Li, R., et al. (2014). The role of corticotropin-releasing hormone receptor 1 in the development of colitis-associated cancer in mouse model. *Endocr. Relat. Cancer* 21, 639–651. doi: 10.1530/erc-14-0239

McNamee, E. N., Masterson, J. C., Veny, M., Collins, C. B., Jedlicka, P., Byrne, F. R., et al. (2015). Chemokine receptor CCR7 regulates the intestinal TH1/TH17/Treg balance during Crohn's-like murine ileitis. *J. Leukoc. Biol.* 97, 1011–1022. doi: 10.1189/jlb.3HI0614-303R

Mirkov, M. U., Verstockt, B., and Cleynen, I. (2017). Genetics of inflammatory bowel disease: beyond NOD2. *Lancet Gastroenterol. Hepatol.* 2, 224–234. doi: 10.1016/s2468-1253(16)30111-x

Mlecnik, B., Tosolini, M., Charoentong, P., Kirilovsky, A., Bindea, G., Berger, A., et al. (2010). Biomolecular network reconstruction identifies T-cell homing factors associated with survival in colorectal cancer. *Gastroenterology* 138, 1429–1440. doi: 10.1053/j.gastro.2009.10.057

Molodecky, N. A., Soon, I. S., Rabi, D. M., Ghali, W. A., Ferris, M., Chernoff, G., et al. (2012). Increasing incidence and prevalence of the inflammatory bowel diseases with time, based on systematic review. *Gastroenterology* 142, 46–54.e42. doi: 10.1053/j.gastro.2011.10.001

Moon, C. M., Kim, S. W., Ahn, J. B., Ma, H. W., Che, X., Kim, T. I., et al. (2018). Deep resequencing of ulcerative colitis-associated genes identifies novel variants in candidate genes in the korean population. *Inflamm. Bowel. Dis.* 24, 1706–1717. doi: 10.1093/ibd/izy122

Ng, S. C., Shi, H. Y., Hamidi, N., Underwood, F. E., Tang, W., Benchimol, E. I., et al. (2018). Worldwide incidence and prevalence of inflammatory bowel disease in the 21st century: a systematic review of population-based studies. *Lancet* 390, 2769–2778. doi: 10.1016/s0140-6736(17)32448-0

Peters, L. A., Perrigoue, J., Mortha, A., Iuga, A., Song, W. M., Neiman, E. M., et al. (2017). A functional genomics predictive network model identifies regulators of inflammatory bowel disease. *Nat. Genet.* 49, 1437–1449. doi: 10.1038/ng.3947

Pujada, A., Walter, L., Patel, A., Bui, T. A., Zhang, Z., Zhang, Y., et al. (2017). Matrix metalloproteinase MMP9 maintains epithelial barrier function and preserves mucosal lining in colitis associated cancer. *Oncotarget* 8, 94650–94665. doi: 10.18632/oncotarget.21841

Ritchie, M. E., Phipson, B., Wu, D., Hu, Y., Law, C. W., Shi, W., et al. (2015). limma powers differential expression analyses for RNA-sequencing and microarray studies. *Nucleic Acids Res.* 43:e47. doi: 10.1093/nar/gkv007

Schwiebs, A., Herrero San Juan, M., Schmidt, K. G., Wiercinska, E., Anlauf, M., Ottenlinger, F., et al. (2019). Cancer-induced inflammation and inflammation-induced cancer in colon: a role for S1P lyase. *Oncogene* doi: 10.1038/s41388-019-0758-x [Epub ahead of print].

Senchenkova, E., Seifert, H., and Granger, D. N. (2015). Hypercoagulability and platelet abnormalities in inflammatory bowel disease. *Semin. Thromb. Hemost.* 41, 582–589. doi: 10.1055/s-0035-1556590

Shukla, P. K., Chaudhry, K. K., Mir, H., Gangwar, R., Yadav, N., Manda, B., et al. (2016). Chronic ethanol feeding promotes azoxymethane and dextran sulfate sodium-induced colonic tumorigenesis potentially by enhancing mucosal inflammation. *BMC Cancer* 16:189. doi: 10.1186/s12885-016-2180-x

Szklarczyk, D., Morris, J. H., Cook, H., Kuhn, M., Wyder, S., Simonovic, M., et al. (2017). The STRING database in 2017: quality-controlled protein-protein association networks, made broadly accessible. *Nucleic Acids Res.* 45, D362–D368. doi: 10.1093/nar/gkw937

Tang, S. W., Bilke, S., Cao, L., Murai, J., Sousa, F. G., Yamade, M., et al. (2015). SLFN11 is a transcriptional target of EWS-FLI1 and a determinant of drug response in ewing sarcoma. *Clin. Cancer Res.* 21, 4184–4193. doi: 10.1158/1078-0432.Ccr-14-2112

Tatiya-Aphiradee, N., Chatuphonprasert, W., and Jarukamjorn, K. (2018). Immune response and inflammatory pathway of ulcerative colitis. *J. Basic Clin. Physiol. Pharmacol.* 30, 1–10. doi: 10.1515/jbcpp-2018-0036

Thaker, A. I., Rao, M. S., Bishnupuri, K. S., Kerr, T. A., Foster, L., Marinshaw, J. M., et al. (2013). IDO1 metabolites activate beta-catenin signaling to promote cancer cell proliferation and colon tumorigenesis in mice. *Gastroenterology* 145, 416–25.e1-4. doi: 10.1053/j.gastro.2013.05.002

Uhlig, H. H., and Muise, A. M. (2017). Clinical genomics in inflammatory bowel disease. *Trends Genet.* 33, 629–641. doi: 10.1016/j.tig.2017.06.008

Wang, Y., Li, J. X., Ji, G. J., Zhai, K., Wang, H. H., and Liu, X. G. (2016). The involvement of Ca(2+) signal pathways in distal colonic myocytes in a rat model of dextran sulfate sodium-induced colitis. *Chin. Med. J.* 129, 1185–1192. doi: 10.4103/0366-6999.181968

Wu, X. F., Ouyang, Z. J., Feng, L. L., Chen, G., Guo, W. J., Shen, Y., et al. (2014). Suppression of NF-kappaB signaling and NLRP3 inflammasome activation in macrophages is responsible for the amelioration of experimental murine colitis by the natural compound fraxinellone. *Toxicol. Appl. Pharmacol.* 281, 146–156. doi: 10.1016/j.taap.2014.10.002

Xu, Z., Zhu, C., Chen, C., Zong, Y., Feng, H., Liu, D., et al. (2018). CCL19 suppresses angiogenesis through promoting miR-206 and inhibiting Met/ERK/Elk-1/HIF-1alpha/VEGF-A pathway in colorectal cancer. *Cell Death Dis.* 9:974. doi: 10.1038/s41419-018-1010-2

Zamanian-Azodi, M., and Rezaei-Tavirani, M. (2019). Investigation of health benefits of cocoa in human colorectal cancer cell line, HT-29 through interactome analysis. *Gastroenterol. Hepatol. Bed Bench* 12, 67–73.

Zhang, X., Wei, L., Wang, J., Qin, Z., Wang, J., Lu, Y., et al. (2017). Suppression colitis and colitis-associated colon cancer by anti-S100a9 antibody in mice. *Front. Immunol.* 8:1774. doi: 10.3389/fimmu.2017.01774

Zhou, Y., Zhou, B., Pache, L., Chang, M., Khodabakhshi, A. H., Tanaseichuk, O., et al. (2019). Metascape provides a biologist-oriented resource for the analysis of systems-level datasets. *Nat. Commun.* 10:1523. doi: 10.1038/s41467-019-09234-6

13

Formal Modeling of mTOR Associated Biological Regulatory Network Reveals Novel Therapeutic Strategy for the Treatment of Cancer

Zurah Bibi[1], Jamil Ahmad[1], Amnah Siddiqa[1], Rehan Z. Paracha[1], Tariq Saeed[1], Amjad Ali[2], Hussnain Ahmed Janjua[2], Shakir Ullah[3], Emna Ben Abdallah[4] and Olivier Roux[4]*

[1] Research Centre for Modeling and Simulation, National University of Sciences and Technology, Islamabad, Pakistan,
[2] Atta-Ur-Rahman School of Applied Biosciences, National University of Sciences and Technology, Islamabad, Pakistan,
[3] School of Business, Stratford University, Falls Church, VA, United States, [4] IRCCyN UMR Centre National de la Recherche Scientifique 6597, BP 92101, Nantes, France

Correspondence:
Jamil Ahmad
jamil.ahmad@rcms.nust.edu.pk

Cellular homeostasis is a continuous phenomenon that if compromised can lead to several disorders including cancer. There is a need to understand the dynamics of cellular proliferation to get deeper insights into the prevalence of cancer. Mechanistic Target of Rapamycin (mTOR) is implicated as the central regulator of the metabolic pathway involved in growth whereas its two distinct complexes mTORC1 and mTORC2 perform particular functions in cellular propagation. To date, mTORC1 is a well defined therapeutic target to inhibit uncontrolled cell division, while the role of mTORC2 is not well characterized. Therefore, the current study is designed to understand the signaling dynamics of mTOR and its partner proteins such as PI3K, PTEN, mTORC2, PKB (Akt), mTORC1, and FOXO. For this purpose, a qualitative model of mTOR-associated Biological Regulatory Network (BRN) is constructed to predict its regulatory behaviors which may not be predictable otherwise. The depleted expression of PTEN and FOXO along with the overexpression of PI3K, mTORC2, mTORC1 and Akt is predicted as a stable steady state which is in accordance with their observed expression levels in the progression of various cancers. The qualitative model also predicts the homeostasis of all the entities in the form of qualitative cycles. The significant qualitative (discrete) cycle is identified by analyzing betweenness centralities of the qualitative (discrete) states. This cycle is further refined as a linear hybrid automaton model with the production (activation) and degradation (inhibition) time delays in order to analyze the real-time constraints for its existence. The analysis of the hybrid model provides a formal proof that during homeostasis the inhibition time delay of Akt is less than the inhibition time delay of mTORC2. In conclusion, our observations characterize that in homeostasis Akt is degraded with a faster rate than mTORC2 which suggests that the inhibition of Akt along with the activation of mTORC2 may be a better therapeutic strategy for the treatment of cancer.

Keywords: mTOR signaling pathway, SMBioNet, Biological regulatory networks (BRNs), René Thomas, Qualitative modeling, Model checking, Cancer

INTRODUCTION

Cells need continuous supply of resources that maintain intracellular energy and require nutrient levels contributing to macromolecular biosynthesis and serving as an upstream regulator of cell size and growth rate (Schmelzle and Hall, 2000; Wullschleger et al., 2006; Avruch et al., 2006; Sonntag et al., 2012). Compromised growth homeostasis can lead to several diseases including metabolic disorders, aging and cancer (Zoncu et al., 2011). A serine/threonine protein kinase mTOR, a member of the phosphatidylinositol kinase related kinases (PIKKs) family (Schmelzle and Hall, 2000), acts as a central regulator of homeostasis during growth and starvation (Zoncu et al., 2011). Recent studies have shown that dysregulation in mTOR signaling could lead to cancer and other pathologies (Menon and Manning, 2008). In these studies, abnormally elevated levels of mTOR have been linked with several human cancers including prostate, pancreas, liver, breast, colorectal, urinary tract, and female reproductive organs. On the other hand, due to excess nutrients supply, hyperactivation of mTOR has also been implicated to cause diabetes (Zoncu et al., 2011). Moreover, being the central regulator of growth, mTOR also monitors the process of aging (Zoncu et al., 2011). mTOR functions in the form of two distinct complexes namely mTOR Complex 1 (mTORC1) and 2 (mTORC2) (Wullschleger et al., 2006; Guertin and Sabatini, 2007). These complexes are distinguished by their unique accessory proteins, i.e., raptor and PRAS40 in case of mTORC1 and rictor, Protor and mSin1 in case of mTORC2 (Hara et al., 2002; Kim et al., 2002; Sarbassov et al., 2004). The function of these accessory proteins is to specify their binding with different substrates and regulators (Hara et al., 2002; Kim et al., 2002; Nojima et al., 2003; Schalm et al., 2003; Wullschleger et al., 2005; Sancak et al., 2007; Pearce et al., 2007). Both mTORC1 and mTORC2 share also some components including mLST8 and Deptor that act as positive and negative regulators, respectively (Loewith et al., 2002).

Signaling of mTOR

The mTOR signaling pathway (**Figure 1**) is initiated by insulin, insulin-like growth factor 1 (IGF1) and Ras (Laplante and Sabatini, 2012) along with others. The binding of insulin with insulin/IGF1 signaling (IIS) receptors causes its autophosphorylation with subsequent recruitment of insulin receptor substrate (IRS) with its cytosolic domain. Activated IRS then activates several downstream effector proteins including PI3K.

The role of PI3K pathway in metabolism and growth is well-established and its dysregulation could result in certain metabolic disorders and cancers (Carracedo and Pandolfi, 2008). In addition to the activation of JNK pathway (Vivanco et al., 2007) that down-regulates PTEN transcription and promotes cellular proliferation by hindering apoptosis, it is also involved in the activation of Akt (Carracedo and Pandolfi, 2008). PI3K phosphorylates and converts phosphatidylinositol (4,5)-bisphosphate (PIP2) to phosphatidylinositol (3,4,5)-trisphosphate to (PIP3) (Engelman et al., 2006; Manning and

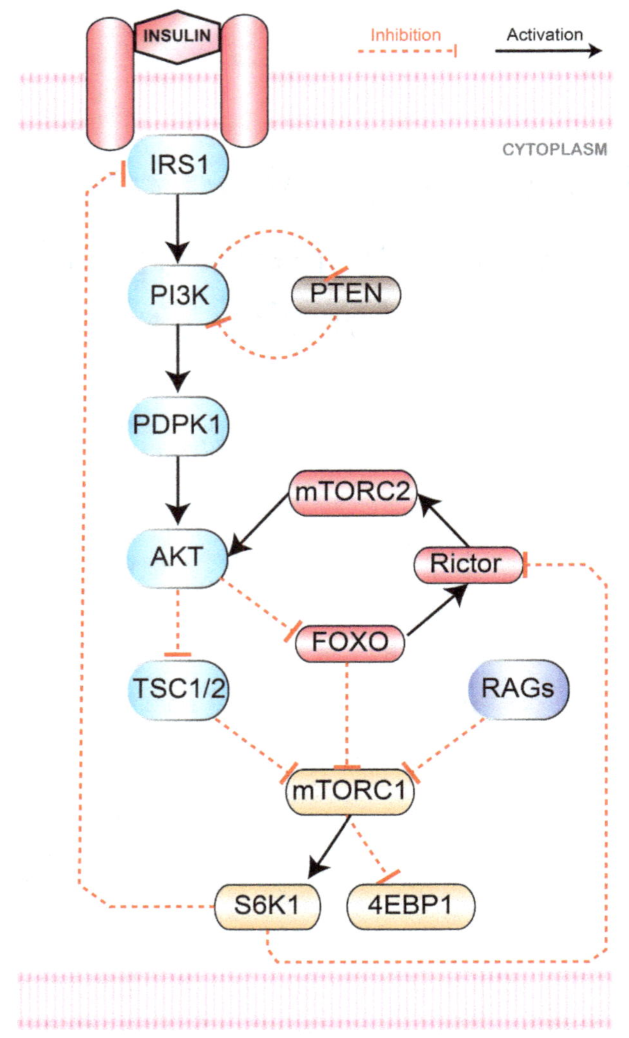

FIGURE 1 | mTOR Signaling Pathway. Collectively growth factors and amino acids (via Rags mediated binding of mTORC1 to Rheb) activate mTORC1. Insulin binds to its IRS1 that activates PI3K and recruits PDPK1 from cell membrane via to PIP3 conversion. PI3K and mTORC2 phoshorylate Akt at Thr308 and Ser473, respectively. Through inhibition of TSC1-TSC2 and FOXO, Akt stimulates mTORC1 to promote mRNA translation and inhibits apoptosis by phosphorylating S6K1 and 4E-BP1. Negative feedback inhibition of IRS1 is initiated by S6K1 to downregulate glucose metabolism. PTEN regulates mutagenic stimulation of PI3K (via PIP3 to PIP2 reconversion) to keep cellular propagation within controlled levels while FOXO is responsible to control hyperactivation of mTORC1.

Cantley, 2007). This event is important for the activation of phosphatidylinositol dependent protein kinase 1 (PDPK1) that eventually stimulates Akt. The activation of Akt is achieved through phosphorylation at two sites i.e., Thr308 and Ser473. Activated PDPK1 phosphorylates Akt at position Thr308 whereas another protein mTORC2 phosphorylates it at Ser473 (Alessi et al., 1997; Sarbassov et al., 2005). Both these phosphorylation events are essential for the complete activation of Akt. Thobe et. al. examined the influence of PI3K pathway kinases on mTORC2 and found PI3K mediated regulation essential for mTORC2 recruitment and further activation Thobe et al. (2017).

Akt regulates several downstream proteins such as Tuberous Sclerosis proteins 1 and 2 (TSC1/TSC2) and FOXO. The heterodimer of TSC1 (hamartin) and TSC2 (tuberin) primarily inhibits the activity of mTORC1 via conversion of active Ras homolog enriched in brain (Rheb)-GAP into inactive Guanosine diphosphate (GDP)-bound Rheb (Inoki et al., 2003; Tee et al., 2003). Akt phoshorylates and inhibits TSC1/TSC2 in order to activate mTORC1 (Inoki et al., 2002; Manning et al., 2002; Potter et al., 2002; Roux et al., 2004; Ma et al., 2005). Akt also elevates the expression of mTORC1 indirectly through the inhibition of FOXO (Guertin et al., 2006; Chen et al., 2010; Zoncu et al., 2011). FOXO acts a homeostatic regulator of cellular energy production and consumption processes under energy stress conditions. Another role of FOXO is to increase the activation of Rictor (a major component of mTORC2) and subsequently mTORC1.

PI3K signaling is mainly buffered through PTEN (Carracedo et al., 2008). PTEN serves as a tumor suppressor and mostly found mutated in its phosphatase domain (Eng, 2003) in several cancers (Li and Sun, 1997; Steck et al., 1997) causing overactive PI3K signaling. PTEN hydrolyzes phosphatidylinositol (3,4,5)-trisphosphate (PIP3) to phosphatidylinositol (4,5)-bisphosphate (PIP2) (**Figure 1**) . In this way, PTEN inhibits PIP3 dependent downstream signaling events like membrane recruitment and activation of AKT to prevent cell growth and proliferation. Hence, PTEN holds critical position in maintaining homeostasis through the inhibition of oncogenic transformation (Carracedo and Pandolfi, 2008).

Finally, the activated mTORC1 activates several downstream effectors mainly eukaryotic translation initiation factor 4E (eIF4E)-binding protein 1 (4E-BP1) and S6 kinase 1 (S6K1), that represses autophagy and promotes protein synthesis. S6K1 phosphorylates rictor causing mTORC2 disassembly (Dibble et al., 2009; Julien et al., 2010; Treins et al., 2010) and also degrades IRS proteins (Harrington et al., 2004; Shah et al., 2004) which dampens the PI3K mediated signaling cascade.

Mutations in the genes encoding for the proteins of mTOR associated BRN can lead to different types of cancers including sporadic cancers, hamartoma syndromes or phakomatoses, cowden syndrome (PTEN), neurofibromatosis (NF1, NF2) and peutz–Jeghers syndrome (LKB1) (Menon and Manning, 2008). Deregulation of entities in mTOR associated BRN result in certain other complications like insulin resistance and type 2 diabetes. Moreover, mTOR pathway can also be hyper-stimulated (e.g., in adipose tissues) under situation of excessive nutrients that can ultimately lead to the same complications (Um et al., 2004; Khamzina et al., 2005; Tremblay et al., 2007).

Computational Modeling

Gene expression is a complex process and its regulation determines the overall cellular dynamics (De Jong, 2002). Computational techniques in systems biology facilitate to explore the role of genes, proteins and overall dynamics of the system (Glass and Kauffman, 1973). Qualitative modeling framework is one of the established methods to analyze gene expression dynamics (Thomas, 1978; Thomas and d'Ari, 1990; De Jong et al., 2004) in the form of biological regulatory networks (BRNs) (Lewin, 2000). A BRN is modeled by a directed graph where vertices represent biological entities e.g., DNA, RNA, proteins and other biological molecules whereas edges correspond to regulatory interactions (i.e., activation and inhibition) (Bernot et al., 2007). The design of the study is illustrated in **Figure 2**.

Contributions

The main objective of this study is to build a refined computational model of mTOR regulation that could predict therapeutic targets to inhibit the progression of cancer. A BRN of mTOR and its interacting proteins (PI3K, PTEN, mTORC2, Akt, mTORC1 and FOXO) has been abstracted from the pathway (**Figure 1**) in order to explore the dynamics based on the logical formalism of René Thomas (Peres and Jean-Paul, 2003; Bernot et al., 2004, 2007). The unknown parameters in the logical model are inferred based on biological observations formally encoded as CTL (Computational Tree Logic) formulas in SMBioNet (Selection of Models of Biological Networks) tool (Mcadams

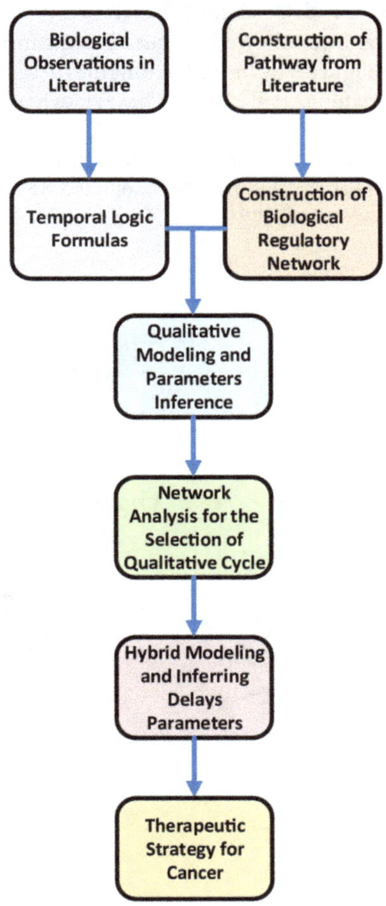

FIGURE 2 | Workflow Design of the study of the therapeutic strategy for cancer.

and Shapiro, 1995). The qualitative model (State Graph) of the BRN infers the dynamics such as homeostasis in the form of qualitative cycles and stable behavior in the form of stable state (SS). The most significant qualitative cycle is selected based on the centrality values of the qualitative states in the model. A linear hybrid automaton of the selected cycle is constructed using Hytech model checker (Henzinger et al., 1997) with new parameters for production and degradation time delays. Hytech inferred the values of these parameters in the form of linear constraints. These constraints are further analyzed to infer the pairwise relations between any possible pair of delays of genes. These relations show only one significant relation between AKT and mTORC2 in terms of delays. The analysis of the hybrid model provides a formal proof that during homeostasis the inhibition time delay of Akt is less than the inhibition time delay of mTORC2. This enforces that in homeostasis Akt is degraded with a faster rate than mTORC2 which suggests that the inhibition of Akt along with the activation of mTORC2 may be a better therapeutic strategy for the treatment of cancer.

METHODS

Reduction of Signaling Pathway

The signaling pathway shown in **Figure 1** is further reduced to a BRN shown in **Figure 3** by the reduction rules described in (Naldi et al., 2009; Saadatpour et al., 2013). These rules have already been applied to reduce the TLR4 and JAK/STAT signaling pathways to a BRN with all possible regulatory feedback circuits (Paracha et al., 2014). The abstracted mTOR-associated BRN is composed of six proteins which are PI3K, PTEN, mTORC2, Akt, mTORC1, and FOXO.

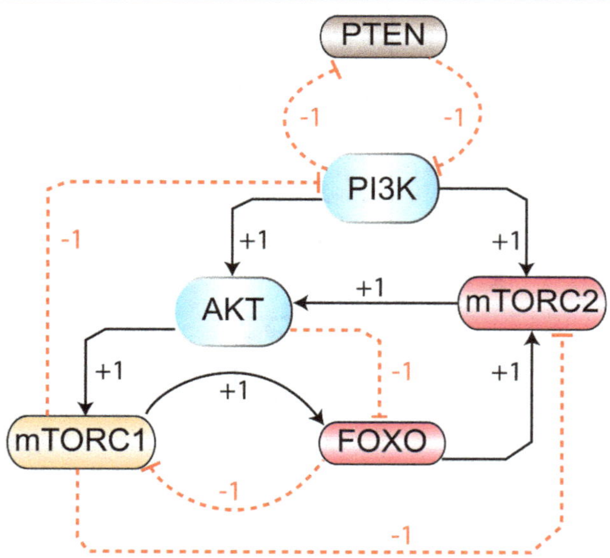

FIGURE 3 | The mTOR-associated BRN: abstraction of mTOR signaling pathway (**Figure 1**) in BRN. Positive (activation) and negative (inhibition) regulations are represented by "+" and "−" signs respectively.

Qualitative Modeling

Biological regulations (production and degradation) are subjected to expression levels of entities in BRN. An entity *p*1 activates or inhibits another entity *p*2, at a specific threshold. A qualitative threshold can be described as a discrete level (first, second, third etc.). René Thomas proposed a modeling framework which assumes qualitative thresholds and parameters to derive the dynamics of a BRN. Several methods are in use to model the behavior of biological systems (Peres and Jean-Paul, 2003; Bernot et al., 2004, 2007). Continuous modeling frameworks based on ordinary and partial differential equations are widely used. These frameworks rely on precise quantitative values, which in many cases are not known. This limitation led to the development of qualitative modeling framework. Kauffman et al., introduced a logical formalism based on Boolean logic where each entity was considered as "ON" (1) or "OFF" (0) to represent its activation or inhibition, respectively (Kauffman, 1969, 1993; Somogyi et al., 1997). This approach was further extended to kinetic logic formalism by Thomas to incorporate multi-valued (0,1,2,3,...) expression levels of entities. Formal methods such as model-checking approach can help to infer the parameters of complex systems (Bernot et al., 2007). BRNs are complex systems and their parameters can be inferred with such approaches.

This study is based on the kinetic logical formalism developed by René Thomas (Thieffry and Thomas, 1995) to model the biological regulatory network (BRN) of mTOR using GENOTECH tool Ahmad (2009) (available at https://github.com/DrJamilAhmad/GENOTECH/blob/master/GenoTechE.jar). An important feature of kinetic modeling is positive or negative feedback circuits. An entity favors the activation of another entity in the BRN through positive feedback and is necessary to generate multi-stationarity (stable states), whereas an entity favoring the inhibition of another entity through negative feedback is a necessary condition to generate oscillatory behavior (homeostasis) (Thomas, 1981). Number of studies performed on genetic networks that incorporated analysis of positive and negative feedbacks with formal methods can be found in Kauffman (1993), Somogyi and Sniegoski (1996), and Szallasi and Liang (1998). Formal definitions provided in Aslam et al. (2014) and Paracha et al. (2014) can be obtained for detailed description.

Parameters Inference using Model Checking

Qualitative dynamics of Thomas networks depend on the values of logical parameters which are unknown a priori. These parameters are used to render system dynamics as a directed state graph (discrete or qualitative model), which incorporates important behaviors such as cycles or stable states. The inference of biologically coherent parameters is an important aspect of qualitative modeling. In this direction, Bernot et al., introduced an approach to infer these logical parameters using a formal method approach called *model checking*. This approach is implemented in SMBioNet (Selection of Models of Biological

Networks) tool. It performs an exhaustive enumeration of models and selects those set of parameters which are consistent with experimental observations expressed as temporal logic formulas. Similar parameter estimation approach (by using SMBioNet tool) has been employed to study qualitative behavior of several biological systems including immunity control mechanism in lambda phage network (Mcadams and Shapiro, 1995), pathogenesis and clearance mechanism of dengue virus (Aslam et al., 2014), MAL-Associated network of Cerebral Malaria (Ahmad et al., 2012) and the role of OGT in Cancer progression (Saeed et al., 2016).

Network Analysis

Graph-theoretic approaches have been successfully applied on large protein networks (Barabasi and Oltvai, 2004; Stelniec-Klotz et al., 2012). The state graph can be further analyzed using network analysis techniques in terms of graph connectivity (Junker and Schreiber, 2011) by sorting it on the basis of maximum betweenness centrality (Freeman, 1977). The states with higher betweenness centralities represent higher chances of their occurrences. This may in terms of biological phenomenon represent the entities with frequent expressions. The qualitative states in the model with high betweenness centralities are compared to the rest of the state space in order to identify most favorable cycle (Tareen et al., 2015; Saeed et al., 2016).

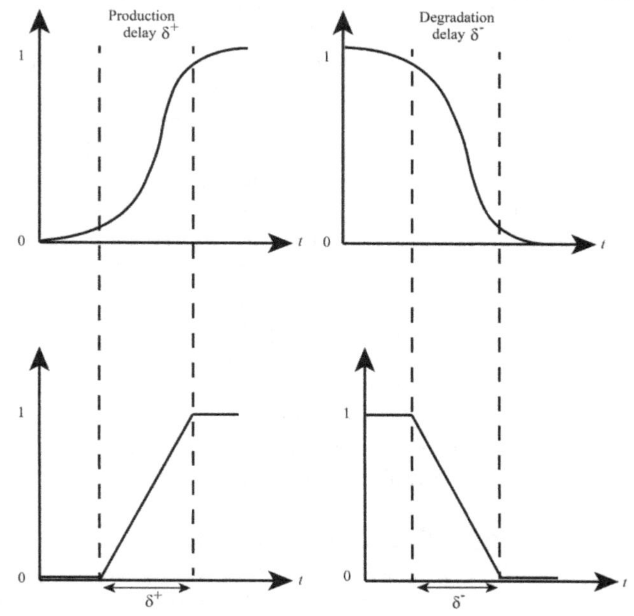

FIGURE 4 | Time delays in expression evolution Ahmad et al. (2012). The evolution of qualitative states is characterized by time delays: δ^+ represents production delay or time required to pass from low level to next high level whereas δ^- is the time delay required for a gene to pass from high level to low level (degradation delay).

Hybrid Modeling

René Thomas' framework provides useful insights into the discrete qualitative behavior of a biological system. However, naturally, the expression levels of proteins evolve in a continuous manner. Hybrid modeling combines discrete changes of a system with continuous changes (differential equation) in a single formalism Bio-Linear Hybrid Automaton (Bio-LHA) has been proposed for the hybrid modeling of qualitative BRNs (Ahmad et al., 2007). Bio-LHA uses time delays along with continuous variables (clocks) to compute production and degradation time of gene expressions. Production (δ^+) or degradation (δ^-) delay is the time required for a gene expression to reach from a lower level to a higher level or vice versa (**Figure 4**). In this approach, a clock variable (h) is associated with each entity which is initially set to zero and it evolves with rate 1 when the expression evolves. A clock is reset when it measures a production or degradation delay as shown in **Figure 5**. Hybrid model checking tool such as HyTech (Henzinger et al., 1997) can be used to infer the values of delays in the form of linear delay constraints for behaviors (paths toward stable states and cycles) observed in the qualitative model. Invariance kernel (Ahmad et al., 2007; Ahmad and Roux, 2010) represents cycles in the hybrid models which can also be characterized with delay constraints. These delay constraints are further converted into the relation matrix in order to find constraints between any two types of delays (production or degradation) of all entities. This modeling approach has been successfully applied to model a variety of BRNs (Ahmad et al., 2007, 2008, 2012; Ahmad, 2009; Aslam et al., 2014; Bibi et al., 2016).

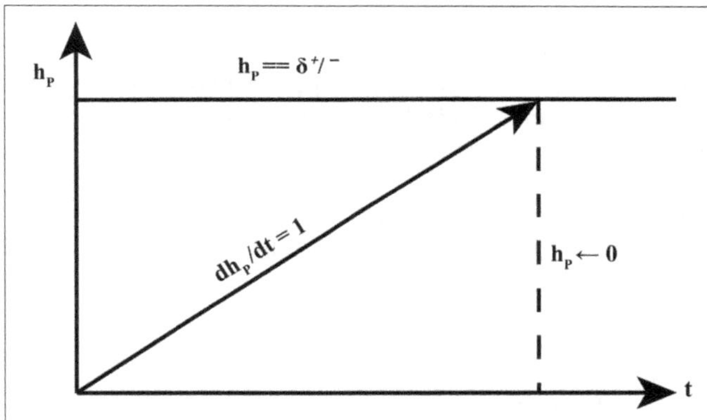

FIGURE 5 | The production and degradation time delays $\delta^{+/-}$ associated with an entity p. The clock h_p measures the production or degradation time delays.

RESULTS

Parameters Inference

To construct qualitative model of the mTOR associated BRN, SMBioNet tool has been employed to correctly estimate logical parameters according to biologicalobservations in literature (Chen et al., 2010; Zoncu et al., 2011; Laplante and Sabatini, 2012). This tool takes Computation Tree Logic (CTL) formulas representing biological observations and BRN as inputs and selects those sets of parameters which verify these formulas. In BRN modeling these parameters are used to incorporate behaviors in the form of paths, cycles and stable states (SS) as specified in the CTL formulas (**Table 1**). Formula 1 in **Table 1** represents that in a particular homeostatic behavior (represented by CTL operator *E*) all entities with 0 expression levels after next qualitative state (represented by CTL operator *X*) finally reach the same expression levels in future (represented by CTL operator *F*). Formula 2 represents the biological observation that the overexpression of PTEN, FOXO, PI3K, mTORC1, and inactivation of Akt gradually leads to (represented by CTL operator ⇒) a steady carcinogenic state (represented by CTL operators *F* and *G*) with the overexpression of Akt, mTORC1, mTORC2, PI3K, and inactivation of PTEN and FOXO. The effect of PTEN inhibition on Akt/mTORC1 pathway eventually leads to a SS where FOXO and PTEN are not expressed. This behavior is encoded by Formula 3. On the basis of CTL formulas, SMBiogenerated eight sets of logical parameters for mTOR associated BRN (see **Supplementary Files 1, 2**).

Selection of a Qualitative Model

The eight qualitative models of these sets were further analyzed for cycle(s) and SS(s) using GENOTECH tool. Almost all the parameter sets provide comparable results, revealing similar cycles and SS(s). First four models were selected on the basis of biological plausible SS $(1, 0, 1, 1, 1, 0)$ representing the activation and inactivation states of entities in order of PI3K, PTEN, mTORC2, Akt, mTORC1 and FOXO, respectively. This SS represents the activation of PI3K, mTORC2, Akt and mTORC1 along with the inactivation of PTEN and FOXO. Subsequently, these 4 models were further compared for the logical parameter values which are coherent with biological observations. The set of logical parameters for this model (**Supplementary File 3**) is given in the last column of **Table 2**. The selected model (**Figure 3**) also shows eight cycles along with one SS $(1, 0, 1, 1, 1, 0)$.

Several states lead the BRN directly into SS which represent critical divergence toward disease. All such states that eventually progress toward deadlock state do not possess functional PTEN or FOXO while having cellular proliferatory elements fully activated, e.g., (1,1,1,1,1,0), (1,0,1,1,1,1) as represented in (**Figure 6**). Thus, the down regulation of these tumor suppressor genes (PTEN and FOXO) bring this deadlock (SS) where no regulator is present to perform its function. The states (1,0,1,1,0,0), (0,0,1,1,1,0), (1,0,0,1,1,0), and (1,0,1,0,1,0) with temporary inhibition of PI3K, mTORC2, Akt, or mTORC1 are restrained in proceeding states resulting in their full and uncontrollable activation. This impact of tumor suppressor gene can be observed in cyclic state (1,1,1,1,1,0) that progresses into (0,1,1,1,1,0) (**Figure 6**) where PI3K is down-regulated through the inhibitory effect of PTEN to slow down further increase in cell mass and number. So the pre-occupation of PTEN is desired to recover the system into homeostatic state (0,1,1,1,1,0) that otherwise could divert into SS (1,0,1,1,1,0). The selected cyclic trajectory along with its respective constraints is given in **Figure 8**, specifies the stay conditions for each cyclic state and its violation would activate counter mechanism of autophagic inhibition by mTORC1 leading to cancer.

Validation of Qualitative Model with ASP

We applied exhaustive model-checking to validate the qualitative model of this study as proposed in Ben Abdallah et al. (2015). In this approach, the authors present a logical approach (using

TABLE 1 | CTL formulas.

No.	CTL Formulas	References
1	$(PI3K = 0 \wedge FOXO = 0 \wedge mTORC2 = 0, \wedge Akt = 0 \wedge mTORC1 = 0 \wedge PTEN = 0) \rightarrow, (EX(EF(PI3K = 0 \wedge FOXO = 0 \wedge mTORC2 = 0 \wedge Akt = 0 \wedge mTORC1 = 0)))$	Zoncu et al., 2011
2	$(PTEN = 1 \wedge FOXO = 1 \wedge Akt = 0 \wedge PI3K = 1 \wedge mTORC1 = 1 \wedge mTORC2 = 1) \rightarrow (EF(AG(Akt = 1 \wedge PTEN = 0 \wedge FOXO = 0 \wedge mTORC1 = 1 \wedge mTORC2 = 1 \wedge PI3K = 1)))$	Carracedo and Pandolfi, 2008; Chen et al., 2010; Zoncu et al., 2011; Laplante and Sabatini, 2012
3	$(PI3K = 1 \wedge FOXO = 0 \wedge Akt = 1 \wedge mTORC1 = 1) \rightarrow (EF(AG(Akt = 1 \wedge FOXO = 0 \wedge PTEN = 0)))$	Carracedo and Pandolfi, 2008; Zoncu et al., 2011

These CTL formulas are used in SMBioNet tool to infer the set of logical parameters. Formula 1 is designed to observe homeostasis while the other two formulas are used for observing stable steady state(s).

TABLE 2 | Selection of logical parameters.

Parameter	Resource(s)	Range of Values	Selected Parameters
K_{PI3K}	{}	0	0
K_{PI3K}	{mTORC1}	0,1	1
K_{PI3K}	{PTEN}	0,1	1
K_{PI3K}	{mTORC1, PTEN}	0,1	1
K_{PTEN}	{}	0	0
K_{PTEN}	{PI3K}	1	1
K_{mTORC2}	{}	0	0
K_{mTORC2}	{FOXO}	0,1	1
K_{mTORC2}	{mTORC1}	1	1
K_{mTORC2}	{PI3K}	0,1	1
K_{mTORC2}	{FOXO, mTORC1}	1	1
K_{mTORC2}	{FOXO, PI3K}	0,1	1
K_{mTORC2}	{mTORC1, PI3K}	1	1
K_{mTORC2}	{FOXO, mTORC1, PI3K}	1	1
K_{Akt}	{}	0	0
K_{Akt}	{mTORC2}	0	0
K_{Akt}	{PI3K}	0	0
K_{Akt}	{mTORC2, PI3K}	1	1
K_{mTORC1}	{}	0	0
K_{mTORC1}	{Akt}	0,1	0
K_{mTORC1}	{FOXO}	1	1
K_{mTORC1}	{Akt, FOXO}	1	1
K_{FOXO}	{}	0	0
K_{FOXO}	{Akt}	1	1
K_{FOXO}	{mTORC1}	0	0
K_{FOXO}	{Akt, mTORC1}	1	1

This table describes the ranges of logical parameter values. Some parameters are fixed to single values 0 or 1 based on biological observations. The last column lists one of the eight selected parameter sets generated by SMBioNet.

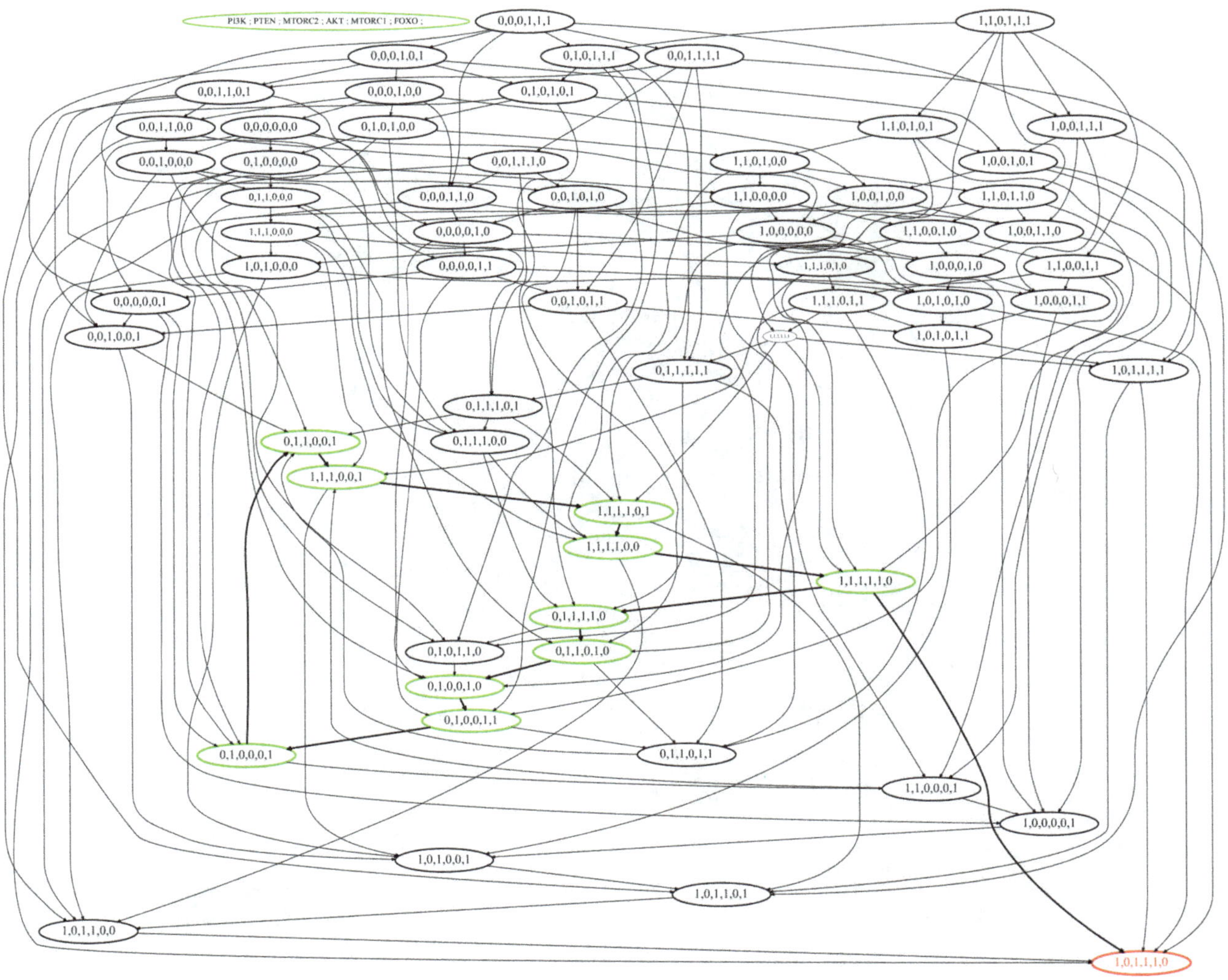

FIGURE 6 | State graph of the mTOR-associated BRN. Nodes of the state graph represent the states of the BRN and edges between states represent the evolution of states. A state in this graph shows the expressions of the entities PI3K, PTEN, mTORC2, Akt, mTORC1, and FOXO respectively. The stable steady state (1,0,1,1,1,0) represents high expression levels of all entities except tumor suppressors. Cycle having maximum betweenness centrality is represented in green color with bold arrows, also showing bifurcation toward stable state (1,0,1,1,1,0).

the Answer Set Programming language (ASP) Baral, 2003) to simulate and exhaustively analyze the dynamics of multivalued biological regulatory networks. The ASP method searches the attractor basins (stable states) which the region from which it is not possible to exit. By translating the model of **Figure 3** to an automata network (**Supplementary Files 6–9**) and giving it as an input to the method of Ben Abdallah et al. (2015), we found that the set of all the attractor basins is reduced to a single stable state: $(PI3K = 1, AKT = 1, PTEN = 0, MTORC2 = 1, FOXO = 0, MTORC1 = 1)$. This result is effectively coherent with the qualitative model given in **Figure 6**.

Selection of Cycle

Since the model shows eight cycles therefore it is important to identify the most probable biological cycle. Thus, on the basis of betweenness centrality a cycle was computed by using Cytoscape tool (Shannon et al., 2003) that sorts all the states on the basis of their betweenness centralities (Freeman, 1977; Tareen et al., 2015), as presented in **Figure 7** (**Supplementary File 4**). The nodes with larger diameter represent states with higher betweenness centrality. The cycle with maximum betweenness centrality: $(1,1,1,0,0,1) \rightarrow (1,1,1,1,0,1) \rightarrow (1,1,1,1,0,0) \rightarrow (1,1,1,1,1,0) \rightarrow (0,1,1,1,1,0) \rightarrow (0,1,1,0,1,0) \rightarrow (0,1,0,0,1,0) \rightarrow (0,1,0,0,1,1) \rightarrow (0,1,0,0,0,1) \rightarrow (0,1,1,0,0,1) \rightarrow (1,1,1,0,0,1)$ shows oscilation of all entities except PTEN. The cycle reveals that the constant activation of PTEN is required for homoeostasis. Any diversion from this cycle would either lead toward carcinogenic SS (1,0,1,1,1,0). All the cyclic trajectories represented in **Figure 6** show expression of PTEN that positively regulates PI3K and enforces the model to

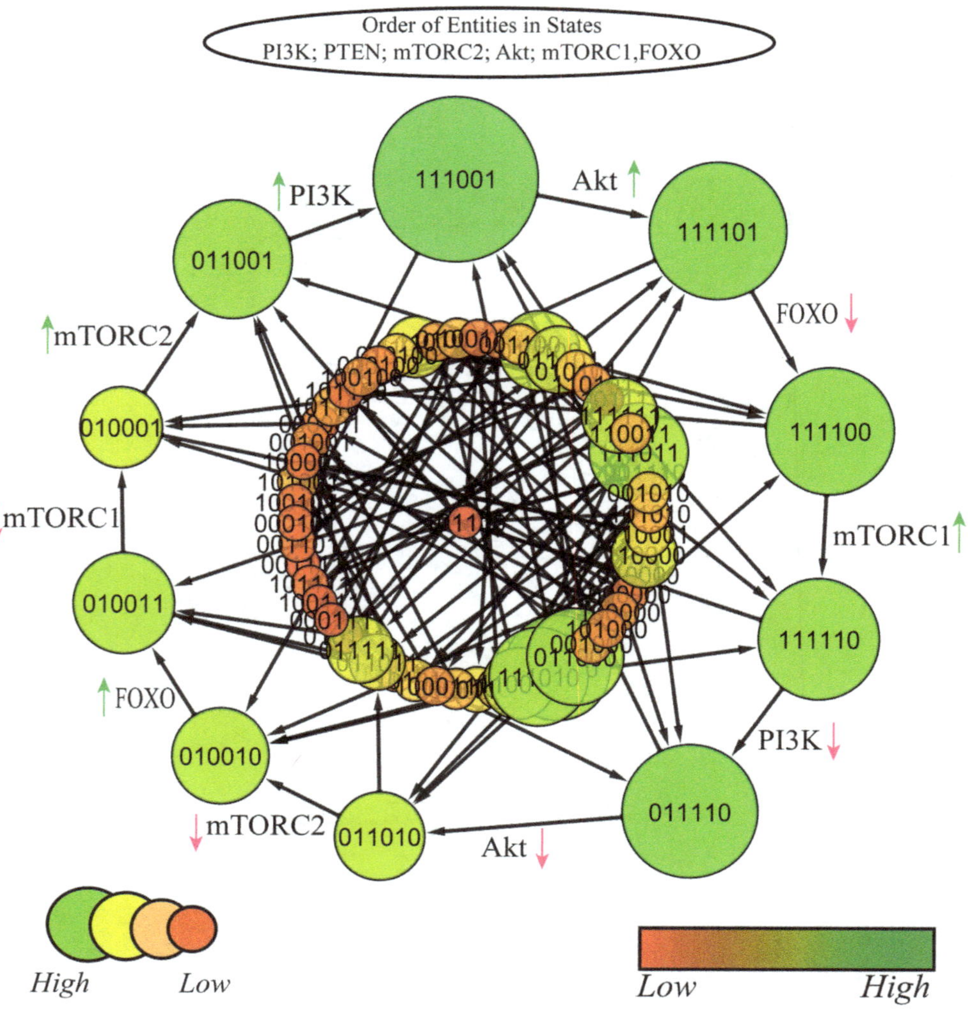

FIGURE 7 | State graph of mTOR associated BRN: size and color of nodes are scaled on the basis of betweenness centrality, larger nodes represent higher centralities with variable shades of green color (darker the color, higher is the centrality). The graph comprises of 64 states and 192 edges. Cycle with maximum betweenness centrality is extracted out at top layer. Red and green arrows represent degradation and production of entities, respectively.

remain in homeostasis. On the contrary, uncontrolled expression of PI3K and subsequent stimulation of cellular proliferative machinery mainly Akt and mTORC1 would either cause diabetic disorders or more severe circumstances like oncogenesis.

Hybrid Model

The cycle in **Figure 7** shows homeostatic biological regulation of entities in the form of the switching of their low and high expression levels. In the cycle, the stable high expression of PTEN gene is revealed as a mandatory condition in all the states to maintain homeostasis (represented by 1 expression level in all cyclic states) while the expression of other entities oscillate in relation to each other. The Bio-LHA model in **Figure 8** of this cycle was implemented in HyTech tool (**Supplementary File 5**) in order to predict its underlying causality relations of delays by analyzing the invariance kernel (Ahmad et al., 2008). The invariance kernel represents a set of viable cyclic trajectories in the state space of the Bio-LHA. Delay constraints characterizing the invariance kernel of the selected cycle were computed by HyTech tool (**Table 3**). In **Table 3**, the notation π is used to represent the sum of production and degradation delays as period (Ahmad, 2009). Conjunctions of all these constraints (1–9) constitute a necessary and sufficient condition for the existence of the invariance kernel and hence the qualitative cycle. Violation of any constraint would result in a null invariance kernel and eventually the qualitative cycle will no more exist. It is therefore sufficient that all the constraints should be valid (true) for the existence of the invariance kernel or qualitative cycle. For example, in **Table 3**, constraint 1 ($\delta^{+}_{FOXO} \leq |\delta^{-}_{mTORC1}| + |\delta^{-}_{Akt}|$) shows that the production (activation) of FOXO is required before the degradation of Akt and mTORC1 and hence constitute a necessary condition for cycle (homeostasis). Again constraint 2 establishes another necessary condition for the existence of

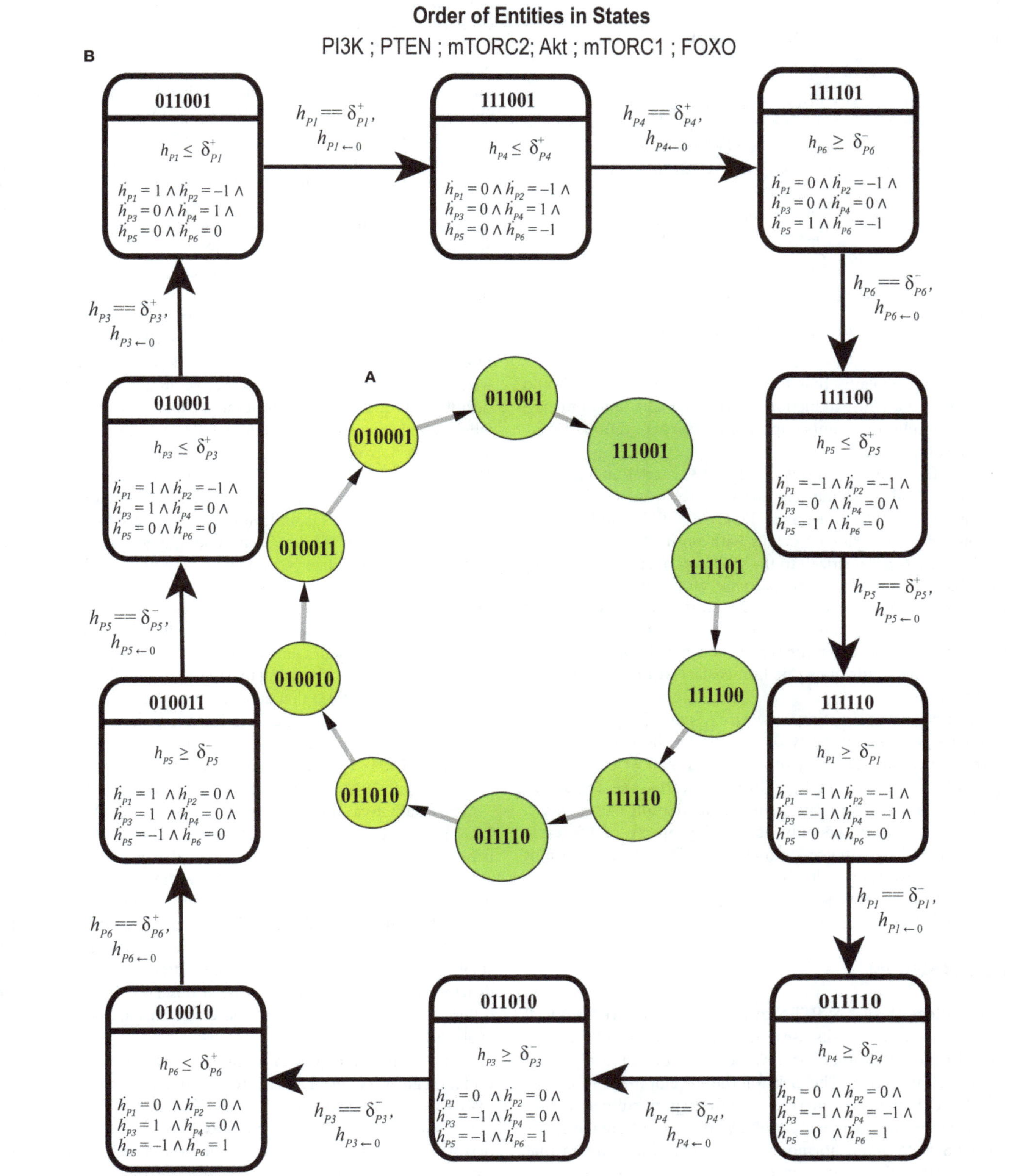

FIGURE 8 | (A) Discrete representation of cycle selected on the basis of centrality, larger circles represent higher centrality states. **(B)** Bio Linear Hybrid Automata of selected cycle: Each square symbol represents a hybrid location by capturing the discrete expression dynamics (top) and the continuous evolution of all clocks. Clock value *h* resets to 0 after each transition. P1 = PI3K, P2 = PTEN, P3 = mTORC2, P4 = Akt, P5 = mTORC1, P6 = FOXO.

TABLE 3 | Delay constraints.

Number	Delay Constraints
1	$\delta^{+}_{FOXO} \leq \vert\delta^{-}_{mTORC1}\vert + \vert\delta^{-}_{Akt}\vert$
2	$\vert\delta^{-}_{FOXO}\vert \leq \delta^{+}_{Akt} + \delta^{+}_{mTORC1}$
3	$\vert\delta^{-}_{PI3K}\vert \leq \delta^{+}_{mTORC1} + \vert\delta^{-}_{Akt}\vert$
4	$\pi(FOXO) + \vert\delta^{-}_{PI3K}\vert \leq, \pi(Akt) + \pi(mTORC1)$
5	$\pi(FOXO) + \pi(PI3K) \leq \pi(Akt) + \pi(mTORC1) + \delta^{+}_{mTORC2}$
6	$\delta^{+}_{FOXO} + \vert\delta^{-}_{PI3K}\vert \leq \pi(mTORC1) + \vert\delta^{-}_{Akt}\vert$
7	$\pi(FOXO) + \pi(PI3K) \leq \pi(mTORC2) + \delta^{+}_{Akt} + \delta^{+}_{mTORC1}$
8	$\delta^{+}_{PI3K} + \delta^{+}_{FOXO} \leq \delta^{+}_{Akt} + \pi(mTORC2)$
9	$\pi(PI3K) + \delta^{+}_{FOXO} \leq \delta^{+}_{Akt} + \pi(mTORC2) + \delta^{+}_{mTORC1}$

Delay Constraints of the selected cycle characterizing its invariance kernel. δ^{+} represents production (activation) delay while δ^{-} represents degradation (inhibition) delay. Notation $\pi(e)$ refers to the sum of production and degradation delays of the entity e.

the cycle that explains that the degradation of FOXO should occur earlier than the production of mTORC1 and Akt. Similarly, other remaining constraints imposes necessary conditions for the existence of the cycle.

From the delay constraints in **Table 3**, a relation matrix is derived in **Table 4** containing pairwise relations of delays of the entities FOXO, PI3K, mTORC1, mTORC2, and Akt. A relation between a pair of delays with both $\leq$ and $\geq$ reveals that the cycle is desensitized to the violation of such constraints. The table contains only one pairwise constraint between the degradation delays of Akt and mTORC2. It is important to note that these relationships are enforcing homeostasis represented by the qualitative cycle. From the results, it can be implicated that if cellular systems tends to escape homeostasis it may lead toward pathogenesis.

The only pairwise relation between δ^{-}_{Akt} and δ^{-}_{mTORC2} (**Table 4**) reveals a significant property of the selected homeostatic cycle where the degradation delay of Akt is less than or equal to the degradation delay of mTORC2. In other words, the degradatin of AKT occurs at faster rate than the degrdation of mTORC2. Interestingly, this is the only observed property of the cycle that enforces its existence dramatically. Thus, this constraint provides a governing rule that if violated may bifurcate the trajectory toward stable steady state (1,0,1,1,1,0) (represented by red colored state in **Figure 6**).

DISCUSSION

The pathological roles of PTEN, mTOR, and Akt have been well established in different diseases including diabetes and different types of cancer (Altomare and Testa, 2005; Zoncu et al., 2011; Hopkins et al., 2014). The risk for the development of cancer in diabetic patients is increased with hyperinsulinemia and oxidative stress (Vigneri et al., 2009). With nutrient uptake, levels of growth factors and hormones rise in the blood stream that triggers certain biochemical processes. Feeding promotes insulin levels in the bloodstream that binds to its particular receptors causing stimulation of PI3K downstream signaling. Deregulation of PI3k/Akt mediated mTOR signaling pathway contributes to insulin resistance and associated conditions (Harrington et al., 2004; Shah et al., 2004). PI3K tends to stimulate mTORC2 and both of these proteins initiate activation of Akt (Alessi et al., 1997; Sarbassov et al., 2005). Subsequently, Akt favors mTORC1 activation by phosphorylating TSC1/TSC2 complex (Zoncu et al., 2011). mTORC1 is able to impair insulin signaling via its substrates S6K1 which then phosphorylates serine residues of IRS1 causing downregulation of PI3K/Akt pathway (Harrington et al., 2004; Shah et al., 2004). In this way, mTORC1 activity can contribute to insulin resistance. Therefore, it is important to identify therapeutically favorable regulatory event in mTOR-associated BRN that plays a major role in triggering pathological signaling cascade (Vigneri et al., 2009).

Formal methods are widely applicable for the correctness of ICT Systems due to their computational ability of rigorous testing. For the last few decades, formal methods have been successfully used for the modeling and verification of complex biological systems (Kitano, 2002). Kinetic Logic formalism is a well-known approach for the qualitative modeling of a BRN that deciphers its qualitative dynamics in the form of a directed graph, where a node represents a qualitative state and an edge represents an evolution from one state to its successor state (Thomas, 1979; Thomas and d'Ari, 1990; Thomas et al., 1995). Since the qualitative model ignores the time in the evolution of expression levels, a hybrid model is built in order to ensure that evolutions due to activation or inhibition are taking place after production and degradation delays (Ahmad et al., 2007, 2008; Ahmad, 2009). Of course, these delays are un-known and are treated as unvalued parameters in the hybrid model. Consequently, any behavior captured in the qualitative model (cycle or path) can be temporally verified against the production and degradation time delay parameters by using the hybrid model checker HyTech (Henzinger et al., 1997) that automatically synthesizes the values of parameters (delays) in the form linear parametric constraints. Moreover, this approach has been successfully applied on a variety of BRNs for the temporal analysis of their behaviors (Ahmad et al., 2012; Aslam et al., 2014; Saeed et al., 2016).

The qualitative model (state graph) of the mTOR-associated BRN predicted cycles and a stable state. The most biologically probable cycle was selected that shows the oscillation of PI3K, mTORC2, Akt, mTORC1, and FOXO while PTEN is constantly expressed (level 1). On the other side, simultaneous deactivation of PTEN and FOXO along with the activation of Akt, PI3K, mTORC1 and mTORC2 tends to maintain the system in a stable state $(1, 0, 1, 1, 1, 0)$. The same pattern of activation and deactivation of entities has also been observed in diabetes and different types of cancers (Altomare and Testa, 2005; Hopkins et al., 2014).

Genes' expression goes through various levels (low and high) under regulatory mechanism to maintain homeostasis. The regulation of the expressions of PI3K is under the regulatory mechanism of PTEN and mTORC1 that has been found perturbed in almost all cancer types (Hopkins et al., 2014). Downregulated PTEN has deleterious impacts on cell cycle regulation, growth and survival. In the stable state of the qualitative model PTEN is downregulated while PI3K is found overexpressed. In recent studies, PTEN has been demonstrated to downregulate the activity of mTORC1 through various pathways

TABLE 4 | Relation matrix.

	δ^+_{FOXO}	$\lvert\delta^-_{FOXO}\rvert$	δ^+_{PI3K}	$\lvert\delta^-_{PI3K}\rvert$	δ^+_{mTORC1}	δ^-_{mTORC1}	δ^+_{mTORC2}	$\lvert\delta^-_{mTORC2}\rvert$	δ^+_{Akt}	$\lvert\delta^-_{Akt}\rvert$
δ^+_{FOXO}	=									
$\lvert\delta^-_{FOXO}\rvert$	≤, ≥	=								
$\lvert\delta^-_{PI3K}\rvert$	≤, ≥	≤, ≥	=							
δ^+_{PI3K}	≤, ≥	≤, ≥	≤, ≥	=						
δ^+_{mTORC1}	≤, ≥	≤, ≥	≤, ≥	≤, ≥	≤, ≥	=				
$\lvert\delta^-_{mTORC1}\rvert$	≤, ≥	≤, ≥	≤, ≥	≤, ≥	≤, ≥	=				
δ^+_{mTORC2}	≤, ≥	≤, ≥	≤, ≥	≤, ≥	≤, ≥	≤, ≥	=			
$\lvert\delta^-_{mTORC2}\rvert$	≤, ≥	≤, ≥	≤, ≥	≤, ≥	≤, ≥	≤, ≥	≤, ≥	=		
δ^+_{Akt}	≤, ≥	≤, ≥	≤, ≥	≤, ≥	≤, ≥	≤, ≥	≤, ≥	≤, ≥	=	
$\lvert\delta^-_{Akt}\rvert$	≤, ≥	≤, ≥	≤, ≥	≤, ≥	≤, ≥	≤, ≥	≤, ≥	≤	≤, ≥	=

Relation matrix of the selected cycle that shows the pairwise relationships of delays of the entities FOXO, PI3K, mTORC1, mTORC2 and Akt.

(Sonntag et al., 2012) which is also evident in the qualitative cycle. However, in the stable state of the qualitative model, PTEN is constantly downregulated and mTORC1 is thus overexpressed. These findings opens up various aspects of future exploration for the role of PTEN in hyperinsulinimia.

The hybrid model of the selected cycle predicted the time delays of the entities to maintain homeostasis. The pairwise relationships of delays suggest one unique pattern of faster Akt degradation than mTORC2 degradation for maintaining homoeostasis. It also suggests that therapeutics must be designed based on the fact that Akt must be cleared out of the system as soon as it performs its function along with keeping a slower degradation rate for mTORC2. This also eliminates the risk of prolong Akt activation that may hyper-activate downstream signaling cascade. Another important fact that is perceived through this constraint relationship is that mTORC1 has to be suppressed (under cancerous circumstances) to reduce its inhibitory effect upon mTORC2 which would prevent early degradation of mTORC2 as compared to Akt. This trend would keep an equilibrium between cellular proliferative elements PI3K, Akt, mTORC1, and that of apoptotic factors (e.g., FOXO). Based on these observations, further wet-lab exploration for the roles of PTEN, mTORC1, mTORC2, and Akt is required in the perspective of targeting cancer cell proliferation.

CONCLUSION

In last few decades, understanding of the glucose metabolism in both proliferating cancer and normal cells is studied extensively. PI3K, Akt and mTOR play significant roles in metabolism and their deregulation can lead to different cancers. In this context, the regulatory network of these entities has been modeled and analyzed to explore its dynamics. Discrete and hybrid models have been constructed to predict the qualitative and timed dependent behaviors. In the qualitative model, cycles representing homeostasis and a stable state representing the disease state have been predicted. The most biologically probable cycle represents that the expression levels of the entities except PTEN should oscillate to maintain homeostasis. Moreover, the cycle states show the constant expression (level 1) of PTEN. On the other hand in the stable state, PI3K, mTORC2, Akt, and mTORC1 are always overexpressed while PTEN and FOXO are constantly down regulated which can ultimately lead to cancer. The hybrid model revealed the time delay constraints of the most biologically probable cycle. Further analysis of the constraints predicted the pairwise relations between the production and degradation time delays of all the entities. One relation highlighted that during homeostasis, the inhibition time delay of Akt is less than the inhibition time delay of mTORC2. In conclusion, our observations characterize that during homeostasis, Akt is degraded with a faster rate than mTORC2 which further suggests that this inhibition of Akt along with the activation of mTORC2 may be exploited for a better therapeutic strategy against cancer.

AUTHORS CONTRIBUTIONS

ZB and JA conceived and designed the experiments, performed the experiments, analyzed the data, contributed reagents/materials/analysis tools, wrote the paper, prepared figures and/or tables, reviewed drafts of the paper. AS and RP analyzed the data, prepared figures and/or tables, wrote the paper, reviewed drafts of the paper. TS, AA, HJ, and SU analyzed the data, reviewed drafts of the paper, technical Support. EB, and OR analyzed the data, contributed reagents/materials/analysis tools, wrote the paper, reviewed drafts of the paper.

SUPPLEMENTARY MATERIAL

Supplementary File 1 | Qualitative models with logical parameters (SMBioNet code).

Supplementary File 2 | SMBioNet output file.

Supplementary File 3 | mTOR BRN (implemented in GENOTECH).

Supplementary File 4 | Cytoscape file (State graph sorted on the basis of betweenness centrality).

Supplementary File 5 | HyTech input file.

Supplementary File 6 | mTOR model represented with Automata Network (AN) formalism.

Supplementary File 7 | mTOR Automata network figure.

Supplementary File 8 | Automata Network (AN) file of mTOR BRN in Answer Set Programming (ASP).

Supplementary File 9 | Answer Set Programming (ASP) results.

REFERENCES

Ahmad, J. (2009). *Modélisation Hybride et Analyse des Dynamiques des Réseaux de Régulations Biologiques en Tenant Compte des délais*, Ph.D. thesis, Ecole Centrale de Nantes, Nantes.
Publisher: Ecole Centrale de Nantes

Ahmad, J., Bernot, G., Comet, J.-P., Lime, D., and Roux, O. (2007). Hybrid modelling and dynamical analysis of gene regulatory networks with delays. *ComPlexUs* 3, 231–251. doi: 10.1159/000110010

Ahmad, J., Niazi, U., Mansoor, S., Siddique, U., and Bibby, J. (2012). Formal modeling and analysis of the mal-associated biological regulatory network: insight into cerebral malaria. *PLoS ONE* 7:e33532. doi: 10.1371/journal.pone.0033532

Ahmad, J., and Roux, O. (2010). Invariance kernel of biological regulatory networks. *Int. J, Data Mining Bioinformat.* 4, 553–570. doi: 10.1504/IJDMB.2010.035900

Ahmad, J., Roux, O., Bernot, G., and Comet, J.-P. (2008). Analysing formal models of genetic regulatory networks with delays. *Int. J. Bioinformat. Res. Appli.* 4, 240–262. doi: 10.1504/IJBRA.2008.019573

Alessi, D. R., James, S. R., Downes, C. P., Holmes, A. B., Gaffney, P. R., Reese, C. B., et al. (1997). Characterization of a 3-phosphoinositide-dependent protein kinase which phosphorylates and activates protein kinase bα. *Curr. Biol.* 7, 261–269. doi: 10.1016/S0960-9822(06)00122-9

Altomare, D. A., and Testa, J. R. (2005). Perturbations of the akt signaling pathway in human cancer. *Oncogene* 24, 7455–7464. doi: 10.1038/sj.onc.1209085

Aslam, B., Ahmad, J., Ali, A., Paracha, R. Z., Tareen, S. H. K., Niazi, U., et al. (2014). On the modelling and analysis of the regulatory network of dengue virus pathogenesis and clearance. *Computat. Biol. Chem.* 53, 277–291. doi: 10.1016/j.compbiolchem.2014.10.003

Avruch, J., Hara, K., Lin, Y., Liu, M., Long, X., Ortiz-Vega, S., et al. (2006). Insulin and amino-acid regulation of mtor signaling and kinase activity through the rheb gtpase. *Oncogene* 25, 6361–6372. doi: 10.1038/sj.onc.1209882

Barabasi, A.-L., and Oltvai, Z. N. (2004). Network biology: understanding the cell's functional organization. *Nat. Rev. Genet.* 5, 101–113. doi: 10.1038/nrg1272

Baral, C. (2003). *Knowledge Representation, Reasoning and Declarative Problem Solving*. Cambridge: Cambridge University Press.

Ben Abdallah, E., Folschette, M., Roux, O., and Magnin, M. (2015). "Exhaustive analysis of dynamical properties of biological regulatory networks with answer set programming," in *Bioinformatics and Biomedicine (BIBM), 2015 IEEE International Conference on* (IEEE), 281–285.

Bernot, G., Cassez, F., Comet, J.-P., Delaplace, F., Müller, C., and Roux, O. (2007). Semantics of biological regulatory networks. *Elect. Notes Theor. Comput. Sci.* 180, 3–14. doi: 10.1016/j.entcs.2004.01.038

Bernot, G., Comet, J.-P., Richard, A., and Guespin, J. (2004). Application of formal methods to biological regulatory networks: extending thomas' asynchronous logical approach with temporal logic. *J. Theor. Biol.* 229, 339–347. doi: 10.1016/j.jtbi.2004.04.003

Bibi, Z., Ahmad, J., Ali, A., Siddiqa, A., Shahzad, S., Tareen, S. H., et al. (2016). On the modeling and analysis of the biological regulatory network of nf-{\kappa} κ b activation in hiv-1 infection. *Complex Adapt. Syst. Model.* 4:1. doi: 10.1186/s40294-015-0013-4

Carracedo, A., and Pandolfi, P. (2008). The pten–pi3k pathway: of feedbacks and cross-talks. *Oncogene* 27, 5527–5541. doi: 10.1038/onc.2008.247

Carracedo, A., Salmena, L., and Pandolfi, P. P. (2008). Snapshot: Pten signaling pathways. *Cell* 133:550. doi: 10.1016/j.cell.2008.04.023

Chen, C.-C., Jeon, S.-M., Bhaskar, P. T., Nogueira, V., Sundararajan, D., Tonic, I., et al. (2010). Foxos inhibit mtorc1 and activate akt by inducing the expression of sestrin3 and rictor. *Develop. Cell* 18, 592–604. doi: 10.1016/j.devcel.2010.03.008

De Jong, H. (2002). Modeling and simulation of genetic regulatory systems: a literature review. *J. Comput. Biol.* 9, 67–103. doi: 10.1089/10665270252833208

De Jong, H., Gouzé, J.-L., Hernandez, C., Page, M., Sari, T., and Geiselmann, J. (2004). Qualitative simulation of genetic regulatory networks using piecewise-linear models. *Bull. Math. Biol.* 66, 301–340. doi: 10.1016/j.bulm.2003.08.010

Dibble, C. C., Asara, J. M., and Manning, B. D. (2009). Characterization of rictor phosphorylation sites reveals direct regulation of mtor complex 2 by s6k1. *Mol. Cell. Biol.* 29, 5657–5670. doi: 10.1128/MCB.00735-09

Eng, C. (2003). Pten: one gene, many syndromes. *Hum. Mutat.* 22, 183–198. doi: 10.1002/humu.10257

Engelman, J. A., Luo, J., and Cantley, L. C. (2006). The evolution of phosphatidylinositol 3-kinases as regulators of growth and metabolism. *Nat. Rev. Genet.* 7, 606–619. doi: 10.1038/nrg1879

Freeman, L. C. (1977). A set of measures of centrality based on betweenness. *Sociometry* 35–41. doi: 10.2307/3033543

Glass, L., and Kauffman, S. A. (1973). The logical analysis of continuous, non-linear biochemical control networks. *J. Theor. Biol.* 39, 103–129. doi: 10.1016/0022-5193(73)90208-7

Guertin, D. A., and Sabatini, D. M. (2007). Defining the role of mtor in cancer. *Cancer Cell* 12, 9–22. doi: 10.1016/j.ccr.2007.05.008

Guertin, D. A., Stevens, D. M., Thoreen, C. C., Burds, A. A., Kalaany, N. Y., Moffat, J., et al. (2006). Ablation in mice of the mtorc components raptor, rictor, or mlst8 reveals that mtorc2 is required for signaling to akt-foxo and pkcα, but not s6k1. *Developmental Cell* 11, 859–871. doi: 10.1016/j.devcel.2006.10.007

Hara, K., Maruki, Y., Long, X., Yoshino, K.-I., Oshiro, N., Hidayat, S., et al. (2002). Raptor, a binding partner of target of rapamycin (tor), mediates tor action. *Cell* 110, 177–189. doi: 10.1016/S0092-8674(02)00833-4

Harrington, L. S., Findlay, G. M., Gray, A., Tolkacheva, T., Wigfield, S., Rebholz, H., et al. (2004). The tsc1-2 tumor suppressor controls insulin–pi3k signaling via regulation of irs proteins. *J. Cell Biol.* 166, 213–223. doi: 10.1083/jcb.200403069

Henzinger, T. A., Ho, P.-H., and Wong-Toi, H. (1997). "Hytech: a model checker for hybrid systems," in *International Conference on Computer Aided Verification* (Berlin; Heidelberg: Springer), 460–463.

Hopkins, B. D., Hodakoski, C., Barrows, D., Mense, S. M., and Parsons, R. E. (2014). Pten function: the long and the short of it. *Trends Biochem. Sci.* 39, 183–190. doi: 10.1016/j.tibs.2014.02.006

Inoki, K., Li, Y., Xu, T., and Guan, K.-L. (2003). Rheb gtpase is a direct target of tsc2 gap activity and regulates mtor signaling. *Genes Develop.* 17, 1829–1834. doi: 10.1101/gad.1110003

Inoki, K., Li, Y., Zhu, T., Wu, J., and Guan, K.-L. (2002). Tsc2 is phosphorylated and inhibited by akt and suppresses mtor signalling. *Nat Cell Biol.* 4, 648–657. doi: 10.1038/ncb839

Julien, L.-A., Carriere, A., Moreau, J., and Roux, P. P. (2010). mtorc1-activated s6k1 phosphorylates rictor on threonine 1135 and regulates mtorc2 signaling. *Mol. Cell. Biol.* 30, 908–921. doi: 10.1128/MCB.00601-09

Junker, B. H., and Schreiber, F. (2011). *Analysis of Biological Networks, Vol. 2.* Hoboken, NJ: John Wiley & Sons.

Kauffman, S. A. (1969). Metabolic stability and epigenesis in randomly constructed genetic nets. *J. Theor. Biol.* 22, 437–467. doi: 10.1016/0022-5193(69)90015-0

Kauffman, S. A. (1993). *The Origins of Order: Self-organization and Selection in Evolution*. New York, NY: Oxford University Press.

Khamzina, L., Veilleux, A., Bergeron, S., and Marette, A. (2005). Increased activation of the mammalian target of rapamycin pathway in liver and skeletal muscle of obese rats: possible involvement in obesity-linked insulin resistance. *Endocrinology* 146, 1473–1481. doi: 10.1210/en.2004-0921

Kim, D.-H., Sarbassov, D. D., Ali, S. M., King, J. E., Latek, R. R., Erdjument-Bromage, H., et al. (2002). mtor interacts with raptor to form a nutrient-sensitive complex that signals to the cell growth machinery. *Cell* 110, 163–175. doi: 10.1016/S0092-8674(02)00808-5

Kitano, H. (2002). Computational systems biology. *Nature* 420, 206–210. doi: 10.1038/nature01254

Laplante, M., and Sabatini, D. M. (2012). mtor signaling in growth control and disease. *Cell* 149, 274–293. doi: 10.1016/j.cell.2012.03.017

Lewin, B. (2000). *Genes seven*. Orford: Oxford University Press.

Li, D.-M., and Sun, H. (1997). Tepl, encoded by a candidate tumor suppressor locus, is a novel protein tyrosine phosphatase regulated by transforming growth factor β. *Cancer Res.* 57, 2124–2129.

Loewith, R., Jacinto, E., Wullschleger, S., Lorberg, A., Crespo, J. L., Bonenfant, D., et al. (2002). Two tor complexes, only one of which is rapamycin sensitive, have distinct roles in cell growth control. *Mol. Cell* 10, 457–468. doi: 10.1016/S1097-2765(02)00636-6

Ma, L., Chen, Z., Erdjument-Bromage, H., Tempst, P., and Pandolfi, P. P. (2005). Phosphorylation and functional inactivation of tsc2 by erk: implications for tuberous sclerosisand cancer pathogenesis. *Cell* 121, 179–193. doi: 10.1016/j.cell.2005.02.031

Manning, B. D., and Cantley, L. C. (2007). Akt/pkb signaling: navigating downstream. *Cell* 129, 1261–1274. doi: 10.1016/j.cell.2007.06.009

Manning, B. D., Tee, A. R., Logsdon, M. N., Blenis, J., and Cantley, L. C. (2002). Identification of the tuberous sclerosis complex-2 tumor suppressor gene product tuberin as a target of the phosphoinositide 3-kinase/akt pathway. *Mol. Cell* 10, 151–162. doi: 10.1016/S1097-2765(02)00568-3

Mcadams, H. H., and Shapiro, L. (1995). Circuit simulation of genetic networks. *Science* 269, 650–656. doi: 10.1126/science.7624793

Menon, S., and Manning, B. D. (2008). Common corruption of the mtor signaling network in human tumors. *Oncogene* 27, S43–S51. doi: 10.1038/onc.2009.352

Naldi, A., Remy, E., Thieffry, D., and Chaouiya, C. (2009). "A reduction of logical regulatory graphs preserving essential dynamical properties," in *International Conference on Computational Methods in Systems Biology* (Berlin; Heidelberg: Springer), 266–280.

Nojima, H., Tokunaga, C., Eguchi, S., Oshiro, N., Hidayat, S., Yoshino, K.-I., et al. (2003). The mammalian target of rapamycin (mtor) partner, raptor, binds the mtor substrates p70 s6 kinase and 4e-bp1 through their tor signaling (tos) motif. *J. Biol. Chem.* 278, 15461–15464. doi: 10.1074/jbc.C200665200

Paracha, R. Z., Ahmad, J., Ali, A., Hussain, R., Niazi, U., Tareen, S. H. K., et al. (2014). Formal modelling of toll like receptor 4 and jak/stat signalling pathways: insight into the roles of socs-1, interferon-β and proinflammatory cytokines in sepsis. *PLoS ONE* 9:e108466. doi: 10.1371/journal.pone.0108466

Pearce, L., Huang, X., Boudeau, J., Pawlowski, R., Wullschleger, S., Deak, M., et al. (2007). Identification of protor as a novel rictor-binding component of mtor complex-2. *Biochem. J.* 405, 513–522. doi: 10.1042/BJ20070540

Peres, S., and Jean-Paul, C. (2003). "Contribution of computational tree logic to biological regulatory networks: example from pseudomonas aeruginosa," in *Computational Methods in Systems Biology*, Vol. 2602, of *Lecture Notes in Computer Science*, ed C. Priami (Berlin;Heidelberg: Springer), 47–56.

Potter, C. J., Pedraza, L. G., and Xu, T. (2002). Akt regulates growth by directly phosphorylating tsc2. *Nat. Cell Biol.* 4, 658–665. doi: 10.1038/ncb840

Roux, P. P., Ballif, B. A., Anjum, R., Gygi, S. P., and Blenis, J. (2004). Tumor-promoting phorbol esters and activated ras inactivate the tuberous sclerosis tumor suppressor complex via p90 ribosomal s6 kinase. *Proc. Natl. Acad. Sci. U.S.A.* 101, 13489–13494. doi: 10.1073/pnas.0405659101

Saadatpour, A., Albert, R., and Reluga, T. C. (2013). A reduction method for boolean network models proven to conserve attractors. *SIAM J. Appl. Dyn. Syst.* 12, 1997–2011. doi: 10.1137/13090537X

Saeed, M. T., Ahmad, J., Kanwal, S., Holowatyj, A. N., Sheikh, I. A., Paracha, R. Z., et al. (2016). Formal modeling and analysis of the hexosamine biosynthetic pathway: role of o-linked n-acetylglucosamine transferase in oncogenesis and cancer progression. *PeerJ* 4:e2348. doi: 10.7717/peerj.2348

Sancak, Y., Thoreen, C. C., Peterson, T. R., Lindquist, R. A., Kang, S. A., Spooner, E., et al. (2007). Pras40 is an insulin-regulated inhibitor of the mtorc1 protein kinase. *Mol. Cell* 25, 903–915. doi: 10.1016/j.molcel.2007.03.003

Sarbassov, D. D., Ali, S. M., Kim, D.-H., Guertin, D. A., Latek, R. R., Erdjument-Bromage, H., et al. (2004). Rictor, a novel binding partner of mtor, defines a rapamycin-insensitive and raptor-independent pathway that regulates the cytoskeleton. *Curr. Biol.* 14, 1296–1302. doi: 10.1016/j.cub.2004.06.054

Sarbassov, D. D., Guertin, D. A., Ali, S. M., and Sabatini, D. M. (2005). Phosphorylation and regulation of akt/pkb by the rictor-mtor complex. *Science* 307, 1098–1101. doi: 10.1126/science.1106148

Schalm, S. S., Fingar, D. C., Sabatini, D. M., and Blenis, J. (2003). Tos motif-mediated raptor binding regulates 4e-bp1 multisite phosphorylation and function. *Curr. Biol.* 13, 797–806. doi: 10.1016/S0960-9822(03)00329-4

Schmelzle, T., and Hall, M. N. (2000). Tor, a central controller of cell growth. *Cell* 103, 253–262. doi: 10.1016/S0092-8674(00)00117-3

Shah, O. J., Wang, Z., and Hunter, T. (2004). Inappropriate activation of the tsc/rheb/mtor/s6k cassette induces irs1/2 depletion, insulin resistance, and cell survival deficiencies. *Curr. Biol.* 14, 1650–1656. doi: 10.1016/j.cub.2004.08.026

Shannon, P., Markiel, A., Ozier, O., Baliga, N. S., Wang, J. T., Ramage, D., et al. (2003). Cytoscape: a software environment for integrated models of biomolecular interaction networks. *Genome Res.* 13, 2498–2504. doi: 10.1101/gr.1239303

Somogyi, R., Fuhrman, S., Askenazi, M., and Wuensche, A. (1997). The gene expression matrix: toward the extraction of genetic network architectures. *Nonlinear Anal. Theory Methods Appl.* 30, 1815–1824. doi: 10.1016/S0362-546X(97)00217-4

Somogyi, R., and Sniegoski, C. (1996). Modeling the complexity of genetic networks: Understanding multigenic and pleiotropic regulation. *Complexity* 1, 45–63. doi: 10.1002/cplx.6130010612

Sonntag, A. G., Dalle Pezze, P., Shanley, D. P., and Thedieck, K. (2012). A modelling–experimental approach reveals insulin receptor substrate (irs)-dependent regulation of adenosine monosphosphate-dependent kinase (ampk) by insulin. *Febs J.* 279, 3314–3328. doi: 10.1111/j.1742-4658.2012.08582.x

Steck, P. A., Pershouse, M. A., Jasser, S. A., Yung, W. A., Lin, H., Ligon, A. H., et al. (1997). Identification of a candidate tumour suppressor gene, mmac1, at chromosome 10q23. 3 that is mutated in multiple advanced cancers. *Nat. Genet.* 15, 356–362. doi: 10.1038/ng0497-356

Stelniec-Klotz, I., Legewie, S., Tchernitsa, O., Witzel, F., Klinger, B., Sers, C., et al. (2012). Reverse engineering a hierarchical regulatory network downstream of oncogenic kras. *Mol. Syst. Biol.* 8:601. doi: 10.1038/msb.2012.32

Szallasi, Z., and Liang, S. (1998). Modeling the normal and neoplastic cell cycle with 'realistic boolean genetic networks': their application for understanding carcinogenesis and assessing therapeutic strategies. *Pac. Symp. Biocomput.* 3, 66–76.

Tareen, S. H. K., Ahmad, J., and Roux, O. (2015). Parametric linear hybrid automata for complex environmental systems modeling. *Front. Environ. Sci.* 3:47. doi: 10.3389/fenvs.2015.00047

Tee, A. R., Manning, B. D., Roux, P. P., Cantley, L. C., and Blenis, J. (2003). Tuberous sclerosis complex gene products, tuberin and hamartin, control mtor signaling by acting as a gtpase-activating protein complex toward rheb. *Curr. Biol.* 13, 1259–1268. doi: 10.1016/S0960-9822(03)00506-2

Thieffry, D., and Thomas, R. (1995). Dynamical behaviour of biological regulatory networks-ii. immunity control in bacteriophage lambda. *Bull. Math. Biol.* 57, 277–297.

Thobe, K., Sers, C., and Siebert, H. (2017). Unraveling the regulation of mtorc2 using logical modeling. *Cell Communic. Signal.* 15:6. doi: 10.1186/s12964-016-0159-5

Thomas, R. (1978). Logical analysis of systems comprising feedback loops. *J. Theor. Biol.* 73, 631–656. doi: 10.1016/0022-5193(78)90127-3

Thomas, R. (1979). Kinetic logic: a boolean approach to the analysis of complex regulatory systems. *Lecture Notes Biomath.* 29:507. doi: 10.1007/978-3-642-49321-8

Thomas, R. (1981). "On the relation between the logical structure of systems and their ability to generate multiple steady states or sustained oscillations," in *Numerical Methods in the Study of Critical Phenomena*, Vol. 9 of *Springer Series in Synergetics*, eds J. Dora, J. Demongeot, and B. Lacolle (Berlin; Heidelberg: Springer), 180–193.

Thomas, R., and d'Ari, R. (1990). *Biological Feedback*. Boca Raton, FL: CRC press.

Thomas, R., Thieffry, D., and Kaufman, M. (1995). Dynamical behaviour of biological regulatory networks–ii. biological role of feedback loops and practical use of the concept of the loop-characteristic state. *Bull. Math. Biol.* 57, 247–276. doi: 10.1007/BF02460618

Treins, C., Warne, P., Magnuson, M., Pende, M., and Downward, J. (2010). Rictor is a novel target of p70 s6 kinase-1. *Oncogene* 29, 1003–1016. doi: 10.1038/onc.2009.401

Tremblay, F., Brûlé, S., Um, S. H., Li, Y., Masuda, K., Roden, M., et al. (2007). Identification of irs-1 ser-1101 as a target of s6k1 in nutrient-and obesity-induced insulin resistance. *Proc. Natl. Acad. Sci. U.S.A.* 104, 14056–14061. doi: 10.1073/pnas.0706517104

Um, S. H., Frigerio, F., Watanabe, M., Picard, F., Joaquin, M., Sticker, M., et al. (2004). Absence of s6k1 protects against age-and diet-induced obesity while enhancing insulin sensitivity. *Nature* 431, 200–205. doi: 10.1038/nature02866

Vigneri, P., Frasca, F., Sciacca, L., Pandini, G., and Vigneri, R. (2009). Diabetes and cancer. *Endocrine Related Cancer* 16, 1103–1123. doi: 10.1677/ERC-09-0087

Vivanco, I., Palaskas, N., Tran, C., Finn, S. P., Getz, G., Kennedy, N. J., et al. (2007). Identification of the jnk signaling pathway as a functional target of the tumor suppressor pten. *Cancer Cell* 11, 555–569. doi: 10.1016/j.ccr.2007.04.021

Wullschleger, S., Loewith, R., and Hall, M. N. (2006). Tor signaling in growth and metabolism. *Cell* 124, 471–484. doi: 10.1016/j.cell.2006.01.016

Wullschleger, S., Loewith, R., Oppliger, W., and Hall, M. N. (2005). Molecular organization of target of rapamycin complex 2. *J. Biol. Chem.* 280, 30697–30704. doi: 10.1074/jbc.M505553200

Zoncu, R., Efeyan, A., and Sabatini, D. M. (2011). mtor: from growth signal integration to cancer, diabetes and ageing. *Nat. Rev. Mol. Cell Biol.* 12, 21–35. doi: 10.1038/nrm3025

14

Non-invasive Imaging and Modeling of Liver Regeneration After Partial Hepatectomy

Sara Zafarnia[1†], Anna Mrugalla[1†], Anne Rix[1], Dennis Doleschel[1], Felix Gremse[1], Stephanie D. Wolf[2], Johannes F. Buyel[3,4‡], Ute Albrecht[2], Johannes G. Bode[2], Fabian Kiessling[1] and Wiltrud Lederle[1]*

[1]Institute for Experimental Molecular Imaging, Medical Faculty, RWTH Aachen University, Aachen, Germany, [2]Department of Gastroenterology, Hepatology and Infectious Diseases, Medical Faculty, Heinrich-Heine-University Düsseldorf, Düsseldorf, Germany, [3]Fraunhofer Institute for Molecular Biology and Applied Ecology IME, Aachen, Germany, [4]Institute for Molecular Biotechnology, RWTH Aachen University, Aachen, Germany

Correspondence:
Wiltrud Lederle
wlederle@ukaachen.de

†These authors have contributed equally to this work

‡orcid.org/0000-0003-2361-143X

The liver has a unique regenerative capability upon injury or partial resection. The regeneration process comprises a complex interplay between parenchymal and non-parenchymal cells and is tightly regulated at different scales. Thus, we investigated liver regeneration using multi-scale methods by combining non-invasive imaging with immunohistochemical analyses. In this context, non-invasive imaging can provide quantitative data of processes involved in liver regeneration at organ and body scale. We quantitatively measured liver volume recovery after 70% partial hepatectomy (PHx) by micro computed tomography (μCT) and investigated changes in the density of CD68$^+$ macrophages by fluorescence-mediated tomography (FMT) combined with μCT using a newly developed near-infrared fluorescent probe. In addition, angiogenesis and tissue-resident macrophages were analyzed by immunohistochemistry. Based on the results, a model describing liver regeneration and the interactions between different cell types was established. *In vivo* analysis of liver volume regeneration over 21 days after PHx by μCT imaging demonstrated that the liver volume rapidly increased after PHx reaching a maximum at day 14 and normalizing until day 21. An increase in CD68$^+$ macrophage density in the liver was detected from day 4 to day 8 by combined FMT-μCT imaging, followed by a decline towards control levels between day 14 and day 21. Immunohistochemistry revealed the highest angiogenic activity at day 4 after PHx that continuously declined thereafter, whereas the density of tissue-resident CD169$^+$ macrophages was not altered. The simulated time courses for volume recovery, angiogenesis and macrophage density reflect the experimental data describing liver regeneration after PHx at organ and tissue scale. In this context, our study highlights the importance of non-invasive imaging for acquiring quantitative organ scale data that enable modeling of liver regeneration.

Keywords: non-invasive imaging, modeling, liver regeneration, partial hepatectomy, macrophages, angiogenesis, FMT-μCT

INTRODUCTION

The liver is known for its high regenerative potential being able to restore up to 70% of its mass after injury or partial resection (Minuk, 2003). The regeneration process constitutes a complex interplay of various cell types and signaling pathways (Taub, 2004). Depending on the circumstances, two different modes of regeneration are known to be activated. In case of an impaired hepatocyte proliferation, as for instance following severe or chronic liver injury, liver stem cells (also known as oval cells in rodents) become activated as a mechanism of the liver to regenerate and recover its function (Itoh and Miyajima, 2014). In contrast, after partial resection or moderate liver damage, complete liver regeneration is achieved by proliferation of the remaining parenchymal and non-parenchymal cells. Hepatocytes are the first cells to grow and proliferate after partial resection followed by Kupffer cells, biliary epithelial cells, and stellate cells. The process is accompanied by the induction of angiogenesis that is also crucially involved in liver regeneration (Drixler et al., 2002; Uda et al., 2013). Besides other cell types, macrophages have been shown to play a stimulatory role in liver regeneration by producing molecular factors that are pivotal in the regeneration process (Abshagen et al., 2007; Li and Hua, 2017). Depletion of resident macrophages (Kupffer cells) as well as an impaired macrophage recruitment from the periphery and bone marrow results in a delayed regeneration demonstrating the stimulatory function of both resident and infiltrating macrophages (Takeishi et al., 1999; Abshagen et al., 2007; Melgar-Lesmes and Edelman, 2015; Nishiyama et al., 2015). The most frequently used model to study liver regeneration is the model of partial hepatectomy (PHx) described first by Higgins and Anderson (1931) in rats. Mitchell and Willenbring recently developed a modified protocol of a standardized surgical technique for PHx in mice (Mitchell and Willenbring, 2008). In both models, approximately two-thirds of the liver are surgically removed. The regeneration process starts immediately leading to full recovery of liver mass within 7–10 days (Taub, 2004; Nishiyama et al., 2015). The advantage of a surgical model in comparison with toxic injury models is the fact that the regeneration process after PHx is not associated with massive necrosis and necrosis-induced acute inflammation so that all changes observed after PHx can be ascribed to the physiological regeneration process (Michalopoulos, 2010). In a clinical context, this physiological regeneration process becomes important in patients who underwent partial liver resection, in donors and recipients following living-donor liver transplantation and in patients with acute liver failure.

Liver regeneration is a complex process involving the interactions of different cell types on various levels. Thus, we followed an approach using multi-scale methods (Castiglione et al., 2014) including non-invasive imaging and histological analyses in order to investigate liver regeneration after pHx. Non-invasive imaging is a useful tool since it enables a longitudinal and quantitative assessment of morphological, functional, and molecular parameters at the organ and whole body level. Liver volume recovery was measured *via* micro computed tomography (μCT), and the density of CD68⁺ macrophages was determined by combined fluorescence-mediated tomography and μCT (FMT-μCT) using a newly developed near-infrared fluorescent (NIRF) probe. The *in vivo* results were validated by immunohistochemical analyses of CD68⁺ and F4/80⁺ macrophages. At the tissue level, the contribution of tissue-resident macrophages and angiogenesis was investigated by additional immunohistochemical analyses. Based on the experimental data, a simple model describing liver regeneration and the interrelation between volume recovery, macrophages, and angiogenesis was generated.

MATERIALS AND METHODS

Generation and Purification of the Near-Infrared Fluorescent CD68 Probe

The NIRF probe targeting CD68⁺ macrophages was generated by coupling an amine-reactive NIR fluorochrome (NHS ester), VivoTag 680 (excitation peak 665 ± 5 nm, emission peak 688 ± 5 nm) (Perkin-Elmer), to a rat anti-mouse CD68 antibody (AbDSerotec) according to manufacturer's instructions. In brief, VivoTag 680 was dissolved in dry dimethyl sulfoxide (Sigma-Aldrich) at a concentration of 10 mg/ml. Prior to the labeling, the buffer of the antibody was exchanged by dialysis into conjugation buffer (50 mM carbonate/bicarbonate buffer, pH 8.5) using Slide-A-Lyzer dialysis cassettes (AbD Serotec) according to the protocol provided by the manufacturer. After buffer exchange, 30 μl of VivoTag 680 was added to the rat anti-mouse CD68 antibody. Following 1 h of incubation at room temperature protected from the light, the NIRF CD68 probe (approximately 151 kDa) was separated from free fluorescent dye (approximately 1 kDa) and antibody oligomers (larger than 300 kDa) by fast protein liquid chromatography using a Superdex 200 resin in a pre-packed 10/300 GL column (GE Healthcare). Probe concentration was determined using a BCA Protein Assay Kit (Uptima) according to the protocol provided by the manufacturer.

In vitro Binding of the Near-Infrared Fluorescent CD68 Probe

Binding specificity of the NIRF CD68 probe was tested *in vitro* by incubating the macrophage cell line J774A.1 (CLS Cell Lines Service) with the NIRF CD68 probe (10 nM, 2 or 4 h, 37°C). For competitive binding analyses, J774A.1 cells were incubated with 10 nM of the NIRF CD68 probe and a 10-fold molar excess of unlabeled CD68 antibody (100 nM, 2 or 4 h, 37°C). Fluorescent microphotographs were acquired with the Axio Imager M2 (Zeiss) and a high-resolution camera (AxioCamMRm Rev.3; Zeiss) using a Cy5.5 filter and a fixed exposure time. The signal intensities were determined using the software ImageJ 1.47v (W. Rasband, National Institutes of Health). For quantification, the mean fluorescent signal intensity at 695 nm was determined by analyzing five microscopic images per well (n = 3 wells per culture condition).

Animal Studies

All animal experiments were performed according to German legal requirements and animal protection laws and were approved by the Authority for Environment Conservation and Consumer Protection of the State of North Rhine-Westphalia (LANUV).

Biodistribution and *in vivo* Specificity of the Near-Infrared Fluorescent CD68 Probe

Biodistribution and *in vivo* specificity of the NIRF CD68 probe were analyzed in male C57BL/6 J mice (Charles River) (n = 5 per group). The mice were fed a chlorophyll-free diet (ssniff Spezialdiäten GmbH) 7 days before imaging, and the scanning area was depilated prior to the scans. For macrophage imaging, 2.6 μg of the NIRF CD68 probe dissolved in 0.9% w/v NaCl was injected intravenously (i.v.). To analyze the biodistribution, animals were scanned longitudinally immediately before and 1, 3, 6, 12, 24, and 48 h after probe injection by FMT-μCT. *In vivo* specificity of the probe was examined by competitive binding analysis injecting a 5-fold mass excess of unlabeled CD68 antibody (13 μg) intraperitoneally (i.p.) 1 h before i.v. injection of the NIRF CD68 probe (2.6 μg). Directly after the last FMT-μCT measurement, the mice were sacrificed, and the liver was resected and cryoconserved in Tissue-Tek (Sakura) for immunohistochemical analyses.

In vivo Determination of Macrophage Density and Volume Recovery During Liver Regeneration After Partial Hepatectomy

Liver regeneration was analyzed in male C57BL/6 J mice (Charles River) after PHx and sham surgery. One hour before surgery, mice were treated with carprofen [subcutan (s.c.) 5 mg/kg] (Pfizer Animal Health SA). PHx and sham surgeries were performed under sterile conditions as previously described by Mitchell and Willenbring (2008). In brief, mice were anesthetized with isoflurane (2% v/v isoflurane in oxygen-enriched air) and positioned on a temperature-controlled pad to regulate body temperature. For PHx, after midline laparotomy, the left lateral lobe was ligated as close to the base of the lobe as possible. The secondary knot was placed above the gall bladder of the median lobe but not closer than 2 mm from the suprahepatic vena cava. The ligated liver lobes were surgically resected. At the end of the surgery, the abdomen was rinsed with saline solution, and the abdominal wall and the skin were sutured separately. For sham surgery, a midline laparotomy was performed with gentle palpation and manipulation of the liver without resection of the liver lobes. Directly after surgery, mice received a s.c. injection of 10 mg/kg enrofloxacin (Bayer). Afterwards, analgesia was continued by s.c. injection of 5 mg/kg carprofen (Pfizer Animal Health SA) once per day for 3 days.

CD68$^+$ macrophages and volume recovery were monitored by FMT-μCT and contrast-enhanced μCT at different time points (4, 8, 14, and 21 days) after PHx and sham surgery. As an additional control, untreated mice were measured. Twelve hours before each FMT-μCT measurement, mice were injected i.v. with 5.7 μg of the NIRF CD68 probe diluted in 0.9% w/v NaCl. In addition, 45 min before the FMT-μCT scans, the mice received an i.v. injection (150 μl) of the contrast agent Imeron 400 (Bracco Imaging) to enable a better segmentation of the liver. Directly after each FMT-μCT measurement, mice were sacrificed, and the liver was resected and cryoconserved in Tissue-Tek (Sakura) for immunohistochemical analyses. The group size was as follows: for assessment of macrophage density: untreated mice: n = 10; mice after PHx: n = 5 for day 4, n = 4 for day 8, n = 4 for day 14, n = 4 for day 21; sham-operated mice: n = 3 for day 4, n = 3 for day 8, n = 3 for day 14, n = 6 for day 21. For volume recovery analysis: n = 5 for each time point.

Imaging Protocols

Three-dimensional (3D) FMT-μCT scans were conducted as described by Kunjachan et al. (2013). For the measurements, mice were anesthetized and positioned in a μCT- and FMT-compatible mouse bed. For anatomical information, mice were scanned in a dual-energy μCT system (TomoScope 30s Duo, CT Imaging GmbH). For biodistribution and *in vivo* competitive binding, analyses scans were performed using the scan protocol SQD-6565-360-29, which acquires 720 projections with 516 × 506 pixels requiring a scanning time of 29 s per subscan. For the assessment of macrophage density and liver volume, the HQD-6565-360-90 protocol was applied, which acquires 720 projections with 1,032 × 1,012 pixels requiring a scanning time of 90 s per subscan. Directly after acquiring the μCT scans, the mouse bed was transferred to the FMT system (FMT 2500LX, PerkinElmer), and FMT scans were performed at 680 nm using 120 excitation positions (3 mm distance). Data fusion and reconstruction of the fluorescence distribution were performed as described (Gremse et al., 2014). Based on the μCT data, organs were manually segmented, and the liver volume and probe concentration in the segmented organs were determined using the Imalytics Preclinical software (ExMI/Gremse-IT) (Gremse et al., 2016). To assess the variability of the organ segmentations, several organs (liver, lung, heart, kidney, and bladder) were segmented in five representative scans by two different persons. The organ volumes of the two analyses correlated strongly (R^2 = 0.996, p < 0.05) between the users. DICE scores, which describe similarity between segmentations, were also high (0.92 ± 0.045), showing good reproducibility of the manual organ segmentation. To further confirm the accuracy of manual organ segmentation, we performed an additional correlation analysis between segmented organ volumes and weights of excised organs. Organ weights (heart, liver, kidneys, spleen, and tumors) and contrast-enhanced μCT scans (n = 6) were available from a previous study (Rosenhain et al., 2018). The analysis resulted in a strong correlation between segmented organ volumes from contrast-enhanced μCT scans and the organ weights (R^2 = 0.976). The slope of the regression line was 0.84, i.e., below 1, which can be explained by the loss of blood during the organ excision and harvesting procedure (thus lower values for the organ weights as compared to the segmented volumes).

Antibodies

The following primary antibodies were used to stain macrophages/Kupffer cells: rat anti-mouse CD68 antibody (AbDSerotec), rat anti-mouse F4/80 antibody (AbDSerotec), and rat anti-mouse CD169 antibody (AbDSerotec). To stain endothelial cells, rat anti-mouse CD31 antibody (BD Biosciences) was applied. Goat anti-mouse VEGFR2 antibody (R and D Systems) was used to determine the VEGFR2 density. Secondary IgG antibodies (donkey anti-rat Alexa Fluor 488, donkey anti-rat Cy-3 and donkey anti-goat Cy-3) were obtained from Dianova. Cell nuclei were counterstained with 4′,6-diamidino-2-phenylindole (DAPI; Merck KGaA).

Indirect Immunohistochemistry

For immunohistochemical analysis, frozen organs were cut into 8-μm slices. Fixation and staining of the cryosections were performed as previously described (Lederle et al., 2010). Per section, five to seven fluorescent microphotographs were acquired with the Axio Imager M2 (Zeiss) and a high-resolution camera (AxioCamMRm Rev.3; Zeiss). The number of $CD68^+$, $F4/80^+$, $CD169^+$ and $DAPI^+$ cells per microphotograph was counted manually using the ImageJ 1.47v software (W. Rasband, National Institutes of Health), and the percentage of $CD68^+$, $F4/80^+$ and $CD169^+$ cells per $DAPI^+$ cells was calculated, respectively. Quantitative analysis of microvessel density and angiogenic activity was done using the AxioVisionRel 4.8 software (Zeiss). The microvessel density was determined by quantifying the $CD31^+$ area fraction, and the angiogenic activity was assessed by determining the proportion of the $VEGFR2^+$ area fraction to the $CD31^+$ area fraction. The group size was as follows: untreated mice: $n = 10$ (CD169: $n = 5$); mice after PHx: $n = 5$ for day 4, $n = 4$ for day 8, $n = 4$ for day 14, $n = 4$ for day 21; sham-operated mice: $n = 4$ for day 4, $n = 6$ (CD169: $n = 3$) for day 8, $n = 3$ for day 14, $n = 7$ for day 21.

Numeric Modeling

Stimulation and growth of liver cell compartments (hepatocytes, Kupffer cells, macrophages, and endothelial cells) were described by differential equations in a simplified model. Based on data from literature, relative proportions of these cell types in healthy livers were assumed to be 0.8, 0.06, 0.06, and 0.08, respectively (Vekemans and Braet, 2005). To simulate PHx, these values were multiplied by 0.3 at the initial state of simulation to account for the reduced total cell amount. The first derivative of each cell compartment fraction was assumed to depend linearly on the amount, excess, or lack of other cell compartments, with six coefficients describing the strength of the corresponding effect. The parameters k_{HE} and k_{ME} describe the stimulation and support of vessel growth by a hepatocyte lack and macrophage excess, respectively. k_{HM} describes attraction of macrophages by a lack of hepatocytes. k_{HK} describes stimulation of Kupffer cell growth by a lack of hepatocytes. k_{EH} describes the connection of blood vessel and hepatocyte growth, because the latter is limited by nutrition supply and structural alignment requirements. A parameter $k_{homeostasis}$ describes other effects not covered by our simplified model, and it drives the four cell compartments slowly toward the homeostatic situation. Therefore, the derivatives of the four compartments are the weighted sums of the affecting coefficients and expressions for relative or absolute lack as described in the following:

$$dH/dt = k_{homeostasis}(1 - H/0.8) + k_{HE}(0.8/0.08 - H/E)$$

$$dK/dt = k_{homeostasis}(1 - K/0.06) + k_{HK}(0.8 - H)$$

$$dM/dt = k_{homeostasis}(1 - M/0.06) + k_{HM}(0.8 - H)$$

$$dE/dt = k_{homeostasis}(1 - E/0.08) + k_{HE}(0.8 - H) + k_{ME}\left(M/(H + K + M + E) - 0.06\right)$$

The simulation was performed using fourth-order Runge-Kutta integration with the time interval of 60 min over a period of 100 days, resulting in four-cell compartment curves. From these, simulated measurement curves were computed, i.e., volume (sum of all compartments), total macrophages (sum of macrophages and Kupffer cells), and Kupffer cells and angiogenesis (derivative of endothelial growth). The six parameters were iteratively adjusted until simulated and measured curves matched.

Statistical Analysis

Statistical analysis was performed using Prism 5.0 (GraphPad software). Results are shown as mean ± standard deviation. All statistical analyses were performed using one-way analysis of variance (ANOVA) followed by Bonferroni correction for multiple comparisons ($^*p < 0.05$, $^{**}p < 0.01$, $^{***}p < 0.001$).

RESULTS

In vitro Binding Specificity of the Near-Infrared Fluorescent CD68 Probe

For non-invasive imaging of macrophages by FMT-μCT, a NIRF probe targeting $CD68^+$ macrophages was generated and evaluated *in vitro* and *in vivo*. The binding specificity of the NIRF CD68 probe was evaluated *in vitro* by competitive binding analysis using the macrophage cell line J774A.1. After 2 and 4 h of incubation with the NIRF CD68 probe alone, a strong fluorescent signal in the cells was observed (**Figure 1A**). Incubation of the cells with the NIRF CD68 probe together with a 10-fold excess of unlabeled anti-CD68 antibody resulted in a strongly reduced signal at both time points. Quantification of the fluorescent images revealed an increase in signal intensity from 2 to 4 h and confirmed a significantly lower mean signal intensity in the cells of the competitive binding group as compared to the cells incubated with the NIRF CD68 probe alone ($p < 0.001$) (**Figure 1B**).

Biodistribution and *in vivo* Specificity of the Near-Infrared Fluorescent CD68 Probe

The biodistribution of the NIRF CD68 probe was analyzed longitudinally in healthy mice by FMT-μCT 1, 3, 6, 12, 24,

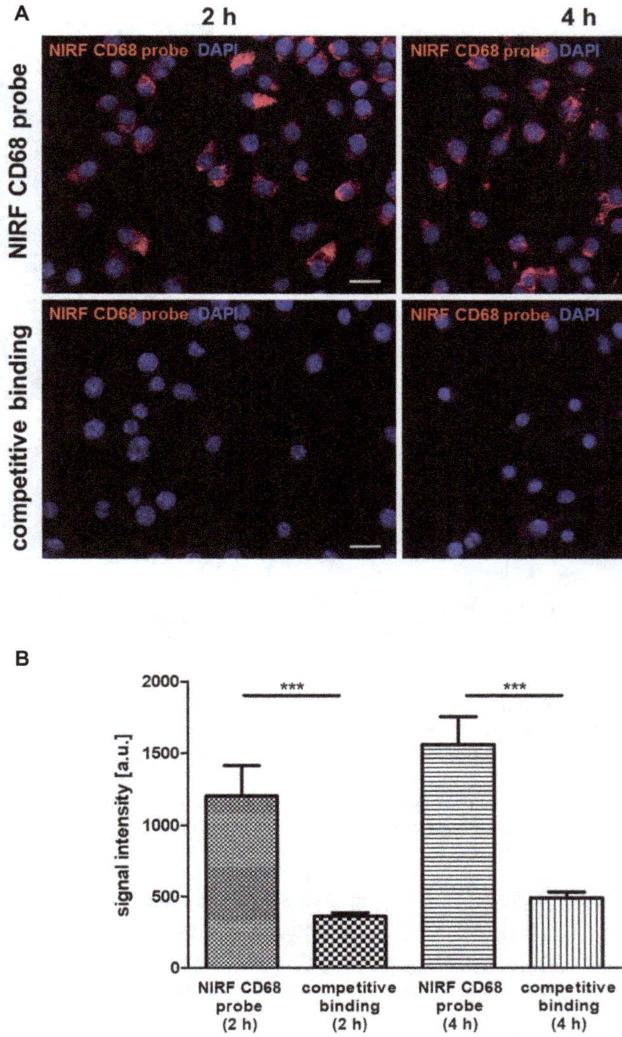

FIGURE 1 | *In vitro* competitive binding analysis of the NIRF CD68 probe. To test the binding specificity of the NIRF CD68 probe, J774A.1 macrophages were incubated for 2 and 4 h with the NIRF CD68 probe alone (NIRF CD68 probe) or with the NIRF CD68 probe and a 10-fold molar excess of unlabeled anti-CD68 antibody (competitive binding). **(A)** Fluorescence images show a high fluorescent signal at 695 nm in macrophages after 2 and 4 h of incubation with the NIRF CD68 probe. Competitive binding results in a strongly reduced signal. NIRF CD68 probe in red, counterstaining of the nuclei with DAPI in blue, scale bar = 20 μm. **(B)** Quantitative analysis of mean fluorescent signal intensities in the NIRF CD68 probe group and in the competitive binding group shows a significantly lower signal intensity as a result of competitive binding (***$p < 0.001$; data are presented as mean values ± SD). a.u., arbitrary units.

and 48 h after injection. Quantitative analysis of the NIRF CD68 probe accumulation in the liver, lung, and kidneys revealed a significantly higher mean concentration in the liver as compared to the kidneys and the lung at all measuring time points ($p < 0.001$ for all time points, respectively) (**Figure 2A**). The concentration in the kidneys and the lung was constantly low without significant changes over time. In the liver, the mean concentration increased after probe injection reaching a maximum concentration at 12 h after injection. Thereafter, the mean probe concentration in the liver declined to a value similar to that observed at 1 h after injection (**Figures 2A,C**; representative 3D rendering of reconstructed FMT-μCT data shown in **Figure 2B**).

The *in vivo* specificity of the NIRF CD68 probe was analyzed in a competitive binding experiment in which a 5-fold excess of unlabeled CD68 antibody was injected 1 h prior to injection of the NIRF CD68 probe (competitive binding group). In the liver, starting from 3 h after probe injection, a lower mean probe concentration was measured in the competitive binding group at each time point compared to the concentration measured after injection of the NIRF CD68 probe alone (control group) (**Figure 3A**; representative transversal FMT-μCT fusion images of competitive binding and control mice are shown in **Figure 3B**). The difference in the mean concentration of NIRF CD68 probe in the liver was significant 12 h after injection.

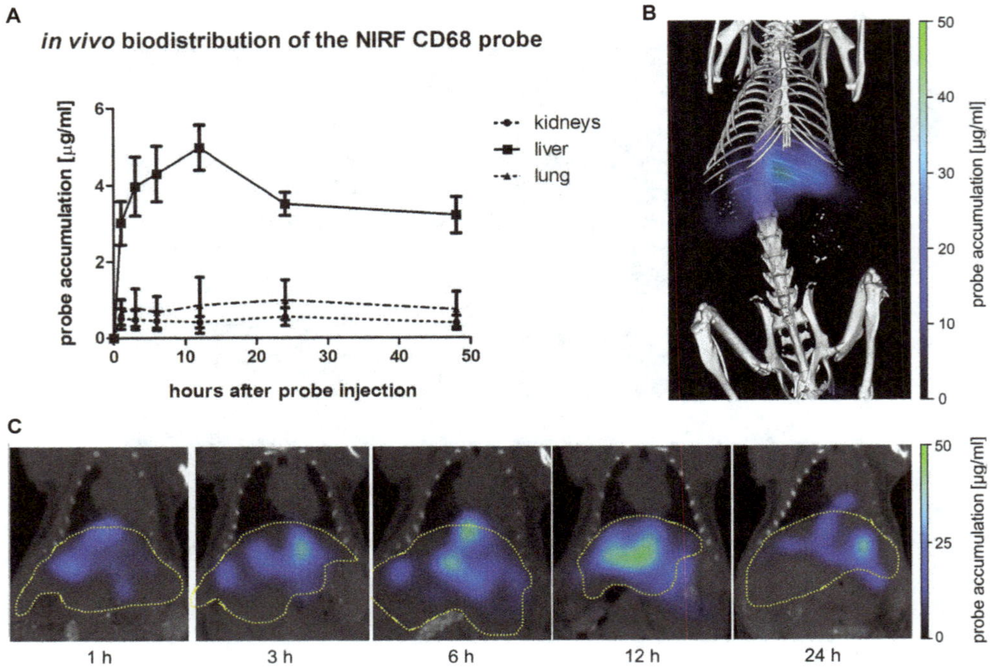

FIGURE 2 | *In vivo* biodistribution of the NIRF CD68 probe. To analyze the biodistribution of the NIRF CD68 probe, the accumulation in different organs was measured longitudinally over 48 h in healthy mice by FMT-µCT. **(A)** Quantitative analysis of the NIRF CD68 probe concentration in the kidneys, liver, and lung revealed a significantly higher concentration in the liver compared to the kidneys and the lung at all measuring time points ($p < 0.001$ for each time point, data are presented as mean values ± SD). **(B)** Representative 3D rendering of reconstructed FMT-µCT data of a mouse 12 h after NIRF CD68 probe injection. **(C)** Representative frontal plane images of reconstructed FMT-µCT data at different time points after NIRF CD68 probe injection show an increasing fluorescent signal intensity in the liver until 12 h after injection, followed by a decline (dashed yellow line indicates the liver).

Volumetric Recovery of the Liver After Partial Hepatectomy

To investigate liver regrowth after PHx by non-invasive imaging, the volume of the liver was measured *via* contrast-enhanced µCT. Quantitative analysis revealed that >70% of the total liver volume was reached at day 4 and > 80% was regained at day 8 after PHx (**Figure 4A**; representative 3D rendered CT images with segmented organs of an untreated control mouse and mice after PHx are shown in **Figure 4B**). The mean value determined at day 14 was slightly above the mean volume of the liver of untreated control mice. The mean volume at day 21 after PHx was comparable to control values.

In vivo Monitoring of CD68⁺ Macrophage Density During Liver Regeneration

Macrophages play an important stimulatory role during liver regeneration (Takeishi et al., 1999; Abshagen et al., 2007; Nishiyama et al., 2015). Thus, we investigated the time course of macrophage density after PHx by non-invasive FMT-µCT imaging. $CD68^+$ macrophages were monitored at day 4, 8, 14, and 21 after PHx and sham surgery using the NIRF CD68 probe. As an additional control, untreated mice were measured. Quantitative analysis of probe accumulation revealed a higher mean NIRF CD68 probe concentration in the liver at day 8, 14, and 21 after PHx compared to untreated and sham-operated control mice (**Figure 5A**). The mean concentration was highest at day 8 and 14 after PHx followed by a decline between day 14 and 21 indicating a transient increase in the density of $CD68^+$ macrophages. No major changes in the mean NIRF CD68 probe concentration were measured in the liver of sham-operated mice during the whole observation period. Representative frontal plane FMT-µCT fusion images of an untreated control mouse and mice after PHx are shown in **Figure 5B**.

Immunohistochemical Analysis of Macrophage Subpopulations During Liver Regeneration

To validate the *in vivo* results, the density of $CD68^+$ macrophages in the liver of untreated and sham-operated control mice and mice after PHx was determined by immunohistochemical analyses. Quantification of the density of $CD68^+$ macrophages confirmed the trend of the *in vivo* findings showing a significant increase in the mean values after PHx until day 8 followed by a decline to levels observed in untreated control animals at day 21 (**Figure 6A**, $p < 0.001$). The mean density in the liver of sham-operated animals remained similar to that of untreated control animals without significant changes over time.

For further validation, we performed an immunohistochemical analysis of cells expressing F4/80, a generic macrophage marker that is independent of CD68 expression. Quantitative analysis of the density of $F4/80^+$ macrophages showed a similar trend over

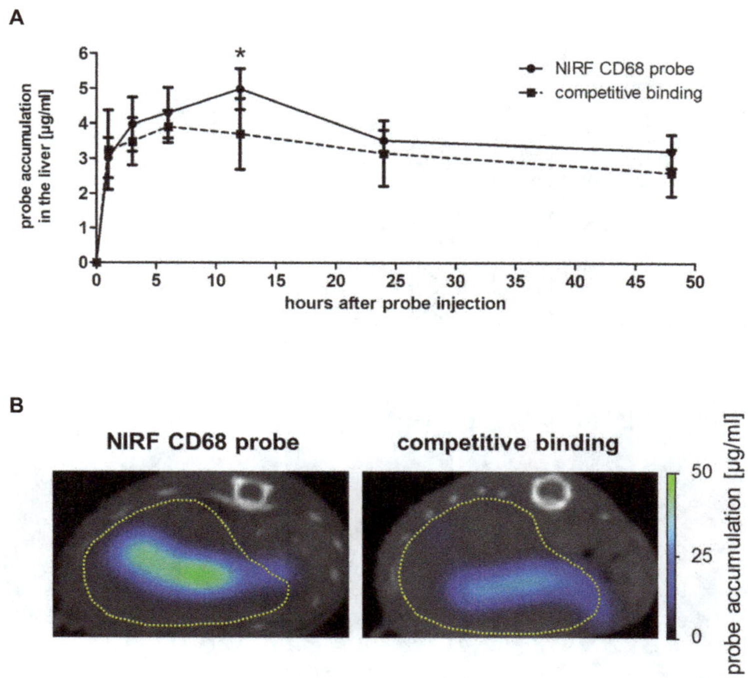

FIGURE 3 | *In vivo* specificity of the NIRF CD68 probe. To analyze the *in vivo* specificity of the NIRF CD68 probe, a competitive binding experiment was performed in which a 5-fold excess of unlabeled CD68 antibody was injected 1 h prior to the injection of the NIRF CD68 probe (competitive binding group). Probe accumulation in the liver was compared to the concentration measured after injection of the NIRF CD68 probe alone (control group). **(A)** Quantitative analysis of probe accumulation in the liver showed a significant difference in the mean concentration 12 h after injection (*$p < 0.05$; data are presented as mean values ± SD). **(B)** Transversal FMT-µCT fusion images of representative mice 12 h after injection show a high fluorescent signal in the liver of the control mouse and a strongly reduced signal in the liver as a result of competitive binding (dashed yellow line indicates the liver).

time as compared to CD68$^+$ macrophages with a significant transient increase and highest mean values at day 8 after PHx (**Figure 6B**, $p < 0.001$). Again, the mean density of F4/80$^+$ in the liver of sham-operated animals was comparable to that of untreated control animals and did not significantly change over time.

An increased density of macrophages during liver regeneration can be a result of tissue-resident Kupffer cell proliferation or caused by an infiltration of macrophages from the blood circulation. Both Kupffer cells and infiltrating macrophages have been shown to play an important role during liver regeneration (Takeishi et al., 1999; Abshagen et al., 2007; Melgar-Lesmes and Edelman, 2015; Nishiyama et al., 2015). To investigate the contribution of tissue-resident macrophages to the increased macrophage density, we analyzed the expression of CD169 by immunohistochemical analysis. In contrast to CD68$^+$ and F4/80$^+$ macrophages, no significant differences in the density of CD169$^+$ macrophages were observed in the liver of untreated and sham-operated control mice and mice after PHx (**Figure 6C**).

Immunohistochemical Analysis of Angiogenesis During Liver Regeneration

Angiogenesis is a crucial process involved in liver regeneration, and macrophages have been shown to stimulate endothelial cell activation and to regulate vessel growth (Melgar-Lesmes and Edelman, 2015). To investigate the interrelation between macrophage density and angiogenesis, we analyzed the microvessel density and angiogenic activity in the liver of untreated control mice and in mice after PHx and sham surgery using immunohistochemistry.

Microvessel density was not significantly different between mice after PHx, untreated and sham-operated control mice (**Figure 7A**). However, the angiogenic activity, as assessed by the proportion of the VEGFR2$^+$ area fraction to the CD31$^+$ area fraction, was markedly increased on day 4 after PHx followed by a continuous decrease until day 21 (**Figure 7B**). In sham-operated and untreated mice, no significant changes were found over time.

Modeling of Liver Regeneration After Partial Hepatectomy

The *in vivo* and immunohistochemical results revealed different time courses of volume recovery, macrophage density and endothelial cell activation (angiogenesis). A simplified mathematical model was developed including different cell compartments of the liver (hepatocytes, Kupffer cells, recruited macrophages, and endothelial cells), and the growth and interplay of these compartments after PHx was simulated (**Figures 8A,B**). Based on the resulting cell compartment curves (**Figure 8B**), simulated measurement curves were computed describing liver volume (sum of all compartments), total macrophages (sum of recruited macrophages and Kupffer cells), and Kupffer cells and angiogenesis (derivative of endothelial growth) (**Figure 8C**).

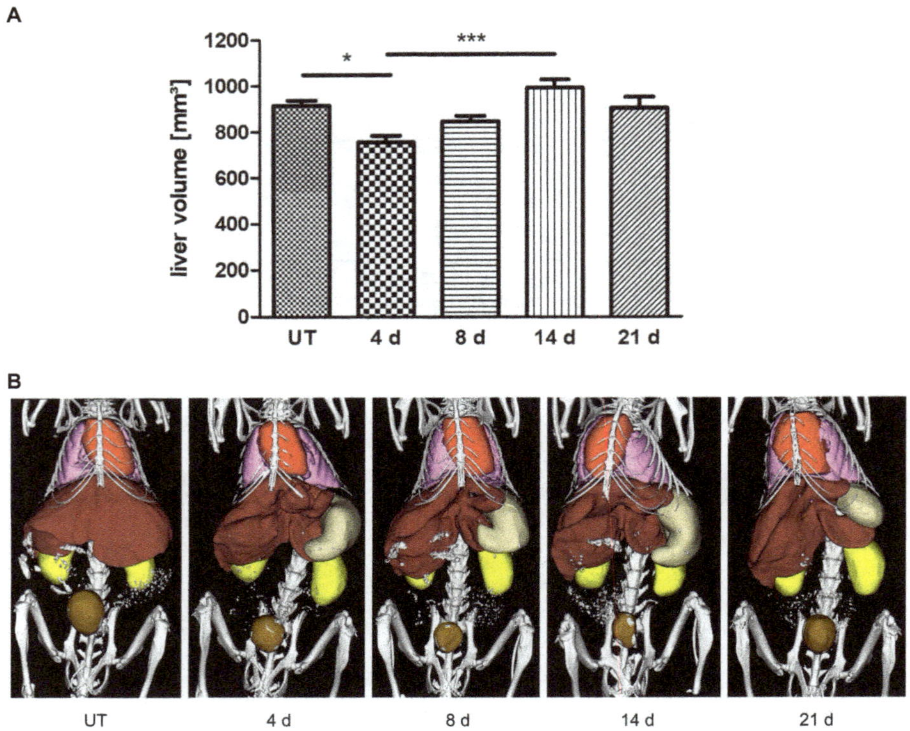

FIGURE 4 | Liver volume recovery after PHx. Liver volume was determined non-invasively at day 4, 8, 14, and 21 after PHx and in untreated control mice by contrast-enhanced µCT. **(A)** Quantitative analysis showed that >70% and > 80% of the total liver volume were regained at day 4 and day 8 after PHx, respectively ($^{*}p < 0.05$, $^{***}p < 0.001$; data are presented as mean values ± SD). **(B)** Representative 3D rendered CT images with segmented organs of an untreated control mouse and mice after PHx show the growth of the remaining liver lobes during regeneration (red, heart; pink, lungs; brown, liver; beige, stomach; ochre, bladder). UT, untreated mice.

After parameter adjustment, the time courses of the numerical model matched the experimental data of angiogenesis, macrophages, and liver volume obtained by non-invasive imaging and immunohistochemical analyses (**Figures 8C,D**). In detail, there was an early onset of angiogenesis, which was followed by an increase in the overall macrophage density peaking on day 8. The liver volume increased rapidly after PHx reaching levels above healthy liver on day 14 before normalization.

DISCUSSION

Liver regeneration after injury or partial resection comprises a complex interplay of different cell types and is tightly regulated at various scales (Taub, 2004; Michalopoulos, 2010; Li and Hua, 2017). To address alterations during liver regeneration after PHx at different levels, we used non-invasive imaging in combination with immunohistochemistry and developed a simple mathematical model describing the interrelations between different cell types involved in liver regeneration, angiogenesis and liver volume recovery.

Liver volume recovery was non-invasively monitored by µCT imaging. The measurements revealed that >70% of the total liver volume were regained within 4 days. However, normalization of the liver volume was not reached until day 21 due to an increased volume observed on day 14. The increased volume can be explained by edema formation that sometimes occurs during liver regeneration (Pleskovic et al., 1996).

Since macrophages are known to play an important stimulatory role during liver regeneration, we investigated the density of different macrophage populations after PHx by non-invasive imaging and immunohistochemistry. For non-invasive imaging, we used combined FMT-µCT imaging and generated a NIRF probe targeting CD68. Specific binding of the NIRF probe to $CD68^{+}$ macrophages was confirmed by competition analyses *in vitro* and *in vivo*. Quantitative *in vivo* FMT-µCT imaging after PHx and sham surgery revealed an increased mean concentration of the CD68 probe in the liver at day 8 and 14 after PHx indicating a transient increase in the density of $CD68^{+}$ macrophages. Immunohistochemical analyses of $CD68^{+}$ and $F4/80^{+}$ macrophages showed the same trend with a significantly higher macrophage density on day 8 after PHx as compared to untreated and sham-operated control mice. However, the immunohistochemical data were more distinct than the results obtained by FMT-µCT imaging. The difference in precision can be explained by the lower spatial resolution of the FMT (about 2 mm). Small changes in the density of macrophages are more difficult to determine by FMT-µCT

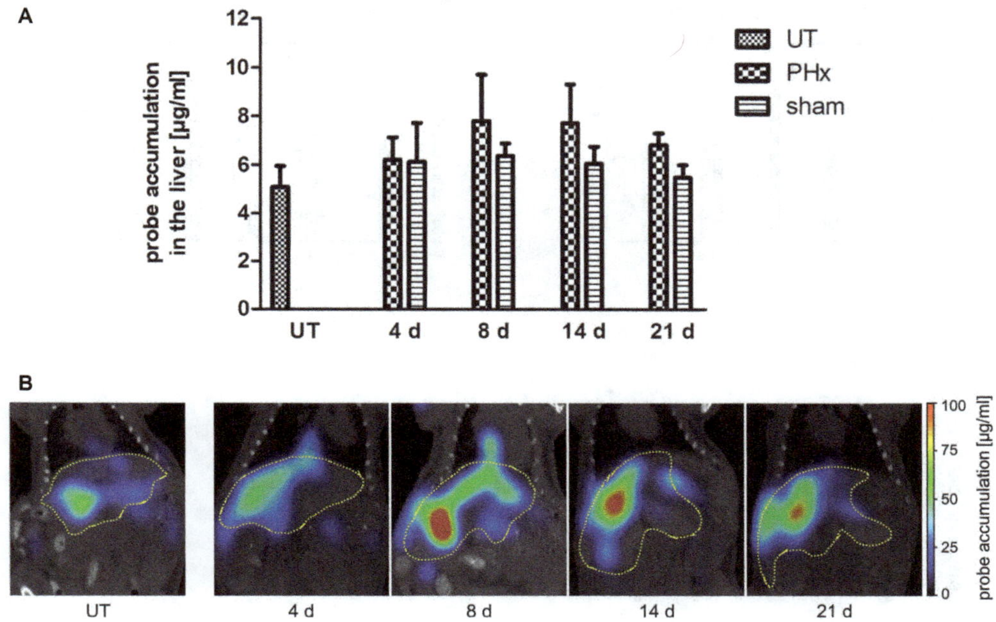

FIGURE 5 | *In vivo* assessment of CD68⁺ macrophages in untreated control mice, sham-operated mice and mice after PHx. CD68⁺ macrophages were non-invasively monitored by FMT-µCT at day 4, 8, 14, and 21 after PHx and sham surgery and in untreated control mice. **(A)** Quantitative analysis showed a higher mean NIRF CD68 probe concentration in the liver at day 8, 14, and 21 after PHx compared to untreated and sham-operated control mice. The highest mean concentration was reached at day 8 (data are presented as mean values ± SD). **(B)** Representative frontal plane FMT-µCT fusion images of an untreated control mouse and mice after PHx show a higher fluorescent signal in the liver of mice at day 8, 14 and 21 after PHx (dashed yellow line indicates the liver). UT, untreated mice.

than *via* immunofluorescence microscopy. Furthermore, although absorption and scattering of the photons are taken into account in the fluorescence reconstruction algorithms, numerical limitations of the complex diffuse optical behavior can still affect the accuracy of the data, especially in deeper lying organs and in organs with a high blood volume, such as the liver, since blood is the main near-infrared absorber *in vivo* (Gremse et al., 2014). Moreover, the blood pool of the circulating probe and the unspecific hepatic uptake of foreign substances such as probes and contrast agents can lead to an unspecific probe signal. Antibodies are known to have a long blood half-life (Freise and Wu, 2015). Since we used an antibody as targeting molecule, we cannot exclude that the blood pool of the imaging probe has influenced the measurements. To reduce the impact of the blood pool, a different targeting molecule could be chosen, e.g., a nanobody, that has a shorter blood half-life.

To analyze the contribution of tissue-resident Kupffer cells in liver regeneration after PHx, we investigated the expression of CD169 by immunohistochemical analysis. Quantification revealed no significant differences in the density of CD169⁺ macrophages in the liver of untreated and sham-operated control mice and mice after PHx. Thus, while the overall density of macrophages in the liver increased significantly after PHx, the density of tissue-resident CD169⁺ Kupffer cells did not. This is in line with previous findings showing that the number of Kupffer cells correlates with liver restoration rate (Melgar-Lesmes and Edelman, 2015). Therefore, the results provide further evidence for the involvement of macrophages recruited from the blood circulation in liver regeneration after PHx (Melgar-Lesmes and Edelman, 2015; Nishiyama et al., 2015; Wen et al., 2015). However, further investigation is needed to unravel the details of resident Kupffer cell and infiltrating macrophage contribution to liver regeneration.

Angiogenesis is an important process involved in liver regeneration after hepatectomy and mutual interactions have been described between hepatocytes, Kupffer cells/macrophages and endothelial cells during liver regeneration (Drixler et al., 2002; Uda et al., 2013; Castiglione et al., 2014). Therefore, we analyzed the angiogenic endothelial cell activity and microvessel density in the liver after PHx by immunohistochemistry. A markedly increased mean angiogenic activity was detected at day 4 after PHx that decreased steadily until day 21 which is in accordance with previously published data (Alizai et al., 2017). Quantitative analysis of the microvessel density showed no significant differences between mice after PHx and control mice. This finding is not in line with results published by other groups that showed an increase in the microvessel density following PHx (Drixler et al., 2002, 2003). The discrepancy can be explained by different quantification methods. While we included larger arterioles and venules in the quantification, they were excluded by the other groups. Larger vessels contribute more to the overall CD31⁺ area fraction than very small vessels. Thus, changes in the density of these small vessels do not have a major effect on the overall vessel density.

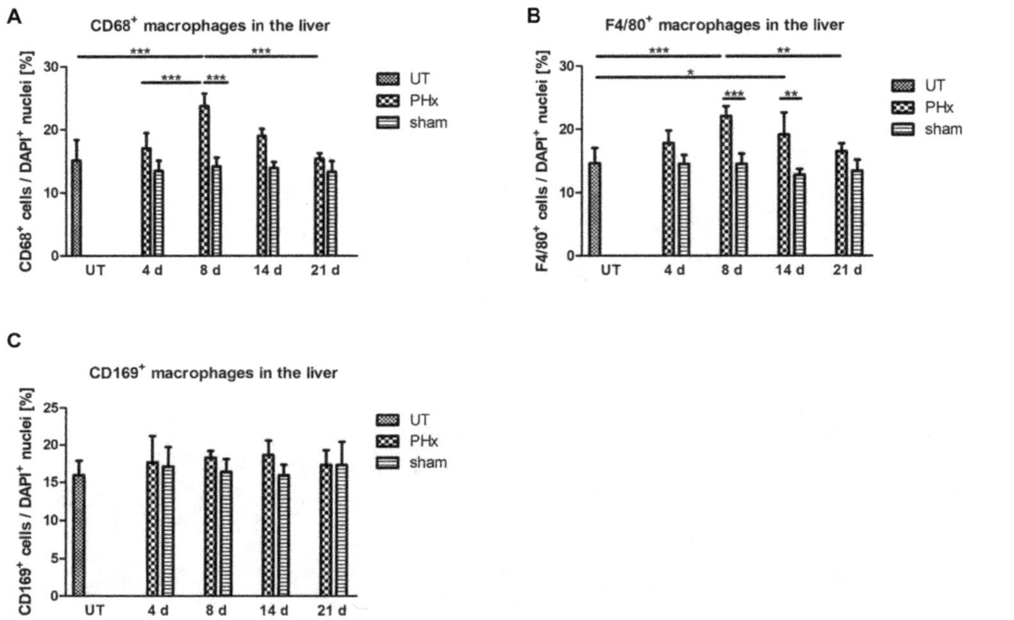

FIGURE 6 | Immunohistochemical analysis of CD68+, F4/80+ and CD169+ macrophages in the liver of untreated and sham-operated control mice and mice after PHx. The density of CD68+, F4/80+, and CD169+ macrophages was determined by immunohistochemical analyses in liver sections taken from mice at day 4, 8, 14, and 21 after PHx and sham surgery and from untreated control mice ($^*p < 0.05$, $^{**}p < 0.01$, $^{***}p < 0.001$; data are presented as mean values ± SD). **(A,B)** Quantitative analysis of the density of CD68+ **(A)** and F4/80+ **(B)** macrophages showed an increase in the mean values after PHx with a maximum at day 8. **(C)** Quantitative analysis of the density of CD169+ macrophages showed no significant differences in the liver of untreated and sham-operated control mice and mice after PHx. UT, untreated mice.

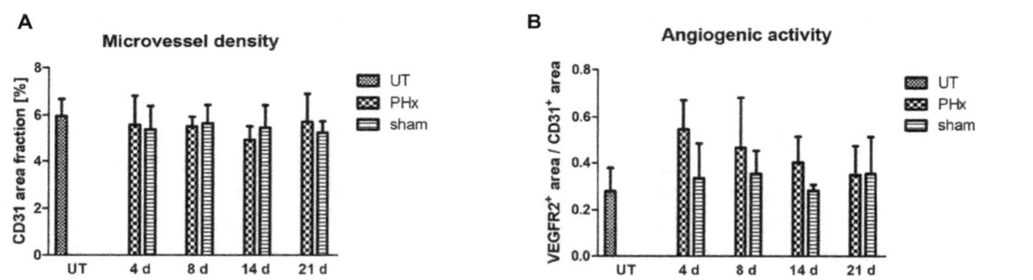

FIGURE 7 | Immunohistochemical analysis of the microvessel density and angiogenic activity in the liver of untreated and sham-operated control mice and mice after PHx. The microvessel density and angiogenic activity were determined by immunohistochemical analysis of liver sections taken from mice at day 4, 8, 14, and 21 after PHx and sham surgery and from untreated control mice (data are presented as mean values ± SD). **(A)** Quantitative analysis of the microvessel density showed no significant differences between untreated and sham-operated control mice and mice after PHx. **(B)** Quantitative analysis of the angiogenic activity showed a markedly increased mean activity at day 4 after PHx that decreased steadily until day 21. UT, untreated mice.

The *in vivo* and immunohistochemical results revealed differences in the time courses for volume recovery, macrophage density and angiogenic endothelial cell activity, nevertheless, all three time courses show a progression towards levels of healthy situation over time. To describe the interrelation between volume recovery, macrophage density and angiogenesis occurring at different scales, we developed a numerical model that describes the growth and interplay of the involved liver cell compartments (hepatocytes, Kupffer cells, recruited macrophages, and endothelial cells). A numerical model serves to bridge the gap between hidden parameters (e.g., k_{HE}) and observable measurements. The model may contain many direct interactions between cell types which are simple by themselves but result in a complicated situation altogether, which cannot be described by closed formulas but require numerical approaches instead. Our simulated measurements generally reflect the experimental data obtained by non-invasive imaging and immunohistochemical analyses. Differences remain in the earlier increase of the macrophage and Kupffer cell populations in our model as compared to the measurements. The maximum in angiogenic activity precedes the peak of macrophage density and normalization of liver volume. This shows that the model can

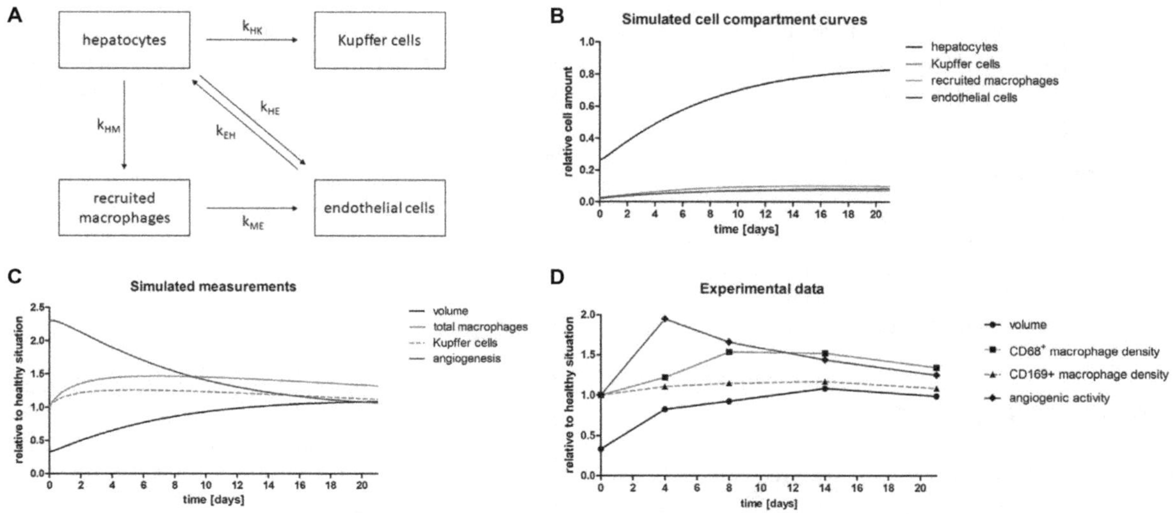

FIGURE 8 | Mathematical model describing liver regeneration. A mathematical model has been developed describing liver regeneration at organ and tissue scale. **(A)** The scheme shows the interrelations between liver cell compartments (hepatocytes, Kupffer cells, recruited macrophages, and endothelial cells) during liver regeneration. **(B)** The simulated cell compartment curves show the normalization of relative cell amounts after PHx. **(C)** The simulated measurement curves were computed based on the simulated cell compartment curves. After iterative adjustment the simulated curves describing liver volume, total macrophages, Kupffer cells, and angiogenesis showed similar time courses as the experimental data. **(D)** Diagram showing the time courses for liver volume, CD68+ macrophage density, CD169+ macrophages, and angiogenic activity of the experimental data acquired in mice after PHx.

describe liver regeneration at organ and tissue scale, and that the model substantially benefits from experimental quantitative non-invasive imaging data. Nevertheless, higher sample numbers would improve the stability and reliability of the model. At tissue scale, different mathematical models with considerable higher complexity than our model have been established that describe and predict specific important processes involved in liver regeneration. Recently, a mathematical model revealed a crucial role of hybrids consisting of hepatocytes and bone marrow cells that trigger proliferation in the regeneration process (Pedone et al., 2017). For liver regeneration after CCl_4 damage, Hoehme et al. have established a model that describes structural alignments of hepatocytes to sinusoids as a crucial pre-requisite for regaining the complex microarchitecture (Hoehme et al., 2010). Simple algorithmic models like the one proposed here have the advantage of high robustness and thus the suitability for integrating less quantitative *in vivo* data but also face several limitations. The model does not comprise the full complexity of the interrelations between the hepatocytes, macrophages, and endothelial cells that occur during liver regeneration. In addition, it does not describe causal relationships between the involved cell compartments in a detailed mechanistic way. Furthermore, the model does not take into consideration hepatic stellate cells, resident and monocyte-derived liver macrophages, additional immune cells such as lymphocytes or dendritic cells, the biliary system, different blood vessel compartments, hepatic blood flow or portal vein pressure, or the complex microarchitecture of the liver. Nevertheless, our model links information about liver regeneration and the interaction of different cell compartments (hepatocytes, Kupffer cells/macrophages, endothelial cells) from tissue to organ scale data. While our model is simplification as explained above, it can be extended to describe further liver cell compartments such as stellate cells, bile duct cells, and additional immune cells beyond macrophages or different macrophage populations. In addition, hepatocyte subpopulations in different activation states such as quiescent, primed, and replicating cells could be included as described by Furchtgott et al. (2009). A numerical model can also be used to extrapolate additional time points. To enable unambiguous parameter estimation, an increase in model complexity should be accompanied by an increase of measurement values. In our study, we used *in vivo* and immunohistochemical analyses for modeling, resulting in mean time curves and therefore one model per group. If longitudinal *in vivo* measurements are used, a model could be applied to analyze individual mice, enabling statistical comparison of kinetic parameters between groups. Either way a numerical model could be used to investigate and explain the effects of genetic modifications, e.g., *csf1*-knock-out resulting in a reduced number of macrophages (Amemiya et al., 2011), macrophage depletion, or extended liver resection (Christ et al., 2017) on different aspects of liver regeneration and such data could be used to refine, extend, or validate our simplified model. In addition, advanced numerical models could be used to get a comprehensive insight into the interrelations between different cells and signaling pathways in chronic liver disease progression or in response to therapeutic interventions (Cook et al., 2015; Schwen et al., 2016).

In summary, based on non-invasive imaging and immunohistochemical analyses, we have established a mathematical model for liver regeneration describing the interrelations between hepatocytes (volume recovery), macrophages, and endothelial cells (angiogenesis) at organ and tissue scale. In this context, non-invasive imaging and suitable probes targeting cell populations such as macrophages are of great value for data acquisition in the course of liver regeneration at organ scale.

ETHICS STATEMENT

All animal experiments were performed according to German legal requirements and animal protection laws and were approved by the Authority for Environment Conservation and Consumer Protection of the State of North Rhine-Westphalia (LANUV).

AUTHOR CONTRIBUTIONS

SZ and AM performed the experiments, acquired, and analyzed the data and wrote the manuscript. AR and DD participated in the experiments and data analyses. FG performed the modeling and FMT-µCT reconstruction. SW participated in the *in vivo* experiments. JFB participated in probe generation. UA participated in supervision and study design. JGB participated in study design. FK participated in study design, provided supervisory support, and edited the manuscript. WL designed and coordinated the experiments, provided supervisory support, wrote, and edited the manuscript. All authors read and approved the final version of the paper. SZ and AM contributed equally to this work.

FUNDING

This study was supported by the BMBF (German Federal Ministry of Education and Research) Projects "The Virtual Liver Network" (Grant No. 0315743 and 0315731) and LiSyM (Grant No. 031L0041), and the German Research Foundation (GR 5027/2-1).

REFERENCES

Abshagen, K., Eipel, C., Kalff, J. C., Menger, M. D., and Vollmar, B. (2007). Loss of NF-kappaB activation in Kupffer cell-depleted mice impairs liver regeneration after partial hepatectomy. *Am. J. Physiol. Gastrointest. Liver Physiol.* 292, G1570–G1577. doi: 10.1152/ajpgi.00399.2006

Alizai, P. H., Bertram, L., Kroy, D., Kummer, J., Andert, A., Neumann, U. P., et al. (2017). Expression of VEGFR-2 during liver regeneration after partial hepatectomy in a bioluminescence mouse model. *Eur. Surg. Res.* 58, 330–340. doi: 10.1159/000479628

Amemiya, H., Kono, H., and Fujii, H. (2011). Liver regeneration is impaired in macrophage colony stimulating factor deficient mice after partial hepatectomy. The role of M-CSF-induced macrophages. *J. Surg. Res.* 165, 59–67. doi: 10.1016/j.jss.2009.08.008

Castiglione, F., Pappalardo, F., Bianca, C., Russo, G., and Motta, S. (2014). Modeling biology spanning different scales. An open challenge. *Biomed. Res. Int.* 2014:902545. doi: 10.1155/2014/902545

Christ, B., Dahmen, U., Herrmann, K.-H., König, M., Reichenbach, J. R., Ricken, T., et al. (2017). Computational modeling in liver surgery. *Front. Physiol.* 8:906. doi: 10.3389/fphys.2017.00906

Cook, D., Ogunnaike, B. A., and Vadigepalli, R. (2015). Systems analysis of non-parenchymal cell modulation of liver repair across multiple regeneration modes. *BMC Syst. Biol.* 9:71. doi: 10.1186/s12918-015-0220-9

Drixler, T. A., Vogten, J. M., Gebbink, M. F. B. G., Carmeliet, P., Voest, E. E., and Borel Rinkes, I. H. M. (2003). Plasminogen mediates liver regeneration and angiogenesis after experimental partial hepatectomy. *Br. J. Surg.* 90, 1384–1390. doi: 10.1002/bjs.4275

Drixler, T. A., Vogten, M. J., Ritchie, E. D., Vroonhoven, v., Theo, J. M. V., Gebbink, M. F. B. G., et al. (2002). Liver regeneration is an angiogenesis-associated phenomenon. *Ann. Surg.* 236, 703–711. discussion 711-2. doi: 10.1097/00000658-200212000-00002

Freise, A. C., and Wu, A. M. (2015). *In vivo* imaging with antibodies and engineered fragments. *Mol. Immunol.* 67, 142–152. doi: 10.1016/j.molimm.2015.04.001

Furchtgott, L. A., Chow, C. C., and Periwal, V. (2009). A model of liver regeneration. *Biophys. J.* 96, 3926–3935. doi: 10.1016/j.bpj.2009.01.061

Gremse, F., Stärk, M., Ehling, J., Menzel, J. R., Lammers, T., and Kiessling, F. (2016). Imalytics preclinical. Interactive analysis of biomedical volume data. *Theranostics* 6, 328–341. doi: 10.7150/thno.13624

Gremse, F., Theek, B., Kunjachan, S., Lederle, W., Pardo, A., Barth, S., et al. (2014). Absorption reconstruction improves biodistribution assessment of fluorescent nanoprobes using hybrid fluorescence-mediated tomography. *Theranostics* 4, 960–971. doi: 10.7150/thno.9293

Higgins, G. M., and Anderson, R. M. (1931). Experimental pathology of liver: restoration of liver in white rat following partial surgical removal. *Arch. Pathol.* 12, 186–202.

Hoehme, S., Brulport, M., Bauer, A., Bedawy, E., Schormann, W., Hermes, M., et al. (2010). Prediction and validation of cell alignment along microvessels as order principle to restore tissue architecture in liver regeneration. *Proc. Natl. Acad. Sci. USA* 107, 10371–10376. doi: 10.1073/pnas.0909374107

Itoh, T., and Miyajima, A. (2014). Liver regeneration by stem/progenitor cells. *Hepatology* 59, 1617–1626. doi: 10.1002/hep.26753

Kunjachan, S., Gremse, F., Theek, B., Koczera, P., Pola, R., Pechar, M., et al. (2013). Noninvasive optical imaging of nanomedicine biodistribution. *ACS Nano* 7, 252–262. doi: 10.1021/nn303955n

Lederle, W., Linde, N., Heusel, J., Bzyl, J., Woenne, E. C., Zwick, S., et al. (2010). Platelet-derived growth factor-B normalizes micromorphology and vessel function in vascular endothelial growth factor-A-induced squamous cell carcinomas. *Am. J. Pathol.* 176, 981–994. doi: 10.2353/ajpath.2010.080998

Li, N., and Hua, J. (2017). Immune cells in liver regeneration. *Oncotarget* 8, 3628–3639. doi: 10.18632/oncotarget.12275

Melgar-Lesmes, P., and Edelman, E. R. (2015). Monocyte-endothelial cell interactions in the regulation of vascular sprouting and liver regeneration in mouse. *J. Hepatol.* 63, 917–925. doi: 10.1016/j.jhep.2015.05.011

Michalopoulos, G. K. (2010). Liver regeneration after partial hepatectomy. Critical analysis of mechanistic dilemmas. *Am. J. Pathol.* 176, 2–13. doi: 10.2353/ajpath.2010.090675

Minuk, G. Y. (2003). Hepatic regeneration. If it ain't broke, don't fix it. *Can. J. Gastroenterol.* 17, 418–424. doi: 10.1155/2003/615403

Mitchell, C., and Willenbring, H. (2008). A reproducible and well-tolerated method for 2/3 partial hepatectomy in mice. *Nat. Protoc.* 3, 1167–1170. doi: 10.1038/nprot.2008.80

Nishiyama, K., Nakashima, H., Ikarashi, M., Kinoshita, M., Nakashima, M., Aosasa, S., et al. (2015). Mouse CD11b+Kupffer cells recruited from bone marrow accelerate liver regeneration after partial hepatectomy. *PLoS One* 10:e0136774. doi: 10.1371/journal.pone.0136774

Pedone, E., Olteanu, V.-A., Marucci, L., Muñoz-Martin, M. I., Youssef, S. A., de Bruin, A., et al. (2017). Modeling dynamics and function of bone marrow cells in mouse liver regeneration. *Cell Rep.* 18, 107–121. doi: 10.1016/j.celrep.2016.12.008

Pleskovic, A., Demsar, F., and Suput, D. (1996). Assessment of liver regeneration by quantitative MRI analysis. *Pflugers Arch. - Eur. J. Physiol.* 431(Suppl. 6), R307–R308.

Rosenhain, S., Magnuska Zuzanna, A., Yamoah, G. G., Wa'el, A. R., Kiessling, F., and Gremse, F. (2018). A preclinical micro-computed tomography database including 3D whole body organ segmentations. *Sci. Data* 5:180294. doi: 10.1038/sdata.2018.294

Schwen, L. O., Kuepfer, L., and Preusser, T. (2016). Modeling approaches for hepatic spatial heterogeneity in pharmacokinetic simulations. *Drug Discov. Today Dis. Model.* 22, 35–43. doi: 10.1016/j.ddmod.2017.09.002

Takeishi, T., Hirano, K., Kobayashi, T., Hasegawa, G., Hatakeyama, K., and Naito, M. (1999). The role of Kupffer cells in liver regeneration. *Arch. Histol. Cytol.* 62, 413–422.

Taub, R. (2004). Liver regeneration. From myth to mechanism. *Nat. Rev. Mol. Cell Biol.* 5, 836–847. doi: 10.1038/nrm1489

Uda, Y., Hirano, T., Son, G., Iimuro, Y., Uyama, N., Yamanaka, J., et al. (2013). Angiogenesis is crucial for liver regeneration after partial hepatectomy. *Surgery* 153, 70–77. doi: 10.1016/j.surg.2012.06.021

Vekemans, K., and Braet, F. (2005). Structural and functional aspects of the liver and liver sinusoidal cells in relation to colon carcinoma metastasis. *World J. Gastroenterol.* 11, 5095–5102. doi: 10.3748/wjg.v11.i33.5095

Wen, Y., Feng, D., Wu, H., Liu, W., Li, H., Wang, F., et al. (2015). Defective initiation of liver regeneration in osteopontin-deficient mice after partial hepatectomy due to insufficient activation of IL-6/Stat3 pathway. *Int. J. Biol. Sci.* 11, 1236–1247. doi: 10.7150/ijbs.12118

15

The Diurnal Timing of Starvation Differently Impacts Murine Hepatic Gene Expression and Lipid Metabolism – A Systems Biology Analysis Using Self-Organizing Maps

Christiane Rennert[1], Sebastian Vlaic[2], Eugenia Marbach-Breitrück[1,3,4], Carlo Thiel[1], Susanne Sales[5], Andrej Shevchenko[5], Rolf Gebhardt[1] and Madlen Matz-Soja[1]*

[1] Rudolf-Schönheimer-Institute of Biochemistry, Faculty of Medicine, Leipzig University, Leipzig, Germany, [2] Leibniz Institute for Natural Product Research and Infection Biology, Hans-Knöll-Institute, Jena, Germany, [3] Institute of Biochemistry, Charité – Universitätsmedizin Berlin, Berlin, Germany, [4] Berlin Institute of Health, Freie Universität Berlin, Humboldt-Universität zu Berlin, Berlin, Germany, [5] Max Planck Institute of Molecular Cell Biology and Genetics, Dresden, Germany

***Correspondence:**
Madlen Matz-Soja
madlen.matz@medizin.uni-leipzig.de

Organisms adapt their metabolism and draw on reserves as a consequence of food deprivation. The central role of the liver in starvation response is to coordinate a sufficient energy supply for the entire organism, which has frequently been investigated. However, knowledge of how circadian rhythms impact on and alter this response is scarce. Therefore, we investigated the influence of different timings of starvation on global hepatic gene expression. Mice (n = 3 each) were challenged with 24-h food deprivation started in the morning or evening, coupled with refeeding for different lengths and compared with *ad libitum* fed control groups. Alterations in hepatocyte gene expression were quantified using microarrays and confirmed or complemented with qPCR, especially for lowly detectable transcription factors. Analysis was performed using self-organizing maps (SOMs), which bases on clustering genes with similar expression profiles. This provides an intuitive overview of expression trends and allows easier global comparisons between complex conditions. Transcriptome analysis revealed a strong circadian-driven response to fasting based on the diurnal expression of transcription factors (e.g., *Ppara*, *Pparg*). Starvation initiated in the morning produced known metabolic adaptations in the liver; e.g., switching from glucose storage to consumption and gluconeogenesis. However, starvation initiated in the evening produced a different expression signature that was controlled by yet unknown regulatory mechanisms. For example, the expression of genes involved in gluconeogenesis decreased and fatty acid and cholesterol synthesis genes were induced. The differential regulation after morning and evening starvation were also reflected at the lipidome level. The accumulation of hepatocellular storage lipids (triacylglycerides, cholesteryl esters) was significantly higher after the initiation of starvation in the morning compared to the evening. Concerning refeeding, the gene expression pattern after a 12 h refeeding period largely resembled that of the corresponding starvation state but approached the *ad libitum* control state after refeeding for 21 h. Some components of these regulatory circuits are discussed. Collectively, these data illustrate a highly time-dependent starvation response in the liver and suggest that a circadian influence cannot be neglected when starvation is the focus of research or medicine, e.g., in the case of treating victims of sudden starvation events.

Keywords: hepatocyte, circadian regulation, self-organizing map, starvation, refeeding

INTRODUCTION

Organisms handle periods of food deprivation by drawing on reserves and adapting their metabolism. Humans use fasting to lose weight and for spiritual reasons. The liver is the central hub for metabolic processes, including glucose, amino acid, and lipid metabolism. Therefore, the impact of fasting and refeeding is immense, especially on hepatic parameters (Longo and Mattson, 2014). In this study we addressed the question how the circadian regulation influences the hepatic starvation response with a rarely but powerful used approach called self-organizing map (SOM).

Livers in the post-prandial state store excessive metabolites as glycogen and produce fatty acids, which are transiently stored as triacylglycerides (TAGs) or secreted as very low density lipoprotein (VLDL) (Rui, 2014). The liver synthesizes new carbohydrates and produces ketone bodies in periods of prolonged fasting after depletion of glucose stores. Hormones, such as insulin and glucagon, regulate these processes at a systemic level, and transcription factors, such as PPARs (peroxisome proliferator activated receptor), SREBP transcripts (sterol regulatory element binding transcription protein), and ChREBP [carbohydrate-responsive element-binding protein or MLX-interacting protein-like (MLXIPL)] adjust the metabolism at the molecular level.

Besides the impact of feeding state on the liver metabolism, the timing of food supply influences the metabolic state enormously (Wehrens et al., 2017). In general, the mammalian physiology is synchronized by an inner time-keeping mechanism called the circadian clock. The molecular circadian regulation is based on central clock genes expressed in almost all tissues and cells. The translated proteins generate and regulate the circadian rhythm via transcriptional and translational feedback loops. The transcriptional activators ARNTL (aryl hydrocarbon receptor nuclear translocator-like protein 1 or BMAL1) and CLOCK (circadian locomotor output cycles kaput) stimulate the expression of the negative regulators Period (*Per1*, *Per2*, and *Per3*) and Cryprochrome (*Cry1* and *Cry2*), which in turn repress ARNTL/CLOCK activity. The overall circadian rhythm is coordinated by the suprachiasmatic nuclei (SCN) in the hypothalamus (Ralph et al., 1990; Welsh et al., 2010). Synchronized by an optic light/dark signal the SCN generates output signals coupling the central pacemaker with the peripheral tissues. On the basis of oscillating hormonal and endocrine signals (Yang et al., 2007) the peripheral organs, such as the liver, synchronize their own circadian oscillation. Approximately 15% of all genes are transcribed in a circadian manner whereby one big aspect of circadian regulation includes metabolic processes and energy homeostasis in peripheral tissues, especially in liver (Albrecht, 2012). The tight connection between circadian clock and metabolic processes is underlined by the fact that a vast majority of liver genes is expressed rhythmically, including those regulating, e.g., glucose or lipid metabolism (Stratmann and Schibler, 2006; Ferrell and Chiang, 2015). Interestingly, the liver clock was shown not only be entrained by SCN-synchronization, but also by external factors. One of the most prominent influencers of liver circadian rhythms is the feeding regime. The consumed food volume and the starvation intervals between the meals are able to alter the liver clock (Hirao et al., 2010) and restricted feeding can even rapidly uncouple the liver rhythm from that of SCN (Stokkan et al., 2001).

Disturbance of the normal eating patterns of mice using external food restriction alters the entire metabolism (Jensen et al., 2013), which were analyzed previously using different omics approaches (Bauer et al., 2004; Sokolović et al., 2008; Hakvoort et al., 2011). However, knowledge of specific modulations produced by circadian regulation is scarce. Therefore, we analyzed the impact of fasting and refeeding at two different time-points [zeitgeber time (ZT) 3 and ZT 12] on the physiological and metabolic states of primary hepatocytes at a global omics level. Evaluations of transcriptome data were performed using SOMs. SOMs are an alternative approach that allows the identification of global expression trends via clustering of similarly expressed genes. The relative expression of gene groups is color-coded and enables an intuitive and unbiased interpretation of the data (Wirth et al., 2011). The results demonstrated that the timing of food restriction altered the influence of starvation on hepatocytes. A 24-h starvation period produced different gene expression patterns and lipidome profiles in liver cells depending on the starting time. While starvation started in the morning led to the known adaptions like initiation of gluconeogenesis and suppression of fatty acid and cholesterol synthesis, starvation started in the evening decreased gluconeogenesis-associated gene expression and induced fatty acid synthesis genes. Refeeding mice for 12 h after a 24-h long starvation period was not sufficient to restore the gene expression pattern of *ad libitum* fed mice, which was revealed by persistent dysregulation of essential metabolic pathways, such as lipid metabolism and autophagy. However, an extended refeeding period of 21 h approached an expression pattern similar to that of the *ad libitum* state, but some differences persisted.

MATERIALS AND METHODS

Maintenance of the Mice and Feeding

Male C57BL/6N mice were maintained in a pathogen-free facility on a 12:12 h light–dark cycle (light on at 6 a.m = ZT 0, light off at 6 p.m. = ZT 12), according to German guidelines and those of the world medical association declaration of Helsinki for the care and safe use of experimental animals. The animal experiments were approved by the Landesdirektion Sachsen. The mice had free access to regular chow (ssniff® R/M-H V1534; 58%, 33%, 9% calories from carbohydrates, proteins and fat, respectively; metabolisable energy: 12.8 kJ/g; ssniff® Spezialdiaeten GmbH, Germany) and tap water.

Prior to the experimental procedures, animals were randomly segregated into six groups ($n = 3$ each). In a first experiment, starvation was started either at ZT 3 (9 a.m.) or at ZT 12 (6 p.m.) and mice were sacrificed after 24 h at the same times on the next day together with *ad libitum* fed groups (**Figure 1A**). In the refeeding experiment two groups of mice were starved for 24 h started at ZT 15 followed by refeeding for 12 or 21 h until ZT 3 and ZT 12 on the next day, respectively (**Figure 1B**).

Isolation of Primary Mouse Hepatocytes, RNA Isolation, and Quantitative Real-Time PCR (qPCR)

The primary hepatocytes were isolated from male C57BL/6N mice, treated like explained above. Isolation was performed by a collagenase perfusion technique as described before (Gebhardt et al., 2003). The cell suspension was cleared of non-parenchymal cells by differential centrifugation steps (Matz-Soja et al., 2014). Pure hepatocyte fraction was used for further procedures.

Total RNA from hepatocytes was extracted using RNeasy® Mini Kit (Qiagen, Hilden) and the quality was controlled by agarose gel electrophoresis. The reverse transcription was performed with the Proto Script M-MuLV First Strand cDNA Synthesis Kit (New England Biolabs). Gene expression quantification by qPCR was performed in duplicates using the Rotor-Gene SYBR® Green PCR Kit and a Rotor-Gene Q (Qiagen). Gene specific intron-spanning primers were designed with Primer 3 software and are listed in **Supplementary Table 1**. The specific qPCR products were quantified using internal amplification standards; 18S was used as reference gene. Values are plotted as average of biological replicates ($n = 3$) $\pm$ standard deviation. The statistical evaluation was performed with the unpaired Student's t-test (GraphPad Prism 7). The null hypothesis was rejected at $^{*}p < 0.05$, $^{**}p < 0.01$, and $^{***}p < 0.001$ levels.

Illumina Microarray Processing and Data Analysis Using SOM

For each condition, the RNA from three mice was pooled and used as one sample in the microarrays (BeadChip Array MouseRef-8 v2, Illumina). The analysis was performed by the Interdisciplinary Centre for Clinical Research, Leipzig (Faculty of Medicine, Leipzig University). The following link provides the raw data of the microarray[1].

All computational analyses were performed using R software (Ihaka and Gentleman, 1996). Microarrays were annotated using the annotation provided by Illumina and raw expression data were pre-processed using the lumi package (Du et al., 2008). Pre-processing included background correction using the bgAdjust method, variance stabilization transformation, and quantile normalization. Detection calls were performed with default parameters to remove absent beads. Furthermore, the expression values for single beads were mapped to a gene symbol identifier. For each array, multiple bead IDs mapping to the same gene symbol were averaged.

General expression trends in each sample were identified using SOMs as implemented in the oposSOM package (Löffler-Wirth et al., 2015). SOMs are artificial neural networks trained by unsupervised learning (Kohonen, 1982). This machine learning approach allows dimension reduction of high-dimensional data by clustering similarly regulated genes to so-called "metagenes". For each treatment, it can be defined if the expression of a certain metagene is over or under the mean expression of this metagene in the analyzed pool (termed as over- and underexpression), and all groups are compared equivalently. The metagenes, here 20×20, can be visualized in a map where adjacent metagenes have similar expression profiles and more distant ones are expressed differently, with the invariant genes located in the center of the map. Furthermore, a color gradient codes the expression level of the metagenes, maroon indicating the highest expression, blue the lowest expression, and yellow and green intermediate levels (Wirth et al., 2011). This image-based analysis allows an intuitive interpretation and provides an overview of the overall regulation patterns. Apart from the creation of SOMs, the oposSOM package also provided additional analytical methods including the identification of over- or underexpressed spots in the SOMs, clustering of metagenes using k-means (Hartigan and Wong, 1979), and enrichment testing for metagene-cluster and over- or underexpressed spots using Gene Ontology (GO) terms (Ashburner et al., 2000) as provided by the Ensembl database (Aken et al., 2016).

Based on the k-means clustering as performed automatically by the oposSOM package, we performed a gene enrichment analysis (GEA) for all genes with an absolute expression change $\geq$ 1.5-fold and the genes from each cluster using the web-based tool DAVID (Database for Annotation, Visualization and Integrated Discovery Bioinformatics Resources 6.8[2], **RRID**:SCR_001881). We selected *Mus musculus* as the background and filtered the GO terms with a Benjamini–Hochberg corrected p-value < 0.05.

Visualization of single genes for the identified significant GO terms was performed using heatmaps. The expression levels of single genes were displayed as relative expression values compared to the mean expression in all six samples analogous to the metagenes (termed as over- and underexpression). All genes with an absolute expression change $\geq$ 1.5-fold [$\log_2(1.5)$] between at least two of the six groups were considered for further analysis.

The STRING database version 10.5[3] was used to explore the interactions between the studied genes/proteins related to hepatic starvation response (Szklarczyk et al., 2015). The networks were

[1] https://seek.lisym.org/data_files/98?code=YGHGwNPpYhqpiEBnnv4qb%2BchjgjUoYGhH6bc3OQp

[2] https://david.ncifcrf.gov/

[3] http://string-db.org

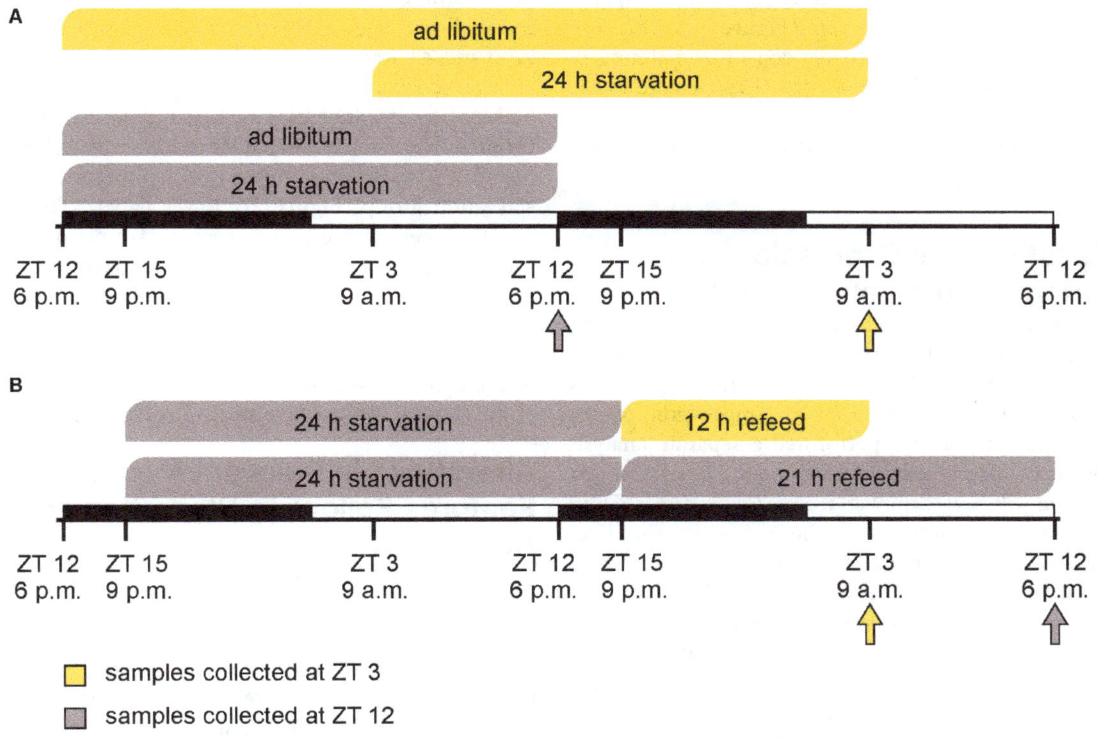

FIGURE 1 | Timeline of feeding/starving cycles and sacrifice. **(A)** Mice were fed *ad libitum* or starved for 24 h prior to sacrifice at ZT 3 (9 a.m.) or ZT 12 (6 p.m.). **(B)** Mice were starved for 24 h from ZT 15 (9 p.m.) to ZT 15 and refed for 12 or 21 h prior sacrifice. The arrows indicate the times of sacrifice.

constructed in the "confidence" mode with a high confidence score (0.7).

Shotgun Lipidomics

Lipids from primary hepatocytes were extracted by a modified protocol of Folch (Folch et al., 1957) and analyzed by shotgun mass spectrometry as described previously (Schuhmann et al., 2012). Briefly, hepatocytes (an amount equivalent to 10 μg of total protein) were dissolved in 200 μl ammonium bicarbonate solution (150 mM). For the subsequent quantification 10 μl internal standard mixture were added (20 pmol TAG 12:0-12:0-12:0, 20 pmol DAG 17:0- 17:0, 40 pmol diethyl PC 18:0-18:0, 50 pmol diethyl PE 20:0-20-0, 10 pmol PG 17:0-17-0, 40 pmol PS 12:0-12:0, 50 pmol PI 16:0-16-0, 40 pmol LPC 12:0, 40 pmol LPE 14:0, 30 pmol SM d18:1-12:0, 90 pmol CE 12:0, 20 pmol Cer d18:1-12:0, 50 pmol cholesterol d7; Avanti Polar Lipids, Inc., Alabaster, AL, United States). Then, 265 μl of methanol and 730 μl of chloroform were added and the mixture was vortexed for 1 h at 4°C. The lower organic phase was collected, dried in a vacuum centrifuge and the lipid extracts were re-dissolved in 120 μl chloroform:methanol [1:2 (v/v)] mixture. The analysis was performed in both, negative, and positive ion mode. For negative mode analyses, 10 μl extract were mixed with either 12 μl of 13 mM ammonium acetate in isopropanol or 0.1% (v/v) triethylamine in methanol. For positive mode analyses, 10 μl extract were mixed with 90 μl of 6.5 mM ammonium acetate in isopropanol before infusion. The analyses were performed on a Q Exactive mass spectrometer (Thermo Fisher Scientific, Germany) equipped with a robotic nanoflow ion source TriVersa NanoMate (Advion BioSciences, Ithaca, NY, United States). High resolution (140,000 at m/z 200) FT-MS spectra were acquired for 1 min within the range of m/z 420–1000 in negative and 450–1000 in positive mode. Cholesterol was quantified as previously described (Liebisch et al., 2006). Briefly, 30 μl of extract were dried under vacuum, then 75 μl acetyl chloride:chloroform [1:2 (v/v)] were added, incubated for 1 h at room temperature, dried under vacuum and re-dissolved in 60 μl chloroform:methanol [1:2 (v/v)]. 10 μl extract were mixed with 90 μl of 6.5 mM ammonium acetate in propanol before infusion and analyzed in positive ion mode. The following lipid classes were identified and quantified using the LipidXplorer software (Herzog et al., 2011): tri- and diacylglycerides (TAG/DAG), cholesteryl esters (CE), sphingomyelins (SM), phosphatidylethanolamines (PEs), phosphatidylcholines (PCs), and cholesterol. The concentrations are plotted in pmol lipid per μg total protein as average of the biological replicates ($n = 3$) ± standard deviation.

RESULTS

Feeding procedures immensely affect an organism's metabolism. The present study examined alterations in the physiology and the metabolism of murine hepatocytes following a 24-h starvation period initiated at ZT 3 (morning) or ZT 12 (evening) compared to hepatocytes from mice fed *ad libitum* (**Figure 1A**). Our data indicated that the effects strongly depended on the timing of starvation. We also compared hepatocytes in refed state to the corresponding starvation group and *ad libitum* fed mice to evaluate whether 12 or 21 h of refeeding were sufficient to restore the *ad libitum* expression profile (**Figure 1B**).

Global Hepatic Gene Expression Is Influenced by Feeding and Timing

Illumina microarrays, analyzed, and visualized using SOMs, delivered an overview of the hepatic alterations induced by different feeding regimes. A GEA of all regulated genes (**Supplementary Table 2A**) produced an impression of the involved GO terms. Further we performed a separate analysis for each cluster to distinguish between them. Based on the SOMs of the *ad libitum* samples from ZT 3 and ZT 12 it strikes that a large amount of the genes in the liver were expressed in a circadian manner (**Figure 2A**), since the expression of almost all metagenes differed. ZT 3 showed two overexpression spots at the left margin, annotated as clusters A and B by a k-means clustering of the SOMs (**Figure 2D** and **Supplementary Table 2B**). Cluster A is associated with immune system processes ('complement activation,' classical pathway,' 'innate immune response') and many GO terms in regard to extracellular space and membrane ('extracellular region,' 'plasma membrane,' 'cell surface'), while cluster B contains many lipid metabolism associated GO terms ('fatty acid metabolic process,' 'acyl-CoA metabolic process') and the GO term 'autophagy.' The large underexpression spot in the upper right corner partly covered by cluster J contains many cholesterol and steroid associated GO terms ('cholesterol metabolic process,' 'steroid metabolic process,' 'fatty acid metabolic process'). In comparison to ZT 3, ZT 12 exhibited a mean expression in the area of clusters B and J (**Figures 2A,D**). But ZT 12 had a small overexpressed area in the upper left corner (cluster H) related to the GO term 'metabolic process' and an underexpression spot in the lower right corner (cluster F) containing GO terms associated with protein binding and degradation ('chaperone binding,' 'endoplasmic reticulum,' 'proteasome accessory complex').

Starvation started at both ZT 3 and ZT 12 immensely changed the expression profiles of the metagenes in the SOMs compared to the related *ad libitum* state (**Figure 2B**). Additionally, comparing ZT 3 and ZT 12 starvation no congruence is visible, which implies a diurnal-driven response to fasting. The 24-h starvation period at ZT 3 began during the day followed by a whole night of fasting (**Figure 1A**), which changed the size and shape of the overexpression spot in the lower left corner and the underexpression spot in the upper right corner (clusters B and J), regions associated with lipid and steroid metabolism (**Figures 2B,D**). In contrast, the ZT 12 starvation period started in the night followed by a whole day of fasting (**Figure 1A**) and resulted in a totally changed metagene expression, where the whole left margin is underexpressed, while the right margin shows an overexpression (**Figure 2B**). The regions (clusters B and J) where GO terms related to autophagy, lipid and steroid metabolism are localized have an opposed expression comparing ZT 3 and ZT 12 starvation.

The refeeding experiment (**Figure 1B**) revealed disparate SOMs after refeeding mice for 12 h and the ZT 3 *ad libitum* group (**Figure 2C**). However, the SOM of 12 h refeed (**Figure 2C**, upper panel) showed high similarity with the corresponding ZT 12 starvation group (**Figure 2B**, lower panel). The mice sampled at ZT 12 were starved for the same 24-h period, but were refed for 21 h prior sacrifice. This prolonged refeed period produced a somehow mixture of expression profiles from ZT 12 *ad libitum* and starvation state (**Figure 2C**). While clusters F and H resemble that of ZT 12 *ad libitum* (**Figure 2A**, lower panel), the regions where lipid and steroid metabolism are localized (clusters B and J) still showed the starvation pattern (**Figure 2B**, lower panel).

Alterations in Relevant Metabolic Features Following Starvation and Refeeding

SOM analysis identified differently regulated metabolic alterations produced by the various feeding regimes. A list of all regulated genes detected by the microarrays is compiled in **Supplementary Table 3**. The present study focused on the expression of genes related to intermediary metabolism (glucose and lipid metabolism), steroid metabolism, insulin signaling, and autophagy. We also analyzed central clock gene expression because the circadian aspect of the feeding regimes was particularly interesting. The interactions of the involved genes/proteins were visualized within a protein interaction network, illustrating the mutual connections (**Supplementary Figure 1**).

Circadian Regulation

Diurnal influence

Being the first order clock genes, *Arntl* and *Clock* gene products activate the expression of different target genes, including *Per1/2/3* homolog and *Cry*. PER and CRY, in turn, repress their own expression by interacting with ARNTL and CLOCK (Partch et al., 2014). Consequently to these regulations the expression of *Arntl/Clock* and *Per* occurs in antiphase, which is seen in **Figure 3** (*ad libitum*). In the *ad libitum* state *Arntl* and *Clock* were overexpressed at ZT 3 and underexpressed at ZT 12, *Per1* and *Per2* were regulated vice versa. *Nr1d2* (Rev-erb beta), another gene of the negative feedback loop, exhibited a typical rhythmic regulation with a higher expression at ZT 12 than at ZT 3. These results were verified by qPCR and used to validate the microarray (data not shown).

Starvation

Expression of central clock genes were primarily regulated in a diurnal manner (**Figure 3**). However, fasting also influenced central circadian genes. A 24-h starvation period initiated at ZT 3 or ZT 12 increased *Arntl* and *Clock* expression levels, but the typical diurnal regulation of these genes remained. The opponent *Per2* was down-regulated after starvation initiated at ZT 3 and up-regulated in the ZT 12 starvation mice compared to the corresponding *ad libitum* samples. The *Per1* expression was only

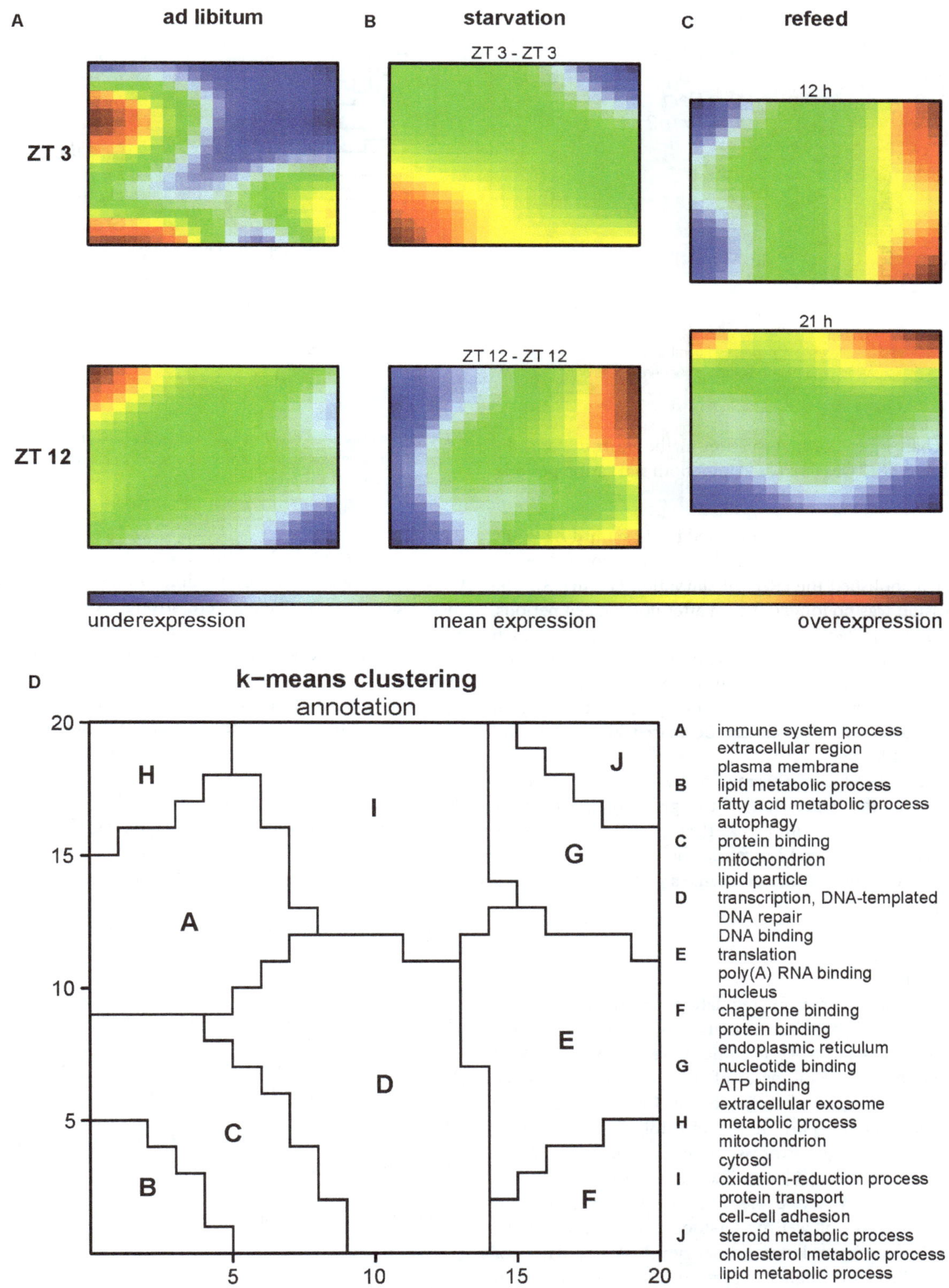

FIGURE 2 | Global hepatic gene expression dependent on feeding patterns and timing. **(A–C)** Self organizing maps (SOMs) illustrating the expression of metagenes (20 × 20); maroon indicates an overexpression, blue an underexpression. Mice were sacrificed at ZT 3 and ZT 12 after **(A)** fed *ad libitum*, **(B)** starved for 24 h or **(C)** starved for 24 h and refed for 12 h until ZT 3 or 21 h until ZT 12. **(D)** Annotation of the SOMs using k-means clustering and following gene-enrichment analysis. Selected GO terms are shown. A full list is available in **Supplementary Table 2B**.

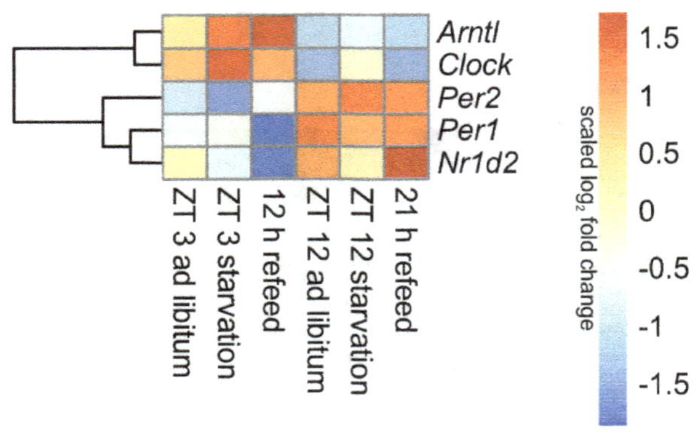

FIGURE 3 | Heatmap of differentially expressed central circadian genes. Red indicates an overexpression, and blue indicates an underexpression.

marginally changed by 24-h starvation in the morning and the evening, while *Nr1d2* was decreased after both starvation periods.

Refeed

When mice were fasted for 24 h and refed for 12 h until ZT 3, the *Arntl* expression was highly increased, while a prolonged refeed period of 21 h abolished the effect of starvation (**Figure 3**). The *Clock* expression was no longer altered after both refeed periods. *Per1* expression was decreased after a 12 h refeed, but the 21 h refeed already restored the *ad libitum* expression. *Per2* expression was higher after both refeed periods in comparison to *ad libitum*. The expression of *Nr1d2* showed big changes after both refeed periods, the expression was further decreased after 12 h and increased after 21 h refeed.

All in all, a 21 h refeeding seemed to be sufficient to abolish the alterations in the expression of the genes of the primary negative-feedback loop (*Arntl*, *Clock*, *Per1*, and *Per2*) caused by starving the mice. But after 12 h refeed the expression of *Arntl*, *Per1*, and *Per2* still showed major changes compared to the *ad libitum* sample.

Insulin Signaling

Diurnal influence

Insulin is one of the master regulators of the metabolism and its effects are partially mediated by insulin receptor signaling (Boucher et al., 2014). The microarray analyses revealed diurnal regulation of several genes of this pathway (**Figure 4**). For example, *Pik3r1* (phosphatidylinositol 3-kinase, regulatory subunit, polypeptide 1), part of the inositol phosphorylation complex, showed a lower expression in the morning (ZT 3) compared to the evening (ZT 12). The same regulation occurs for *Mup4* (major urinary protein 4) whose influence on energy metabolism is not well understood yet. However, *Pdk4* (pyruvate dehydrogenase kinase, isoenzyme 4), regulator of glucose metabolism, was higher expressed in the morning than in the evening.

Starvation

The 24-h starvation period initiated in the morning produced strong overexpression of central hepatic insulin signaling genes

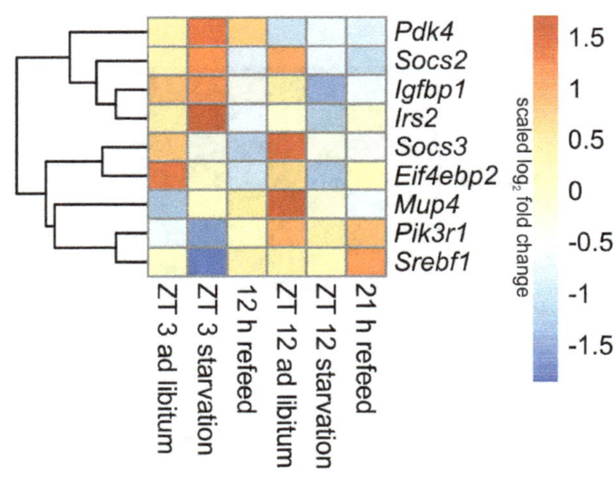

FIGURE 4 | Heatmap of differentially expressed genes related to insulin signaling. Red indicates an overexpression, and blue indicates an underexpression.

[e.g., *Pdk4*, *Mup4*, *Irs2* (insulin receptor substrate 2) and *Igfbp1* (insulin like growth factor binding protein 1)]. Notably, all of these genes, except *Pdk4*, were strongly down-regulated after starvation initiated at ZT 12. The expression of *Pik3r1* and *Eif4ebp2* (eukaryotic translation initiation factor 4E binding protein 2), which is a regulator of translation, was lowered in both starvation periods (**Figure 4**). The transcription factor *Srebf1c* was down-regulated only due to starvation started at ZT 3, and it was unaffected by evening starvation (**Figure 6**).

Socs2 and *Socs3* (suppressor of cytokine signaling), which were not regulated diurnally in *ad libitum* fed mice, are associated to the negative regulation of insulin signaling. The data for *Socs2* and *Socs3* revealed a change from an overexpression in ZT 12 *ad libitum* sample to a strong underexpression due to starvation started at ZT 12. *Socs3* expression also slightly decreased when starvation was initiated at ZT 3, but *Socs2* expression slightly increased (**Figure 4**).

Refeed

The expression of nearly all detected genes of insulin receptor signaling did not recover during the 12 h refeeding and resembled the expression of the ZT 12 starvation mice (**Figure 4**). Exceptions included *Pdk4*, which almost reached *ad libitum* levels, and *Srebf1c*, which was highly induced during refeeding. The gene expression levels of *Pdk4*, *Eif4ebp2*, *Pik3r1*, and *Irs2* after a refeeding period of 21 h were similar to the corresponding *ad libitum* levels. The *Socs2* and *Socs3* genes were considerably underexpressed after both refeeding periods.

Autophagy

Diurnal influence

In *ad libitum* fed mice, central genes of the mammalian autophagy pathway, such as *Ulk2* (unc-51 like kinase 2) and *Uvrag* (UV radiation resistance associated gene), were lower expressed in the morning compared to evening. However, *Sqstm1*

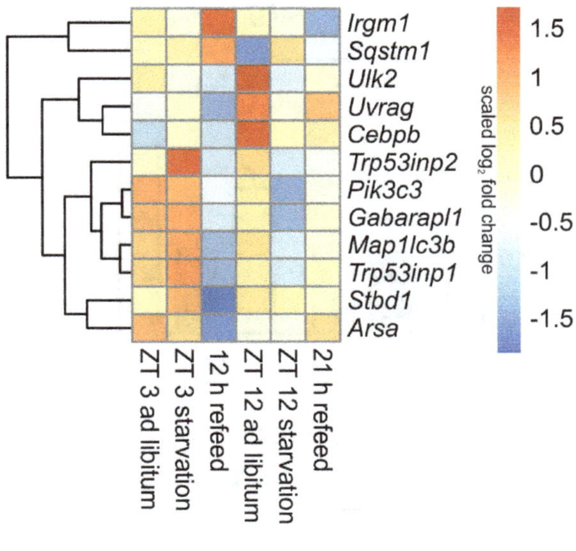

FIGURE 5 | Heatmap of differentially expressed genes related to autophagy. Red indicates an overexpression, and blue indicates an underexpression.

(sequestosome 1), which is required for the recognition of protein aggregates by the autophagy machinery (Bjorkoy et al., 2005), was significantly down-regulated at ZT 12 compared to ZT 3 *ad libitum*. A regulator of autophagy, *Cebpb* (CCAAT/enhancer binding protein beta) was higher expressed in the evening than in the morning (**Figure 5**).

Starvation

When starvation was started at ZT 3 expression of many of the autophagy-associated genes [e.g., *Ulk2, Uvrag, Sqstm1, Pik3c3* (phosphatidylinositol 3-kinase catalytic subunit type 3), *Trp53inp1* (transformation related protein 53 inducible nuclear protein 1), *Gabarapl1* (gamma-aminobutyric acid A receptor-associated protein-like 1), *Map1lc3b* (microtubule-associated protein 1 light chain 3 beta)] was not altered (**Figure 5**). Only *Trp53inp2*, which is essential for autophagosome formation, was markedly up-regulated during the ZT 3 starvation period.

This observation dramatically changed when the starvation period of 24-h was started at ZT 12. The above-mentioned central autophagy genes, with the exception of *Sqstm1*, were dramatically down-regulated during this fasting period, which was especially prominent for *Ulk2* expression. The transcription factor *Cebpb* was up-regulated after food deprivation started at ZT 3 and down-regulated in the evening (**Figure 5**).

Refeed

Our study revealed that the dramatic down-regulation of central autophagy genes due to the initiation of starvation in the evening remained during a refeeding period of 12 h (**Figure 5**). The expression of *Uvrag, Trp53inp1, Stbd1* (starch binding domain 1) and *Arsa* (arylsulfatase A) was further reduced. However, *Sqstm1* and *Irgm1* (immunity-related GTPase family M member 1), which are involved in autophagic protein degradation (Traver et al., 2011), were up-regulated during the 12 h refeeding period. After a prolonged refeeding of 21 h, most autophagy-related genes approached the ZT 12 *ad libitum* expression levels, but did not reach it. *Cebpb* was expressed at the *ad libitum* level after the 12 h refeed, but its expression was lowered after the 21 h refeed (**Figure 5**).

Intermediary Metabolism

Diurnal influence

Many genes associated with intermediary metabolism (lipid and glucose metabolism) showed a time-dependent expression. The transcription factors that mainly regulate intermediary metabolism, such as *Ppara, Pparg,* and *Hnf4a* (hepatocyte nuclear factor 4 alpha), were higher expressed at ZT 12 than at ZT 3, *Mlxipl* (ChREBP) exhibits a vice versa regulation (**Figures 6, 7**). *Srebf1* transcripts showed no diurnal changes (**Figure 6**). The members of the Elovl (elongation of very long chain fatty acids protein) family (*Elovl2, Elovl3,* and *Elovl5*), which are involved in lipid metabolism, were higher expressed at ZT 3 compared to ZT 12, but *Elovl6* exhibited an inverse regulation (**Figure 7**).

Starvation

The regulation of hepatic lipid and glucose metabolisms is based on different transcription factors. The expression of *Ppara, Pparg,* and *Hnf4a* was elevated after starvation initiation at ZT 3 compared to the *ad libitum* group (**Figures 6, 7**).

Notably, starvation initiated at ZT 12 decreased the expression of *Pparg* by significantly by more than 40% and *Ppara* and *Hnf4a* were only marginally regulated. *Hes6*, which is an interaction partner of HNF4a, exhibited diminished expression during starvation started at ZT 3 and increased expression under ZT 12 starvation. *Fgf21* (fibroblast growth factor 21), which is another regulatory element that is closely connected to the PPAR family and the starvation response, exhibited an expression increase by approximately 20-fold after starvation initiated at ZT 3, but this increase was much lower in the ZT 12 group (**Figure 6**). *Mlxipl* was strongly down-regulated after starvation in the morning and was not altered in the evening group. The *Srebf1c* mRNA levels decreased by more than threefold after food deprivation started ZT 3 but were not affected in the ZT 12 group.

The liver ensures the synthesis of sufficient amounts of acetyl coenzyme A (CoA), especially during starvation. Therefore, beta-oxidation is increased due to starvation by the up-regulated expression of many of the involved enzymes, including *Cpt2* (carnitine palmitoyltransferase 2), *Hadhb* (hydroxyacyl-CoA dehydrogenase/3-ketoacyl-CoA thiolase/enoyl-CoA hydratase), *Ehhadh, Acaa1b* (acetyl-CoA acyltransferase 1B), *Acsl1* (acyl-CoA synthetase long-chain family member 1) and *Decr1* (2,4-dienoyl CoA reductase 1) (**Figure 7**). However, this increase was much greater when starvation was initiated at ZT 3 rather than at ZT 12. Members of the *Acsl* family are responsible for the activation of long fatty acids and exhibited different regulation. While *Acsl1* strongly increased by starvation started at ZT 3, *Acsl3* and *Acsl5* strongly decreased. In contrast, starting starvation of mice at ZT 12, *Acsl1* and *Acsl5* expression was not altered and *Acsl3* increased.

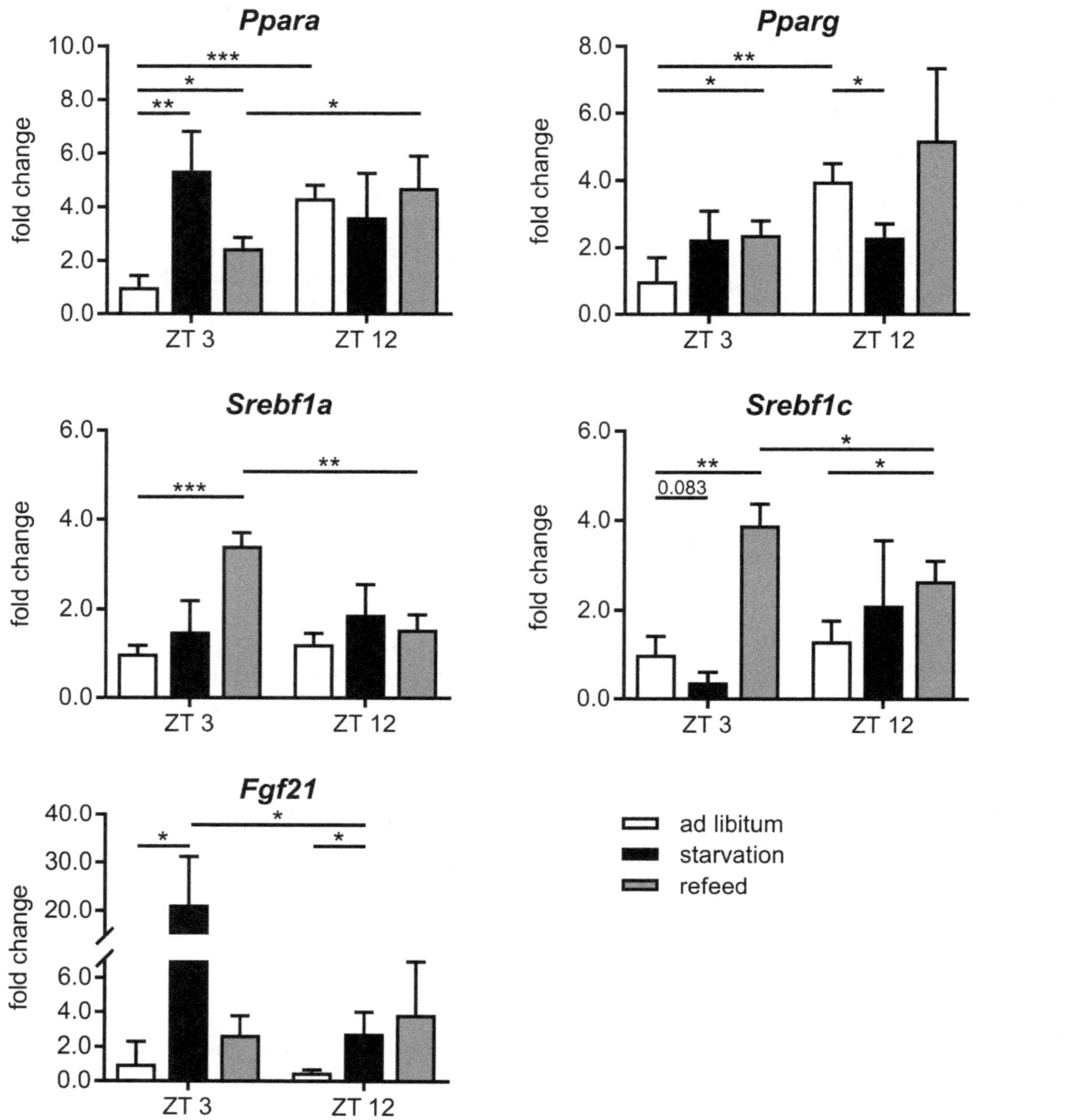

FIGURE 6 | Response of regulatory factors to starvation and refeeding in a diurnal manner. Expression of *Ppara*, *Pparg*, *Srebf1a*, *Srebf1c,* and *Fgf21* in primary hepatocytes of mice fed *ad libitum* (white bars), starved 24 h (black bars) or starved 24 h and refed 12 h (until ZT 3) and 21 h (until ZT 12) (gray bars) quantified using qPCR ($n = 3$). Data are plotted as mean ± standard deviation relative to ZT 3 *ad libitum*, $^{*}p < 0.05$, $^{**}p < 0.01$, and $^{***}p < 0.001$.

Ketogenesis is an essential metabolic pathway to generate ketone bodies during starvation. Genes for the two essential enzymes of ketone body formation, *Hmgcs2* (3-hydroxy-3-methylglutaryl-CoA synthase 2) and *Hmgcl* (3-hydroxymethyl-3-methylglutaryl-CoA lyase), were highly increased after 24-h starvation started at ZT 3, but regulation was only marginal at ZT 12. *Hmgcs2, Hmgcl, Ehhadh, Hadhb,* and *Acaa1b* are also involved in the degradation of the amino acids valine, isoleucine, and leucine. The up-regulation of all enzymes after starvation initiated at ZT 3 ensured an efficient supply of acetyl-CoA (**Figure 7**).

The key enzyme of fatty acid synthesis, *Fasn* (fatty acid synthase), was decreased by 24-h starvation started at ZT 3 and, surprisingly, increased in the ZT 12 group. The gene expression of enzymes involved in elongation and formation of unsaturated fatty acids [e.g., *Scd1* (stearoyl-CoA desaturase 1), *Fads1* (fatty acid desaturase 1), *Hsd17b12* (hydroxysteroid-17-beta dehydrogenase 12), *Thrsp* (thyroid hormone responsive), and

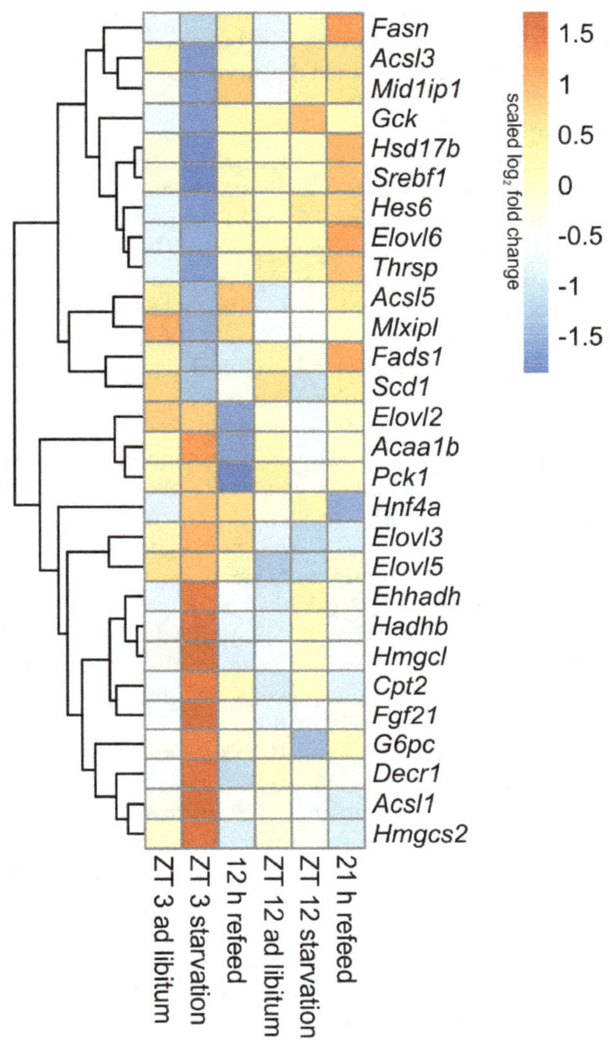

FIGURE 7 | Heatmap of differentially expressed genes related to intermediary metabolism. Red indicates an overexpression, and blue indicates an underexpression.

Mid1ip1 (Mid1 interacting protein 1)] were predominantly down-regulated after starvation initiated at ZT 3 (**Figure 7**). In contrast, starvation initiated at ZT 12 elevated *Scd1* and *Mid1ip1* expression and did not change *Fads1, Hsd17b12,* and *Thrsp*. The members of the Elovl family showed only a regulation when starvation was started at ZT 3, but were not influenced at ZT 12. The *Elovl6* level strongly decreased at ZT 3 starvation, whereas *Elovl3* increased (**Figure 7**).

By gluconeogenesis the liver can synthesize glucose, which is an essential pathway during starvation. As expected, *Pck1* (phosphoenolpyruvate carboxykinase 1), the enzyme for the rate-limiting step of gluconeogenesis, and *G6pc* (glucose-6-phosphatase catalytic subunit), essential to release glucose in the last step of gluconeogenesis, were both increased due to starvation started at ZT 3, but decreased at ZT 12. *Gck* (glucokinase), catalyzing the opposite reaction, shows an inverse regulation (**Figure 7**).

Taken together, the expression patterns at ZT 3 predominantly corresponded to the known starvation responses of the liver. However, the initiation of fasting at ZT 12 revealed unknown regulatory events that produced more subtle and inversely regulated expression levels.

Refeeding

Refeeding mice after a 24 h starvation challenges the liver. The depleted stores must be refilled, and the metabolism should return to a normal feeding state. The transcription factors *Ppara* and *Pparg* remained elevated after the 12 h refeeding compared to the *ad libitum* group, but *ad libitum* expression was nearly restored after refeeding for 21 h. *Fgf21* expression remained increased after both refeeding periods (**Figure 6**). By contrast, *Hnf4a* expression after the 12 h refeeding was comparable to that after starvation started at ZT 12 and decreased after the 21 h refeeding compared to *ad libitum*. *Mlxipl* expression was restored after the 12 h refeeding (**Figure 7**). The expression of *Srebf1c* increased significantly after both refeeding periods (**Figure 6**).

Hepatocytes exhibited a strong up-regulation of *Fasn* expression, especially after the 21 h refeed; while after 12 h refeed the increase was comparable with starvation started at ZT 12. The genes *Scd1, Acsl5, Elovl6, Hsd17b12, Fads1,* and *Thrsp* showed a similar regulation pattern as *Fasn*. However, the expression of other enzymes, such *Acsl1, Acsl3, Elovl2,* and *Elovl3* resembled the corresponding *ad libitum* sample after 12 and 21 h refeed (**Figure 7**). Expression of the enzymes of beta-oxidation and mitochondrial fatty acid synthesis were restored (*Cpt2, Ehhadh, Hadhb, Decr1*) or remained decreased (*Acaa1b*) after both refeeding periods (**Figure 7**).

The synthesis of ketone bodies and degradation of amino acids are no longer a necessary energy source when sufficient amounts of nutrients are available. Accordingly, the expression of *Hmgcs2* was slightly decreased after 12 and 21 h of refeeding compared to the corresponding *ad libitum* samples, and *Hmgcl* exhibited the same expression as the *ad libitum* state. The level of *Pck1* strongly decreased after the 12 h refeeding compared to *ad libitum* and was slightly reduced after refeeding for 21 h. Both refeeding times restored *G6pc* expression to *ad libitum* levels (**Figure 7**).

Steroid Metabolism

Diurnal influence

Steroid metabolism, especially cholesterol synthesis, is another important function of the liver, and it is partially regulated diurnally (**Figure 8A**). Comparing ZT 3 and ZT 12 *ad libitum Pmvk* (phosphomevalonate kinase), *Mvd* (mevalonate decarboxylase), *Ebp* (phenylalkylamine Ca^{2+} antagonist binding protein), *Sc5d* (sterol-C5-desaturase), and *Cyp17a1* (cytochrome P450, family 17, subfamily a, polypeptide 1) exhibited a higher expression in the morning than in the evening. The regulators of SREBP1, *Scap* (SREBP cleavage-activating protein) and *Insig1/2* (insulin induced gene), were also expressed higher at ZT 3 than at ZT 12. In accordance with enhanced synthesis over the day, the amount of hepatic cholesterol is 1.3-fold higher in the evening

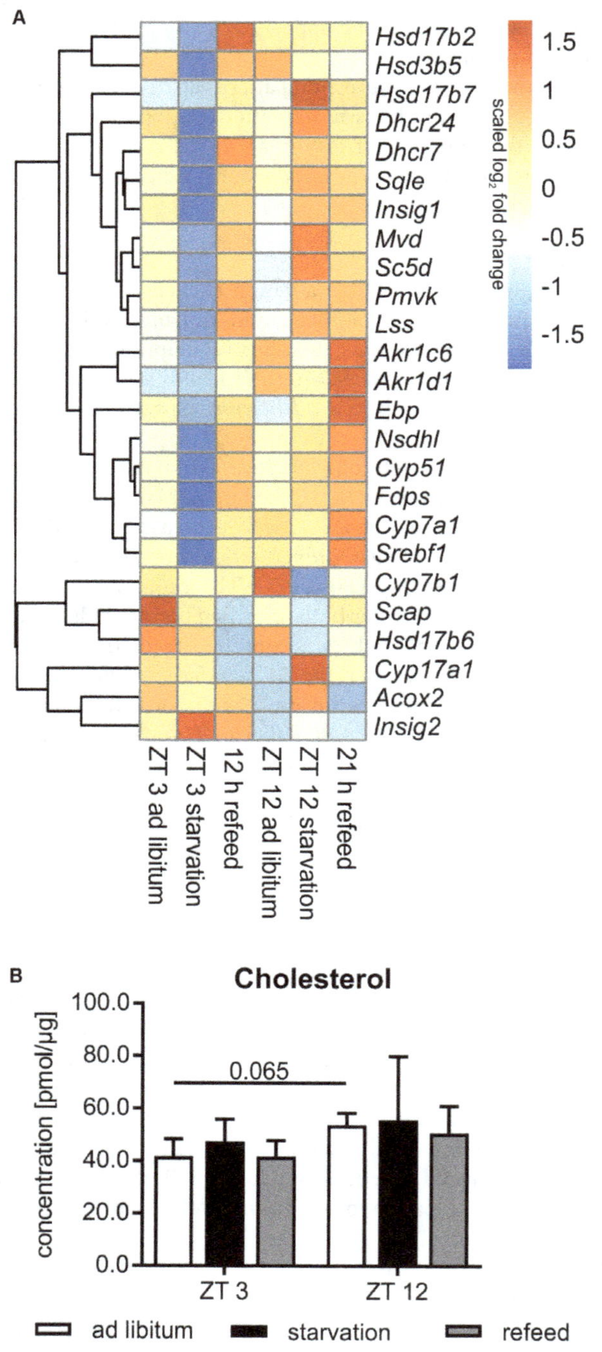

FIGURE 8 | Regulation of steroid metabolism. **(A)** Heatmap of differentially expressed genes related to steroid metabolism. Red indicates an overexpression, and blue indicates an underexpression. **(B)** Concentration of cholesterol in primary hepatocytes of mice fed *ad libitum* (white bars), starved 24 h (black bars) or starved 24 h and refed 12 h (until ZT 3) and 21 h (until ZT 12) (gray bars) (n = 3). Data are plotted as mean ± standard deviation.

than in the morning (**Figure 8B**). Concerning steroidogenesis and cholesterol conversion, the hydroxysteroid dehydrogenases *Hsd3b5* and *Hsd17b2* showed a higher expression in the evening.

The expression of many enzymes [*Cyp7a1*, *Cyp7b1*, *Akr1d1*, *Akr1c6* (aldo-keto reductase family 1, member D1/C6)] involved in steroid degradation by formation of bile acids were also higher expressed in the evening than in the morning.

Starvation

Already in the early fifties it was shown that the synthesis rate of cholesterol is markedly decreased by starvation. This metabolic profile was true in mice starved from ZT 3, in which most genes encoding cholesterol synthesizing enzymes [*Pmvk*, *Mvd*, *Fdps* (farnesyl diphosphate synthetase), *Sqle* (squalene epoxidase), *Lss* (lanosterol synthase), *Dhcr24* (24-dehydrocholesterol reductase), *Cyp51*, *Nsdhl* (NAD(P) dependent steroid dehydrogenase-like), *Hsd17b7*, *Ebp*, *Sc5d*, and *Dhcr7*] exhibited reduced expression compared to *ad libitum* mice (**Figure 8A**). By contrast, the shift of starvation time to the evening produced a reverse regulation and a primarily elevated expression of these genes. Notably, 24 h starvation did not significantly alter the cholesterol content (**Figure 8B**). The regulatory transcription factor of cholesterol synthesis, *Srebf1a*, was not significantly altered following starvation (**Figure 6**). Due to starvation initiated at ZT 3, *Insig1* and *Insig2* exhibited a reciprocal expression, reflecting published data (Ye and DeBose-Boyd, 2011), while the evening starvation period resulted in an equal increase in *Insig1* and *Insig2* expression. *Scap* expression was slightly lower after starvation in both periods (**Figure 8A**).

Cytochrome P450 enzymes (CYPs) and hydroxysteroid dehydrogenases (HSDs) synthesize steroid hormones with cholesterol as starting compound. The expression of *Cyp17a1* (steroid 17α-monooxygenase), which is a key enzyme of steroidogenesis, was highly induced after starvation started at ZT 12 and not altered in ZT 3 mice. By contrast, Hsd expression (*Hsd3b5*, *Hsd17b2,* and *Hsd17b6*) was more or less down-regulated after both starvation periods (**Figure 8A**).

The breakdown of cholesterol is performed by the synthesis of bile acids in the liver. *Cyp7a1*, which is the rate-limiting enzyme, was dramatically down-regulated following starvation initiated at ZT 3 and unchanged in ZT 12 mice compared to *ad libitum*. *Cyp7b1* was almost unaffected after starvation started at ZT 3 and highly decreased in ZT 12 mice. *Akr1c6* is another enzyme of bile acid synthesis and was down-regulated after both starvation periods. *Akr1d1* was marginally altered. *Acox2* was unchanged after starvation initiated at ZT 3, but it was increased in ZT 12 mice (**Figure 8A**).

Cholesterol metabolism exhibits a similar regulation in response to fasting like the lipid metabolism: cholesterol synthesis was regulated in the known manner in ZT 3 mice, but its synthesis exhibited unknown regulation in ZT 12 mice.

Refeeding

The genes of cholesterol synthesis (*Pmvk*, *Mvd*, *Sqle*, *Lss*, *Dhcr24*, *Hsd17b7*, and *Scd5*) remained elevated after the 21 h refeeding period compared to ZT 12 *ad libitum* (**Figure 8A**). *Fdps*, *Cyp51*, *Nsdhl*, and *Ebp* were even higher expressed after 21 h refeeding compared to the corresponding starvation period at ZT 12. The expression of almost all above-mentioned genes was elevated after the 12 h refeed compared to ZT 3 *ad libitum* and was very similar to that under ZT 12 starvation. Only *Ebp* and *Scd5* exhibited restored expression after 12 h refeeding (**Figure 8A**). Expression of the regulator *Srebf1a* was highly induced after the 12 h refeeding compared to ZT 3 *ad libitum*, and it was restored after refeeding for 21 h (**Figure 6**). *Scap* and *Insig2* exhibited a similar expression after 21 h refeed and at ZT 12 *ad libitum*. After 12 h refeed the expression of *Insig1* was slightly increased and *Insig2* was elevated much more, whereas *Scap* was decreased (**Figure 8A**).

Cyp17a1 expression remained increased after the 21 h refeeding and decreased after 12 h compared to the corresponding *ad libitum* samples. *Hsd17b6* expression was lower after 12 and 21 h refeed than in the *ad libitum* samples. *Hsd3b5* remained down-regulated after 21 h refeeding. *Hsd17b2* expression increased after 12 h refeed (**Figure 8A**).

The key enzyme of bile acid synthesis *Cyp7a1* was up-regulated after both refeeding times. *Akr1d1* and *Akr1c6* were also up-regulated, especially after the 21 h refeed. *Acox2*

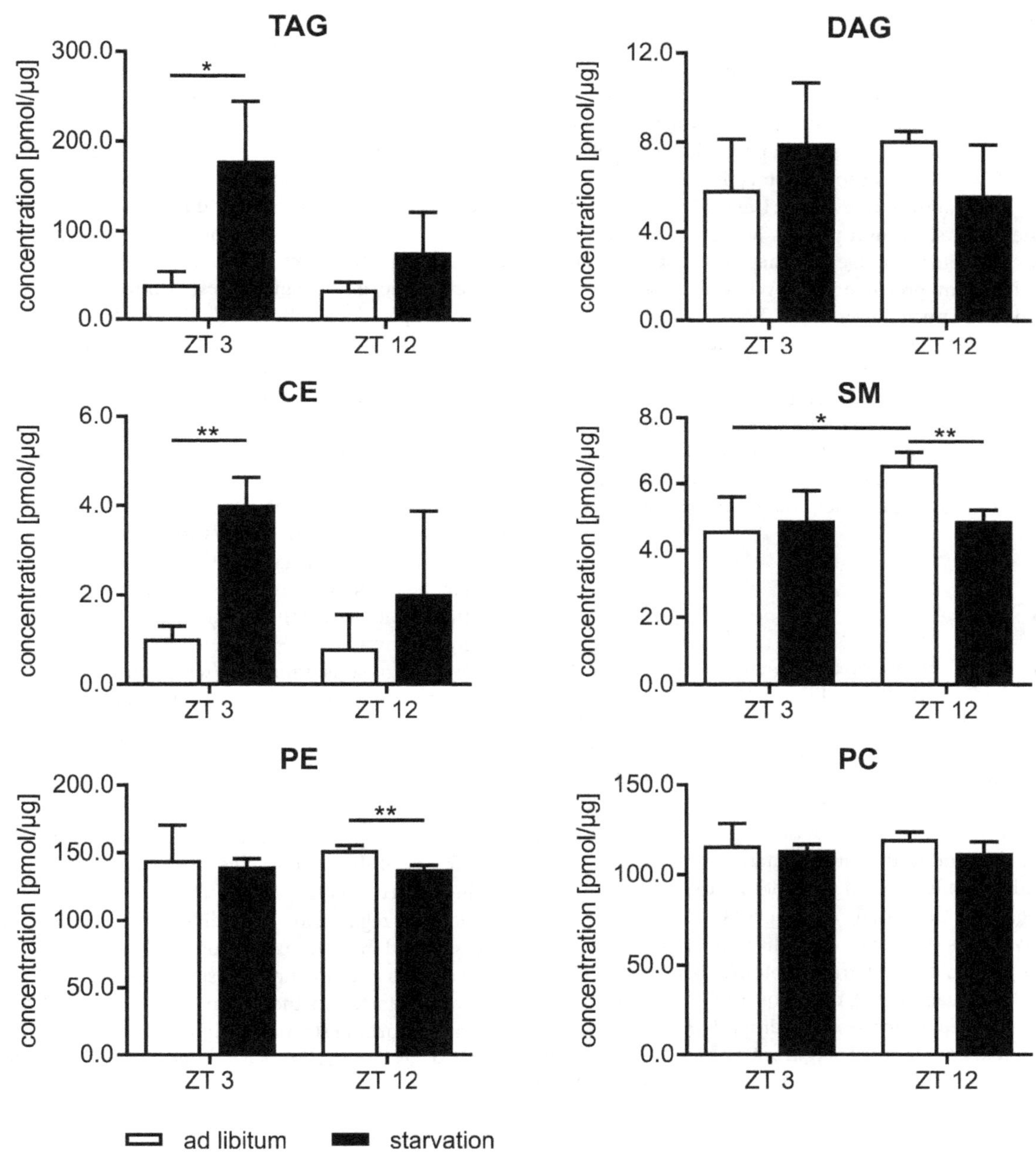

FIGURE 9 | Lipidome profile of primary hepatocytes. Mice were fed *ad libitum* (white bars) or starved 24 h (black bars). Concentration of tri- and diacylglycerides (TAG/DAG), cholesteryl esters (CE), sphingomyelins (SM), phosphatidylethanolamines (PE), and phosphatidylcholines (PC) ($n = 3$). Data are plotted as mean ± standard deviation, *$p < 0.05$ and **$p < 0.01$.

expression was restored after refeeding (12 and 21 h), but *Cyp7b1* remained down-regulated after 21 h of refeeding (**Figure 8A**).

Lipidome Analysis of Hepatocytes

Beside the evaluation of the gene expression, we analyzed the lipidome profile of the hepatocytes via mass spectrometry (**Figure 9**). The amount of lipids in mice fed *ad libitum* exhibited a basal level and no diurnal changes, with the exception of sphingomyelin (SM), where the content was 1.4-fold higher in ZT 12 than in ZT 3 mice. However, hepatic lipids used for storage, such as TAGs and cholesteryl esters (CEs), were strongly elevated in starving mice, and this regulation is highly time-dependent. Starvation started at ZT 3 produced a greater than fourfold increase in TAGs and CEs compared to *ad libitum* mice. By contrast, 24 h starvation initiated at ZT 12 produced only an approximately twofold increase. Polyunsaturated TAG species primarily reflected these differences in TAG levels (**Supplementary Figure 2**). However, TAGs with a high saturation level (50:1 and 52:2) were equally increased after both starvation periods because these TAGs are less reactive and remain longer in the cells. Diacylglycerides (DAGs) are transient precursor of TAG, and these molecules are produced at a much lower level. Both starvation periods slightly altered DAG levels. The membrane components SM and phosphatidylethanolamines (PE) were significantly reduced when starvation was initiated at ZT 12. The PC content did not change (**Figure 9**). Hepatic TAG exhibited still a 2.5-fold increase after the 12 h refeeding compared to *ad libitum* mice. However, the 21 h refeeding normalized the TAG concentration. Refeeding did not significantly alter the other lipid classes (**Supplementary Figure 3**).

DISCUSSION

The results of our study revealed a strong circadian-driven response to fasting in the liver (**Figure 10**). Twenty-four hour starvation initiated and terminated in the morning (ZT 3 to ZT 3) induced the expression of genes involved in metabolic pathways that produce energy-rich substrates for the organism. The gene expression of energy-consuming and temporary expendable processes diminished. However, starvation started in the evening (ZT 12 to ZT 12) produced a totally different hepatic expression signature, with partially opposing regulations, e.g., genes involved in gluconeogenesis decreased, while genes of fatty acid and cholesterol synthesis were induced. These novel findings were unraveled by the analysis of transcriptome data using SOMs. SOMs perfectly visualized the opposing expression profiles of the above-mentioned processes by comparing ZT 3 and ZT 12 starvation (clusters B and J, **Figure 2**). These differences in the expression of metabolic enzymes and their regulators are discussed below in detail.

Metabolic Adaptions Upon Starvation

So far, it was assumed that starvation adapts liver metabolism in two ways: (i) by activating processes producing energy-rich metabolites and (ii) by suppressing energy-consuming pathways. However, our study revealed new diurnal-dependent aspects of these mechanisms. Acetyl-CoA and glucose or equivalents are essential energy-rich substrates produced by the liver upon starvation. Our study confirmed the strong induction of the expression of genes responsible for beta-oxidation, especially when starvation was initiated at ZT 3. However, this induction was much lower at ZT 12. Expression levels of essential enzymes of gluconeogenesis (*Pck1* and *G6pc*) and ketone body synthesis (*Hmgcs2* and *Hmgcl*) were distinctly decreased after food deprivation started in the evening and increased in the morning in the known way (Potthoff et al., 2009). Because both processes use similar starting compounds, IRS2 and PDK4 balance the rate of gluconeogenesis and ketone body synthesis in the liver upon fasting, respectively. Our microarray demonstrated increased *Irs2* and *Pdk4* expression when food deprivation began at ZT 3, as shown previously (Wu et al., 2000; Ide et al., 2004), whereas evening starvation did not affect *Pdk4* expression and decreased *Irs2*. Another process of delivering energy is autophagy, whereby, especially during starvation, expendable or dysfunctional cellular components are degraded and recycled (Yin et al., 2008). As a consequence of starvation started at ZT 12, however, the autophagic genes exhibited a lower expression level compared to ZT 12 *ad libitum* conditions. This result was consistent with the strongly decreased expression of a potent activator of autophagy, *Cebpb*, after starvation in the evening. In contrast, upon starvation in the morning, *Cebpb* exhibited induced expression, although most autophagic genes were not relevantly altered. It was published that the activation of autophagy is based on a changed phosphorylation pattern (Shang et al., 2011), but our results indicate a transcriptional regulation as well, which needs to be further investigated. The transcriptional data suggest a so far unknown down-regulation of energy-supplying processes after starvation started in the evening, while morning starvation led to the known activation of those pathways.

For energy-consuming and temporary expendable metabolic processes, we discovered similar diurnal regulation differences by starvation. The synthesis of fatty acids, manly carried out by fatty acid synthase, seems to be increased based on the elevated expression of *Fasn* after food deprivation in the evening. This observation was contrary to the decreased *Fasn* expression detected after starvation started in the morning and the published knowledge of diminished lipogenesis upon fasting (Horton et al., 1998). The hypothesis of the opposing lipogenesis regulation after different starvation periods was strengthened by the expression of *Gck*, forming the carbon source (pyruvate) for lipogenesis, which was also induced after starvation started in the evening and decreased in the known way after morning starvation (Iynedjian et al., 1987). Cholesterol synthesis is another process known to be diminished while starving. However, enzymes of cholesterol synthesis exhibited elevated gene expression following starvation initiated at ZT 12. Food deprivation initiated at ZT 3 reduced the expression levels of most down-stream genes encoding cholesterol synthesizing enzymes, which indicates diminished cholesterol synthesis, as previously shown (Tomkins and Chaikoff, 1952), even if expression of the rate-limiting enzyme of cholesterol synthesis,

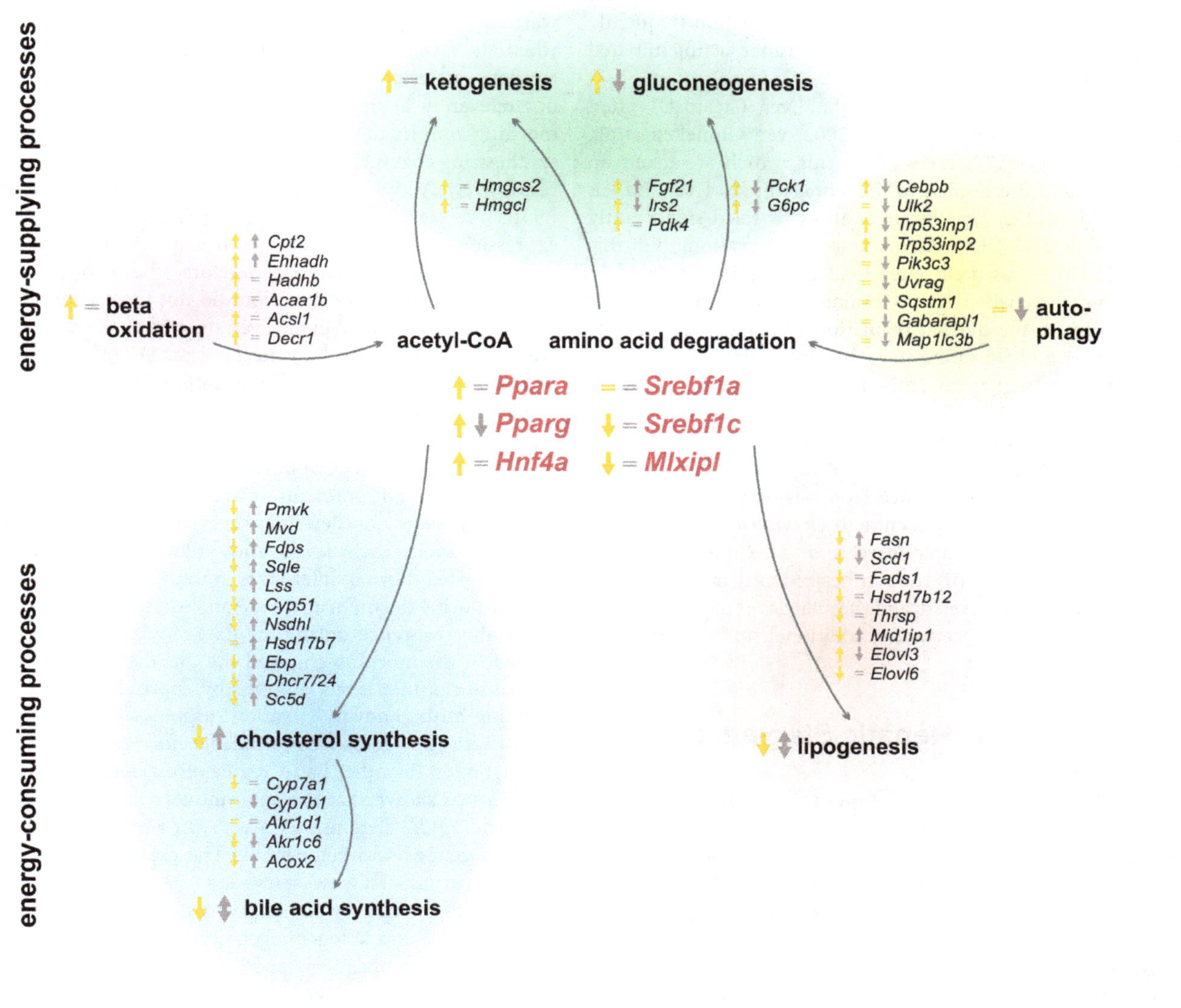

FIGURE 10 | Summary of expression changes after 24 h starvation. Arrows indicate higher (↑) or lower (↓) expression after starvation initiated at ZT 3 (yellow) and ZT 12 (brown) compared to the corresponding *ad libitum* samples. Equality signs (=) indicate no expression changes after starvation.

Hmgcr (3-hydroxy-3-methyl-glutaryl-coenzyme A reductase), was not found in our microarray. Bile acids are secreted into the intestine to increase the solubility of hydrophobic molecules and allow their absorption (Hofmann and Borgström, 1964) and have a poorly understood function as potent signaling compounds (Chiang, 2017). Our study revealed a higher expression of genes involved in bile acid synthesis in the evening than in the morning in *ad libitum* fed mice. This result was consistent with the known diurnal expression of the rate-limiting enzyme CYP7A1, which is highest when the greatest amount of food is consumed (Gooley, 2016). Mice are nocturnal and consume approximately three times more food during scotophase than during photophase (Kurokawa et al., 2000). Bile acid production is a redundant process during starvation, and our analysis revealed a lower expression of *Cyp7a1* after food deprivation at ZT 3. However, starvation in the evening did not alter *Cyp7a1* expression. Several groups reported a similar pattern of *Cyp7a1* expression after starvation (Noshiro et al., 1990; Li et al., 2012), but other studies demonstrated an induction (De Fabiani et al., 2003; Shin et al., 2003). The timing and length of the starvation period used by different groups may explain these diverse results and illustrate the importance of our study. Steroid hormone synthesis is generally localized in the gonads and adrenal glands, but the adult liver also performs steroidogenesis under specific conditions (Grasfeder et al., 2009; Rennert et al., 2017). *Cyp17a1* expression, which is a central steroidogenic enzyme, was induced following evening starvation. This result confirms previous work and strengthens the idea of steroids as mediators of starvation responses (Bauer et al., 2004; Grasfeder et al., 2009). Our data show a novel regulation of energy-consuming processes after starvation started in the evening, contrary to the established down-regulation frequently published as the hepatic starvation response after fasting initiated in the morning.

The accumulation of lipids in the liver (steatosis) often accompanies starvation (Kok et al., 2003; van Ginneken et al., 2007). Adipose tissues secrete fatty acids, which are taken up by hepatocytes and esterified to the storage lipids TAG and CE or secreted as VLDL. Lipidomics analysis revealed significantly elevated TAG and CE contents due to starvation, but this increase was twice as great after food deprivation initiated in the morning than when it was initiated in the evening. This may be based on the diurnal regulation of adipose triglyceride lipase (ATGL) and hormone-sensitive lipase (HSL), which are the lipolysis pacemaker enzymes in adipose tissue and direct targets of CLOCK/ARNTL (Shostak et al., 2013). The lower level of TAG and CE after starvation started in the evening appears inconsistent with the increased expression of *Fasn*. Two possible explanations are (i) since *Fasn* was only detected at the mRNA level, the synthesis of enough enzyme protein and the accumulation of a measurable increase of TAG may be delayed for several hours and/or (ii) the synthesized fatty acids were not stored in the liver but secreted, and the analysis could not capture them. To unravel this uncertainty, additional studies have to be performed.

Regulation of the Hepatic Starvation Response

Additionally, for the transcription factors regulating the observed starvation-induced transcriptional alterations, our study exhibited novel diurnal expression profiles. A main activator of the energy-supplying processes is the PPAR family. Elevated expression of *Ppara* and *Pparg* in the liver upon fasting induces beta-oxidation, stimulating lipid uptake and fatty acid storage (Kersten et al., 1999; Gavrilova et al., 2003; Tanaka et al., 2005). However, we detected this up-regulated expression only when starvation was initiated at ZT 3 and not at ZT 12, which explains the weak induction of beta-oxidation, the decreased gluconeogenesis and ketogenesis and the lower amount of TAG accumulation in the liver after evening starvation. Furthermore, HNF4A contributes to this regulation due to additional activation of *Ppara* and diminishment of the repressor *Hes6* (Martinez-Jimenez et al., 2010). Our data nicely reflected this mechanism after starvation started in the morning. However, after evening starvation, *Hnf4a* was unchanged and the *Hes6* level increased.

The SREBP1 family and ChREBP (*Mlxipl*) are transcription factors more responsible for the post-prandial state and are supposed to be down-regulated during starvation to not activate energy-consuming pathways. For *Mlxipl*, we detected a transcriptional response with a strong down-regulation after starvation in the morning, but no changes were observed when starvation was initiated in the evening. This was contrary to the published regulation carried out only at the post-translational level via phosphorylation (Iizuka and Horikawa, 2008) and requires a more focused study. *Srebf1c* expression was reduced only after food deprivation initiation in the morning, and its expression was unchanged following starvation in the evening, which may explain the induced expression of the target *Fasn* when starvation was started at ZT 12. SREBP-1a is known to regulate cholesterol synthesis, but even if its expression was not relevantly altered, neither after starvation initiated in the morning nor in the evening, the genes encoding cholesterol synthesizing enzymes responded with a down- or up-regulation, respectively. Additionally, the influence of the SREBP1 inhibitors, INSIG1/2, seemed to depend on diurnality, since *Insig1/2* expression was elevated after both starvation periods, but the regulatory output differed. Therefore, the known regulatory mechanisms of *Srebf1* expression did not seem applicable when starvation was initiated in the evening, and further investigations are needed to delineate these mechanisms. All in all, the diurnally regulated expression of the transcription factors *Ppara*, *Pparg*, *Mlxipl*, *Srebf1a*, and *Srebf1c* following starvation likely underlie many of the observed metabolic alterations.

Concerning the regulation of the fed and starved state, two hormones are omnipresent: insulin and glucagon. Since the hormones were not determined in our study, we can only speculate about their levels and influence. Shi et al. (2013) demonstrated diurnal differences in mice with enhanced insulin activity during the night and a metabolism that was characterized by insulin resistance during the day. However, 24 h starvation started in the morning changed the diurnal insulin regulation, and serum insulin levels dropped by approximately two-thirds, resulting in the known starvation responses (Ahrén and Havel, 1999), but no data were available for evening starvation. Glucagon, on the other hand, regulates metabolism in the fasted state. It was shown that glucagon induces the expression of the hormone *Fgf21* (Berglund et al., 2010), which in turn activates gluconeogenesis and ketogenesis. The expression of *Fgf21* was much more induced when starvation was started in the morning than in the evening, which explains the diurnal differences in gluconeogenic and ketogenic gene expression and suggests that the glucagon response also depends on the timing of starvation.

The overall regulators of circadian rhythm are the core clock genes *Arntl*, *Clock* and *Per*, which were elevated after both starvation periods but maintained their typical diurnal expression pattern. This result was consistent with a previous study that demonstrated induced *Arntl* expression due to raised glucagon levels (Sun et al., 2015). Since the transcriptional analysis was performed in hepatocytes, a screen of other organs would help to fully understand the regulatory differences following starvation started in the morning and in the evening.

Metabolic Adaptions and Regulations Upon Refeed

Peripheral tissues first refill their glucose stores when an organism switches from a starved to a refed state, and the liver subsequently synthesizes and stores glycogen, fatty acids, and cholesterol (Berg et al., 2002). Our experimental setting investigated the effects of two refeeding durations (12 and 21 h) after the same starvation period (**Figure 11**). The already mentioned clusters B and J in the SOMs, where most genes of intermediary and steroid metabolism were localized, exhibited similar expression profiles

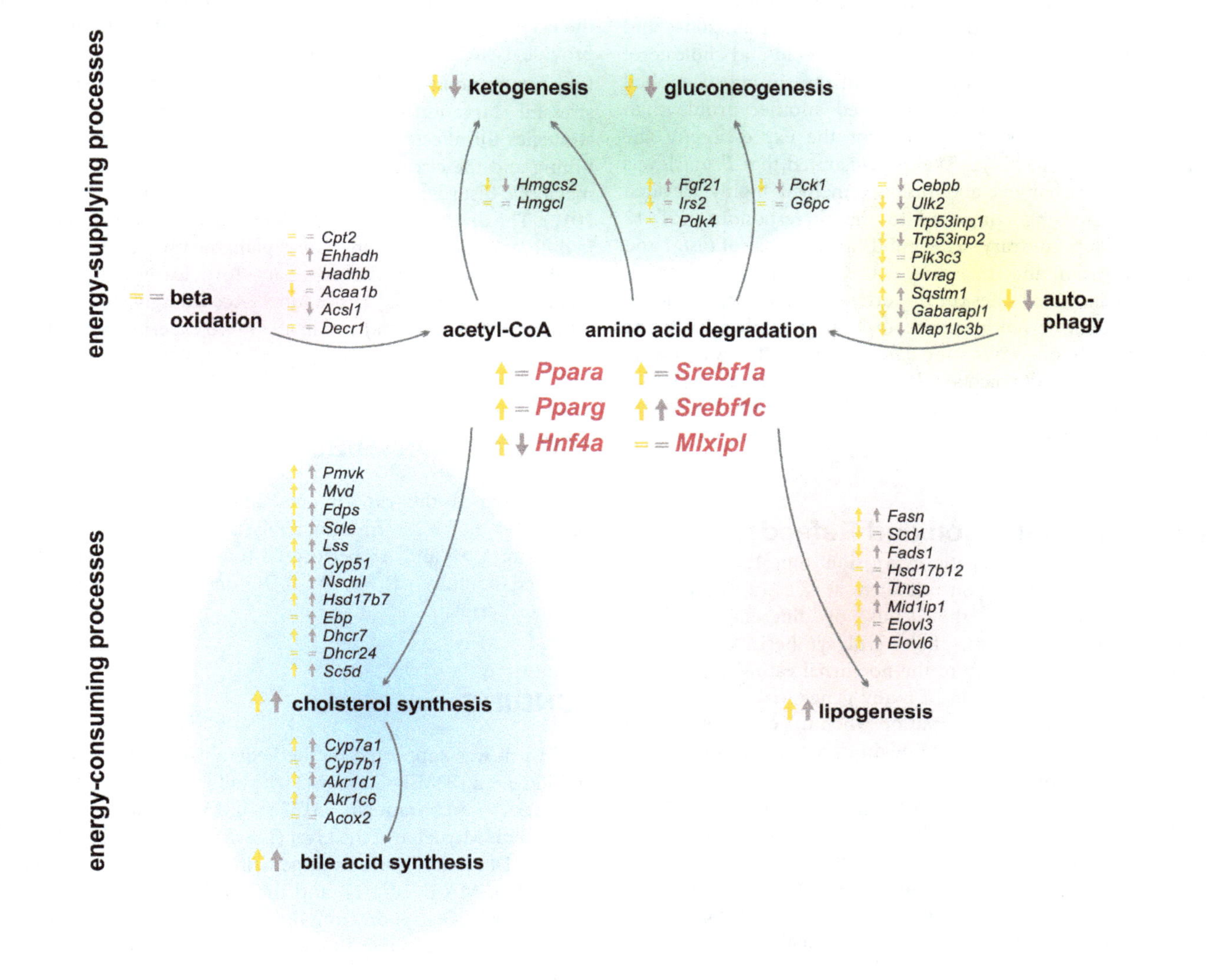

FIGURE 11 | Summary of expression changes following 12 and 21 h refeeding after 24 h starvation. Arrows indicate higher (↑) or lower (↓) expression after refeeding for 12 h until ZT 3 (yellow) and 21 h until ZT 12 (brown) compared to the corresponding *ad libitum* samples. Equality signs (=) indicate a restored *ad libitum* expression levels.

after both refeeding periods, which were totally different from the *ad libitum* groups. The expression levels in other regions of the SOM after 21 h refeeding partially resembled the *ad libitum* group, which indicated a return to the untreated state.

Since food intake delivers all essential metabolites, the liver (i) activates the energy-consuming metabolism and (ii) the production of energy-rich substrates returns to normal. The liver no longer synthesizes ketone bodies and glucose after refeeding, and the expression of the relevant genes reached *ad libitum* or decreased levels. The genes of beta-oxidation were expressed at *ad libitum* levels as well. Early findings demonstrated that refeeding suppressed autophagy (Mortimore et al., 1983), which was confirmed since most of the autophagic genes exhibited a much lower expression after 12 h refeeding compared to starvation, and these genes returned to an approximately *ad libitum* level after 21 h. In contrast, the synthesis of fatty acids and steroids is induced by refeeding. Our study demonstrated that the expression of *Fasn* was highly increased to a maximum after the 21 h refeed. The genes encoding cholesterol synthesizing enzymes were elevated after 12 and 21 h of refeeding as well. This led to an induced synthesis of fatty acids and cholesterol to refill the emptied stores. Bile acid synthesis is associated with the food consumption, and it increased due to elevated expression levels of *Cyp7a1*, as reported previously (Li et al., 2012). The lipidome profile revealed that TAG content remained increased after 12 h refeeding but reached *ad libitum* levels after 21 h. Previous studies demonstrated a normalization of liver lipid content after 48 h of refeeding (Kok et al., 2003).

Since SREBF1 stimulates lipogenesis and cholesterol synthesis, the expression of the transcription factors *Srebf1a* and *Srebf1c* was highly induced after 12 h refeeding, which was consistent with previous results (Horton et al., 1998; Ide et al., 2004) and resulted in the observed induction of fatty acid and cholesterol synthesis. Resulting from differences in the timing of applied starvation periods, our results revealed another profile than what has been suggested thus far for the expression of the inhibitors *Insig1* and *Insig2*. We demonstrated that *Insig1* levels were almost unchanged and *Insig2* remained highly elevated after 12 h refeeding compared to the corresponding ZT 12 starvation group, contrary to the published decrease of *Insig1* and *Insig2a* expression after refeeding (Attie, 2004; Lee et al., 2017). This discrepancy illustrates the importance of further knowledge of the circadian-driven response to fasting in the liver. The transcription factors, *Ppara* and *Pparg*, remained elevated after the 12 h refeeding but reached *ad libitum* levels after 21 h. Geisler et al. (2016) demonstrated a similar decline in *Ppara* levels with advanced refeeding times.

Linkage of Starvation and Refeed

SOMs that the overall hepatic expression after 12 h refeeding highly resembled starvation initiated at ZT 12, which was confirmed according to the details of different metabolic pathways (e.g., lipogenesis, cholesterol synthesis, autophagy). This may be a consequence of the nocturnal eating behavior of mice, because the expression of many genes may be decreased as a direct consequence of starvation when mice were sacrificed after 24 h starvation in the morning directly after the scotophase when they typically consume their major meal. By contrast, when mice are sacrificed in the evening, the previous period was the photophase during which they consume less food, and the diurnal regulation of mice anticipating food may predominate. Furthermore, mice in which starvation was started in the evening consumed only small amounts of food in the prior period because it was daytime, and the fasting period was actually longer and the stores may be more depleted. These differences may also explain the differences in TAG content. We can only speculate on these points because refeeding in our experiments was only initiated in the evening and not in the morning. We also cannot distinguish between the effects of the longer refeeding period and circadian regulation because samples were taken during another circadian time.

CONCLUSION

Our experiments convincingly demonstrate that the response to starvation periods differed depending on the timing of starvation initiation and report valuable new information about expression levels based on the initiation and termination of starvation in the evening. Performing analogous experiments in humans may provide useful information of the metabolic state after differently timed starvation periods, which may lead to better understanding stressful starvation conditions and develop medical treatment strategies for affected patients. In chronic disturbances of meal timing and the circadian rhythm, e.g., upon shift work, various metabolic disorders are known (Canuto et al., 2013; James et al., 2017). The diverse timings and lengths of starvation periods used in different research groups may explain the variance in published results and support the necessity for clearly designed and recorded experimental procedures. Accordingly, the circadian influence must be considered in all *in vivo* experiments including starvation.

AUTHOR CONTRIBUTIONS

CR performed the experiments and analyzed the data. SV performed the bioinformatical analysis. EM-B and CT collected the samples. SS and AS performed the lipidomics analysis. RG designed the study. CR, SV, EM-B, RG, and MM-S wrote or edited the manuscript.

FUNDING

This work was supported by the Federal Ministry of Education and Research (BMBF, Germany) within the projects Virtual Liver Network (VLN) (Grant No. 0315735, 0315736, and 0315775) and the Systems Medicine of the Liver (LiSyM) (Grant No. 031L0054), by the Deutsche Forschungsgemeinschaft (DFG, Germany) (Grant No. MA 6610/2-1), and the Joachim Herz Foundation. We acknowledge support from the German Research Foundation (DFG) and Leipzig University within the program of Open Access Publishing.

ACKNOWLEDGMENTS

We thank PD Dr. Knut Krohn for Illumina microarray analysis from the Interdisciplinary Centre for Clinical Research Leipzig (Faculty of Medicine, Leipzig University). We cordially thank Kerstin Heise and Doris Mahn for excellent technical assistance. Further, we would like to thank Petra Hirrlinger, Petra Fink-Sterba, and Sigrid Weisheit from the Experimental Centre of the Faculty of Medicine (Leipzig University) for taking excellent care of the mice.

REFERENCES

Ahrén, B., and Havel, P. J. (1999). Leptin increases circulating glucose, insulin and glucagon via sympathetic neural activation in fasted mice. *Int. J. Obes. Relat. Metab. Disord.* 23, 660–665. doi: 10.1038/sj.ijo.0800899

Aken, B. L., Ayling, S., Barrell, D., Clarke, L., Curwen, V., Fairley, S., et al. (2016). The Ensembl gene annotation system. *Database* 2016:baw093. doi: 10.1093/database/baw093

Albrecht, U. (2012). Timing to perfection: the biology of central and peripheral circadian clocks. *Neuron* 74, 246–260. doi: 10.1016/j.neuron.2012.04.006

Ashburner, M., Ball, C. A., Blake, J. A., Botstein, D., Butler, H., Cherry, J. M., et al. (2000). Gene ontology: tool for the unification of biology. The gene ontology consortium. *Nat. Genet.* 25, 25–29. doi: 10.1038/75556

Attie, A. D. (2004). Insig: a significant integrator of nutrient and hormonal signals. *J. Clin. Invest.* 113, 1112–1114. doi: 10.1172/JCI200421450

Bauer, M., Hamm, A. C., Bonaus, M., Jacob, A., Jaekel, J., Schorle, H., et al. (2004). Starvation response in mouse liver shows strong correlation with life-span-prolonging processes. *Physiol. Genomics* 17, 230–244. doi: 10.1152/physiolgenomics.00203.2003

Berg, J. M., Tymoczko, J. L., Stryer, L., and Clarke, N. D. (2002). *Biochemistry*. New York, NY: W. H. Freeman.

Berglund, E. D., Kang, L., Lee-Young, R. S., Hasenour, C. M., Lustig, D. G., Lynes, S. E., et al. (2010). Glucagon and lipid interactions in the regulation of hepatic AMPK signaling and expression of PPARalpha and FGF21 transcripts in vivo. *Am. J. Physiol. Endocrinol. Metab.* 299, E607–E614. doi: 10.1152/ajpendo.00263.2010

Bjorkoy, G., Lamark, T., Brech, A., Outzen, H., Perander, M., Overvatn, A., et al. (2005). p62/SQSTM1 forms protein aggregates degraded by autophagy and has a protective effect on huntingtin-induced cell death. *J. Cell Biol.* 171, 603–614. doi: 10.1083/jcb.200507002

Boucher, J., Kleinridders, A., and Kahn, C. R. (2014). Insulin receptor signaling in normal and insulin-resistant states. *Cold Spring Harb. Perspect. Biol.* 6:a009191. doi: 10.1101/cshperspect.a009191

Canuto, R., Garcez, A. S., and Olinto, M. T. A. (2013). Metabolic syndrome and shift work: a systematic review. *Sleep Med. Rev.* 17, 425–431. doi: 10.1016/j.smrv.2012.10.004

Chiang, J. Y. L. (2017). Bile acid metabolism and signaling in liver disease and therapy. *Liver Res.* 1, 3–9. doi: 10.1016/j.livres.2017.05.001

De Fabiani, E., Mitro, N., Gilardi, F., Caruso, D., Galli, G., and Crestani, M. (2003). Coordinated control of cholesterol catabolism to bile acids and of gluconeogenesis via a novel mechanism of transcription regulation linked to the fasted-to-fed cycle. *J. Biol. Chem.* 278, 39124–39132. doi: 10.1074/jbc.M305079200

Du, P., Kibbe, W. A., and Lin, S. M. (2008). Lumi: a pipeline for processing Illumina microarray. *Bioinformatics* 24, 1547–1548. doi: 10.1093/bioinformatics/btn224

Ferrell, J. M., and Chiang, J. Y. L. (2015). Circadian rhythms in liver metabolism and disease. *Acta Pharm. Sin. B* 5, 113–122. doi: 10.1016/j.apsb.2015.01.003

Folch, J., Lees, M., and Sloane Stanley, G. H. (1957). A simple method for the isolation and purification of total lipides from animal tissues. *J. Biol. Chem.* 226, 497–509.

Gavrilova, O., Haluzik, M., Matsusue, K., Cutson, J. J., Johnson, L., Dietz, K. R., et al. (2003). Liver peroxisome proliferator-activated receptor gamma contributes to hepatic steatosis, triglyceride clearance, and regulation of body fat mass. *J. Biol. Chem.* 278, 34268–34276. doi: 10.1074/jbc.M300043200

Gebhardt, R., Hengstler, J. G., Müller, D., Glöckner, R., Buenning, P., Laube, B., et al. (2003). New hepatocyte in vitro systems for drug metabolism: metabolic capacity and recommendations for application in basic research and drug development, standard operation procedures. *Drug Metab. Rev.* 35, 145–213. doi: 10.1081/DMR-120023684

Geisler, C. E., Hepler, C., Higgins, M. R., and Renquist, B. J. (2016). Hepatic adaptations to maintain metabolic homeostasis in response to fasting and refeeding in mice. *Nutr. Metab.* 13:62. doi: 10.1186/s12986-016-0122-x

Gooley, J. J. (2016). Circadian regulation of lipid metabolism. *Proc. Nutr. Soc.* 75, 440–450. doi: 10.1017/S0029665116000288

Grasfeder, L. L., Gaillard, S., Hammes, S. R., Ilkayeva, O., Newgard, C. B., Hochberg, R. B., et al. (2009). Fasting-induced hepatic production of DHEA is regulated by PGC-1alpha, ERRalpha, and HNF4alpha. *Mol. Endocrinol.* 23, 1171–1182. doi: 10.1210/me.2009-0024

Hakvoort, T. B. M., Moerland, P. D., Frijters, R., Sokoloviæ, A., Labruyère, W. T., Vermeulen, J. L. M., et al. (2011). Interorgan coordination of the murine adaptive response to fasting. *J. Biol. Chem.* 286, 16332–16343. doi: 10.1074/jbc.M110.216986

Hartigan, J. A., and Wong, M. A. (1979). Algorithm AS 136: a K-means clustering algorithm. *Appl. Stat.* 28, 100–108. doi: 10.2307/2346830

Herzog, R., Schwudke, D., Schuhmann, K., Sampaio, J. L., Bornstein, S. R., Schroeder, M., et al. (2011). A novel informatics concept for high-throughput shotgun lipidomics based on the molecular fragmentation query language. *Genome Biol.* 12:R8. doi: 10.1186/gb-2011-12-1-r8

Hirao, A., Nagahama, H., Tsuboi, T., Hirao, M., Tahara, Y., and Shibata, S. (2010). Combination of starvation interval and food volume determines the phase of liver circadian rhythm in Per2::Luc knock-in mice under two meals per day feeding. *Am. J. Physiol. Gastrointest. Liver Physiol.* 299, G1045–G1053. doi: 10.1152/ajpgi.00330.2010

Hofmann, A. F., and Borgström, B. (1964). The intraluminal phase of fat digestion in man: the lipid content of the micellar and oil phases of intestinal content obtained during fat digestion and absorption. *J. Clin. Invest.* 43, 247–257. doi: 10.1172/JCI104909

Horton, J. D., Bashmakov, Y., Shimomura, I., and Shimano, H. (1998). Regulation of sterol regulatory element binding proteins in livers of fasted and refed mice. *Proc. Natl. Acad. Sci. U.S.A.* 95, 5987–5992. doi: 10.1073/pnas.95.11.5987

Ide, T., Shimano, H., Yahagi, N., Matsuzaka, T., Nakakuki, M., Yamamoto, T., et al. (2004). SREBPs suppress IRS-2-mediated insulin signalling in the liver. *Nat. Cell Biol.* 6, 351–357. doi: 10.1038/ncb1111

Ihaka, R., and Gentleman, R. (1996). R: a language for data analysis and graphics. *J. Comput. Graph. Stat.* 5, 299–314. doi: 10.2307/1390807

Iizuka, K., and Horikawa, Y. (2008). ChREBP: a glucose-activated transcription factor involved in the development of metabolic syndrome. *Endocr. J.* 55, 617–624. doi: 10.1507/endocrj.K07E-110

Iynedjian, P. B., Ucla, C., and Mach, B. (1987). Molecular cloning of glucokinase cDNA. Developmental and dietary regulation of glucokinase mRNA in rat liver. *J. Biol. Chem.* 262, 6032–6038.

James, S. M., Honn, K. A., Gaddameedhi, S., and van Dongen, H. P. A. (2017). Shift work: disrupted circadian rhythms and sleep-implications for health and well-being. *Curr. Sleep Med. Rep.* 3, 104–112. doi: 10.1007/s40675-017-0071-6

Jensen, T. L., Kiersgaard, M. K., Sørensen, D. B., and Mikkelsen, L. F. (2013). Fasting of mice: a review. *Lab. Anim.* 47, 225–240. doi: 10.1177/0023677213501659

Kersten, S., Seydoux, J., Peters, J. M., Gonzalez, F. J., Desvergne, B., and Wahli, W. (1999). Peroxisome proliferator-activated receptor alpha mediates the adaptive response to fasting. *J. Clin. Invest.* 103, 1489–1498. doi: 10.1172/JCI6223

Kohonen, T. (1982). Self-organized formation of topologically correct feature maps. *Biol. Cybern.* 43, 59–69. doi: 10.1007/BF00337288

Kok, T., Wolters, H., Bloks, V. W., Havinga, R., Jansen, P. L. M., Staels, B., et al. (2003). Induction of hepatic ABC transporter expression is part of the PPARalpha-mediated fasting response in the mouse. *Gastroenterology* 124, 160–171. doi: 10.1053/gast.2003.50007

Kurokawa, M., Akino, K., and Kanda, K. (2000). A new apparatus for studying feeding and drinking in the mouse. *Physiol. Behav.* 70, 105–112. doi: 10.1016/S0031-9384(00)00226-2

Lee, J.-H., Kang, H. S., Park, H. Y., Moon, Y.-A., Kang, Y. N., Oh, B.-C., et al. (2017). PPARα-dependent Insig2a overexpression inhibits SREBP-1c processing during fasting. *Sci. Rep.* 7:9958. doi: 10.1038/s41598-017-10523-7

Li, T., Francl, J. M., Boehme, S., Ochoa, A., Zhang, Y., Klaassen, C. D., et al. (2012). Glucose and insulin induction of bile acid synthesis: mechanisms and implication in diabetes and obesity. *J. Biol. Chem.* 287, 1861–1873. doi: 10.1074/jbc.M111.305789

Liebisch, G., Binder, M., Schifferer, R., Langmann, T., Schulz, B., and Schmitz, G. (2006). High throughput quantification of cholesterol and cholesteryl ester by electrospray ionization tandem mass spectrometry (ESI-MS/MS). *Biochim. Biophys. Acta* 1761, 121–128. doi: 10.1016/j.bbalip.2005.12.007

Löffler-Wirth, H., Kalcher, M., and Binder, H. (2015). oposSOM: r-package for high-dimensional portraying of genome-wide expression landscapes on bioconductor. *Bioinformatics* 31, 3225–3227. doi: 10.1093/bioinformatics/btv342

Longo, V. D., and Mattson, M. P. (2014). Fasting: molecular mechanisms and clinical applications. *Cell Metab.* 19, 181–192. doi: 10.1016/j.cmet.2013.12.008

Martinez-Jimenez, C. P., Kyrmizi, I., Cardot, P., Gonzalez, F. J., and Talianidis, I. (2010). Hepatocyte nuclear factor 4alpha coordinates a transcription factor network regulating hepatic fatty acid metabolism. *Mol. Cell. Biol.* 30, 565–577. doi: 10.1128/MCB.00927-09

Matz-Soja, M., Aleithe, S., Marbach, E., Böttger, J., Arnold, K., Schmidt-Heck, W., et al. (2014). Hepatic Hedgehog signaling contributes to the regulation of IGF1 and IGFBP1 serum levels. *Cell Commun. Signal.* 12:11. doi: 10.1186/1478-811X-12-11

Mortimore, G. E., Hutson, N. J., and Surmacz, C. A. (1983). Quantitative correlation between proteolysis and macro- and microautophagy in mouse hepatocytes during starvation and refeeding. *Proc. Natl. Acad. Sci. U.S.A.* 80, 2179–2183. doi: 10.1073/pnas.80.8.2179

Noshiro, M., Nishimoto, M., and Okuda, K. (1990). Rat liver cholesterol 7 alpha-hydroxylase. Pretranslational regulation for circadian rhythm. *J. Biol. Chem.* 265, 10036–10041.

Partch, C. L., Green, C. B., and Takahashi, J. S. (2014). Molecular architecture of the mammalian circadian clock. *Trends Cell Biol.* 24, 90–99. doi: 10.1016/j.tcb.2013.07.002

Potthoff, M. J., Inagaki, T., Satapati, S., Ding, X., He, T., Goetz, R., et al. (2009). FGF21 induces PGC-1alpha and regulates carbohydrate and fatty acid metabolism during the adaptive starvation response. *Proc. Natl. Acad. Sci. U.S.A.* 106, 10853–10858. doi: 10.1073/pnas.0904187106

Ralph, M. R., Foster, R. G., Davis, F. C., and Menaker, M. (1990). Transplanted suprachiasmatic nucleus determines circadian period. *Science* 247, 975–978. doi: 10.1126/science.2305266

Rennert, C., Eplinius, F., Hofmann, U., Johänning, J., Rolfs, F., Schmidt-Heck, W., et al. (2017). Conditional loss of hepatocellular Hedgehog signaling in female mice leads to the persistence of hepatic steroidogenesis, androgenization and infertility. *Arch. Toxicol.* 91, 3677–3687. doi: 10.1007/s00204-017-1999-5

Rui, L. (2014). Energy metabolism in the liver. *Compr. Physiol.* 4, 177–197. doi: 10.1002/cphy.c130024

Schuhmann, K., Almeida, R., Baumert, M., Herzog, R., Bornstein, S. R., and Shevchenko, A. (2012). Shotgun lipidomics on a LTQ Orbitrap mass spectrometer by successive switching between acquisition polarity modes. *J. Mass Spectrom.* 47, 96–104. doi: 10.1002/jms.2031

Shang, L., Chen, S., Du, F., Li, S., Zhao, L., and Wang, X. (2011). Nutrient starvation elicits an acute autophagic response mediated by Ulk1 dephosphorylation and its subsequent dissociation from AMPK. *Proc. Natl. Acad. Sci. U.S.A.* 108, 4788–4793. doi: 10.1073/pnas.1100844108

Shi, S.-Q., Ansari, T. S., McGuinness, O. P., Wasserman, D. H., and Johnson, C. H. (2013). Circadian disruption leads to insulin resistance and obesity. *Curr. Biol.* 23, 372–381. doi: 10.1016/j.cub.2013.01.048

Shin, D.-J., Campos, J. A., Gil, G., and Osborne, T. F. (2003). PGC-1alpha activates CYP7A1 and bile acid biosynthesis. *J. Biol. Chem.* 278, 50047–50052. doi: 10.1074/jbc.M309736200

Shostak, A., Meyer-Kovac, J., and Oster, H. (2013). Circadian regulation of lipid mobilization in white adipose tissues. *Diabetes Metab. Res. Rev.* 62, 2195–2203. doi: 10.2337/db12-1449

Sokolović, M., Sokolović, A., Wehkamp, D., van Loren Themaat, E., de Waart, D. R., Gilhuijs-Pederson, L. A., et al. (2008). The transcriptomic signature of fasting murine liver. *BMC Genomics* 9:528. doi: 10.1186/1471-2164-9-528

Stokkan, K. A., Yamazaki, S., Tei, H., Sakaki, Y., and Menaker, M. (2001). Entrainment of the circadian clock in the liver by feeding. *Science* 291, 490–493. doi: 10.1126/science.291.5503.490

Stratmann, M., and Schibler, U. (2006). Properties, entrainment, and physiological functions of mammalian peripheral oscillators. *J. Biol. Rhythms* 21, 494–506. doi: 10.1177/0748730406293889

Sun, X., Dang, F., Zhang, D., Yuan, Y., Zhang, C., Wu, Y., et al. (2015). Glucagon-CREB/CRTC2 signaling cascade regulates hepatic BMAL1 protein. *J. Biol. Chem.* 290, 2189–2197. doi: 10.1074/jbc.M114.612358

Szklarczyk, D., Franceschini, A., Wyder, S., Forslund, K., Heller, D., Huerta-Cepas, J., et al. (2015). STRING v10: protein-protein interaction networks, integrated over the tree of life. *Nucleic Acids Res.* 43, D447–D452. doi: 10.1093/nar/gku1003

Tanaka, T., Masuzaki, H., Ebihara, K., Ogawa, Y., Yasue, S., Yukioka, H., et al. (2005). Transgenic expression of mutant peroxisome proliferator-activated receptor gamma in liver precipitates fasting-induced steatosis but protects against high-fat diet-induced steatosis in mice. *Metab. Clin. Exp.* 54, 1490–1498. doi: 10.1016/j.metabol.2005.05.015

Tomkins, G. M., and Chaikoff, I. L. (1952). Cholesterol synthesis by liver. I. Influence of fasting and of diet. *J. Biol. Chem.* 196, 569–573.

Traver, M. K., Henry, S. C., Cantillana, V., Oliver, T., Hunn, J. P., Howard, J. C., et al. (2011). Immunity-related GTPase M (IRGM) proteins influence the localization of guanylate-binding protein 2 (GBP2) by modulating macroautophagy. *J. Biol. Chem.* 286, 30471–30480. doi: 10.1074/jbc.M111.251967

van Ginneken, V., Verhey, E., Poelmann, R., Ramakers, R., van Dijk, K. W., Ham, L., et al. (2007). Metabolomics (liver and blood profiling) in a mouse model in response to fasting: a study of hepatic steatosis. *Biochim. Biophys. Acta* 1771, 1263–1270. doi: 10.1016/j.bbalip.2007.07.007

Wehrens, S. M. T., Christou, S., Isherwood, C., Middleton, B., Gibbs, M. A., Archer, S. N., et al. (2017). Meal timing regulates the human circadian system. *Curr. Biol.* 27, 1768–1775.e3. doi: 10.1016/j.cub.2017.04.059

Welsh, D. K., Takahashi, J. S., and Kay, S. A. (2010). Suprachiasmatic nucleus: cell autonomy and network properties. *Annu. Rev. Physiol.* 72, 551–577. doi: 10.1146/annurev-physiol-021909-135919

Wirth, H., Löffler, M., von Bergen, M., and Binder, H. (2011). Expression cartography of human tissues using self organizing maps. *BMC Bioinformatics* 12:306. doi: 10.1186/1471-2105-12-306

Wu, P., Blair, P. V., Sato, J., Jaskiewicz, J., Popov, K. M., and Harris, R. A. (2000). Starvation increases the amount of pyruvate dehydrogenase kinase in several mammalian tissues. *Arch. Biochem. Biophys.* 381, 1–7. doi: 10.1006/abbi.2000.1946

Yang, X., Lamia, K. A., and Evans, R. M. (2007). Nuclear receptors, metabolism, and the circadian clock. *Cold Spring Harb. Symp. Quant. Biol.* 72, 387–394. doi: 10.1101/sqb.2007.72.058

Ye, J., and DeBose-Boyd, R. A. (2011). Regulation of cholesterol and fatty acid synthesis. *Cold Spring Harb. Perspect. Biol.* 3:a004754. doi: 10.1101/cshperspect.a004754

Yin, X.-M., Ding, W.-X., and Gao, W. (2008). Autophagy in the liver. *Hepatology* 47, 1773–1785. doi: 10.1002/hep.22146

16

Computational Modeling in Liver Surgery

Bruno Christ[1‡], Uta Dahmen[2‡], Karl-Heinz Herrmann[3‡], Matthias König[4‡], Jürgen R. Reichenbach[3‡], Tim Ricken[5†‡], Jana Schleicher[2, 6‡], Lars Ole Schwen[7‡], Sebastian Vlaic[8‡] and Navina Waschinsky[5‡]*

[1] Molecular Hepatology Lab, Clinics of Visceral, Transplantation, Thoracic and Vascular Surgery, University Hospital Leipzig, University of Leipzig, Leipzig, Germany, [2] Experimental Transplantation Surgery, Department of General, Visceral and Vascular Surgery, University Hospital Jena, Jena, Germany, [3] Medical Physics Group, Institute for Diagnostic and Interventional Radiology, University Hospital Jena, Friedrich Schiller University Jena, Jena, Germany, [4] Department of Biology, Institute for Theoretical Biology, Humboldt University of Berlin, Berlin, Germany, [5] Mechanics, Structural Analysis, and Dynamics, TU Dortmund University, Dortmund, Germany, [6] Department of Bioinformatics, Friedrich Schiller University Jena, Jena, Germany, [7] Fraunhofer MEVIS, Bremen, Germany, [8] Leibniz Institute for Natural Product Research and Infection Biology, Hans Knöll Institute, Jena, Germany

***Correspondence:**
Bruno Christ
bruno.christ@medizin.uni-leipzig.de

The need for extended liver resection is increasing due to the growing incidence of liver tumors in aging societies. Individualized surgical planning is the key for identifying the optimal resection strategy and to minimize the risk of postoperative liver failure and tumor recurrence. Current computational tools provide virtual planning of liver resection by taking into account the spatial relationship between the tumor and the hepatic vascular trees, as well as the size of the future liver remnant. However, size and function of the liver are not necessarily equivalent. Hence, determining the future liver volume might misestimate the future liver function, especially in cases of hepatic comorbidities such as hepatic steatosis. A systems medicine approach could be applied, including biological, medical, and surgical aspects, by integrating all available anatomical and functional information of the individual patient. Such an approach holds promise for better prediction of postoperative liver function and hence improved risk assessment. This review provides an overview of mathematical models related to the liver and its function and explores their potential relevance for computational liver surgery. We first summarize key facts of hepatic anatomy, physiology, and pathology relevant for hepatic surgery, followed by a description of the computational tools currently used in liver surgical planning. Then we present selected state-of-the-art computational liver models potentially useful to support liver surgery. Finally, we discuss the main challenges that will need to be addressed when developing advanced computational planning tools in the context of liver surgery.

Keywords: Liver resection, risk assessment, systems medicine, multi-scale modeling, function prediction, liver regeneration, liver metabolism, liver surgical planning

FROM SYSTEMS BIOLOGY VIA SYSTEMS MEDICINE TO SYSTEMS SURGERY OF THE LIVER

Systems biology is characterized by the application of computational models and methods to a biological question, focusing on entire biological systems and the complex interactions therein. In systems biology, an iterative cycle of model building and validation based on experimental data generation and analysis is pursued. The key purpose of computational models is the integration of biological knowledge into a mathematical representation of the underlying processes allowing *in silico* testing of new hypotheses. Systems biology applied to human diseases is an interdisciplinary approach broadening our understanding of mechanisms involved in disease development and progression. Thus, mathematical models of human diseases can enable us to discover new therapy strategies and targets.

Using the systems biology approach in a clinical setting is termed systems medicine (Wolkenhauer et al., 2013). In systems medicine, computational models are applied for disease diagnosis, prediction of disease progression, and for guidance to select suitable therapeutic strategies. In addition, computational models provide the opportunity for individualization. Patients differ in their individual anatomy, physiology, genetic background, and personal history, all of which influence the severity and course of the disease and determine the specific response of the patient. Therefore, in medicine and especially in surgery, a modeling approach is needed, which permits a patient-specific perspective on disease development and progression, taking preexisting patient-specific conditions into consideration.

Computational surgery refers to the use of computational support in the context of surgery (Garbey et al., 2012; Bass and Garbey, 2014). Computational models can guide surgery to optimize intervention and improve outcome. Such models are applied in surgery for (a) preoperative risk assessment of a patient to guide surgical planning, (b) adjustments of the procedure during a surgical intervention, e.g., by using image-based technologies, and (c) prediction of the surgical outcome accompanied by decision guiding for postoperative therapy. Computational approaches have been developed to guide surgeries for, e.g., heart failures (Kayvanpour et al., 2015; Meoli et al., 2015), brain tumors (Rockne et al., 2010; Baldock et al., 2013), and liver resections (Soler et al., 2014).

Surgical planning, especially for liver resection, benefits from computational support. The preoperative planning needs to be accurate and predictive, but also fast and easy to cope with the growing number of patients. More individualized surgical planning will be required to push the limits in liver surgery toward operating more patients with more advanced malignant tumors, higher age, and preexisting liver damage. With increasing severity of disease, the risk of postoperative liver failure rises. Here, computational support in the future will enable better risk assessment and highly individualized surgical planning for the patients requiring liver surgery, allowing to perform more successful procedures in higher-risk patients with improved outcome.

Current computational support in hepatic surgery focuses on anatomical assessment. To do so, the patient's individual hepatic anatomy is taken into account to enable preoperative surgical planning. This ensures an optimal compromise between an oncologically radical resection and a remnant liver of sufficient size, see **Figure 1**. A radical resection involves surgically removing the tumor including a large safety margin and mitigates the risk of recurrence at the cost of an increased risk of failure. In contrast, a small safety margin maximizes the size of the liver remnant and thus reduces the risk of failure, but involves a higher risk of recurrence. Computational support of today utilizes sophisticated preoperative imaging in combination with surgical planning tools. This approach allows to assess the patient-specific anatomical condition, but does not consider the functional state of the liver. Neglecting the functional state, however, represents a serious limitation, because the success of liver surgery strongly depends on the functional quality of the remnant liver after operation, i.e., the metabolic and proliferative capacity, as well as on the adequate stress response to the surgical injury.

Future computational support must include such functional aspects. Surgical planning could be optimized by prediction of the hepatic stress response, postoperative recovery of metabolic functions, and regeneration of the future remnant liver. Both anatomical and functional assessments are needed to better predict the impact of surgical interventions. Computational support combining anatomical assessment with a risk assessment of liver (dys-)function could provide many benefits for patients undergoing liver surgery, including faster recovery, less infections, and reduced mortality, altogether leading to improved patient outcome.

Employing models from systems biology in the context of surgery, thus aiming at considering all relevant biological processes by the means of predictive computational models, is an approach that could be termed as "Systems Surgery." Numerous computational models simulating selected hepatic functions have been developed in the field of systems biology. These models were primarily developed to improve the understanding of hepatic physiology, but their integration into current surgical planning tools is lacking so far. Extending these tools by integrating computational models involving the hepatic stress response, metabolic function, and liver regeneration would allow better prediction of the surgical risk and the postoperative course and outcome.

In this review, we provide an overview of mathematical liver modeling and its prospective application to computational liver surgery. Following a comprehensive summary of the biological and medical background relevant for liver surgery, we present an overview of state-of-the-art computational approaches supporting current liver surgical planning. Next, we provide an outline of selected liver-specific models from the field of systems biology with a special focus on their relevance for liver surgery. Finally, we identify the main challenges associated with the application of computational models in liver surgery.

UNIQUE CHALLENGES OF LIVER RESECTION

The liver is a highly complex organ. It is characterized by (a) its multi-scale architecture, (b) its special perfusion system with two parallel inflows (hepatic artery and portal vein) and one outflow (hepatic vein), (c) its multitude of functions including metabolic homeostasis, synthesis of essential compounds, detoxification, and excretion of toxic substances, and (d) its high regenerative capacity after injury. Despite the seemingly regular microstructure of the liver, perfusion, functional, and regenerative capacity are distributed heterogeneously in the

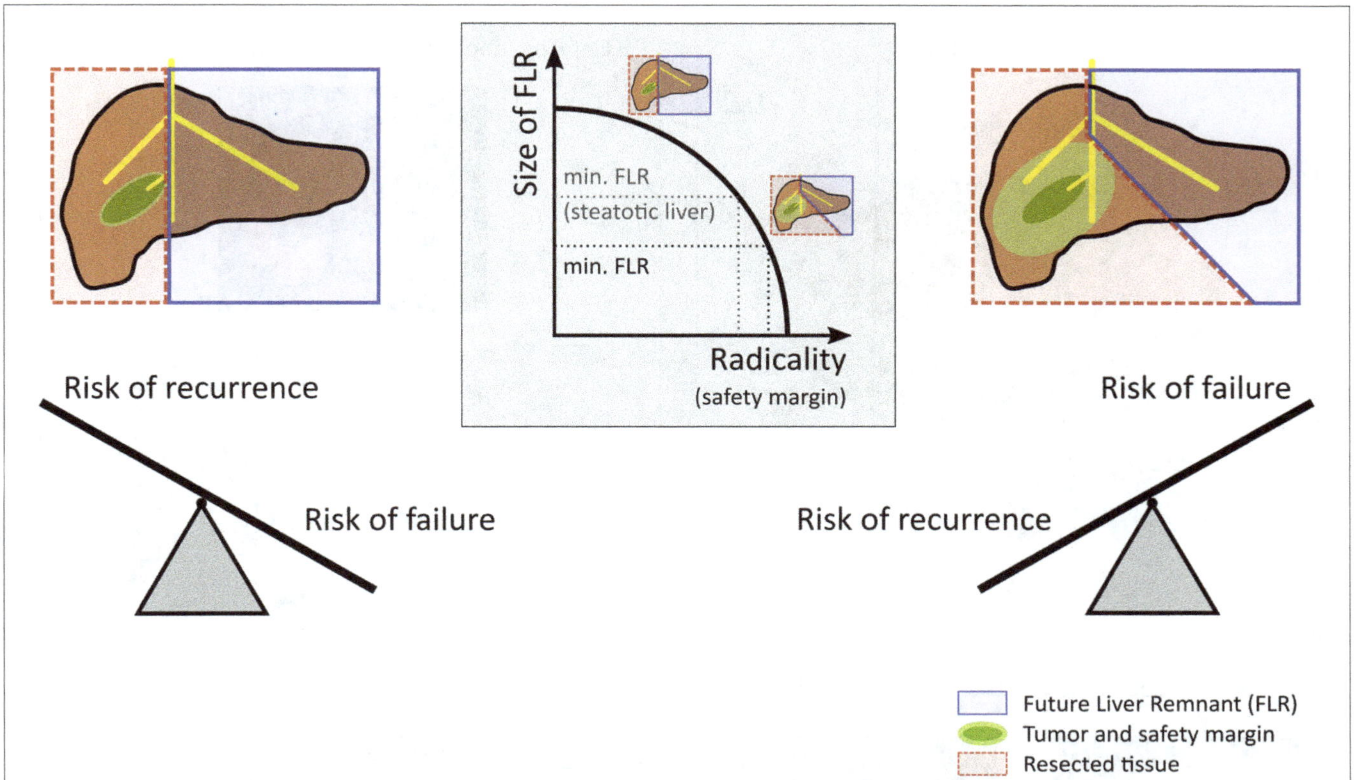

FIGURE 1 | Risk assessment and decision making in hepatic resection. Planning for a safe resection of a liver tumor with a large future liver remnant (FLR) reduces the risk for postoperative liver failure but increases the risk of recurrence. In contrast, planning for an oncologic radical surgery requires a safety margin. Extending the safety margin (e.g., 10 vs. 1 mm) in case of a centrally located tumor leads to a substantially extended resection leaving a rather small future liver remnant behind, which increases the risk of postoperative liver failure. Preexisting liver disease such as steatosis increases the risk for postoperative liver failure and might therefore call for a smaller safety margin compared to livers without preexisting diseases.

organ at different spatial scales, see **Figure 2**. Liver diseases can impair the hepatic structure, microcirculation, metabolic function, and the regenerative capacity, all potentially increasing the risk of postoperative liver failure.

Anatomy and Physiology

Multi-scale Architecture and Hepatic Perfusion

The multi-scale structure of the liver consists of cells, lobules, segments, and lobes (Boyer et al., 2011). Organization of the liver in lobes and segments is based on portal supply via the two main (right and left portal vein) and eight segmental branches of the portal vein. In contrast, hepatic drainage is ensured via the three main hepatic veins (right, median, and left hepatic vein).

Hepatocytes, the main cell type of the liver, are organized in cords along the hepatic sinusoids, the capillary-like small blood vessels in the liver. This alignment of hepatocytes supports efficient functioning by (a) separating opposing pathways in spatially separated zones, (b) preventing substrate competition between different metabolic pathways, and (c) connecting consecutive pathways.

Sinusoids draining into the same central vein form the liver lobule, the functional unit of the liver on the tissue level. Perfusion of the liver lobules, also called hepatic microcirculation, is unique since the sinusoidal network receives both oxygenated blood from the hepatic artery (~20%) and (partially) deoxygenated blood from the portal vein (~80%). Alterations in the sinusoidal morphology (**Figures 2C,D**) lead to changes and heterogeneity in the microcirculation.

Liver lobules in the region supplied by the same segmental branch of the portal vein form one of eight segments of the liver, the so-called Couinaud segments (Couinaud, 1957), cf. **Figure 2A**. In contrast, each of the three main branches of the hepatic vein drains two adjacent segments (and each segment has multiple draining hepatic veins). The interplay of vascular anatomy and flow resistances at the microcirculatory (sinusoidal) level leads to heterogeneous liver perfusion (**Figure 2B**). This complex and highly individual anatomy makes surgical planning difficult.

Metabolism

The liver is crucial for maintaining metabolic homeostasis. This is achieved via synthesis, degradation, and storage of metabolites (e.g., glucose, glycogen, fatty acids, or amino acids) (Boyer et al., 2011). For instance, constant glucose levels are maintained via gluconeogenesis and glycogenolysis to continuously supply the brain and other tissues between meals

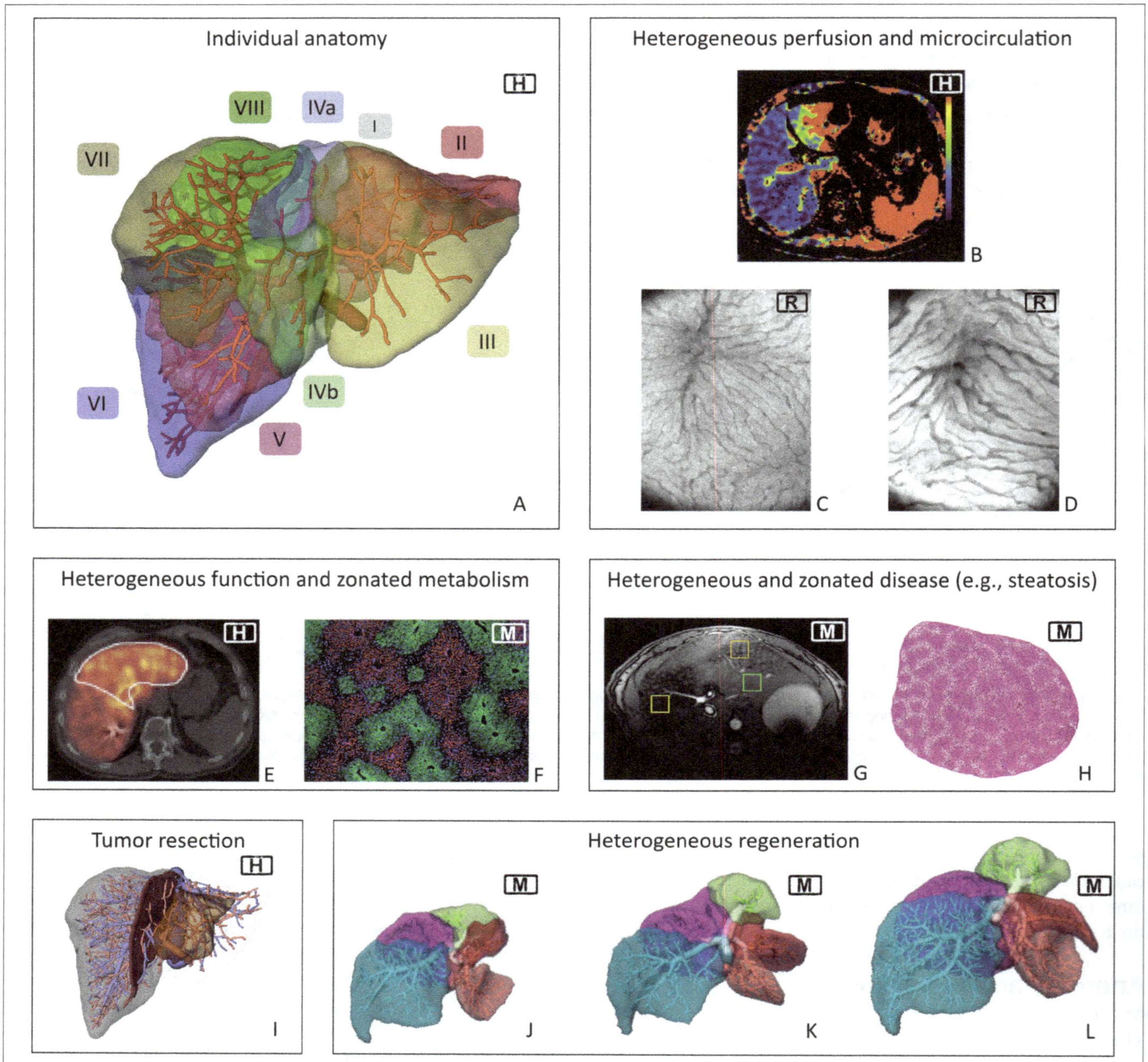

FIGURE 2 | Spatial heterogeneity in liver physiology. Visualization of human individual hepatic vascular and parenchymal anatomy (**A**, the labels indicate the different Couinaud segments) is the basis of current surgical planning **(I)**. Planning currently does not take any functional heterogeneity into account. However, heterogeneity exists on the macro- and microscale in terms of hepatic perfusion (**B**, clinical perfusion CT*) and microcirculation [**C,D**, orthogonal polarization spectroscopy image from **(C)** normal rat liver and **(D)** rat liver after 90%PHx]. Heterogeneity also occurs in terms of regional distribution of functional activity (**E**, Mebrofenin scan of human liver**) and of metabolic zonation in mouse liver (**F**, periportal expression of E-cadherin and perivenous expression of CYP2E1). Furthermore, inhomogeneous distribution also occurs in case of morphologic changes due to global liver disease, here shown regional heterogeneity of fat distribution (**G,** MRT of steatotic mouse liver) as well as zonated distribution of fat accumulation in periportal hepatocytes in a mouse liver **(H)**. Current planning focuses on visualizing tumor location **(I)**. Monitoring of liver regeneration is mostly restricted to experimental or clinical studies and revealed inhomogeneous growth of the remnant lobes in mice **(J–L)**. H, human; M, mouse; R, rat. *Reprinted from Cieslak et al. (2016), with permission from Elsevier. **Reprinted from Wang et al. (2013), with permission from Elsevier.

(König et al., 2012). Other crucial tasks are the synthesis and excretion of bile acids, the synthesis of plasma proteins (e.g., enzymes, coagulation factors, and complement proteins), and the metabolization and detoxification of xenobiotic compounds (e.g., most drugs and toxins are cleared by the liver) (Boyer et al., 2011).

The function of individual hepatocytes depends on their position in the liver lobule, a phenomenon called metabolic zonation. Hepatocytes close to the portal field (periportal) receive oxygen-rich blood from the hepatic artery and nutrient-rich blood from the portal vein and are specialized in oxidative metabolism comprising gluconeogenesis, β-oxidation of fatty acids, and cholesterol synthesis. In contrast, hepatocytes close to the central vein (pericentral) receive lower oxygen and nutrient levels and perform glycolysis, lipogenesis, bile acid synthesis, and drug detoxification by cytochrome P450 (CYP) enzymes (Kietzmann, 2017). This zonation is mainly a consequence of differential protein expression along the sinusoid, e.g., the restricted periportal expression of E-cadherin and perivenous expression of CYP2E1 depicted in **Figure 2F**.

Metabolic zonation is the reason for predominantly zonal damage in response to specific challenges. For example, systemic metabolic diseases like Type 2 Diabetes mainly impact the regional specialization of periportal hepatocytes, e.g., periportal hepatocytes expressing the key gluconeogenic enzyme phosphoenolpyruvate carboxykinase (Yang et al., 2009). Similarly, initiation and progression of fibrosis during pathogenesis of liver cirrhosis affects primarily the periportal areas, since deposition of extracellular matrix originates from mesenchymal cells resident or recruited to the portal area of the liver lobule (Bataller and Brenner, 2005). In contrast, intoxication, e.g., with acetaminophen, mainly affects pericentral hepatocytes, which express the cytochrome P450 enzymes needed for metabolization of the drug (Woolbright and Jaeschke, 2017).

The metabolic functions of the liver are the result of a complex interplay between metabolism on the cellular scale, tissue structure, and perfusion of the tissue/organ. As a result of multiple heterogeneous phenomena, functional hepatocellular activity is distributed heterogeneously in the liver (**Figure 2F**). Consequently, important questions before liver resection are: How does a surgical intervention impact the metabolic functions of the liver? i.e., what is the remaining functional capacity of the liver for metabolic tasks after resection? Is this sufficient to support volume regeneration and functional recovery?

Surgery and Recovery

Resection

The incidence of liver tumors is increasing with the age of the patients. The demographic change with a constantly increasing elderly population leads to a growing number of patients in need of liver surgery (Liu et al., 2017).

Liver resection is the most common liver surgery and consists of removal of liver tissue due to focal lesions, most often malignant tumors (Abdeldayem, 2013). Malignant tumors, like hepato- or cholangiocellular carcinoma, or liver metastases, but also living liver donation, often require extended partial liver resections of more than two thirds of the liver. The extent of resection is determined by the size and location of the focal lesion and the estimated function of the future liver remnant. The function of the liver remnant depends on several factors including its volume, the size of in- or outflow compromised territories, the impairment of hepatic micro- and macro-circulation induced by resection (Nilsson et al., 2014), and the severity of any preexisting damage aggravating the microcirculatory impairment (Hossain et al., 2006).

Reduction of hepatic liver mass results in portal hypertension and portal hyperperfusion. After resection, all blood from the intestine has to pass through the reduced vascular bed resulting in an increased perfusion pressure and flow rate. Portal hyperperfusion leads to decreased arterial perfusion due to the hepatic arterial buffer response (Lautt et al., 1984). The impaired microcirculation challenges the liver remnant with a high metabolic and regenerative demand, thereby increasing the risk of liver failure.

Transecting hepatic parenchyma requires transecting branches of both the portal and the hepatic vein. Due to the anatomical disparity of two portal veins supplying, but three hepatic veins draining the liver, a certain focal in- or outflow obstruction is inevitable. The impairment of hepatic perfusion and microcirculation may cause hepatocyte dysfunction and pericentral confluent necrosis, further reducing the functional liver mass (Lee et al., 2001).

Prior to liver resection, surgeons have to assess the patient's individual risk for postoperative liver dysfunction. In case of malignant tumors, surgeons have to identify the surgical strategy best suited to allow radical oncological removal without putting the patient at risk of postoperative liver failure due to excessive removal of liver mass (**Figure 1**) (see also, van Dam et al., 2014; Kang and Ahn, 2017). Depending on the size, etiology, and location of the tumor, the surgeon has to define the best strategy in terms of the resection surface, but also in terms of the surgical technique such as the use of vascular occlusion to minimize blood loss. Both together determine the total parenchymal loss and the extent of damage to the remnant liver (**Figure 2I**). Deciding on the resection surface determines the safety margin around the tumor and the vessels which have to be transected. Therefore, a key challenge in planning liver resection is to ensure adequate vascular supply and venous drainage, both of which are essential for normal liver function. Small changes in placing the resection surface can have large effects on the size of the compromised portal/arterial inflow and venous outflow territories. In addition to the loss of liver mass by resection, compromised territories further reduce the remaining functional liver tissue, increasing the risk of the procedure.

Stress Response

Resection causes tissue damage and induces a stress response in hepatic cells. An adequate stress response to the injury, consisting of modulation of gene expression and various signaling pathways, is imperative for the patient's survival and recovery. Particularly, the impairment of hepatic microcirculation after resection, which is accompanied by an altered substrate delivery via blood to the hepatocytes (Siu et al., 2014; Dold et al., 2015), makes an adaptation of the metabolic activity necessary. Here, a sufficient supply with oxygen for oxidative processes is required, but local hypoxia caused by the impaired perfusion leads to an increased production of reactive oxygen species (ROS) upon reperfusion (Bhogal et al., 2010). Physiologically, ROS are signaling molecules involved in mediating an adequate stress response to tissue injury by modulating metabolic adaptations and activating the innate immune system. Pathophysiologically, however, excess ROS may cause cell damage. Particularly, if vascular exclusion is used during liver resection to minimize blood loss (Garcea et al., 2006), the level of ROS production raises, ultimately resulting in vast cell damage, decreased metabolic function, and ischemia/reperfusion injury (Zhang et al., 2007). This hampers the function of the remnant liver, again contributing to the risk for postoperative liver failure. Subsequently, the surgeon is faced with a critical trade-off between the advantage of reduced blood loss and the risk of ischemia/reperfusion injury (van Riel et al., 2016).

The hepatic stress response also triggers, besides metabolic adaptations, an activation of the regenerative process (Michalopoulos, 2017) and a local inflammatory response (Alazawi et al., 2016). The latter is not only important for removal of damaged and necrotic cells and triggering regeneration, but also to prevent infections. After surgery, patients are faced with increased risk for complications, such as focal infections, the systemic inflammatory response syndrome, or sepsis (Alazawi et al., 2016). This risk increases with postoperative hepatic dysfunction, which is ultimately determined by the remnant liver volume (Schindl et al., 2005). The levels of inflammatory cytokines, such as IL-6, IL-8, and MCP-1 (monocyte chemotactic protein-1) correlate with the degree of tissue damage and reflect the early response to surgical injury (Badia et al., 1998; Strey et al., 2011; Friedman et al., 2012).

Regeneration

The liver possesses a high regenerative capacity (Fausto et al., 2012). This unique capability ensures restoration of size and function after surgical, physical, or chemical injury (**Figures 2J,K,L**). In principle, two different types of damage require restoration of the liver mass: (a) cell death due to systemic injury of the liver, predominantly occurring in a zonated manner, and (b) tissue loss due to removal of liver segments or lobes via resection.

Original liver mass after resection is restored by mature hepatocytes in the residual liver undergoing oscillating cell divisions (Miyaoka and Miyajima, 2013). The first wave of division encompasses about 60% of the hepatocytes, followed by waves of considerably less proliferation (Zou et al., 2012; Miyaoka and Miyajima, 2013). The immediate regenerative response after resection is mediated by HGF and IL-6, the so-called priming factors of liver regeneration allowing hepatocytes to re-enter the cell cycle (Fausto and Campbell, 2003). As part of the stress response of liver cells to tissue injury, the process of liver growth is highly controlled by a variety of signaling molecules involving, among others, cytokines, growth factors (Böhm et al., 2010), and hormones (Marino et al., 1992).

Substantial recovery of the liver mass occurs within 10 days, and 80 to 90% of the original liver mass is reached within 6–12 months following 70% resection (Nadalin et al., 2004; Kele et al., 2012). In contrast, reports about the recovery of liver function are highly variable, as this depends on the specific aspect under investigation. For instance, liver biochemical parameters [bilirubin, international normalized ratio (indicator of blood coagulation)] return to normal within 10 days, whereas cholinesterase, albumin, and galactose elimination capacity recover within 90 days (Nadalin et al., 2004).

The liver accumulates lipids during regeneration (Michalopoulos, 2007; Zou et al., 2012; Miyaoka and Miyajima, 2013). These lipids derive from an increased adipose tissue lipolysis and provide energy substrates for the proliferation of hepatocytes in the liver (Farrell, 2004; Fausto, 2004; Walldorf et al., 2010). While this "physiological" post-resection steatosis is beneficial, excess lipid accumulation in hepatocytes causes hepatocyte death and impaired liver regeneration. This is of special interest after extended liver resections, because a small liver remnant has lower lipid storage capacity, and thus a higher risk of lipid overload and organ dysfunction, than a larger remnant. Since obviously the liver is unable to regulate the amount of lipid uptake in relation to its size after resection, extended resections lead to a pathophysiological shift from utilization during regeneration to excess storage (Shteyer et al., 2004; Hamano et al., 2014; Tautenhahn et al., 2016).

Ultimately, the course of liver regeneration depends on the functional capacity of hepatocytes in the liver remnant. The loss of liver tissue puts an additional stress on the residual parenchyma to take over the metabolic tasks previously accomplished by the whole liver prior to resection. This is critical in situations where hepatocyte function is already impaired by preexisting damage, like, e.g., hepatic steatosis as discussed below.

Preexisting Diseases

Preexisting global liver diseases can increase the risk of liver surgery. Liver diseases affecting the whole organ comprise metabolic, inflammatory and autoimmune, or infectious diseases. Such diseases compromise architecture, function, and regeneration of the liver and are often associated with or may lead to steatosis, cholestasis, and fibrosis. In the following, we focus on hepatic steatosis to delineate how one exemplary liver disease may aggravate liver surgery.

Hepatic steatosis is defined as an excessive accumulation of fat in the hepatocytes. Steatosis starts with development of small droplets (microvesicular steatosis) progressing to large droplet formation (macrovesicular steatosis). Depending on the etiology, fat accumulation often starts in one specific zone, e.g., in the pericentral zone in case of ethanol-induced toxic etiology. Besides zonal accentuation (**Figure 2H**), fat distribution can also be subject to regional variations, resulting in substantial heterogeneity in the regional fat content (**Figure 2G**; Capitan et al., 2012; Idilman et al., 2016; Schwen et al., 2016).

Patients with steatosis have a higher surgical risk than patients without steatosis (Kooby et al., 2003; Clavien et al., 2007; McCormack et al., 2007). Several reasons contribute to the risk: (a) Steatosis causes an alteration of hepatic architecture leading to an inhomogeneous impairment of perfusion and to an increase in portal pressure (Seifalian et al., 1998). Impaired perfusion is at least partially caused by swollen fatty hepatocytes and sinusoidal "capillarization" (Brock and Dorman, 2007) and reduces oxygen and nutrient supply, contributing to the impaired regenerative response (Yarbrough et al., 1991). (b) Steatosis induces metabolic impairment, which aggravates post-resection lipid overload. Preexisting steatosis is the result of the pathologic shift of lipid metabolism from utilization to storage due to regulatory impairment. This impairment is not resolved after PHx. Therefore, fat further accumulates instead of is being utilized for regeneration. This extends lipotoxic exposure for each single hepatocyte, thus augmenting cell death by, e.g., ROS as described below. Hence, preexisting steatosis exacerbates the reduction of the functional capacity of the liver after resection. (c) Steatosis aggravates hepatic ischemia/reperfusion injury. The increased metabolic supply and the impaired microcirculation in the fatty liver "disrupt hepatic oxygen homeostasis," ultimately leading to local tissue hypoxia (Suzuki et al., 2014). This preoperative condition makes fat-loaded hepatocytes particularly vulnerable to ischemia/reperfusion due to an increased level of oxidative stress. Thus, aberrant lipid accumulation in hepatocytes sensitizes them against ischemia/reperfusion injury, which occurs during the surgical procedure of partial liver resection and transplantations (El-Badry et al., 2011; Kimura et al., 2016).

Taken together, flow restrictions due to excessive lipid accumulation, hepatocyte impairment of lipid metabolism in association with oxidative stress, and cell death impair liver regeneration after resection in case of preexisting fatty liver diseases. This is corroborated by clinical and experimental studies indicating that preoperative metabolic interventions improve the impaired regenerative response of the steatotic liver (Liu et al., 2013). In mice fed with a high fat diet, which induced hepatic steatosis, omega-3 polyunsaturated fatty acids given 1 h prior to operation, ameliorated liver regeneration after both two thirds and 86% partial liver resection by attenuating hepatic steatosis and ischemia/reperfusion injury (Linecker et al., 2017).

In summary, preexisting liver diseases such as hepatic steatosis increase the surgical risk for liver resection in multiple aspects. Currently, this multi-dimensional risk is difficult to quantify preoperatively for the individual patient. Therefore, tools are needed to promote an integrated risk-assessment based on different assessment modalities taking as many aspects as possible into consideration.

COMPUTATIONAL-AIDED SURGERY FOR LIVER RESECTION

Current computational tools primarily support surgical planning and intraoperative guidance based on images of the individual patient anatomy, but do not include functional aspects (see **Figure 3**). Surgical planning needs to address questions (Hansen et al., 2014) related to (a) anatomic resectability, (b) safety margin widths around lesions, and (c) resection strategy, but also to (d) the functional capacity of the future remnant liver.

Medical Imaging Techniques for Liver Surgery

A variety of imaging techniques is available for the detection and differential diagnosis of liver pathologies, the assessment of liver anatomy, and more lately also for the spatially resolved evaluation of liver function. The armamentarium includes ultrasonography, computed tomography (CT) and magnetic resonance imaging (MRI) as well as nuclear medical imaging modalities. The latter, for instance, play an important role in detecting microvascular invasion of carcinoma preoperatively using ^{18}F fluorodeoxyglucose (FDG) PET-CT (Kobayashi et al., 2016), but also allow to assess hepatic perfusion and excretory function based on hepatobiliary sequence scintigraphy (Cieslak et al., 2015, 2016) using different tracers, such as ^{99m}Tc (technetium), ^{99m}Tc-galactosyl, or ^{99m}Tc-mebrofenin.

CT is a core technology for tumor staging and volumetric evaluation of the liver. It enables precise visualization of the tumor location with respect to the intrahepatic vascular anatomy. In fact, the first computational planning tools considering the individual hepatic anatomy were developed on the basis of CT imaging (Radtke et al., 2007; Lehmann et al., 2008). Currently, CT is the most common first-line imaging modality for staging and monitoring of liver diseases (Pinato et al., 2017) as well as postoperative risk prediction based on future remnant liver volume (Vauthey et al., 2002; Truant et al., 2007). Advantages

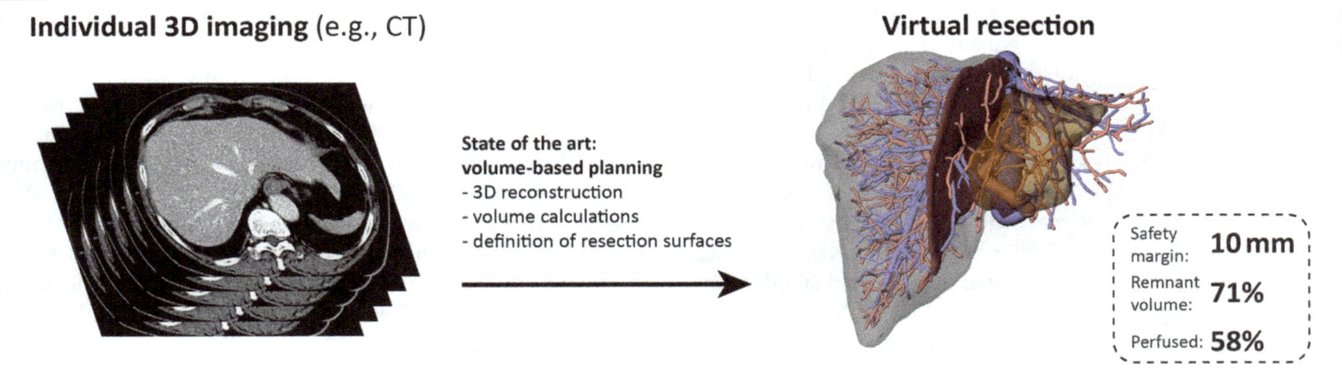

FIGURE 3 | Preoperative surgical planning of today. Current surgical planning tools allow visualization of the individual liver volumes, hepatic vascular anatomy and the corresponding portal venous and hepatic venous territories. Interactive tools allow to perform virtual liver resections and the (perfused) volume of the future liver remnant can be calculated for the selected resection surface. The resection surface can be modified according to the width of the safety margin. The state of the art of surgical planning for liver resection is based on the assumption that all liver volume is functionally equal without any heterogeneity. Such an approach does not take functional aspects into account. The stack of CT images on the left was adapted from (Figure 1B in Chung et al., 2013), image license: CC-BY (https://creativecommons.org/licenses/by/3.0/).

of CT include low cost, high availability, and fast scan times. With perfusion CT, functional assessment of the liver is made possible by performing dynamic CT acquisitions following intravenous administration of contrast agent to extract blood supply characteristics into the tissue (Wang et al., 2013).

More recently, liver ultrasonography (US) and MRI have gained ground with regard to their use in the detection, characterization, and assessment of the response to treatment of focal and diffuse liver diseases (van Beers et al., 2015).

Ultrasonography allows early diagnosis, treatment management, and monitoring therapy outcome (Matos et al., 2015). Recent developments in dynamic contrast-enhanced US (Lencioni et al., 2007) and US-based elastography (Serai et al., 2017; Wang et al., 2017) have facilitated dedicated and specific liver pathology assessment. Contrast-enhanced US promises great potential to evaluate tumor vascularization in real time (Rübenthaler et al., 2017b) and has meanwhile evolved to a minimally invasive imaging modality for evaluating unclear liver lesions (Bartolotta et al., 2016; Rübenthaler et al., 2017a). However, there are still several open issues concerning standardization, operator dependency, 3D capabilities, and the potential for quantitative perfusion. US-based elastography allows predicting postoperative liver failure based on the elasticity of the tissue (Shen et al., 2017).

MRI stands out for its superior soft tissue contrast and the absence of ionizing radiation. MRI makes it possible to evaluate different tissue properties, including fat content, restriction of water diffusion, or increased T_2-relaxation times, all of which support lesion detection. Furthermore, in combination with a liver-specific contrast agent such as gadoxetic acid (Gd-EOB-DTPA), monitoring the perfusion dynamics and the uptake of the agent allows functional assessment of the liver (Imbriaco et al., 2017; Szklaruk et al., 2017; Zhou et al., 2017), thereby improving the detection of liver carcinoma and classification of microvascular invasion in hepatocellular carcinoma. Thus, MRI is a versatile modality for creating detailed, anatomically accurate models for computationally aided liver surgery (Oshiro and Ohkohchi, 2017; Rutkowski et al., 2017). In addition, it offers further potential in form of magnetic resonance cholangiography or contrast enhanced magnetic resonance angiography allowing comprehensive assessment of a patient's biliary and vascular status and possible complications (Boraschi et al., 2008).

Localized magnetic resonance spectroscopy is a non-invasive method to quantify the relative fat fractions of liver tissue, thus providing an elegant means to assess preexisting steatosis (Chiang et al., 2016; Di Martino et al., 2016; Krishan et al., 2016; Kramer et al., 2017). It is often used as gold standard for determining the proton density fat fraction with the potential to replace liver biopsy and takes advantage of the so-called chemical shift, which is based on magnetic field shielding by the molecules' electrons. The different chemical shifts between hydrogen bound to water and lipids can also be utilized by fat-water quantification imaging sequences (Hedderich et al., 2017; Jhaveri et al., 2017), which offer more detailed insight into the spatially inhomogeneous distribution of fat deposits in a steatotic liver (Jang et al., 2017). This way, image-based MR methods may overcome some of the limitations of magnetic resonance spectroscopy associated with restricted spatial coverage and subjective positioning of the volume of interest, which may adversely affect accuracy.

As mentioned before, nuclear medicine also offers very specific imaging methods to support liver surgery. Using the radio-fluorinated carbohydrate (Mun, 2013) 2-[(18)F]fluoro-2-deoxy-D-galactose and PET-CT detection to assess galactose clearance, improved detection of hepatocellular carcinoma has been demonstrated (Horsager et al., 2016). For patients undergoing a major resection, risk assessment and prediction of remnant and future liver function based on hepatobiliary scintigraphy using ^{99m}Tc-mebrofenin has been shown to provide better sensitivity, specificity, and positive/negative prediction values compared to conventional remnant liver volume-based risk assessments (de Graaf et al., 2010; Cieslak et al., 2016). Though this method is currently used only in explorative studies at a small number of sites, combining ^{99m}Tc scintigraphy with the liver-specific functionalization agent mebrofenin appears fairly promising for spatially resolved, accurate functional assessment of the liver.

Taken together, a diversity of imaging modalities and methods is currently available which, however, are not evenly spread and readily available at all centers for daily routine yet. While basic CT, US, and MRI are ubiquitously performed, particularly the more recently developed methods in magnetic resonance imaging and spectroscopy, contrast-enhanced US and nuclear medicine, despite being very promising, are so far largely limited to specialized centers.

Current Virtual Resection Tools

Presently, most computational models supporting liver resection planning are based on individual patient anatomy (see **Figure 3**), in particular the spatial relationship between tumor location and hepatic vascular systems (e.g., Fishman et al., 1996; Marescaux et al., 1998; Lang et al., 2005). Accurate visualization of this spatial relationship is important for the surgical success of a liver resection (Saito et al., 2005), and can be achieved by 3D imaging and appropriate visualization techniques (e.g., Fishman et al., 1996).

More advanced approaches support the planning of the resection by virtual resection tools. HepaVision (now MeVis LiverAnalyzer; Schenk et al., 1999) and LiverPlanner (Reitinger et al., 2006) provide a patient-specific resection planning proposal and highlight different safety margins sizes and affected vascular structures as well as the remaining total and perfused liver volume. Thus, the surgeon can adjust the desired safety margin, which influences the resection proposal. Such planning software is implemented in clinical routine for extended liver resection planning.

Recent developments integrate additional biophysical properties of the liver. Liversim (Oshiro et al., 2015) is a novel virtual hepatectomy simulation software tool, which additionally captures motion and deformation of the liver caused by the intervention. A soft-tissue deformation model including hyperelasticity, porosity, and viscosity of hepatic tissue allows simulating realistic liver deformations and intrahepatic displacements in real time for surgery training (Marchesseau et al., 2010) and planning. Modern medical imaging coupled with computational fluid dynamics (CFD) modeling also facilitates predicting patient-specific alterations in hepatic hemodynamics in response to partial hepatectomy (Rutkowski et al., 2017).

Volume-Based Risk Assessment in Clinical Routine

Optimizing the surgical planning phase by computer-assisted risk analysis can enhance surgery success. In case of hepatic cancer, liver resections can be supported by a preoperative, computer-based calculation of the remnant liver volume (Lang et al., 2005). Hepatic volume estimation by a surgical planning software tool revealed enhanced accuracy compared to the radiologist's volume estimations based on planimetry of a single CT/MR slice (DuBray et al., 2011). The ratio of pre- and postoperative liver tissue volumes, as a rough approximation of postoperative liver function, has been included in virtual surgical planning systems (e.g., Glombitza et al., 1999a,b; Simpson et al., 2014; Hallet et al., 2015; Oshiro and Ohkohchi, 2017).

The aim of liver tumor resection is the complete removal of the cancer. The surgical planning phase encompasses the determination of an optimal safety margin width around the tumor locations (Vandeweyer et al., 2009). Here, a trade-off exists between adequate remnant liver function and sufficient safety margin width. Some computer-based resection planning tools that link visualization of liver structures with an additional volume-margin function support precise operation planning (Glombitza et al., 1999b; Preim et al., 2002; Hansen et al., 2009), thereby enhancing the awareness of the surgical risk and supporting the decision for a smaller resection volume compared to surgical planning based only on conventional 2D/3D viewer application (Hansen et al., 2014).

The Challenge of Function-Based Risk Assessment

Current surgical planning tools focus on the estimation of liver volume as a surrogate predictor of remnant liver function. The underlying assumption is that all hepatocytes contribute equally to liver function. This, however, neglects the spatial heterogeneity of liver metabolism and perfusion, potential alterations of hepatic function in the presence of a liver disease, or individual variations in metabolic function due to genetic variants, or as a consequence of lifestyle.

Consequently, accurate assessment of the preoperative risk requires improved evaluation of the individual functional capacity and prediction of this capacity for the future liver remnant. Such an improved assessment is essential for the ultimate goal of prevention and early detection of postoperative liver failure (Daylami et al., 2016). The measured changes in metabolic function associated with liver surgery and disease depends on the substance used in the function test. However, as outlined above, the liver is a multifunctional organ, for which a single functional assay only provides information about one specific aspect of hepatic function.

Only few diagnostic tools are currently available for measuring metabolic function of the liver. Information about the metabolic functional capacity can be obtained by means of dynamic quantitative liver function tests, which measure the clearance of selected substances specifically metabolized by the liver such as, e.g., the clearance of caffeine (Fuhr et al., 1996), indocyanine green (De Gasperi et al., 2016), or methacetin (LiMAx test, Jara et al., 2015). The metabolic clearance of a selected compound is hereby used to approximate global metabolic liver function as a cumulative effect. Hence, it is necessary to understand the underlying metabolism of the relevant substances and its alteration due to disease and surgery.

This approach cannot provide information about spatial heterogeneity such as, e.g., inhomogeneously distributed steatosis throughout the organ resulting in areas with higher and lower functional activity. Furthermore, such approaches cannot discriminate between the influences of cellular metabolic activity and altered perfusion or liver size after surgery. Here, novel methods are needed to accurately reflect severity, distribution, and composition of fat accumulation and, even more importantly, the resulting spatially resolved functional impairment.

A comprehensive function-based risk assessment requires consideration of all relevant clinical information. Such an assessment needs to integrate information about resection volume/amount, preoperative metabolic impairment in case of preexisting liver disease, intraoperative damage to the future liver remnant as well as metabolic and regenerative capacity of the future liver remnant. To achieve this, multi-scale computational approaches are needed for integrating all relevant processes into one comprehensive risk prediction. Currently, however, only some of the required features are already available (see section below on "Computational Modeling of Liver Diseases Relevant for Surgeries"), but not within one comprehensive risk assessment tool.

One first attempt to extend surgical planning beyond mere visualization and volume estimation has been provided recently by a model, which simulates postoperative liver regeneration in a patient-specific manner (Yamamoto et al., 2016). This model provides predictions of the duration of the postoperative recovery period and possible complications.

COMPUTATIONAL LIVER MODELS RELEVANT FOR LIVER SURGERIES

Regulation and maintenance of liver function involves complex biological processes spanning multiple spatial and temporal scales. Spatial scales range from the intracellular level up to the level of the organism, whereas temporal scales have to reflect time periods of seconds to years (e.g., metabolism in seconds to days, regeneration over weeks, or disease progression over months). Various biological processes play a role for hepatic function in liver surgery, particularly important are the hepatic stress response, metabolic adaptations, and regeneration.

Thus, multi-scale-oriented modeling approaches are especially suited to provide a more comprehensive understanding of hepatic processes and mechanisms. Multi-scale-oriented modeling consists of developing "simple" separate models of certain sub-aspects or scales of the function of interest. Subsequent model integration links input and output variables of these separate models and leads to a more comprehensive combined model, possibly spanning multiple scales. This so-called hierarchical modeling approach (Cedersund and Strålfors, 2009; Nyman et al., 2011) allows adapting the model resolution to the corresponding research question (Kirschner et al., 2014). Current computational models can simulate a variety of selected liver functions, see **Tables 1–3** and reviews (Bogle et al., 2012; Hetherington et al., 2012; Sumner et al., 2012; Fisher et al., 2014; Petta et al., 2016).

The following sections present selected models/modeling approaches for addressing liver functions, which might be essential for future multi-scale models supporting liver resection: (a) the hepatic stress response following physical damage, (b) the metabolic pathways affected by surgery, as well as (c) the regeneration of liver volume and function recovery.

TABLE 1 | Selection of existing computational models to address the stress response with potential relevance for surgical planning, sorted according to spatial scale (*cell to organism*).

Scale	Modeling Approaches
Cell	*Intracellular signaling to adjust hepatic function to external conditions, e.g.,* • Dietary composition—**ODE** (Woller et al., 2016) • Reactive oxygen species production—**ODE** (Selivanov et al., 2009, 2012; Gauthier et al., 2013; Smith and Shanley, 2013; Markevich and Hoek, 2015) • Hepatocyte growth factor network—**ODE** (D'Alessandro et al., 2015b) *Local inflammatory reaction due to tissue damage (i.e., activation of the immune response)* • IL-1 and IL-6 signaling network—**Boolean network** (Ryll et al., 2011) • Hepatic stellate cell activation (signaling)—**PetriNet** (Kuttippurathu et al., 2014)
Lobule	*Inter- and intracellular interactions* • To trigger liver regeneration—**ODE** (Cook et al., 2015) • Involved in signal propagation—**ODE** (Verma et al., 2016) *Establishment of zonation patterns* • Wnt/ß signaling—**ODE** (Kogan et al., 2012; Benary et al., 2013) • Hedgehog signaling— **fuzzy-logic-based** (Schmidt-Heck et al., 2015)
Organ	*Simulating patient's immune response (immune cells, blood concentrations of various signal molecules, blood pressure, tissue damage)* • To pathogen infection—**ODE** (Clermont et al., 2004) (*in silico* clinical trials to predict outcome of sepsis) • To surgical trauma and hemorrhagic shock—**ODE** (Chow et al., 2005; Lagoa et al., 2006)
Organism	(none)
Multi-Scale Integration	(none)

ODE, Ordinary differential equations.

Stress Response Induced by Physical Damage

Resection induces a hepatic stress response, which involves a modulation of signaling pathways and gene expressions. Understanding the signaling network of the liver and how the signaling affects metabolism, inflammatory processes, and regeneration is important to assess the overall hepatic stress response to resection. Signaling pathways are interconnected in a non-linear fashion, involving complex interactions as well as feedforward and feedback loops (D'Alessandro et al., 2015a). An intuitive understanding of the signaling network is impossible due to this intricate dynamic behavior. Here, mathematical modeling can be used to disentangle the complex crosstalk between signaling pathways. Based on this knowledge, further mathematical models can be developed, which connect the degree of surgical injury with liver function, inflammatory response, and regenerative capacity. Such models enable predictions of the hepatic response to surgical intervention and possible postoperative complications in regard to an impaired metabolism or regeneration based on the degree and/or location of surgical damage. Here, understanding the relation between remnant liver volume, hepatic metabolic function, and the local immune response is important to optimize liver resections planning (Schindl et al., 2005).

In the following, we provide a short overview of existing computational models of hepatic signaling pathways to illustrate the current state of knowledge. Then, we focus on ROS as important signaling molecules (Dickinson and Chang, 2011; Ray et al., 2012) and as a source of cellular damage impairing hepatic metabolism and activating inflammatory processes after surgical injury. Finally, we take a closer look at current models considering the inflammatory response and the activation of the innate immune system. A summary of selected models available to address the hepatic stress response, which might be relevant for surgical planning, is given in **Table 1**.

Models of Signaling Pathways

A variety of mathematical models of hepatic signaling processes were developed, mostly using ordinary differential equations (ODEs). Aspects covered by such models include, e.g., the origin of zonation patterning (e.g., Wnt/β-catenin signaling pathway, Kogan et al., 2012; Benary et al., 2013), the propagation of calcium waves at the lobular scale involved in the regulation of diverse hepatic functions (Verma et al., 2016), or the link between the circadian clock and hepatic metabolism (Woller et al., 2016). These models elucidate important features in the regulation and signaling of hepatic function. One example is a fuzzy-logic based model of the GLI-code, the set of three transcription factors linking hedgehog signaling with regulation of metabolic zonation as well as lipid and drug metabolism in hepatocytes (Schmidt-Heck et al., 2015). This relation was also used to explain the link between hedgehog signaling and steatosis (Matz-Soja et al., 2016).

Mathematical models of signaling pathways relevant for liver surgery are necessary to predict, how the liver responds to interventions. One promising approach is the hybrid modeling strategy (D'Alessandro et al., 2015b), which links interaction graph modeling of the signaling network with ODEs, thus

TABLE 2 | Selection of existing computational models addressing metabolism with potential relevance for surgical planning, sorted according to spatial scale (*cell to organism*).

Scale	Modeling Approaches
Cell	*Metabolization of drugs* • Toxicity and timescale analysis, acetaminophen detoxification—**ODE** (Reddyhoff et al., 2015; Sluka et al., 2016) *Glucose metabolism* • Glucose homeostasis and hormonal regulation—**ODE** (König and Holzhütter, 2012; König et al., 2012) *Lipid metabolism*—**ODE** • Steatosis development (Schleicher et al., 2014) • Insulin resistance & high intake diets (Ashworth W. et al., 2016) • Beta-oxidation (van Eunen et al., 2013) *Genome scale metabolism*—**FBA** • Flux predictions under various conditions (Gille et al., 2010; Jerby et al., 2010; Agren et al., 2014; Naik et al., 2014) • Gain and loss of enzymes (Pagliarini et al., 2016) • Integration of transcriptomics & metabolic data (Hyötyläinen et al., 2016) • Alterations of pathways in NAFLD (Mardinoglu et al., 2014)
Lobule	*Perfusion* • Resolved hepatic microvascular system—**PDE** (Rani et al., 2006) • Anisotropic permeability—**multiphase-PDE** (Ricken et al., 2010, 2013) • Role of vascular septa—**PDE** (Debbaut et al., 2014) • Multilevel approach CFD—**PDE** (Peeters et al., 2015) • CFD boundary conditions—**PDE** (Aramburu et al., 2016) *Perfusion + glucose metabolism* • Glycogen patterns & zonation—**multiphase-PDE + ODE** (Ricken et al., 2015) • Zonated glucose metabolism—**ODE** (Chalhoub et al., 2007; Ashworth W. B. et al., 2016) *Perfusion + lipid metabolism* • Zonated lipid metabolism—**ODE** (Schleicher et al., 2014) • Zonated damage & steatosis—**ODE** (Ashworth W. et al., 2016) *Perfusion + drug clearance* • Sinusoidal unit/representative sinusoid—**PDE+ODE** (Schwen et al., 2015) *Perfusion + ammonia detoxification* • CCl4 damage—**AB+ODE** (Schliess et al., 2014; Ghallab et al., 2016)
Organ	*Perfusion + Metabolization* • Well-stirred compartments for acetaminophen detoxification (Reddyhoff et al., 2015)—**ODE** • Spatially resolved porous medium (Schwen et al., 2014)—**PDE+ODE**
Organism	*Pharmacokinetics* • Physiologically based whole-body PK, coupling GEMs to PK/PD—**FBA+ODE** (Bordbar et al., 2011; Krauss et al., 2012; Naik et al., 2014) • Lumped compartment PK models, e.g. acetaminophen liver model in PK/PD—**ODE** (Geenen et al., 2013) • With inter-individual differences (Krauss et al., 2013)—parameter adaption
Multi-Scale Integration	• Cellular metabolic network model integrated in whole-body PBPK model (Krauss et al., 2012)—**FBA+ODE** • Representative sinusoid: contains cells, contributes to organ, embedded in organism—**PDE+ODE** (Schwen et al., 2015) • Glucose regulation (sinusoidal models & PK/PD)—**ODE** (Ashworth W. B. et al., 2016) • Acetaminophen detoxification on multiple scales—**ODE** (Sluka et al., 2016)

AB, Agent-based; CFD, computational fluid dynamics; FBA, flux-balance analysis; NAFLD, non-alcoholic fatty liver disease; ODE, ordinary differential equations; PDE, partial differential equations; PK/PD, pharmacokinetic/pharmacodynamic modeling.

permitting time-dependent simulations. In a first step, the minimal model structure of a signaling network is identified by interaction graphs. Then, subsequent analysis of ODE models of this minimal model structure allows the identification of the best model version. Such a modeling strategy helps to disentangle the intracellular signaling network structure and to predict the outcome of disturbances. The strategy was applied to the hepatocyte growth factor-induced signaling network and allows the prediction of the network response to interventions. An accurate and precise prediction of the response of a relevant signaling network to liver resection would allow better assessment of, e.g., course of regeneration, and thus help to optimize surgical procedures or even to decide for or against an operation.

Models of Reactive Oxygen Species

Reactive oxygen species play a prominent role in the signaling network being active after liver resection, and influence, for example, the JNK pathway (Seki et al., 2012). During the first hours after liver resection, an increased level of ROS was observed

TABLE 3 | Selection of existing computational models addressing regeneration processes with potential relevance for surgical planning, sorted according to spatial scale (*cell to organism*).

Scale	Modeling Approaches
Cell	*Proliferation and its regulation* • Identification of molecular mechanisms (Zhou et al., 2014)—**correlation network**
Lobule	*Growth and remodeling* • Continuum mechanical models of soft tissue—**multiphase-PDE** (Ricken and Bluhm, 2009) • Mixture theory—**multiphase-PDE** (Hum2002, BenGor2005, AmbPetRicStyCia2016) • Growth of biological tissues—**multiphase-PDE** (Ateshian and Ricken, 2010) • Onephasic—**multiphase-PDE** (Menzel and Kuhl, 2012) • Biphasic—**multiphase-PDE** (Ricken et al., 2015) • Triphasic—**multiphase-PDE** (Ricken et al., 2007; Ricken and Bluhm, 2010; Waschinsky et al., 2016) *Regulation of regeneration* • After CCl4 intoxication—**agent-based+ODE** (Hoehme et al., 2010) • By perfusion or metabolic load in model sinusoid (1D hepatocyte layer)—**IPS + ODE** (Hohmann et al., 2014)
Organ	*Tissue growth* • Continuum mechanics—**PDE** (Garikipati et al., 2004) *Volume recovery* • Liver size—**ODE** (Shestopaloff and Sbalzarini, 2014) • Liver size taking into account extrahepatic parameters (such as BMI)—**ODE** (Yamamoto et al., 2016) *Regulation of growth* • Molecular species and number/growth of liver cells—**ODE** (Furchtgott et al., 2009; Periwal et al., 2014; Cook et al., 2015) • Role of bone marrow cell migration in damaged tissue—**ODE** (Pedone et al., 2017)
Organism	(none)
Multi-Scale Integration	• Cells in lobule—**AB+ODE** (Hoehme et al., 2010) • Cells at sinusoid—**IPS+ODE** (Hohmann et al., 2014)

AB, Agent-based; IPS, interacting particle system; ODE, ordinary differential equations; PDE, partial differential equations.

(Guerrieri et al., 1999; Lee et al., 1999). This high ROS level is involved in the initiation of regenerative (Fausto, 2000; Tormos et al., 2013) and inflammatory processes (Bhogal et al., 2010; Seki et al., 2012) in response to the injury. Moreover, these oxygen-based radicals are toxic and lead to oxidative stress, which can result in vast cell damage and decreased metabolic function.

Therefore, computational models focusing on ROS linked to relevant signaling pathways may be helpful in understanding (and predicting) the hepatic surgical stress response. Based on ODEs, several computational models have considered various aspects of the production and degradation of ROS (e.g., Selivanov et al., 2009, 2012; Gauthier et al., 2013; Markevich and Hoek, 2015). Furthermore, a mathematical model simulating the complex regulation of insulin signaling by ROS yielded insights into both protective and detrimental effects of ROS (Smith and Shanley, 2013). The comprehensive overview by Pereira et al. (2016) of the intracellular ROS crosstalk, including the previous models, provides a systems-level examination of the complexities of ROS as intracellular signal molecule and toxic compound. However, mathematical models describing ROS signaling pathways relevant for liver surgery are still missing and no specific model of the processes leading to ischemia/reperfusion injury in the liver exists.

Models of Inflammation and the Immune Response

The stress response of the liver involves also a local inflammatory reaction. The signaling process starts with the release of so-called damage-associated molecular patterns (Zhang et al., 2010) from stressed hepatocytes. These signals activate the production of pro-inflammatory cytokines in Kupffer cells, which initiate the recruitment of leukocyte subsets to the injured site (van Golen et al., 2012). Immediately after surgery, the concentration of cytokines provides some hint of the degree of tissue damage (Badia et al., 1998; Strey et al., 2011; Friedman et al., 2012). Genome-wide gene expression measures were used to fit and refine a literature-based Boolean model of interleukin 1 and interleukin 6 signaling as a representation of hepatocellular inflammation and proliferation (Ryll et al., 2011). Novel relations between proliferation-associated processes were identified in this study, which provided better understanding of the stress response after surgery. In addition, the release of interleukin 6 and tumor necrosis factor alpha by activated Kupffer cells triggered the cell cycle entry of hepatocytes and therefore initiates liver regeneration (van Mierlo et al., 2016). An ODE model to simulate the cytokine signaling and the increased metabolic demand as triggers for regeneration has been established (Cook et al., 2015). Depending on signaling patterns, the model showed the existence of different modes of regeneration after resection and emphasized the importance of Kupffer cell cytokine signaling for the regenerative process.

Computational models can help to elucidate important links between hepatic function and the immune response. Postoperative hepatic dysfunction augments the probability to acquire an infection (Schindl et al., 2005). Thus, quantifying the relationship between liver volume, hepatic function, and the immune response is of major importance to enhance the safety of liver resections (Schindl et al., 2005). For example, the Petri net approach was used to clarify the timing and regulation of activation of hepatic stellate cells (Kuttippurathu et al., 2014), an important cell type for the modulation of the innate immune response. Relevant signaling pathways, such as NF-κB and STAT3, were coupled to the regulation of microRNAs and the model elucidated the driving regulatory factors in the process of stellate cell activation. Another modeling framework used a set of ODEs to simulate key inflammatory processes (see Clermont et al., 2004; Chow et al., 2005 for model details) initiated by surgical trauma and hemorrhagic shock to predict global damage and dysfunction as an approximation to patient survival (Lagoa et al., 2006).

Perspective: Stress Response Models in Computational Liver Surgery

In conclusion, computational models coupling signaling and the innate immune response already exist. Their usage has greatly improved the understanding of the immediate hepatic stress response to physical damage. However, mathematical models linking, for example, the postoperative metabolic impairment with ROS-induced cellular damage are still missing. The cell damage caused by an increased level of ROS after an operation affects the function of the remnant liver and, therefore, is relevant for the risk assessment of postoperative liver failure. Future computer-based predictions of the remnant liver function should take into account the preoperative metabolic capacity of the liver as well as the possible postoperative impairment caused by oxidative stress. Also, computationally supported identification of patients at specific risks for developing sepsis or acquiring a serious infection after the intervention is still lacking.

The challenge for modelers in the field of hepatic signaling is now to shift the focus to a surgical perspective. Computational models are needed that incorporate the knowledge of signaling networks and the hepatic stress response, thus linking the degree of surgically caused tissue damage to impairments in metabolism and to the activation of the inflammatory response. This would enable a more precise computer-supported risk assessment before resection. It is conceivable that such a tool predicts the surgical outcome in response to the expected surgical tissue damage and guides the decision of the surgeon for or against a resection and for postoperative therapy strategy.

Metabolism

Removal of functional liver tissue exceeding a critical cut-off leads to a compromised metabolic liver function and ultimately to liver failure. For accurate and quantitative evaluation of the remnant functional capacity, the metabolic function of the remaining volume must be determined. This function depends on alterations of metabolism, perfusion, and morphology in the acute phase after surgical intervention and during regeneration. Computational models of hepatic metabolism can provide a better understanding of the functional capacity of the healthy liver (for an overview see also Cvitanović et al., 2017) and the metabolic alterations occurring with disease, after liver resection, and during regeneration.

In the following, we provide an overview on computational models describing metabolic liver function with a special focus on models incorporating multiple scales and coupling liver morphology and perfusion to metabolism, followed by an outlook on the application of such models to liver surgery. A summary of selected models available to address the hepatic metabolism, which might be relevant for surgical planning, is given in **Table 2**.

Models on the Cellular Scale

A comprehensive view of the various metabolic capabilities of the liver can be obtained via genome-scale metabolic models (GEMs) to analyze the flow of metabolites through hepatic metabolism based on steady state approaches. The most popular approach is Flux Balance Analysis (Orth et al., 2010). Multiple GEMs of the liver have been published (Gille et al., 2010; Jerby et al., 2010; Agren et al., 2014; Naik et al., 2014) and were applied to study central metabolic functions of the liver like the NH_4^+ detoxification (Gille et al., 2010), to predict metabolic fluxes across different hormonal and dietary conditions, or to simulate alterations as a consequence of gain or loss of function of single liver enzymes (Pagliarini et al., 2016). Such GEMs have proven useful as templates for the integration of omics data to understand the genotype-phenotype relationship in a mechanistic manner (Agren et al., 2014). In recent years, GEMs have been applied to stratify HCC patients (Björnson et al., 2015), to chart metabolic activity and functionality in non-alcoholic fatty liver disease (NAFLD) by integrating metabolic flux data and global transcriptomic data from human liver biopsies (Hyötyläinen et al., 2016), or to reveal alterations of metabolic pathways in NAFLD (Mardinoglu et al., 2014).

To date, GEMs have not been applied in the context of liver surgery, but coupling of omics data to analyse the global metabolic changes following liver resection and during regeneration could be an important next step.

An alternative approach is the use of kinetic pathway models based on ODEs. This approach focusses on specific metabolic functions by means of detailed mathematical description of the involved cellular processes and molecular players. Computational models of central liver functions have been developed, e.g., for the hepatic glucose homeostasis (König et al., 2012) providing insights into the switch of glucose pathways and the role of hormonal regulation. Additional examples are a minimal model of lipid metabolism in steatosis development (Schleicher et al., 2014) and a computational model of both hepatic glucose and lipid metabolism (Ashworth W. B. et al., 2016; Ashworth W. et al., 2016) yielding insight in the development of steatosis. Moreover, one possible mechanism involved in hepatic lipid deficiencies was elucidated by a detailed kinetic model of fatty acid beta-oxidation, in which an overload of substrate slowed down lipid degradation (van Eunen et al., 2013). Multiple pathways models for the detoxification of individual drugs have been published, e.g., for acetaminophen (Reddyhoff et al., 2015).

A more data-driven approach to metabolic function is to apply genome-wide omics data for phenomenological modeling of liver-related diseases. A large number of such studies exists, most of them aiming to identify key molecules, biological functions, and pathways relevant for the disease by differential omics analysis or via correlation-based networks and subsequent topological analysis. Omics-based models have been applied in the context of liver-related surgery, such as, e.g., in the analysis of pathobiochemical signatures of cholestatic liver disease after bile duct ligation in mice (Abshagen et al., 2015). Quantitative metabolomics was potentially useful to diagnose early graft dysfunction in liver transplantation (Serkova et al., 2007). Metabolomics data in orthotopic liver transplantation by consecutive liver biopsies revealed hundreds of significant metabolic differences between pre- and post-reperfusion grafts, among others increased urea production and bile acid synthesis (Hrydziuszko et al., 2010). Omics-based models will be an essential tool in understanding the alterations in liver functional capacity after resection and during regeneration.

Models on the Sinusoidal and Lobular Scale

Kinetic pathway models, GEMs and omics approaches provide important information about metabolic functions and their alteration with disease. However, these approaches are limited, because they neither include tissue architecture nor perfusion, two important determinants of liver function especially in the context of liver surgery. Hepatic metabolism involves multiple spatial scales, ranging from metabolic pathways on the cellular scale via lobular zonation of metabolic properties and gradients of relevant compounds to metabolic heterogeneity on the organ level. Various multi-scale modeling approaches have been proposed (Diaz Ochoa et al., 2012; Kuepfer et al., 2012; Sluka et al., 2016) to represent the metabolism of the entire liver and especially the spatial heterogeneity of metabolic function on the lobule and organ scales.

One common approach of coupling metabolism to perfusion is treating the 1D porto-central axis of the sinusoid, consisting of a sinusoid surrounded by hepatocytes, as the repeating unit of the liver. Such ODE-based computational models were used to model the zonated damage and steatosis in NAFLD (Ashworth W. et al., 2016) or to analyze glucose homeostasis (Chalhoub et al., 2007; Ashworth W. B. et al., 2016), lipid metabolism (Schleicher et al., 2014, 2017), hepatic glucose and lipid metabolism (Chalhoub et al., 2007), the detoxification of xenobiotics like acetaminophen (Sluka et al., 2016), or effects of zonated damage on drug metabolism (Schwen et al., 2015, 2016). These sinusoidal unit models can be used as building blocks of whole-liver and whole-body models (for details, cf. Schwen et al., 2015; Sluka et al., 2016).

On the lobule-scale, metabolic pathway models have been integrated with agent-based models of perfusion and ammonia metabolism (Toepfer et al., 2007; Bartl et al., 2010, 2015; Schliess et al., 2014; Ghallab et al., 2016), contributing to a better understanding of how liver function depends on liver structure. In the agent-based approach, individual hepatocytes act as agents with intrinsic metabolism and behavior (like movement and proliferation). Such mathematical models have been applied to investigate the effect of liver damage on metabolic function after CCl_4-induced necrosis (Schliess et al., 2014; Ghallab et al., 2016).

Alternatively, the liver lobule is modeled using homogenized continuum mechanical multiphase approaches, e.g., via the theory of porous media (Ehlers, 2002; Ricken et al., 2010, 2013, 2015; De Boer, 2012). Embedding a coupled system of ODEs in a porous medium model results in a spatio-temporal description of perfusion and metabolism. This approach was used to evaluate an anisotropic relation for the permeability of the liver lobule, the effect of outflow obstruction on liver remodeling and hepatic perfusion (Ricken et al., 2014), or the importance of vascular septa for homogeneous perfusion (Debbaut et al., 2014). Cellular glucose metabolism was coupled to the blood flow through a porous medium leading to an ODE/PDE (partial differential equations) model that helped to better understand glucose homeostasis on the lobule scale (Ricken et al., 2015).

An alternative approach for modeling perfusion is to apply Computational Fluid Dynamics (CFD) using detailed perfusion models in vessel geometries. CFD was applied to the liver to study blood flow in a segment of a lobule consisting of a resolved hepatic microvascular system (Rani et al., 2006). CFD was also used to simulate hemodynamic changes of the macro-circulation in the cirrhotic liver, a multi-scale computational model to simulate perfusion in the human liver on the organ and lobule scale (Peeters et al., 2015), and in liver cancer arterial perfusion models (Aramburu et al., 2016). A 3D multi-scale model of biliary fluid dynamics in the mouse liver lobule predicted drug-induced alterations of bile flow, and demonstrated that bile flow is driven by the osmotic effects of bile secretion and bile canaliculi contractility (Meyer et al., 2017). Until now the integration of metabolic models with CFD and porous medium models is very limited, and application in the context of liver surgery is missing.

Models on the Whole-Liver and Whole-Body Scale

Sinusoid and lobule-scale models allow to represent the entire liver by applying appropriate scaling in a simplified way. Such models are based on the assumption that the organ does not contribute additional heterogeneity (e.g., in Sluka et al., 2016), or use multiple instances of such models "in parallel" to capture organ-scale heterogeneity (e.g., in Schwen et al., 2015). The organ scale has also been addressed directly via an ODE/PDE model of perfusion in the liver vessel tree and drug metabolization (Schwen et al., 2014). Tissue and whole-liver models allow to incorporate metabolic changes due to damage and resection by suitable adaptation of model parameters. With such approaches, effects of necrosis can be simulated on the lobule scale (Schliess et al., 2014) or changes in drug clearance can be predicted in steatotic livers (Schwen et al., 2014).

The liver in the context of the whole body is typically modeled using pharmacokinetic/pharmacodynamic (PK/PD) models (Jones and Rowland-Yeo, 2013) with a model spectrum ranging from detailed physiologically based models (Willmann et al., 2012) to strongly lumped models (Pilari and Huisinga, 2010). Many simplified models of various drugs being detoxified by the liver exist, often modeled via simple one-step reactions or a few reactions in the context of such PK/PD models (e.g., glutathione and acetaminophen metabolism; Geenen et al., 2013). For the liver, GEMs have been integrated into PK/PD models (Bordbar et al., 2011; Krauss et al., 2012; Naik et al., 2014) predicting, e.g., paracetamol clearance (Krauss et al., 2012). Examples of the coupling of sinusoidal metabolic models to PK/PD models are the analysis of glucose regulation (Ashworth W. B. et al., 2016) or acetaminophen detoxification (Sluka et al., 2016).

Perspective: Metabolic Models in Computational Liver Surgery

Computational models of metabolic functions of the liver have been developed, many of them based on multi-scale approaches and integration of perfusion and tissue architecture. However, the application of such models to liver surgery, especially on how the metabolic function is changing after resection and subsequent regeneration, is still in its infancy. By coupling metabolic models to models capable of describing the effects of perfusion and morphology on liver function, a holistic understanding of changes after liver surgery on a local (tissue) and global (organ) scale could be achieved.

Surgical planning using model-based predictions of functional liver volumes could substantially improve clinical outcome. Importantly, computational models of hepatic metabolism could provide insights into the heterogenous distribution of metabolic liver functions like the heterogeneity of fat in NAFLD and its consequences for the regional functional capacity. Multi-scale metabolic models of NAFLD/steatosis would allow to calculate hepatic functional capacity based on given fat content, tissue properties like stiffness and elasticity, and perfusion. Thereby, they would provide important insights into surgical planning. Multi-scale computational models of metabolic functions may also improve evaluation of quantitative liver function tests, like galactose elimination capacity or LiMAx. Integrated with surgical planning tools, computational models of such liver function tests could provide a more accurate prediction of metabolic function after resection and during regeneration.

Integrating omics data with metabolic models for predicting changes after liver surgery seems a promising future direction. Personalizing generic models based on individual omics data, a personalized prediction of metabolic liver function and its alteration after resection could be achieved. This personalization as well as the stratification of patients into subgroups has already been demonstrated (Björnson et al., 2015; Hyötyläinen et al., 2016). The use of omics data, however, is not yet part of clinical routine, but could be important for the prediction of the remnant liver function and thereby surgical planning in the future. For individual function predictions, computational models could be parametrized with a subset of omics data relevant for the respective model.

Regeneration

The liver is capable of regenerating both volume and function after physical damage induced by medical interventions. This includes damage at the lobule scale induced by intoxication with CCl_4 (Weber et al., 2003) or damage at the organ scale due to surgical interventions (Riehle et al., 2011), as well as spatial and functional graft adaptation after transplantation (Taki-Eldin et al., 2012). Once the liver is damaged, loss of hepatic mass leads to an increase in portal blood flow per unit mass followed by metabolic overload in the remaining tissue and an increase in diverse signaling molecules including IL-6, TNFα, HGF, and EGF (Michalopoulos, 2010). These signaling molecules, as well as Hedgehog signaling (Matz-Soja, 2017), jointly orchestrate the tightly controlled process of hepatocellular proliferation. This process is composed of three phases: priming (initiation), proliferation, and termination (Fausto, 2000). Mathematical modeling of the involved biological processes in the different phases of regeneration has the potential to aid in understanding the underlying molecular mechanisms.

In this section, we review existing phenomenological models of biological tissue growth, followed by mechanistic models, which include relations and interactions between the involved biological processes specifically during liver regeneration. A summary of selected models available to address regenerative processes in the liver, which might be relevant for surgical planning, is given in **Table 3**.

Phenomenological Models of Liver Volume Regeneration

Different types of models have been developed to simulate biological growth (see, e.g., the reviews Ambrosi et al., 2011; Jones and Chapman, 2012) and its regulation (Chara et al., 2014), in particular continuum mechanics models of growth (Skalak et al., 1982; Lubarda and Hoger, 2002), for soft tissues (Rodriguez et al., 1994; Garikipati et al., 2004; Himpel et al., 2005), or tumors (Greenspan, 1976). Such models are able to calculate the mechanically induced volumetric growth of tissue without explicitly resolving the underlying biological structures and mechanisms.

A model for volumetric growth of organs including quantitative characteristics and geometric shape of the liver (Shestopaloff and Sbalzarini, 2014) was used to quantitatively estimate patient-specific optimal size and shape of liver transplants. Volume recovery computed from 3D image data, such as shown in Haga et al. (2008), is a typical way of quantifying regeneration and can be used to either calibrate or validate the models and their predictions.

A model predicting postoperative liver volume regeneration from individual quantitative clinical data was recently developed (Yamamoto et al., 2016). This phenomenological model predicted, whether liver size would recover or remain irreversibly reduced, based on preoperative physiological and functional parameters as well as parameters of the surgical procedure.

Mechanistic Models of Liver Volume Regeneration

Temporal Models

Several studies aimed to mathematically model liver regeneration based on known interactions between regeneration-associated biological processes and representative molecules. These models are based on ODEs or delayed differential equations, and thus focus on the temporal scale of the process of regeneration without resolving spatial processes, in particular assuming spatial homogeneity. A model reflecting the interplay of cytokines and growth factors involved in initiating and terminating liver regeneration (Furchtgott et al., 2009) was used to derive different hypotheses for the improvement of liver regeneration. This model was later transferred to modeling of human liver regeneration in living liver transplant donors (Periwal et al., 2014). Further extensions of the model by Furchtgott et al. (2009) was used to emphasize the role of bone marrow cell migration into the liver after resection in mice (Pedone et al., 2017), and to integrate cell growth and its regulation, also in case of model diseases (Cook et al., 2015). The aforementioned models assume that the metabolic overload induces regeneration. However, studies also hypothesize that the increased portal flow per mass unit initiates the process of liver regeneration. The two hypotheses were assessed by comparison of two models reflecting liver regeneration as a consequence of hemodynamic changes or the metabolic overload (Hohmann et al., 2014).

Spatio-Temporal Models

A number of studies also focused on including spatial properties of liver regeneration. Already half a century ago, an ODE-based model for cells at the sinusoidal scale was presented (Sendov and Tsanev, 1968), involving proteins, ribosomes, DNA, and mechanisms predicting cellular death and division. Such models could be used to identify hepatocyte-specific triggers when applying general cell cycle models (see e.g., Kriete et al., 2014). A mechanistic model at the cellular and lobular scale for liver regeneration after CCl_4-induced damage at the lobule scale in mice was used to show that not only hepatocyte proliferation but also coordinated cell orientation as well as cell polarity are critical aspects ensuring restoration of the lobular micro-architecture (Höhme et al., 2007; Hoehme et al., 2010).

One common approach for spatio-temporal continuum models of regeneration is using mixture theory (multiphasic approaches) embedded into a biomechanical framework. This allows the integration of underlying biological mechanisms, see among others (Humphrey, 2003; Amar and Goriely, 2005; Ambrosi et al., 2017). The field of growth and remodeling in biomechanics is covered by one-phasic (Menzel and Kuhl, 2012) as well as bi-phasic (Ricken and Bluhm, 2009) approaches. Remodeling processes are presented in Ricken et al. (2010), where a mechanical biphasic model was developed and the effect of outflow obstruction on liver remodeling and hepatic perfusion was studied. Dealing with coupled solid-fluid interaction, a mixture framework using the finite element method was presented (Ricken et al., 2015). This approach allows calculating tissue growth depending on nutrient supply, e.g., diet high of free fatty acids (Waschinsky et al., 2016).

Network Models

Furthermore, omics-based network models are commonly used for the initial identification of genes and proteins involved in liver regeneration and are thus used to identify key-molecules to be considered in mechanistic models. However, few studies have employed mathematical modeling based on genome-wide transcriptomics data for the identification of liver regeneration-associated molecular mechanisms and biological pathways. A correlation-based model was inferred from genome-wide transcriptomics data for the identification of molecular mechanisms underlying regeneration induced by partial hepatectomy (Zhou et al., 2014). This identified de-regulation of several genes associated with hepatocyte proliferation, inflammation, and DNA replication processes.

Models of Liver Function Recovery

Only few models of recovery of liver function have been reported, most of them being phenomenological. Liver function (in particular the lack thereof) has mostly been addressed in terms of postoperative liver failure. Well-known risk factors for postoperative liver failure are, e.g., preexisting disease, age, nutrition (Hammond et al., 2011). The risk of liver failure can be predicted partly by preoperative tests and risk-defined score models (Clavien et al., 2007) and additionally by postoperative parameters (Yamanaka et al., 1984).

A mechanistic model (Schliess et al., 2014; Ghallab et al., 2016) of function recovery on the tissue scale deals with the recovery of ammonia detoxification and amino acid metabolism during regeneration after CCl_4-induced pericentral necrosis. This model included two selected aspects of liver function and regeneration from damage pattern clearly different from those encountered in surgery, but could be used as a starting point for bridging the cellular and organ scale in regeneration modeling in computational liver surgery.

Perspective: Regeneration Models in Computational Liver Surgery

To our knowledge, currently no mechanistic mathematical model addresses liver regeneration after hepatic surgery. Future models supporting the prediction of regeneration could be integrated in surgical risk assessment and help preventing postoperative complications. The existing predictions of liver failure could be extended to predicting the recovery of liver function based on more advanced and more mechanistic models. The tissue-scale function recovery model (Schliess et al., 2014; Ghallab et al., 2016) could form the basis for a model describing changes in lobular architecture and its impact on more generic function recovery after resection. The main challenge for modeling recovery of liver function is to link tissue regeneration to metabolism, as already described in the previous subsection. Moreover, correlation of volume and function recovery for different diseases (Yamanaka et al., 1993) could be used for phenomenological models of functional recovery.

VISION: SYSTEMS SURGERY OF THE LIVER

Future integrated models of liver metabolism and regeneration should provide function-based risk assessment. Such models need to be accessible via a usable tool for surgery planning. To achieve a more accurate and comprehensive prediction of the functional capacity for Systems Surgery, several medical and computational challenges have to be resolved (Belghiti, 2016).

These challenges involve (a) precise determination of the preoperative state and functional capacity of the liver, taking preexisting disease into account (model input data), (b) estimation of the extent of surgical damage inflicted on the liver during the resection, and (c) prediction of the impact of hepatic tissue loss and surgical damage on the functional capacity of the (diseased) future liver remnant and its recovery process (model output data).

Integrated Planning Tool for Liver Resection

Future surgical planning software should include a workflow for function-based risk assessment. Input data data comprise in addition to the liver anatomical architecture also spatially resolved data assessing hepatic perfusion and function as well as clinical data, e.g., quantitative dynamical liver function tests, and information about existing liver disease as summarized graphically in **Figure 4**. Multi-scale computational models of the liver based on animal models and clinical data will enable to predict *in silico* function and regeneration after resection in respect to variation of resection surface and safety margins.

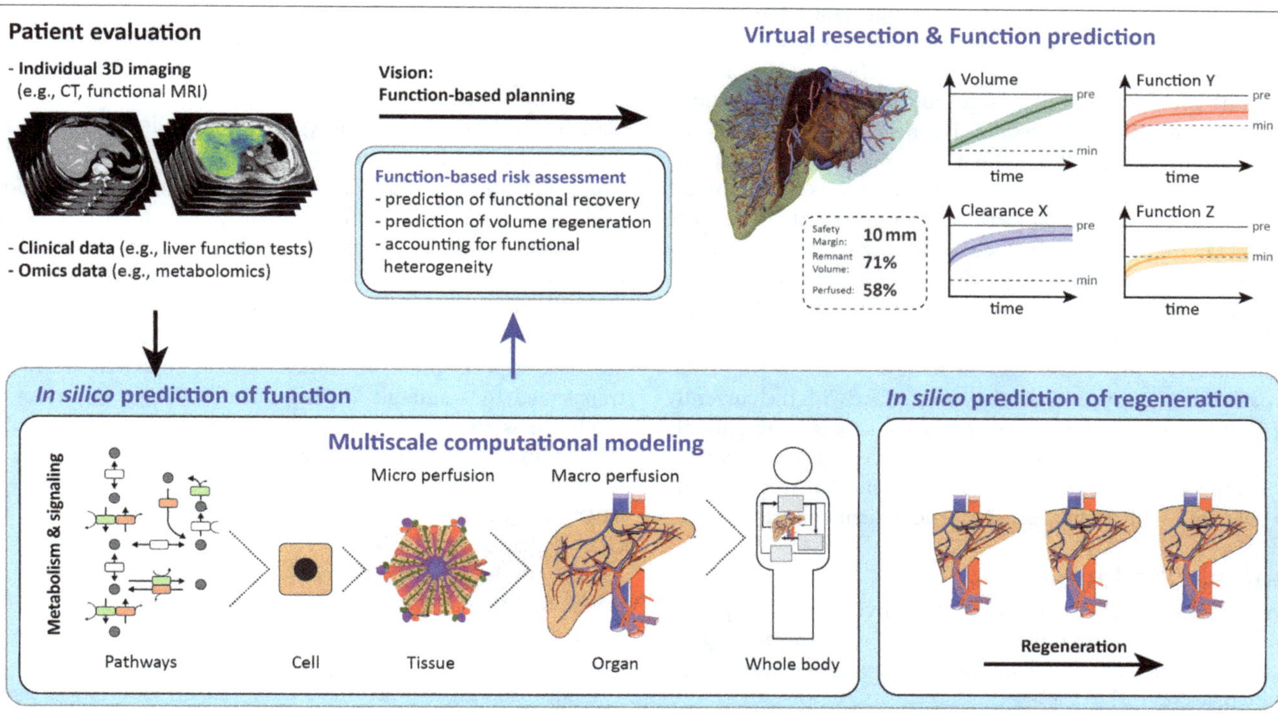

FIGURE 4 | Vision of future liver surgical planning tools. Surgical planning tools of the future will improve risk prediction by accounting for the functional heterogeneity of the healthy and diseased liver and by providing predictions of the functional capacity of the future remnant liver. Multi-scale computational models of the liver will provide the required *in silico* prediction of function and regeneration (blue box). Key information for surgical planning are time-resolved functional recovery curves, e.g., how clearance of certain substances is affected and recovers after resection. Suitable computational models have to be integrated and validated based on animal models and clinical data (for an overview over computational models of the liver applicable in the context of surgical planning see **Tables 1–3**). The input data for such function-based risk assessment includes in addition to the assessment of liver geometry, also the spatially resolved assessment of hepatic perfusion and hepatic function as well as clinical data, e.g., quantitative dynamical liver function tests, and information about existing liver disease. Additional output of the future surgical planning tool includes prediction of selected functions after resection, (e.g., hepatic perfusion, metabolic parameters) and their recovery in respect to variation of resection surface and safety margins. CT image stack adapted from (Figure 1B in Chung et al., 2013), image license: CC-BY (https://creativecommons.org/licenses/by/3.0/).

Functional predictive models need to be integrated into the existing individual 3D planning of the liver representing the vascular structure of the liver and the location of the tumor.

Such an integrated planning tool will improve individualized risk prediction for hepatic surgery and provide important information about the expected liver function after surgical intervention and during subsequent liver regeneration. This tool will ultimately support surgeons in their decision about a patient's operability and the choice of a suitable intervention, but will also make them aware of possible postoperative complications allowing therapy adjustments after resection.

The integrated tool will support risk assessment depending on preexisting liver disease and damage of the liver. This requires integrating underlying pathophysiologic conditions and preexisting risk states on an individual basis. For example, steatosis and other chronic liver diseases (such as cirrhosis already impairing liver function) substantially impact the function of the future liver remnant and its regeneration, and hence increase the risk of postoperative complications and liver failure. Surgeons and patients will benefit from more comprehensive risk predictions taking functional aspects into account without the need of own expertise in multi-scale computational modeling in the implementation.

Future Developments

Further development of such an integrated liver model can be envisioned to obtain better disease- or cohort-specific predictions and to enhance the prognostic power for the individual patient.

Reaching better disease- or cohort -specific predictions would call for including further cohort-specific data to tune the integrated model according to the specific aspect in question. Doing so will contribute to getting a better insight into disease progression and curation. However, this will require to generate considerably more animal experimental data of the specific disease and of course to collect a substantial amount of additional cohort-specific clinical data.

Such data are needed to generate probabilistic disease models, which have to be integrated into the proposed "liver resection and regeneration" model.

Enhancing the prognostic power for the individual patient could be achieved by extending the knowledge-based selection of relevant patient-specific pre-, peri-, and postoperative data considered to be relevant. Additional input data regarding the activity and severity of the complicating liver disease as well as data regarding the general patient condition (e.g., cardiovascular condition) appears extremely useful for this purpose. Similarly, additional outcome data would be necessary, requiring an detailed follow-up of the patient to collect data regarding extra-hepatic surgical and general complications [e.g., abscess formation, postoperative infections and grade their severity (Clavien-Dindo classification)] and reflecting the recovery of the patient's general condition (e.g., days in ICU and in hospital). However, increasing the number of entry variables would call for a higher number of outcome observations.

Alternatively, this could also be achieved using a "big data" approach by focussing on creating an interface with the currently used hospital information systems to have access to all patients and all patient-specific information. Following this approach, a rather large number of patients would be needed to reflect the high data variability as presented in true patient cohorts.

Medical Challenges

Determining the preoperative state of the liver and the expected alterations after surgery must be improved to optimize surgical planning and reduce the probability of postoperative liver failure. This involves several challenges.

Improving Preoperative Diagnostics

Here, the key point is to improve spatial resolution, which will benefit the assessment of morphological and structural alterations due to the underlying preexisting hepatic disease, the assessment of hepatic perfusion, and most importantly, the quantitative assessment of hepatic function.

Identifying Prognostically Relevant Aspects of Hepatic Function and their Spatially Resolved Assessment

Identifying meaningful and relevant diagnostic assays from the multitude of available assays is a major challenge. These assays should be non-invasive and serve as a basis for valid predictions regarding surgical complications, surgical outcome, and changes in liver functions following liver surgery.

Estimating Surgically Induced Damage

It is not sufficient to only quantify the loss of liver volume due to tissue removal, but also necessary to quantify the volume of liver tissue at risk due to alterations of hepatic perfusion. The key challenge is to estimate the loss of functional tissue with respect to the extent of resection, the resection surface, and the resection technique. In addition, preexisting global liver diseases impair hepatic function in a spatially heterogenous way (cf. the section "Hepatic Diseases"), which has to be taken into account during the surgical planning phase.

Predicting Postoperative Function of the Liver Remnant

The functional capacity of the remnant liver should be predicted based on the preoperative disease state and the predicted loss of liver tissue and liver function by resection.

Modeling Challenges

Building a comprehensive model for the prediction of the hepatic functional capacity after resection faces many challenges.

Identifying, Understanding, and Modeling Relevant Processes in Liver Surgery

A prerequisite for building a comprehensive model of functional prediction is the availability of high quality models reflecting those aspects that are important for liver surgery, such as liver function depending on perfusion, liver volume regeneration in case of preexisting damage, or recovery of hepatic metabolic function after resection. The key processes and mechanisms of all these aspects must be understood in sufficient detail and transferred to a suitable mathematical formalism. Part of the challenge is to extend compatible model components and to develop interfaces to bring these building blocks together.

Improving Data Availability and Quality for Computational Models

Besides understanding the processes, further key steps for model building are parameterizing and subsequently validating parametrized models. A key requirement for these steps is the availability of high-quality experimental and clinical data.

Many existing studies have only looked at a single aspect of liver surgery, such as regeneration, liver function, or changes in perfusion. Assembling data from different sources is difficult, since the experimental and clinical conditions are in general vastly different. A multitude of experimental resection studies has been performed in rodents under controlled conditions and with various liver diseases, but using a variety of experimental conditions and read-out parameters. Consequently, comparability is often limited and data integration into a single model questionable. A similar problem is the extrapolation from clinical data measured in one cohort to another cohort with different characteristics, e.g., data from young subjects to old subjects. For similar reasons, translation of results from animal studies to the human situation is even more challenging.

One recurring problem is the quality of experimental and clinical data, e.g., inaccurate or high-variance data, with model predictions strongly depending on the accuracy of the measured patient-specific data. The aforementioned issues with experimental data require new comprehensive and targeted data sets to ensure all needed input data were generated under the same conditions. One key aspect is to perform targeted experiments and studies to collect the information for model parameterization and validation. Alternatively (or in addition), analysis of the effects of the underlying datasets on model predictions and quantification of the resulting uncertainties in the predictions must be performed in order to analyze sensitivity.

Integrating Data with Computational Models

One major challenge is the integration of different types of data (e.g., concentrations, tension, elasticity, image data, omics data, etc.) and to handle the heterogeneity within similar datasets (e.g., from different laboratories, different readers) with computational models. Standardization of data formats and models for simple and reproducible integration of the different data sets into the models is important (König et al., 2016). Especially with the perspective of routine application of such models in Systems Surgery of the liver, standardization of models and experimental data sets will be a major challenge and facilitator.

Developing Large Multi-scale Models

Multi-scale models and models coupling distinct modeling approaches are often not easy to compute. Reasons are that such large computational models require substantial computational resources (e.g., agent-based, porous media, CFD), and that coupling of different modeling is often not supported in simulation software and difficult to implement. Multi-scale computational modeling requires connecting models via clearly defined interfaces between the different scales and sub-models. General challenges of computational modeling like parameter fitting/overfitting, model selection, parameter selection, or parameter identifiability are also major challenges in multi-scale models, often aggravated due to the large number of parameters in models spanning multiple scales.

Performing Model Reduction

Often, model reduction is necessary for efficient model simulation (e.g., integration of a system of ODEs for metabolism in a meso- or macroscale model of whole-liver perfusion) and reduction of the parameter space for analysis. The overall goal is to reduce complexity without compromising the aspects relevant for the question at hand. Different approaches of model reduction have been applied in the field of liver simulations, e.g., representative sinusoids (Schwen et al., 2015), method of proper orthogonal decomposition (Fink and Ehlers, 2015), or the use of an energy function (Holzapfel et al., 2000; Humphrey, 2003; Balzani et al., 2006).

Improving Model Quality and Validating Predictions

Further important challenges are the evaluation of model quality and validation of model predictions, which are two requirements for application of such models in surgical support systems. Validation of models for Systems Surgery of the liver will require prospective clinical trials, which compare the model predictions of liver function after resection and during regeneration with clinical trial data. In the surgical setting, the availability of postoperative data (invasive methods for data measurements are not feasible) limits model validation, so this will need to be done mostly in animal models.

Quantifying Uncertainty and Robustness

Important questions to be answered in the context of model validation are (a) What is the uncertainty in input data and model parameters? and (b) How sensitive is the overall system? Together, this can quantify how robust model predictions are against uncertainty in the generic model parameters and individualized input data. There are various sources of uncertainty, e.g., direct or indirect measurement of biochemical and biophysical parameters, clinically measured physiological and systemic functional parameters, limited resolution, and noise in imaging. An analytic assessment of the sensitivity is only feasible for sub-models of limited complexity. Quantifying the robustness of an integrated multi-scale model will require thorough parameter studies to quantify the sensitivity against uncertainty in individual parameters and, e.g., Monte-Carlo simulations to determine confidence ranges of model predictions under combined parameter uncertainty.

Implementation Challenges

Addressing these clinical and modeling challenges to achieve such model-assisted risk predictions requires a truly multidisciplinary approach involving basic and applied, clinical and computational scientists and engineers. On the one hand, anatomical and physiological phenomena, as well as clinical diagnostic and surgical procedures, need to be accurately described and translated to suitable, improved or novel, computational models. On the other hand, such models must be made available in the form of interactive and user-friendly software and thus usable not only by domain experts in systems biology. Practical usability requires user interactivity, easy and quick handling, automation, minimum of editing, and expert input in the final usage, model adaptation to work on standard workstations available in the clinics, etc. Moreover, interfaces have to be developed, which allow integration of computational models with widely used hospital information systems, e.g., using patient data for the personalization of models and adding model-based risk evaluation to electronic patient records.

CONCLUSION

Already today, patients benefit from computational support in the planning of liver resections. This is, however, limited to an assessment of remnant liver volume and taking into account a number of risk factors for postoperative liver failure. A prediction of liver function recovery is currently not included, but would be particularly useful in case of preexisting liver disease.

Basic biological processes involved in liver metabolism, disease, and regeneration are well-understood, and various computational models for these aspects are available. However, no comprehensive model integrating all these effects on different scales has been presented yet.

With increasing knowledge of disease mechanisms, availability of experimental and clinical data as input for model-based predictions, and expertise in design and integration of computational models, the next logical step is to develop a comprehensive model for predicting liver function and regeneration. This type of outcome prediction will be an indispensable part of a strategy for a patient-tailored optimization of intervention and therapy after liver surgery.

AUTHOR CONTRIBUTIONS

All authors listed have made a substantial, direct and intellectual contribution to the work, and approved it for publication.

FUNDING

MK and LS were supported by the Federal Ministry of Education and Research (BMBF, Germany) within the research network Systems Medicine of the Liver [LiSyM, grant numbers 031L0054 (MK) and 031L0040 (LS)]. JS and UD acknowledge financial support by the German Research Foundation [grant numbers

SCHL 2130/1-1 (JS) and DA 251/10-1 (UD)]. The authors moreover acknowledge support from the German Research Foundation (DFG) and Leipzig University within the program of Open Access Publishing.

ACKNOWLEDGMENTS

The authors would like to thank Andrea Schenk for her support with 3D liver visualizations.

REFERENCES

Abdeldayem, H. (2013). *General Introduction: Advances in Hepatic Surgery*. London: InTech.

Abshagen, K., König, M., Hoppe, A., Müller, I., Ebert, M., Weng, H., et al. (2015). Pathobiochemical signatures of cholestatic liver disease in bile duct ligated mice. *BMC Syst. Biol.* 9:83. doi: 10.1186/s12918-015-0229-0

Agren, R., Mardinoglu, A., Asplund, A., Kampf, C., Uhlen, M., and Nielsen, J. (2014). Identification of anticancer drugs for hepatocellular carcinoma through personalized genome-scale metabolic modeling. *Mol. Syst. Biol.* 10:721. doi: 10.1002/msb.145122

Alazawi, W., Pirmadjid, N., Lahiri, R., and Bhattacharya, S. (2016). Inflammatory and immune responses to surgery and their clinical impact. *Ann. Surg.* 264, 73–80. doi: 10.1097/SLA.0000000000001691

Amar, M. B., and Goriely, A. (2005). Growth and instability in elastic tissues. *J. Mech. Phys. Solids* 53, 2284–2319. doi: 10.1016/j.jmps.2005.04.008

Ambrosi, D., Ateshian, G. A., Arruda, E. M., Cowin, S. C., Dumais, J., Goriely, A., et al. (2011). Perspectives on biological growth and remodeling. *J. Mech. Phys. Solids* 59, 863–883. doi: 10.1016/j.jmps.2010.12.011

Ambrosi, D., Pezzuto, S., Riccobelli, D., Stylianopoulos, T., and Ciarletta, P. (2017). Solid tumors are poroelastic solids with a chemo-mechanical feedback on growth. *J. Elast.* 129, 107–124. doi: 10.1007/s10659-016-9619-9

Aramburu, J., Antón, R., Rivas, A., Ramos, J. C., Sangro, B., and Bilbao, J. I. (2016). Liver cancer arterial perfusion modelling and CFD boundary conditions methodology: a case study of the haemodynamics of a patient-specific hepatic artery in literature-based healthy and tumour-bearing liver scenarios. *Int. J. Numer. Method. Biomed. Eng.* 32:e02764. doi: 10.1002/cnm.2764

Ashworth, W. B., Davies, N. A., and Bogle, I. D. L. (2016). A computational model of hepatic energy metabolism: understanding zonated damage and steatosis in NAFLD. *PLoS Comput. Biol.* 12:e1005105. doi: 10.1371/journal.pcbi.1005105

Ashworth, W., Perez-Galvan, C., Davies, N., and Bogle, I. D. L. (2016). Liver function as an engineering system. *AIChE J.* 62, 3285–3297. doi: 10.1002/aic.15292

Ateshian, G. A., and Ricken, T. (2010). Multigenerational interstitial growth of biological tissues. *Biomech. Model. Mechanobiol.* 9, 689–702. doi: 10.1007/s10237-010-0205-y

Badia, J. M., Ayton, L. C., Evans, T. J., Carpenter, A. J., Nawfal, G., Kinderman, H., et al. (1998). Systemic cytokine response to hepatic resections under total vascular exclusion. *Eur. J. Surg.* 164, 185–190. doi: 10.1080/110241598750004625

Baldock, A. L., Rockne, R. C., Boone, A. D., Neal, M. L., Hawkins-Daarud, A., Corwin, D. M., et al. (2013). From patient-specific mathematical neuro-oncology to precision medicine. *Front. Oncol.* 3:62. doi: 10.3389/fonc.2013.00062

Balzani, D., Neff, P., Schröder, J., and Holzapfel, G. A. (2006). A polyconvex framework for soft biological tissues. Adjustment to experimental data. *Int. J. Solids Struct.* 43, 6052–6070. doi: 10.1016/j.ijsolstr.2005.07.048

Bartl, M., Pfaff, M., Ghallab, A., Driesch, D., Henkel, S. G., Hengstler, J. G., et al. (2015). Optimality in the zonation of ammonia detoxification in rodent liver. *Arch. Toxicol.* 89, 2069–2078. doi: 10.1007/s00204-015-1596-4

Bartl, M., Pfaff, M., Toepfer, S., Zellmer, S., Gebhardt, R., Schuster, S., et al. (2010). "Model-based optimization to explain liver zonation in nitrogen metabolism," in *55th International Scientific Colloquium* (Ilmenau), 235–240

Bartolotta, T. V., Vernuccio, F., Taibbi, A., and Lagalla, R. (2016). Contrast-enhanced ultrasound in focal liver lesions: where do we stand? *Semin. Ultrasound CT MR* 37, 573–586. doi: 10.1053/j.sult.2016.10.003

Bass, B. L., and Garbey, M. (2014). A road map for computational surgery: challenges and opportunities. *J. Comput. Surg.* 1:2. doi: 10.1186/2194-3990-1-2

Bataller, R., and Brenner, D. A. (2005). Liver fibrosis. *J. Clin. Invest.* 115, 209–218. doi: 10.1172/JCI24282

Belghiti, J. (2016). How could we image the future in hepatic surgery. *Hepatob. Surg. Nutr.* 5, 279–280. doi: 10.21037/hbsn.2015.12.07

Benary, U., Kofahl, B., Hecht, A., and Wolf, J. (2013). Modeling Wnt/beta-catenin target gene expression in APC and wnt gradients under wild type and mutant conditions. *Front. Physiol.* 4:21. doi: 10.3389/fphys.2013.00021

Bhogal, R. H., Curbishley, S. M., Weston, C. J., Adams, D. H., and Afford, S. C. (2010). Reactive oxygen species mediate human hepatocyte injury during hypoxia/reoxygenation. *Liver Transpl.* 16, 1303–1313. doi: 10.1002/lt.22157

Björnson, E., Mukhopadhyay, B., Asplund, A., Pristovsek, N., Cinar, R., Romeo, S., et al. (2015). Stratification of hepatocellular carcinoma patients based on acetate utilization. *Cell Rep.* 13, 2014–2026. doi: 10.1016/j.celrep.2015.10.045

Bogle, I. D. L., Jalan, R., Shephard, E., Seymour, R., Finkelstein, A., Sumner, T., et al. (2012). *Systems Biology of the Liver*. Weinheim: Wiley-VCH Verlag GmbH & Co. KgaA.

Böhm, F., Köhler, U. A., Speicher, T., and Werner, S. (2010). Regulation of liver regeneration by growth factors and cytokines. *EMBO Mol. Med.* 2, 294–305. doi: 10.1002/emmm.201000085

Boraschi, P., Donati, F., Gigoni, R., Salemi, S., Urbani, L., Filipponi, F., et al. (2008). Complications after liver transplantation: evaluation with magnetic resonance imaging, magnetic resonance cholangiography, and 3-dimensional contrast-enhanced magnetic resonance angiography in a single session. *Can. Assoc. Radiol. J.* 59, 259–263.

Bordbar, A., Feist, A. M., Usaite-Black, R., Woodcock, J., Palsson, B. O., and Famili, I. (2011). A multi-tissue type genome-scale metabolic network for analysis of whole-body systems physiology. *BMC Syst. Biol.* 5:180. doi: 10.1186/1752-0509-5-180

Boyer, T. D., Wright, T. L., and Manns, M. P. (2011). *Zakim and Boyer's Hepatology, 6th Edn., A Textbook of Liver Disease.* Amsterdam: Elsevier Health Sciences.

Brock, R. W., and Dorman, R. B. (2007). Obesity, insulin resistance and hepatic perfusion. *Microcirculation* 14, 339–347. doi: 10.1080/10739680701282986

Capitan, V., Petit, J.-M., Aho, S., Lefevre, P.-H., Favelier, S., Loffroy, R., et al. (2012). Macroscopic heterogeneity of liver fat: an MR-based study in type-2 diabetic patients. *Eur. Radiol.* 22, 2161–2168. doi: 10.1007/s00330-012-2468-4

Cedersund, G., and Strålfors, P. (2009). Putting the pieces together in diabetes research: towards a hierarchical model of whole-body glucose homeostasis. *Eur. J. Pharmaceut. Sci.* 36, 91–104. doi: 10.1016/j.ejps.2008.10.027

Chalhoub, E., Hanson, R. W., and Belovich, J. M. (2007). A computer model of gluconeogenesis and lipid metabolism in the perfused liver. *Am. J. Physiol. Endocrinol. Metab.* 293, E1676–E1686. doi: 10.1152/ajpendo.00161.2007

Chara, O., Tanaka, E. M., and Brusch, L. (2014). Mathematical modeling of regenerative processes. *Curr. Top. Dev. Biol.* 108, 283–317. doi: 10.1016/B978-0-12-391498-9.00011-5

Chiang, H.-J., Chang, W.-P., Chiang, H.-W., Lazo, M. Z., Chen, T.-Y., Ou, H.-Y., et al. (2016). Magnetic resonance spectroscopy in living-donor liver transplantation. *Transpl. Proc.* 48, 1003–1006. doi: 10.1016/j.transproceed.2015.10.068

Chow, C. C., Clermont, G., Kumar, R., Lagoa, C., Tawadrous, Z., Gallo, D., et al. (2005). The acute inflammatory response in diverse shock states. *Shock* 24, 74–84. doi: 10.1097/01.shk.0000168526.97716.f3

Chung, Y. E., Kim, M.-J., Kim, Y.-E., Park, M.-S., Choi, J. Y., and Kim, K. W. (2013). Characterization of incidental liver lesions: comparison of multidetector CT versus Gd-EOB-DTPA-enhanced MR imaging. *PLoS ONE* 8:e66141. doi: 10.1371/journal.pone.0066141

Cieslak, K. P., Bennink, R. J., de Graaf, W., van Lienden, K. P., Besselink, M. G., Busch, O. R. C., et al. (2016). Measurement of liver function using hepatobiliary scintigraphy improves risk assessment in patients undergoing major liver resection. *HPB* 18, 773–780. doi: 10.1016/j.hpb.2016.06.006

Cieslak, K. P., Olthof, P. B., van Lienden, K. P., Besselink, M. G., Busch, O. R., van Gulik, T. M., et al. (2015). Assessment of liver function using (99m)Tc-Mebrofenin Hepatobiliary Scintigraphy in ALPPS (Associating Liver Partition and Portal Vein Ligation for Staged Hepatectomy). *Case Rep. Gastroenterol.* 9, 353–360. doi: 10.1159/000441385

Clavien, P. A., Petrowsky, H., DeOliveira, M. L., and Graf, R. (2007). Strategies for safer liver surgery and partial liver transplantation. *N. Engl. J. Med.* 356, 1545–1559. doi: 10.1056/NEJMra065156

Clermont, G., Bartels, J., Kumar, R., Constantine, G., Vodovotz, Y., and Chow, C. (2004). *In silico* design of clinical trials: a method coming of age. *Crit. Care Med.* 32, 2061–2070. doi: 10.1097/01.CCM.0000142394.28791.C3

Cook, D., Ogunnaike, B. A., and Vadigepalli, R. (2015). Systems analysis of non-parenchymal cell modulation of liver repair across multiple regeneration modes. *BMC Syst. Biol.* 9:71. doi: 10.1186/s12918-015-0220-9

Couinaud, C. (1957). *Le Foie: Études Anatomiques et Chirurgicales*. Paris: Masson.

Cvitanović, T., Reichert, M. C., Moškon, M., Mraz, M., Lammert, F., and Rozman, D. (2017). Large-scale computational models of liver metabolism: how far from the clinics? *Hepatology* 66, 1323–1334. doi: 10.1002/hep.29268

D'Alessandro, L. A., Hoehme, S., Henney, A., Drasdo, D., and Klingmüller, U. (2015a). Unraveling liver complexity from molecular to organ level: challenges and perspectives. *Prog. Biophys. Mol. Biol.* 117, 78–86. doi: 10.1016/j.pbiomolbio.2014.11.005

D'Alessandro, L. A., Samaga, R., Maiwald, T., Rho, S.-H., Bonefas, S., Raue, A., et al. (2015b). Disentangling the complexity of HGF signaling by combining qualitative and quantitative modeling. *PLoS Comput. Biol.* 11:e1004192. doi: 10.1371/journal.pcbi.1004192

Daylami, R., Schneider, P. D., and Khatri, V. P. (2016). *Liver Function Assessment before and after Hepatic Resection, Vol. 1*. Sharjah: Bentham Science Publisher.

De Boer, R. (2012). *Theory of Porous Media: Highlights in Historical Development and Current State*. Luxemburg: Springer Science & Business Media.

De Gasperi, A., Mazza, E., and Prosperi, M. (2016). Indocyanine green kinetics to assess liver function: ready for a clinical dynamic assessment in major liver surgery? *World J. Hepatol.* 8, 355–367. doi: 10.4254/wjh.v8.i7.355

de Graaf, W., van Lienden, K. P., Dinant, S., Roelofs, J. J., Busch, O. R. C., Gouma, D. J., et al. (2010). Assessment of future remnant liver function using hepatobiliary scintigraphy in patients undergoing major liver resection. *J. Gastrointest. Surg.* 14, 369–378. doi: 10.1007/s11605-009-1085-2

Debbaut, C., Vierendeels, J., Siggers, J. H., Repetto, R., Monbaliu, D., and Segers, P. (2014). A 3D porous media liver lobule model: the importance of vascular septa and anisotropic permeability for homogeneous perfusion. *Comput. Methods Biomech. Biomed. Eng.* 17, 1295–1310. doi: 10.1080/10255842.2012.744399

Di Martino, M., Pacifico, L., Bezzi, M., Di Miscio, R., Sacconi, B., Chiesa, C., et al. (2016). Comparison of magnetic resonance spectroscopy, proton density fat fraction and histological analysis in the quantification of liver steatosis in children and adolescents. *World J. Gastroenterol.* 22, 8812–8819. doi: 10.3748/wjg.v22.i39.8812

Diaz Ochoa, J. G., Bucher, J., Péry, A. R., Zaldivar Comenges, J. M., Niklas, J., and Mauch, K. (2012). A multi-scale modeling framework for individualized, spatiotemporal prediction of drug effects and toxicological risk. *Front. Pharmacol.* 3:204. doi: 10.3389/fphar.2012.00204

Dickinson, B. C., and Chang, C. J. (2011). Chemistry and biology of reactive oxygen species in signaling or stress responses. *Nat. Chem. Biol.* 7, 504–511. doi: 10.1038/nchembio.607

Dold, S., Richter, S., Kollmar, O., von Heesen, M., Scheuer, C., Laschke, M. W., et al. (2015). Portal hyperperfusion after extended hepatectomy does not induce a hepatic arterial buffer response (HABR) but impairs mitochondrial redox state and hepatocellular oxygenation. *PLoS ONE* 10:e0141877. doi: 10.1371/journal.pone.0141877

DuBray, J. B., Levy, R. V., Balachandran, P., Conzen, K. D., Upadhya, G. A., Anderson, C. D., et al. (2011). Novel three-dimensional imaging technique improves the accuracy of hepatic volumetric assessment. *HPB* 13, 670–674. doi: 10.1111/j.1477-2574.2011.00350.x

Ehlers, W. (2002). "Foundations of multiphasic and porous materials," in *Porous Media*, eds W. Ehlers and J. Bluhm (Berlin; Heidelberg: Springer), 3–86.

El-Badry, A. M., Jang, J. H., Elsherbiny, A., Contaldo, C., Tian, Y., Raptis, D. A., et al. (2011). Chemical composition of hepatic lipids mediates reperfusion injury of the macrosteatotic mouse liver through thromboxane A(2). *J. Hepatol.* 55, 1291–1299. doi: 10.1016/j.jhep.2011.04.019

Farrell, G. C. (2004). Probing prometheus: fat fueling the fire? *Hepatology* 40, 1252–1255. doi: 10.1002/hep.20522

Fausto, N. (2000). Liver regeneration. *J. Hepatol.* 32, 19–31. doi: 10.1016/S0168-8278(00)80412-2

Fausto, N. (2004). Liver regeneration and repair: hepatocytes, progenitor cells, and stem cells. *Hepatology* 39, 1477–1487. doi: 10.1002/hep.20214

Fausto, N., and Campbell, J. S. (2003). The role of hepatocytes and oval cells in liver regeneration and repopulation. *Mech. Dev.* 120, 117–130. doi: 10.1016/S0925-4773(02)00338-6

Fausto, N., Campbell, J. S., and Riehle, K. J. (2012). Liver regeneration. *J. Hepatol.* 57, 692–694. doi: 10.1016/j.jhep.2012.04.016

Fink, D., and Ehlers, W. (2015). Application and modification of the POD method and the POD-DEIM for model reduction in porous-media simulations. *PAMM* 15, 385–386. doi: 10.1002/pamm.201510183

Fisher, C. P., Kierzek, A. M., Plant, N. J., and Moore, J. B. (2014). Systems biology approaches for studying the pathogenesis of non-alcoholic fatty liver disease. *World J. Gastroenterol.* 20, 15070–15078. doi: 10.3748/wjg.v20.i41.15070

Fishman, E., Kuszyk, B., Heath, D., Gao, L., and Cabral, B. (1996). Surgical planning for liver resection. *Computer* 29, 64–72. doi: 10.1109/2.481467

Friedman, B. H., Wolf, J. H., Wang, L., Putt, M. E., Shaked, A., Christie, J. D., et al. (2012). Serum cytokine profiles associated with early allograft dysfunction in patients undergoing liver transplantation. *Liver Transpl.* 18, 166–176. doi: 10.1002/lt.22451

Fuhr, U., Rost, K. L., Engelhardt, R., Sachs, M., Liermann, D., Belloc, C., et al. (1996). Evaluation of caffeine as a test drug for CYP1A2, NAT2 and CYP2E1 phenotyping in man by *in vivo* versus *in vitro* correlations. *Pharmacogenetics* 6, 159–176. doi: 10.1097/00008571-199604000-00003

Furchtgott, L. A., Chow, C. C., and Periwal, V. (2009). A model of liver regeneration. *Biophys. J.* 96, 3926–3935. doi: 10.1016/j.bpj.2009.01.061

Garbey, M., Bass, B., and Berceli, S. (2012). Multiscale mechanobiology modeling for surgery assessment. *Acta Mech. Sin.* 28, 1186–1202. doi: 10.1007/s10409-012-0133-4

Garcea, G., Gescher, A., Steward, W., Dennison, A., and Berry, D. (2006). Oxidative stress in humans following the Pringle manoeuvre. *Hepatob. Pancreat. Dis Int.* 5, 210–214.

Garikipati, K., Arruda, E. M., Grosh, K., Narayanan, H., and Calve, S. (2004). A continuum treatment of growth in biological tissue: the coupling of mass transport and mechanics. *J. Mech. Phys. Solids* 52, 1595–1625. doi: 10.1016/j.jmps.2004.01.004

Gauthier, L. D., Greenstein, J. L., Cortassa, S., O'Rourke, B., and Winslow, R. L. (2013). A computational model of reactive oxygen species and redox balance in cardiac mitochondria. *Biophys. J.* 105, 1045–1056. doi: 10.1016/j.bpj.2013.07.006

Geenen, S., Yates, J. W., Kenna, J. G., Bois, F. Y., Wilson, I. D., and Westerhoff, H. V. (2013). Multiscale modelling approach combining a kinetic model of glutathione metabolism with PBPK models of paracetamol and the potential glutathione-depletion biomarkers ophthalmic acid and 5-oxoproline in humans and rats. *Integr. Biol.* 5, 877–888. doi: 10.1039/c3ib20245c

Ghallab, A., Cellière, G., Henkel, S. G., Driesch, D., Hoehme, S., Hofmann, U., et al. (2016). Model-guided identification of a therapeutic strategy to reduce hyperammonemia in liver diseases. *J. Hepatol.* 64, 860–871. doi: 10.1016/j.jhep.2015.11.018

Gille, C., Bölling, C., Hoppe, A., Bulik, S., Hoffmann, S., Hübner, K., et al. (2010). HepatoNet1: a comprehensive metabolic reconstruction of the human hepatocyte for the analysis of liver physiology. *Mol. Syst. Biol.* 6:411. doi: 10.1038/msb.2010.62

Glombitza, G., Evers, H., Hassfeld, S., Engelmann, U., and Meinzer, H. P. (1999a). Virtual surgery in a (tele-)radiology framework. *IEEE Trans. Inf. Technol. Biomed.* 3, 186–196.

Glombitza, G., Lamadé, W., Demiris, A. M., Göpfert, M. R., Mayer, A., Bahner, M. L., et al. (1999b). Virtual planning of liver resections: image processing, visualization and volumetric evaluation. *Int. J. Med. Inform.* 53, 225–237. doi: 10.1016/S1386-5056(98)00162-2

Greenspan, H. P. (1976). On the growth and stability of cell cultures and solid tumors. *J. Theor. Biol.* 56, 229–242. doi: 10.1016/S0022-5193(76)80054-9

Guerrieri, F., Vendemiale, G., Grattagliano, I., Cocco, T., Pellecchia, G., and Altomare, E. (1999). Mitochondrial oxidative alterations following partial hepatectomy. *Free Radic. Biol. Med.* 26, 34–41. doi: 10.1016/S0891-5849(98)00145-2

Haga, J., Shimazu, M., Wakabayashi, G., Tanabe, M., Kawachi, S., Fuchimoto, Y., et al. (2008). Liver regeneration in donors and adult recipients after living donor liver transplantation. *Liver Transpl.* 14, 1718–1724. doi: 10.1002/lt.21622

Hallet, J., Gayet, B., Tsung, A., Wakabayashi, G., Pessaux, P., and 2nd International Consensus Conference on Laparoscopic Liver Resection Group (2015). Systematic review of the use of pre-operative simulation and navigation for hepatectomy: current status and future perspectives. *J. Hepatob. Pancreat. Sci.* 22, 353–362. doi: 10.1002/jhbp.220

Hamano, M., Ezaki, H., Kiso, S., Furuta, K., Egawa, M., Kizu, T., et al. (2014). Lipid overloading during liver regeneration causes delayed hepatocyte DNA replication by increasing ER stress in mice with simple hepatic steatosis. *J. Gastroenterol.* 49, 305–316. doi: 10.1007/s00535-013-0780-7

Hammond, J. S., Guha, I. N., Beckingham, I. J., and Lobo, D. N. (2011). Prediction, prevention and management of postresection liver failure. *Br. J. Surg.* 98, 1188–1200. doi: 10.1002/bjs.7630

Hansen, C., Zidowitz, S., Hindennach, M., Schenk, A., Hahn, H., and Peitgen, H. O. (2009). Interactive determination of robust safety margins for oncologic liver surgery. *Int. J. Comput. Assist. Radiol. Surg.* 4, 469–474. doi: 10.1007/s11548-009-0359-1

Hansen, C., Zidowitz, S., Preim, B., Stavrou, G., Oldhafer, K. J., and Hahn, H. K. (2014). Impact of model-based risk analysis for liver surgery planning. *Int. J. Comput. Assist. Radiol. Surg.* 9, 473–480. doi: 10.1007/s11548-013-0937-0

Hedderich, D. M., Hasenberg, T., Haneder, S., Schoenberg, S. O., Kücükoglu, Ö., Canbay, A., et al. (2017). Effects of bariatric surgery on non-alcoholic fatty liver disease: magnetic resonance imaging is an effective, non-invasive method to evaluate changes in the liver fat fraction. *Obes. Surg.* 27, 1755–1762. doi: 10.1007/s11695-016-2531-3

Hetherington, J., Sumner, T., Seymour, R. M., Li, L., Rey, M. V., Yamaji, S., et al. (2012). A composite computational model of liver glucose homeostasis. I. Building the composite model. *J. R. Soc. Interface* 9, 689–700. doi: 10.1098/rsif.2011.0141

Himpel, G., Kuhl, E., Menzel, A., and Steinmann, P. (2005). Computational modelling of isotropic multiplicative growth. *Comp. Mod. Eng. Sci.* 8, 119–134. doi: 10.3970/cmes.2005.008.119

Hoehme, S., Brulport, M., Bauer, A., Bedawy, E., Schormann, W., Hermes, M., et al. (2010). Prediction and validation of cell alignment along microvessels as order principle to restore tissue architecture in liver regeneration. *Proc. Natl. Acad. Sci. U.S.A.* 107, 10371–10376. doi: 10.1073/pnas.0909374107

Hohmann, N., Weiwei, W., Dahmen, U., Dirsch, O., Deutsch, A., and Voss-Böhme, A. (2014). How does a single cell know when the liver has reached its correct size? *PLoS ONE* 9:e93207. doi: 10.1371/journal.pone.0093207

Höhme, S., Hengstler, J. G., Brulport, M., Schäfer, M., Bauer, A., Gebhardt, R., et al. (2007). Mathematical modelling of liver regeneration after intoxication with CCl4. *Chem. Biol. Interact.* 168, 74–93. doi: 10.1016/j.cbi.2007.01.010

Holzapfel, G. A., Gasser, T. C., and Ogden, R. W. (2000). A new constitutive framework for arterial wall mechanics and a comparative study of material models. *J. Elast. Phys. Sci. Solids* 61, 1–48. doi: 10.1023/A:1010835316564

Horsager, J., Bak-Fredslund, K., Larsen, L. P., Villadsen, G. E., Bogsrud, T. V., and Sørensen, M. (2016). Optimal 2-[(18)F]fluoro-2-deoxy-D-galactose PET/CT protocol for detection of hepatocellular carcinoma. *EJNMMI Res.* 6:56. doi: 10.1186/s13550-016-0206-7

Hossain, M. A., Wakabayashi, H., Izuishi, K., Okano, K., Yachida, S., Tokuda, M., et al. (2006). Improved microcirculatory effect of D-allose on hepatic ischemia reperfusion following partial hepatectomy in cirrhotic rat liver. *J. Biosci. Bioeng.* 101, 369–371. doi: 10.1263/jbb.101.369

Hrydziuszko, O., Silva, M. A., Perera, M. T., Richards, D. A., Murphy, N., Mirza, D., et al. (2010). Application of metabolomics to investigate the process of human orthotopic liver transplantation: a proof-of-principle study. *OMICS* 14, 143–150. doi: 10.1089/omi.2009.0139

Humphrey, J. D. (2003). Continuum biomechanics of soft biological tissues. *Proc. R. Soc. Lond. Ser A Math. Phys. Eng. Sci.* 459, 3–46. doi: 10.1098/rspa.2002.1060

Hyötyläinen, T., Jerby, L., Petäjä, E. M., Mattila, I., Jäntti, S., Auvinen, P., et al. (2016). Genome-scale study reveals reduced metabolic adaptability in patients with non-alcoholic fatty liver disease. *Nat. Commun.* 7:8994. doi: 10.1038/ncomms9994

Idilman, I. S., Ozdeniz, I., and Karcaaltincaba, M. (2016). Hepatic steatosis: etiology, patterns, and quantification. *Semin. Ultras. CT MR* 37, 501–510. doi: 10.1053/j.sult.2016.08.003

Imbriaco, M., De Luca, S., Coppola, M., Fusari, M., Klain, M., Puglia, M., et al. (2017). Diagnostic accuracy of Gd-EOB-DTPA for Detection Hepatocellular Carcinoma (HCC): a comparative study with dynamic contrast enhanced Magnetic Resonance Imaging (MRI) and dynamic contrast enhanced Computed Tomography (CT). *Pol. J. Radiol.* 82, 50–57. doi: 10.12659/PJR.899239

Jang, J. K., Jang, H.-J., Kim, J. S., and Kim, T. K. (2017). Focal fat deposition in the liver: diagnostic challenges on imaging. *Abdom. Radiol.* 42, 1667–1678. doi: 10.1007/s00261-017-1049-z

Jara, M., Bednarsch, J., Valle, E., Lock, J. F., Malinowski, M., Schulz, A., et al. (2015). Reliable assessment of liver function using LiMAx. *J. Surg. Res.* 193, 184–189. doi: 10.1016/j.jss.2014.07.041

Jerby, L., Shlomi, T., and Ruppin, E. (2010). Computational reconstruction of tissue-specific metabolic models: application to human liver metabolism. *Mol. Syst. Biol.* 6:401. doi: 10.1038/msb.2010.56

Jhaveri, K. S., Guo, L., and Guimarães, L. (2017). Current state-of-the-Art MRI for comprehensive evaluation of potential living liver donors. *AJR. Am. J. Roentgenol.* 209, 55–66. doi: 10.2214/AJR.16.17741

Jones, G. W., and Chapman, S. J. (2012). Modeling growth in biological materials. *SIAM Rev.* 54, 52–118. doi: 10.1137/080731785

Jones, H., and Rowland-Yeo, K. (2013). Basic concepts in physiologically based pharmacokinetic modeling in drug discovery and development. *CPT Pharmacomet. Syst. Pharmacol.* 2:e63. doi: 10.1038/psp.2013.41

Kang, K. J., and Ahn, K. S. (2017). Anatomical resection of hepatocellular carcinoma: a critical review of the procedure and its benefits on survival. *World J. Gastroenterol.* 23, 1139–1146. doi: 10.3748/wjg.v23.i7.1139

Kayvanpour, E., Mansi, T., Sedaghat-Hamedani, F., Amr, A., Neumann, D., Georgescu, B., et al. (2015). Towards personalized cardiology: multi-scale modeling of the failing heart. *PLoS ONE* 10:e0134869. doi: 10.1371/journal.pone.0134869

Kele, P. G., de Boer, M., van der Jagt, E. J., Lisman, T., and Porte, R. J. (2012). Early hepatic regeneration index and completeness of regeneration at 6 months after partial hepatectomy. *Br. J. Surg.* 99, 1113–1119. doi: 10.1002/bjs.8807

Kietzmann, T. (2017). Metabolic zonation of the liver: the oxygen gradient revisited. *Redox Biol.* 11, 622–630. doi: 10.1016/j.redox.2017.01.012

Kimura, K., Shirabe, K., Yoshizumi, T., Takeishi, K., Itoh, S., Harimoto, N., et al. (2016). Ischemia-reperfusion injury in fatty liver is mediated by activated NADPH Oxidase 2 in rats. *Transplantation* 100, 791–800. doi: 10.1097/TP.0000000000001130

Kirschner, D. E., Hunt, C. A., Marino, S., Fallahi-Sichani, M., and Linderman, J. J. (2014). Tuneable resolution as a systems biology approach for multi-scale, multi-compartment computational models. *Wiley Interdiscip. Rev. Syst. Biol. Med.* 6, 225–245. doi: 10.1002/wsbm.1270

Kobayashi, T., Aikata, H., Honda, F., Nakano, N., Nakamura, Y., Hatooka, M., et al. (2016). Preoperative fluorine 18 fluorodeoxyglucose positron emission tomography/computed tomography for prediction of microvascular invasion in small hepatocellular carcinoma. *J. Comput. Assis. Tomogr.* 40, 524–530. doi: 10.1097/RCT.0000000000000405

Kogan, Y., Halevi-Tobias, K. E., Hochman, G., Baczmanska, A. K., Leyns, L., and Agur, Z. (2012). A new validated mathematical model of the Wnt signalling pathway predicts effective combinational therapy by sFRP and Dkk. *Biochem. J.* 444, 115–125. doi: 10.1042/BJ20111887

König, M., and Holzhütter, H.-G. (2012). Kinetic modeling of human hepatic glucose metabolism in type 2 diabetes mellitus predicts higher risk of hypoglycemic events in rigorous insulin therapy. *J. Biol. Chem.* 287, 36978–36989. doi: 10.1074/jbc.M112.382069

König, M., Bulik, S., and Holzhütter, H.-G. (2012). Quantifying the contribution of the liver to glucose homeostasis: a detailed kinetic model of human hepatic glucose metabolism. *PLoS Comput. Biol.* 8:e1002577. doi: 10.1371/journal.pcbi.1002577

König, M., Oellrich, A., Waltemath, D., Dobson, R. J., Hubbard, T. J., and Wolkenhauer, O. (2016). "Challenges and opportunities for system biology standards and tools in medical research," in *ODLS* (London), 1–6.

Kooby, D. A., Fong, Y., Suriawinata, A., Gonen, M., Allen, P. J., Klimstra, D. S., et al. (2003). Impact of steatosis on perioperative outcome following hepatic resection. *J. Gastrointest. Surg.* 7, 1034–1044. doi: 10.1016/j.gassur.2003.09.012

Kramer, H., Pickhardt, P. J., Kliewer, M. A., Hernando, D., Chen, G.-H., Zagzebski, J. A., et al. (2017). Accuracy of Liver fat quantification with advanced CT, MRI, and Ultrasound Techniques: prospective comparison with MR spectroscopy. *AJR. Am. J. Roentgenol.* 208, 92–100. doi: 10.2214/AJR.16.16565

Krauss, M., Burghaus, R., Lippert, J., Niemi, M., Neuvonen, P., Schuppert, A., et al. (2013). Using Bayesian-PBPK modeling for assessment of inter-individual variability and subgroup stratification. *In Silico Pharmacol.* 1, 1–11. doi: 10.1186/2193-9616-1-6

Krauss, M., Schaller, S., Borchers, S., Findeisen, R., Lippert, J., and Kuepfer, L. (2012). Integrating cellular metabolism into a multiscale whole-body model. *PLoS Comput. Biol.* 8:e1002750. doi: 10.1371/journal.pcbi.1002750

Kriete, A., Noguchi, E., and Sell, C. (2014). Introductory review of computational cell cycle modeling. *Methods Mol. Biol.* 1170, 267–275. doi: 10.1007/978-1-4939-0888-2_12

Krishan, S., Jain, D., Bathina, Y., Kale, A., Saraf, N., Saigal, S., et al. (2016). Non-invasive quantification of hepatic steatosis in living, related liver donors using dual-echo Dixon imaging and single-voxel proton spectroscopy. *Clin. Radiol.* 71, 58–63. doi: 10.1016/j.crad.2015.10.002

Kuepfer, L., Lippert, J., and Eissing, T. (2012). Multiscale mechanistic modeling in pharmaceutical research and development. *Adv. Exp. Med. Biol.* 736, 543–561. doi: 10.1007/978-1-4419-7210-1_32

Kuttippurathu, L., Parrish, A., and Vadigepalli, R. (2014). Integrated computational model of intracellular signaling and microRNA regulation predicts the network balances and timing constraints critical to the hepatic stellate cell activation process. *Processes* 2, 773–794. doi: 10.3390/pr2040773

Lagoa, C. E., Bartels, J., Baratt, A., Tseng, G., Clermont, G., Fink, M. P., et al. (2006). The role of initial trauma in the host's response to injury and hemorrhage: insights from a correlation of mathematical simulations and hepatic transcriptomic analysis. *Shock* 26, 592–600. doi: 10.1097/01.shk.0000232272.03602.0a

Lang, H., Radtke, A., Hindennach, M., Schroeder, T., Frühauf, N. R., Malagó, M., et al. (2005). Impact of virtual tumor resection and computer-assisted risk analysis on operation planning and intraoperative strategy in major hepatic resection. *Arch. Surg.* 140, 629–638. doi: 10.1001/archsurg.140.7.629

Lautt, W. W., Legare, D. J., and Daniels, T. R. (1984). The comparative effect of administration of substances via the hepatic artery or portal vein on hepatic arterial resistance, liver blood volume and hepatic extraction in cats. *Hepatology* 4, 927–932. doi: 10.1002/hep.1840040524

Lee, F. Y., Li, Y., Zhu, H., Yang, S., Lin, H. Z., Trush, M., et al. (1999). Tumor necrosis factor increases mitochondrial oxidant production and induces expression of uncoupling protein-2 in the regenerating mice [correction of rat] liver. *Hepatology* 29, 677–687. doi: 10.1002/hep.510290320

Lee, S., Park, K., Hwang, S., Lee, Y., Choi, D., Kim, K., et al. (2001). Congestion of right liver graft in living donor liver transplantation. *Transplantation* 71, 812–814. doi: 10.1097/00007890-200103270-00021

Lehmann, K. S., Ritz, J.-P., Valdeig, S., Schenk, A., Holmer, C., Peitgen, H.-O., et al. (2008). Portal vein segmentation of a 3D-planning system for liver surgery–*in vivo* evaluation in a porcine model. *Ann. Surg. Oncol.* 15, 1899–1907. doi: 10.1245/s10434-008-9934-x

Lencioni, R., Della Pina, C., Crocetti, L., Bozzi, E., and Cioni, D. (2007). Clinical management of focal liver lesions: the key role of real-time contrast-enhanced US. *Eur. Radiol.* 17(Suppl. 6), F73–F79. doi: 10.1007/s10406-007-0231-8

Linecker, M., Limani, P., Kambakamba, P., Kron, P., Tschuor, C., Calo, N., et al. (2017). Omega-3 fatty acids protect fatty and lean mouse livers after major hepatectomy. *Ann. Surg.* 266, 324–332. doi: 10.1097/SLA.0000000000001968

Liu, P., Xie, S.-H., Hu, S., Cheng, X., Gao, T., Zhang, C., et al. (2017). Age-specific sex difference in the incidence of hepatocellular carcinoma in the United States. *Oncotarget* 8, 68131–68137. doi: 10.18632/oncotarget.19245

Liu, Q., Izamis, M. L., Xu, H., Berendsen, T., Yarmush, M., and Uygun, K. (2013). Strategies to rescue steatotic livers before transplantation in clinical and experimental studies. *World J. Gastroenterol.* 19, 4638–4650. doi: 10.3748/wjg.v19.i29.4638

Lubarda, V. A., and Hoger, A. (2002). On the mechanics of solids with a growing mass. *Int. J. Solids Struct.* 39, 4627–4664. doi: 10.1016/S0020-7683(02)00352-9

Marchesseau, S., Heimann, T., Chatelin, S., Willinger, R., and Delingette, H. (2010). Fast porous visco-hyperelastic soft tissue model for surgery simulation: application to liver surgery. *Prog. Biophys. Mol. Biol.* 103, 185–196. doi: 10.1016/j.pbiomolbio.2010.09.005

Mardinoglu, A., Agren, R., Kampf, C., Asplund, A., Uhlen, M., and Nielsen, J. (2014). Genome-scale metabolic modelling of hepatocytes reveals serine deficiency in patients with non-alcoholic fatty liver disease. *Nat. Commun.* 5:3083. doi: 10.1038/ncomms4083

Marescaux, J., Clément, J. M., Tassetti, V., Koehl, C., Cotin, S., Russier, Y., et al. (1998). Virtual reality applied to hepatic surgery simulation: the next revolution. *Ann. Surg.* 228, 627–634. doi: 10.1097/00000658-199811000-00001

Marino, M., Mangiantini, M. T., Spagnuolo, S., Luly, P., and Leoni, S. (1992). Signal transduction during liver regeneration: role of insulin and vasopressin. *J. Cell. Physiol.* 152, 403–409. doi: 10.1002/jcp.1041520223

Markevich, N. I., and Hoek, J. B. (2015). Computational modeling analysis of mitochondrial superoxide production under varying substrate conditions and upon inhibition of different segments of the electron transport chain. *Biochim. Biophys. Acta* 1847, 656–679. doi: 10.1016/j.bbabio.2015.04.005

Matos, A. P., Altun, E., Ramalho, M., Velloni, F., AlObaidy, M., and Semelka, R. C. (2015). An overview of imaging techniques for liver metastases management. *Expert Rev. Gastroenterol. Hepatol.* 9, 1561–1576. doi: 10.1586/17474124.2015.1092873

Matz-Soja, M. (2017). Computational modelling of hedgehog signalling in liver regeneration. *Drug Discov. Today Dis. Models.* doi: 10.1016/j.ddmod.2017.06.001

Matz-Soja, M., Rennert, C., Schönefeld, K., Aleithe, S., Boettger, J., Schmidt-Heck, W., et al. (2016). Hedgehog signaling is a potent regulator of liver lipid metabolism and reveals a GLI-code associated with steatosis. *Elife* 5:e13308. doi: 10.7554/eLife.13308

McCormack, L., Petrowsky, H., Jochum, W., Furrer, K., and Clavien, P. A. (2007). Hepatic steatosis is a risk factor for postoperative complications after major hepatectomy: a matched case-control study. *Ann. Surg.* 245, 923–930. doi: 10.1097/01.sla.0000251747.80025.b7

Menzel, A., and Kuhl, E. (2012). Frontiers in growth and remodeling. *Mech. Res. Commun.* 42, 1–14 doi: 10.1016/j.mechrescom.2012.02.007

Meoli, A., Cutrì, E., Krishnamurthy, A., Dubini, G., Migliavacca, F., Hsia, T. Y., et al. (2015). A multiscale model for the study of cardiac biomechanics in single-ventricle surgeries: a clinical case. *Interface Focus* 5:20140079. doi: 10.1098/rsfs.2014.0079

Meyer, K., Ostrenko, O., Bourantas, G., Morales-Navarrete, H., Porat-Shliom, N., Segovia-Miranda, F., et al. (2017). A predictive 3D multi-scale model of biliary fluid dynamics in the liver lobule. *Cell Syst.* 4, 277–290.e9. doi: 10.1016/j.cels.2017.02.008

Michalopoulos, G. K. (2007). Liver regeneration. *J. Cell. Physiol.* 213, 286–300. doi: 10.1002/jcp.21172

Michalopoulos, G. K. (2010). Liver regeneration after partial hepatectomy: critical analysis of mechanistic dilemmas. *Am. J. Pathol.* 176, 2–13 doi: 10.2353/ajpath.2010.090675

Michalopoulos, G. K. (2017). Hepatostat: liver regeneration and normal liver tissue maintenance. *Hepatology* 65, 1384–1392. doi: 10.1002/hep.28988

Miyaoka, Y., and Miyajima, A. (2013). To divide or not to divide: revisiting liver regeneration. *Cell Div.* 8:8. doi: 10.1186/1747-1028-8-8

Mun, J. (2013). Radiofluorinated carbohydrates for positron emission tomography. *Curr. Top. Med. Chem.* 13, 944–950. doi: 10.2174/1568026611313080007

Nadalin, S., Testa, G., Malagó, M., Beste, M., Frilling, A., Schroeder, T., et al. (2004). Volumetric and functional recovery of the liver after right hepatectomy for living donation. *Liver Transpl.* 10, 1024–1029. doi: 10.1002/lt.20182

Naik, A., Rozman, D., and Belič, A. (2014). SteatoNet: the first integrated human metabolic model with multi-layered regulation to investigate liver-associated pathologies. *PLoS Comput. Biol.* 10:e1003993. doi: 10.1371/journal.pcbi.1003993

Nilsson, J., Eriksson, S., Blind, P.-J., Rissler, P., and Sturesson, C. (2014). Microcirculation changes during liver resection–a clinical study. *Microvasc. Res.* 94, 47–51. doi: 10.1016/j.mvr.2014.05.002

Nyman, E., Brännmark, C., Palmér, R., Brugård, J., Nyström, F. H., Strålfors, P., et al. (2011). A hierarchical whole-body modeling approach elucidates the link between *in vitro* insulin signaling and *in vivo* glucose homeostasis. *J. Biol. Chem.* 286, 26028–26041. doi: 10.1074/jbc.M110.188987

Orth, J. D., Thiele, I., and Palsson, B. Ø. (2010). What is flux balance analysis? *Nat. Biotechnol.* 28, 245–248. doi: 10.1038/nbt.1614

Oshiro, Y., and Ohkohchi, N. (2017). Three-dimensional liver surgery simulation: computer-assisted surgical planning with three-dimensional simulation software and three-dimensional printing. *Tissue Eng. Part A* 23, 474–480. doi: 10.1089/ten.tea.2016.0528

Oshiro, Y., Yano, H., Mitani, J., Kim, S., Kim, J., Fukunaga, K., et al. (2015). Novel 3-dimensional virtual hepatectomy simulation combined with real-time deformation. *World J. Gastroenterol.* 21, 9982–9992. doi: 10.3748/wjg.v21.i34.9982

Pagliarini, R., Castello, R., Napolitano, F., Borzone, R., Annunziata, P., Mandrile, G., et al. (2016). *In silico* modeling of liver metabolism in a human disease reveals a key enzyme for histidine and histamine homeostasis. *Cell Rep.* 15, 2292–2300. doi: 10.1016/j.celrep.2016.05.014

Pedone, E., Olteanu, V.-A., Marucci, L., Muñoz-Martin, M. I., Youssef, S. A., de Bruin, A., et al. (2017). Modeling dynamics and function of bone marrow cells in mouse liver regeneration. *Cell Rep.* 18, 107–121. doi: 10.1016/j.celrep.2016.12.008

Peeters, G., Debbaut, C., Cornillie, P., De Schryver, T., Monbaliu, D., Laleman, W., et al. (2015). A multilevel modeling framework to study hepatic perfusion characteristics in case of liver cirrhosis. *J. Biomech. Eng.* 137:051007. doi: 10.1115/1.4029280

Pereira, E. J., Smolko, C. M., and Janes, K. A. (2016). Computational Models of reactive oxygen species as metabolic byproducts and signal-transduction modulators. *Front. Pharmacol.* 7:457. doi: 10.3389/fphar.2016.00457

Periwal, V., Gaillard, J., Needleman, L., and Doria, C. (2014). Mathematical model of liver regeneration in human live donors. *J. Cell. Physiol.* 229, 599–606 doi: 10.1002/jcp.24482

Petta, S., Valenti, L., Bugianesi, E., Targher, G., Bellentani, S., Bonino, F., et al. (2016). A "systems medicine" approach to the study of non-alcoholic fatty liver disease. *Dig. Liver Dis.* 48, 333–342. doi: 10.1016/j.dld.2015.10.027

Pilari, S., and Huisinga, W. (2010). Lumping of physiologically-based pharmacokinetic models and a mechanistic derivation of classical compartmental models. *J. Pharmacokinet. Pharmacodyn.* 37, 365–405. doi: 10.1007/s10928-010-9165-1

Pinato, D. J., Howell, J., Ramaswami, R., and Sharma, R. (2017). Review article: delivering precision oncology in intermediate-stage liver cancer. *Aliment. Pharmacol. Ther.* 45, 1514–1523. doi: 10.1111/apt.14066

Preim, B., Bourquain, H., Selle, D., and Oldhafer, K. J. (2002). *Resection Proposals for Oncologic Liver Surgery Based On Vascular Territories.* Berlin; Heidelberg: Springer, 353–358.

Radtke, A., Nadalin, S., Sotiropoulos, G. C., Molmenti, E. P., Schroeder, T., Valentin-Gamazo, C., et al. (2007). Computer-assisted operative planning in adult living donor liver transplantation: a new way to resolve the dilemma of the middle hepatic vein. *World J. Surg.* 31, 175–185. doi: 10.1007/s00268-005-0718-1

Rani, H. P., Sheu, T. W. H., Chang, T. M., and Liang, P. C. (2006). Numerical investigation of non-Newtonian microcirculatory blood flow in hepatic lobule. *J. Biomech.* 39, 551–563. doi: 10.1016/j.jbiomech.2004.11.029

Ray, P. D., Huang, B. W., and Tsuji, Y. (2012). Reactive oxygen species (ROS) homeostasis and redox regulation in cellular signaling. *Cell. Signal.* 24, 981–990. doi: 10.1016/j.cellsig.2012.01.008

Reddyhoff, D., Ward, J., Williams, D., Regan, S., and Webb, S. (2015). Timescale analysis of a mathematical model of acetaminophen metabolism and toxicity. *J. Theor. Biol.* 386, 132–146. doi: 10.1016/j.jtbi.2015.08.021

Reitinger, B., Bornik, A., Beichel, R., and Schmalstieg, D. (2006). Liver surgery planning using virtual reality. *IEEE Comput. Graph. Appl.* 26, 36–47. doi: 10.1109/MCG.2006.131

Ricken, T., and Bluhm, J. (2009). Evolutional growth and remodeling in multiphase living tissue. *Comput. Mater. Sci.* 45, 806–811. doi: 10.1016/j.commatsci.2008.10.016

Ricken, T., and Bluhm, J. (2010). Remodeling and growth of living tissue: a multiphase theory. *Arch. Appl. Mech.* 80, 453–465. doi: 10.1007/s00419-009-0383-1

Ricken, T., Dahmen, U., and Dirsch, O. (2010). A biphasic model for sinusoidal liver perfusion remodeling after outflow obstruction. *Biomech. Model. Mechanobiol.* 9, 435–450. doi: 10.1007/s10237-009-0186-x

Ricken, T., Dahmen, U., Dirsch, O., and Werner, D. Q. (2013). "A Biphasic 3D-FEM model for the remodeling of microcirculation in liver lobes," in *Computer Models in Biomechanics*, eds G. A. Holzapfel and E. Kuhl (Dordrecht: Springer), 277–292.

Ricken, T., Schwarz, A., and Bluhm, J. (2007). A triphasic model of transversely isotropic biological tissue with applications to stress and biologically induced growth. *Comput. Mater. Sci.* 39, 124–136. doi: 10.1016/j.commatsci.2006.03.025

Ricken, T., Sindern, A., Bluhm, J., Widmann, R., Denecke, M., Gehrke, T., et al. (2014). Concentration driven phase transitions in multiphase porous media with application to methane oxidation in landfill cover layers. *ZAMM* 94, 609–622. doi: 10.1002/zamm.201200198

Ricken, T., Werner, D., Holzhütter, H.-G., König, M., Dahmen, U., and Dirsch, O. (2015). Modeling function–perfusion behavior in liver lobules including tissue, blood, glucose, lactate and glycogen by use of a coupled two-scale PDE–ODE approach. *Biomech. Model. Mechanobiol.* 14, 515–536. doi: 10.1007/s10237-014-0619-z

Riehle, K. J., Dan, Y. Y., Campbell, J. S., and Fausto, N. (2011). New concepts in liver regeneration. *J. Gastroenterol. Hepatol.* 26(Suppl. 1), 203–212. doi: 10.1111/j.1440-1746.2010.06539.x

Rockne, R., Rockhill, J. K., Mrugala, M., Spence, A. M., Kalet, I., Hendrickson, K., et al. (2010). Predicting the efficacy of radiotherapy in individual glioblastoma patients *in vivo*: a mathematical modeling approach. *Phys. Med. Biol.* 55, 3271–3285. doi: 10.1088/0031-9155/55/12/001

Rodriguez, E. K., Hoger, A., and McCulloch, A. D. (1994). Stress-dependent finite growth in soft elastic tissues. *J. Biomech.* 27, 455–467. doi: 10.1016/0021-9290(94)90021-3

Rübenthaler, J., Paprottka, K. J., Hameister, E., Hoffmann, K., Joiko, N., Reiser, M., et al. (2017a). Contrast-enhanced ultrasound (CEUS) prediction of focal liver lesions in patients after liver transplantation in comparison to histopathology results. *Clin. Hemorheol. Microcirc.* 66, 303–310. doi: 10.3233/CH-179104

Rübenthaler, J., Paprottka, K. J., Hameister, E., Hoffmann, K., Joiko, N., Reiser, M., et al. (2017b). Diagnostic accuracy of contrast-enhanced ultrasound (CEUS) in monitoring vascular complications in patients after liver transplantation - diagnostic performance compared with histopathological results. *Clin. Hemorheol. Microcirc.* 66, 311–316. doi: 10.3233/CH-179105

Rutkowski, D. R., Reeder, S. B., Fernandez, L. A., and Roldán-Alzate, A. (2017). Surgical planning for living donor liver transplant using 4D flow MRI, computational fluid dynamics and *in vitro* experiments. *Comput. Methods Biomech. Biomed. Eng.* 1–11. doi: 10.1080/21681163.2017.1278619

Ryll, A., Samaga, R., Schaper, F., Alexopoulos, L. G., and Klamt, S. (2011). Large-scale network models of IL-1 and IL-6 signalling and their hepatocellular specification. *Mol. Biosyst.* 7, 3253–3270. doi: 10.1039/c1mb05261f

Saito, S., Yamanaka, J., Miura, K., Nakao, N., Nagao, T., Sugimoto, T., et al. (2005). A novel 3D hepatectomy simulation based on liver circulation: application to liver resection and transplantation. *Hepatology* 41, 1297–1304. doi: 10.1002/hep.20684

Schenk, A., Breitenborn, J., Selle, D., Schindewolf, T., Böhm, D., Spindler, W., et al. (1999). *ILabMed-Workstation: Eine Entwicklungsumgebung für radiologische Anwendungen.* Heidelberg: Springer, 238–242.

Schindl, M. J., Redhead, D. N., Fearon, K. C., Garden, O. J., Wigmore, S. J., Edinburgh Liver, S., et al. (2005). The value of residual liver volume as a predictor of hepatic dysfunction and infection after major liver resection. *Gut* 54, 289–296. doi: 10.1136/gut.2004.046524

Schleicher, J., Dahmen, U., Guthke, R., and Schuster, S. (2017). Zonation of hepatic fat accumulation: insights from mathematical modelling of nutrient gradients and fatty acid uptake. *J. R. Soc. Interface* 14:20170443. doi: 10.1098/rsif.2017.0443

Schleicher, J., Guthke, R., Dahmen, U., Dirsch, O., Holzhuetter, H. G., and Schuster, S. (2014). A theoretical study of lipid accumulation in the liver-implications for nonalcoholic fatty liver disease. *Biochim. Biophys. Acta* 1841, 62–69. doi: 10.1016/j.bbalip.2013.08.016

Schliess, F., Hoehme, S., Henkel, S. G., Ghallab, A., Driesch, D., Böttger, J., et al. (2014). Integrated metabolic spatial-temporal model for the prediction of ammonia detoxification during liver damage and regeneration. *Hepatology* 60, 2040–2051. doi: 10.1002/hep.27136

Schmidt-Heck, W., Matz-Soja, M., Aleithe, S., Marbach, E., Guthke, R., and Gebhardt, R. (2015). Fuzzy modeling reveals a dynamic self-sustaining network of the GLI transcription factors controlling important metabolic regulators in adult mouse hepatocytes. *Mol. Biosyst.* 11, 2190–2197. doi: 10.1039/C5MB00129C

Schwen, L. O., Homeyer, A., Schwier, M., Dahmen, U., Dirsch, O., Schenk, A., et al. (2016). Zonated quantification of steatosis in an entire mouse liver. *Comput. Biol. Med.* 73, 108–118. doi: 10.1016/j.compbiomed.2016.04.004

Schwen, L. O., Krauss, M., Niederalt, C., Gremse, F., Kiessling, F., Schenk, A., et al. (2014). Spatio-temporal simulation of first pass drug perfusion in the liver. *PLoS Comput. Biol.* 10, 1–18. doi: 10.1371/journal.pcbi.1003499

Schwen, L. O., Schenk, A., Kreutz, C., Timmer, J., Bartolomé Rodríguez, M. M., Kuepfer, L., et al. (2015). Representative sinusoids for hepatic four-scale pharmacokinetics simulations. *PLoS ONE* 10:e0133653. doi: 10.1371/journal.pone.0133653

Seifalian, A. M., Chidambaram, V., Rolles, K., and Davidson, B. R. (1998). *In vivo* demonstration of impaired microcirculation in steatotic human liver grafts. *Liver Transpl. Surg.* 4, 71–77. doi: 10.1002/lt.500040110

Seki, E., Brenner, D. A., and Karin, M. (2012). A liver full of JNK: signaling in regulation of cell function and disease pathogenesis, and clinical approaches. *Gastroenterology* 143, 307–320. doi: 10.1053/j.gastro.2012.06.004

Selivanov, V. A., Cascante, M., Friedman, M., Schumaker, M. F., Trucco, M., Votyakova, T. V., et al. (2012). Multistationary and oscillatory modes of free radicals generation by the mitochondrial respiratory chain revealed by a bifurcation analysis. *PLoS Comput. Biol.* 8:e1002700. doi: 10.1371/journal.pcbi.1002700

Selivanov, V. A., Votyakova, T. V., Zeak, J. A., Trucco, M., Roca, J., and Cascante, M. (2009). Bistability of mitochondrial respiration underlies paradoxical reactive oxygen species generation induced by anoxia. *PLoS Comput. Biol.* 5:e1000619. doi: 10.1371/journal.pcbi.1000619

Sendov, B., and Tsanev, R. (1968). Computer simulation of the regenerative processes in the liver. *J. Theor. Biol.* 18, 90–104. doi: 10.1016/0022-5193(68)90172-0

Serai, S. D., Obuchowski, N. A., Venkatesh, S. K., Sirlin, C. B., Miller, F. H., Ashton, E., et al. (2017). Repeatability of MR elastography of liver: a meta-analysis. *Radiology* 285, 92–100. doi: 10.1148/radiol. 2017161398

Serkova, N. J., Zhang, Y., Coatney, J. L., Hunter, L., Wachs, M. E., Niemann, C. U., et al. (2007). Early detection of graft failure using the blood metabolic profile of a liver recipient. *Transplantation* 83, 517–521. doi: 10.1097/01.tp.0000251649.01148.f8

Shen, Y., Zhou, C., Zhu, G., Shi, G., Zhu, X., Huang, C., et al. (2017). Liver stiffness assessed by shear wave elastography predicts postoperative liver failure in patients with hepatocellular carcinoma. *J. Gastro.Surg.* 21, 1471–1479. doi: 10.1007/s11605-017-3443-9

Shestopaloff, Y. K., and Sbalzarini, I. F. (2014). A method for modeling growth of organs and transplants based on the general growth law: application to the liver in dogs and humans. *PLoS ONE* 9:e99275. doi: 10.1371/journal.pone.0099275

Shteyer, E., Liao, Y., Muglia, L. J., Hruz, P. W., and Rudnick, D. A. (2004). Disruption of hepatic adipogenesis is associated with impaired liver regeneration in mice. *Hepatology* 40, 1322–1332. doi: 10.1002/hep.20462

Simpson, A. L., Geller, D. A., Hemming, A. W., Jarnagin, W. R., Clements, L. W., D'Angelica, M. I., et al. (2014). Liver planning software accurately predicts postoperative liver volume and measures early regeneration. *J. Am. Coll. Surg.* 219, 199–207. doi: 10.1016/j.jamcollsurg.2014.02.027

Siu, J., McCall, J., and Connor, S. (2014). Systematic review of pathophysiological changes following hepatic resection. *HPB* 16, 407–421. doi: 10.1111/hpb.12164

Skalak, R., Dasgupta, G., Moss, M., Otten, E., Dullemeijer, P., and Vilmann, H. (1982). Analytical description of growth. *J. Theor. Biol.* 94, 555–577. doi: 10.1016/0022-5193(82)90301-0

Sluka, J. P., Fu, X., Swat, M., Belmonte, J. M., Cosmanescu, A., Clendenon, S. G., et al. (2016). A liver-centric multiscale modeling framework for xenobiotics. *PLoS ONE* 11:e0162428. doi: 10.1371/journal.pone.0162428

Smith, G. R., and Shanley, D. P. (2013). Computational modelling of the regulation of Insulin signalling by oxidative stress. *BMC Syst. Biol.* 7:41. doi: 10.1186/1752-0509-7-41

Soler, L., Nicolau, S., Pessaux, P., Mutter, D., and Marescaux, J. (2014). Real-time 3D image reconstruction guidance in liver resection surgery. *Hepatobiliary Surg. Nutr.* 3, 73–81. doi: 10.3978/j.issn.2304-3881.2014.02.03

Strey, C. W., Marquez-Pinilla, R. M., Markiewski, M. M., Siegmund, B., Oppermann, E., Lambris, J. D., et al. (2011). Early post-operative measurement of cytokine plasma levels combined with pre-operative bilirubin levels identify high-risk patients after liver resection. *Int. J. Mol. Med.* 27, 447–454. doi: 10.3892/ijmm.2010.592

Sumner, T., Hetherington, J., Seymour, R. M., Li, L., Varela Rey, M., Yamaji, S., et al. (2012). A composite computational model of liver glucose homeostasis. II. Exploring system behaviour. *J. R. Soc. Interface* 9, 701–706. doi: 10.1098/rsif.2011.0783

Suzuki, T., Shinjo, S., Arai, T., Kanai, M., and Goda, N. (2014). Hypoxia and fatty liver. *World J. Gastroenterol.* 20, 15087–15097. doi: 10.3748/wjg.v20.i41.15087

Szklaruk, J., Luersen, G., Ma, J., Wei, W., and Underwood, M. (2017). Gd-EOB-DTPA based magnetic resonance imaging for predicting liver response to portal vein embolization. *World J. Radiol.* 9, 199–205. doi: 10.4329/wjr.v9.i4.199

Taki-Eldin, A., Zhou, L., Xie, H.-Y., and Zheng, S.-S. (2012). Liver regeneration after liver transplantation. *Eur. Surg. Res.* 48, 139–153. doi: 10.1159/000337865

Tautenhahn, H. M., Brückner, S., Baumann, S., Winkler, S., Otto, W., von Bergen, M., et al. (2016). Attenuation of postoperative acute liver failure by mesenchymal stem cell treatment due to metabolic implications. *Ann. Surg.* 263, 546–556. doi: 10.1097/SLA.0000000000001155

Toepfer, S., Zellmer, S., Driesch, D., Woetzel, D., Guthke, R., Gebhardt, R., et al. (2007). "Compartment model of glutamine and ammonia metabolism in liver tissue, "in *Proceedings of the 52nd International Scientific Colloquium, Vol. 2,* (Ilmenau), 107–112.

Tormos, A. M., Taléns-Visconti, R., Nebreda, A. R., and Sastre, J. (2013). p38 MAPK: a dual role in hepatocyte proliferation through reactive oxygen species. *Free Radic. Res.* 47, 905–916. doi: 10.3109/10715762.2013.821200

Truant, S., Oberlin, O., Sergent, G., Lebuffe, G., Gambiez, L., Ernst, O., et al. (2007). Remnant liver volume to body weight ratio $\geq$ 0.5%: a new cut-off to estimate postoperative risks after extended resection in noncirrhotic liver. *J. Am. Coll. Surg.* 204, 22–33. doi: 10.1016/j.jamcollsurg.2006.09.007

van Beers, B. E., Daire, J.-L., and Garteiser, P. (2015). New imaging techniques for liver diseases. *J. Hepatol.* 62, 690–700. doi: 10.1016/j.jhep.2014.10.014

van Dam, R. M., Lodewick, T. M., van den Broek, M. A. J., de Jong, M. C., Greve, J. W., Jansen, R. L. H., et al. (2014). Outcomes of extended versus limited indications for patients undergoing a liver resection for colorectal cancer liver metastases. *HPB* 16, 550–559. doi: 10.1111/hpb.12181

van Eunen, K., Simons, S. M. J., Gerding, A., Bleeker, A., den Besten, G., Touw, C. M. L., et al. (2013). Biochemical competition makes fatty-acid-oxidation vulnerable to substrate overload. *PLoS Comput. Biol.* 9:e1003186. doi: 10.1371/journal.pcbi.1003186

van Golen, R. F., van Gulik, T. M., and Heger, M. (2012). The sterile immune response during hepatic ischemia/reperfusion. *Cytokine Growth Factor Rev.* 23, 69–84. doi: 10.1016/j.cytogfr.2012.04.006

van Mierlo, K. M., Schaap, F. G., Dejong, C. H., and Olde Damink, S. W. (2016). Liver resection for cancer: new developments in prediction, prevention and management of postresectional liver failure. *J. Hepatol.* 65, 1217–1231. doi: 10.1016/j.jhep.2016.06.006

van Riel, W. G., van Golen, R. F., Reiniers, M. J., Heger, M., and van Gulik, T. M. (2016). How much ischemia can the liver tolerate during resection? *Hepatobiliary Surg. Nutr.* 5, 58–71. doi: 10.3978/j.issn.2304-3881.2015.07.05

Vandeweyer, D., Neo, E. L., Chen, J. W., Maddern, G. J., Wilson, T. G., and Padbury, R. T. (2009). Influence of resection margin on survival in hepatic resections for colorectal liver metastases. *HPB* 11, 499–504. doi: 10.1111/j.1477-2574.2009.00092.x

Vauthey, J.-N., Abdalla, E. K., Doherty, D. A., Gertsch, P., Fenstermacher, M. J., Loyer, E. M., et al. (2002). Body surface area and body weight predict total liver volume in Western adults. *Liver Transpl.* 8, 233–240. doi: 10.1053/jlts.2002.31654

Verma, A., Makadia, H., Hoek, J. B., Ogunnaike, B. A., and Vadigepalli, R. (2016). Computational modeling of spatiotemporal Ca(2+) signal propagation along hepatocyte cords. *IEEE Trans. Biomed. Eng.* 63, 2047–2055. doi: 10.1109/TBME.2016.2550045

Walldorf, J., Hillebrand, C., Aurich, H., Stock, P., Hempel, M., Ebensing, S., et al. (2010). Propranolol impairs liver regeneration after partial hepatectomy in C57Bl/6-mice by transient attenuation of hepatic lipid accumulation and increased apoptosis. *Scand. J. Gastroenterol.* 45, 468–476. doi: 10.3109/00365520903583848

Wang, T., Shao, C., Zhang, G., and Xu, Y. (2017). Real-time elastography (RTE): a valuable sonography-based non-invasive method for the assessment of liver fibrosis in chronic hepatitis B. *Abdom. Radiol.* 42, 2632–2638. doi: 10.1007/s00261-017-1186-4.

Wang, X., Xue, H.-D., Jin, Z.-Y., Su, B.-,y., Li, Z., Sun, H., et al. (2013). Quantitative hepatic CT perfusion measurement: comparison of Couinaud's hepatic segments with dual-source 128-slice CT. *Eur. J. Radiol.* 82, 220–226. doi: 10.1016/j.ejrad.2012.09.015

Waschinsky, N., Werner, D., Ricken, T., Dahmen, U., and Dirsch, O. (2016). On a bi-scale and tri-phasic model for the description of growth in biological tissue using the example of the human liver. *PAMM* 16, 109–110. doi: 10.1002/pamm.201610043

Weber, L. W. D., Boll, M., and Stampfl, A. (2003). Hepatotoxicity and mechanism of action of haloalkanes: carbon tetrachloride as a toxicological model. *Crit. Rev. Toxicol.* 33, 105–136. doi: 10.1080/713611034

Willmann, S., Thelen, K., and Lippert, J. (2012). Integration of dissolution into physiologically-based pharmacokinetic models III: PK-Sim®;. *J. Pharm. Pharmacol.* 64, 997–1007. doi: 10.1111/j.2042-7158.2012.01534.x

Wolkenhauer, O., Auffray, C., Jaster, R., Steinhoff, G., and Dammann, O. (2013). The road from systems biology to systems medicine. *Pediatr. Res.* 73, 502–507. doi: 10.1038/pr.2013.4

Woller, A., Duez, H., Staels, B., and Lefranc, M. (2016). A mathematical model of the liver circadian clock linking feeding and fasting cycles to clock function. *Cell Rep.* 17, 1087–1097. doi: 10.1016/j.celrep.2016.09.060

Woolbright, B. L., and Jaeschke, H. (2017). Role of the inflammasome in acetaminophen-induced liver injury and acute liver failure. *J. Hepatol.* 66, 836–848. doi: 10.1016/j.jhep.2016.11.017

Yamamoto, K. N., Ishii, M., Inoue, Y., Hirokawa, F., MacArthur, B. D., Nakamura, A., et al. (2016). Prediction of postoperative liver regeneration from clinical information using a data-led mathematical model. *Sci. Rep.* 6:34214. doi: 10.1038/srep34214

Yamanaka, N., Okamoto, E., Kawamura, E., Kato, T., Oriyama, T., Fujimoto, J., et al. (1993). Dynamics of normal and injured human liver regeneration after hepatectomy as assessed on the basis of computed tomography and liver function. *Hepatology* 18, 79–85. doi: 10.1002/hep.1840180114

Yamanaka, N., Okamoto, E., Kuwata, K., and Tanaka, N. (1984). A multiple regression equation for prediction of posthepatectomy liver failure. *Ann. Surg.* 200:658. doi: 10.1097/00000658-198411000-00018

Yang, J., Reshef, L., Cassuto, H., Aleman, G., and Hanson, R. W. (2009). Aspects of the control of phosphoenolpyruvate carboxykinase gene transcription. *J. Biol. Chem.* 284, 27031–27035. doi: 10.1074/jbc.R109.040535

Yarbrough, J., Cunningham, M., Yamanaka, H., Thurman, R., and Badr, M. (1991). Carbohydrate and oxygen metabolism during hepatocellular proliferation: a study in perfused livers from mirex-treated rats. *Hepatology* 13, 1229–1234. doi: 10.1002/hep.1840130632

Zhang, Q., Raoof, M., Chen, Y., Sumi, Y., Sursal, T., Junger, W., et al. (2010). Circulating mitochondrial DAMPs cause inflammatory responses to injury. *Nature* 464, 104–107. doi: 10.1038/nature08780

Zhang, W., Wang, M., Xie, H. Y., Zhou, L., Meng, X. Q., Shi, J., et al. (2007). Role of reactive oxygen species in mediating hepatic ischemia-reperfusion injury and its therapeutic applications in liver transplantation. *Transplant. Proc.* 39, 1332–1337. doi: 10.1016/j.transproceed.2006.11.021

Zhou, Y., Xu, J., Liu, Y., Li, J., Chang, C., and Xu, C. (2014). Rat hepatocytes weighted gene co-expression network analysis identifies specific modules and hub genes related to liver regeneration after partial hepatectomy. *PLoS ONE* 9:e94868. doi: 10.1371/journal.pone.0094868

Zhou, Z.-P., Long, L.-L., Qiu, W.-J., Cheng, G., Huang, L.-J., Yang, T.-F., et al. (2017). Evaluating segmental liver function using T1 mapping on Gd-EOB-DTPA-enhanced MRI with a 3.0 Tesla. *BMC Med. Imaging* 17, 20. doi: 10.1186/s12880-017-0192-x

Zou, Y., Bao, Q., Kumar, S., Hu, M., Wang, G.-Y., and Dai, G. (2012). Four waves of hepatocyte proliferation linked with three waves of hepatic fat accumulation during partial hepatectomy-induced liver regeneration. *PLoS ONE* 7:e30675. doi: 10.1371/journal.pone.0030675

Permissions

All chapters in this book were first published by Frontiers; hereby published with permission under the Creative Commons Attribution License or equivalent. Every chapter published in this book has been scrutinized by our experts. Their significance has been extensively debated. The topics covered herein carry significant findings which will fuel the growth of the discipline. They may even be implemented as practical applications or may be referred to as a beginning point for another development.

The contributors of this book come from diverse backgrounds, making this book a truly international effort. This book will bring forth new frontiers with its revolutionizing research information and detailed analysis of the nascent developments around the world.

We would like to thank all the contributing authors for lending their expertise to make the book truly unique. They have played a crucial role in the development of this book. Without their invaluable contributions this book wouldn't have been possible. They have made vital efforts to compile up to date information on the varied aspects of this subject to make this book a valuable addition to the collection of many professionals and students.

This book was conceptualized with the vision of imparting up-to-date information and advanced data in this field. To ensure the same, a matchless editorial board was set up. Every individual on the board went through rigorous rounds of assessment to prove their worth. After which they invested a large part of their time researching and compiling the most relevant data for our readers.

The editorial board has been involved in producing this book since its inception. They have spent rigorous hours researching and exploring the diverse topics which have resulted in the successful publishing of this book. They have passed on their knowledge of decades through this book. To expedite this challenging task, the publisher supported the team at every step. A small team of assistant editors was also appointed to further simplify the editing procedure and attain best results for the readers.

Apart from the editorial board, the designing team has also invested a significant amount of their time in understanding the subject and creating the most relevant covers. They scrutinized every image to scout for the most suitable representation of the subject and create an appropriate cover for the book.

The publishing team has been an ardent support to the editorial, designing and production team. Their endless efforts to recruit the best for this project, has resulted in the accomplishment of this book. They are a veteran in the field of academics and their pool of knowledge is as vast as their experience in printing. Their expertise and guidance has proved useful at every step. Their uncompromising quality standards have made this book an exceptional effort. Their encouragement from time to time has been an inspiration for everyone.

The publisher and the editorial board hope that this book will prove to be a valuable piece of knowledge for researchers, students, practitioners and scholars across the globe.

List of Contributors

Svantje Sobotta, Xiaoyun Huang, Anja Jünger, Sebastian Bohl, Lorenza A. D'Alessandro, Stephanie Mueller-Bohl, Martin E. Boehm, Philippe Lucarelli, Sandra Bonefas, Wolf D. Lehmann, Marcel Schilling and Ursula Klingmüller
Division Systems Biology of Signal Transduction, German Cancer Research Center, Heidelberg, Germany

Andreas Raue
Discovery Division, Merrimack Pharmaceuticals, Cambridge, MA, United States

Joep Vanlier and Jens Timmer
Institute of Physics, Albert Ludwigs University of Freiburg, Freiburg, Germany
BIOSS Centre for Biological Signalling Studies, Albert Ludwigs University of Freiburg, Freiburg, Germany

Ute Albrecht, Maximilian J. Hahnel, Stephanie Wolf, Christian Ehlting and Johannes G. Bode
Clinic of Gastroenterology, Hepatology and Infectious Diseases, University Hospital, Heinrich Heine University of Düsseldorf, Düsseldorf, Germany

Nikola S. Mueller
Institute of Computational Biology, Helmholtz Zentrum München, Neuherberg, Germany

Georg Damm and Daniel Seehofer
Department of Hepatobiliary Surgery and Visceral Transplantation, Leipzig University, Leipzig, Germany

Stefan Rose-John
Institute of Biochemistry, University of Kiel, Kiel, Germany

Frank van der Hoeven
Transgenic Service, Center for Preclinical Research, German Cancer Research Center, Heidelberg, Germany

Norbert Gretz
Medical Research Center, Medical Faculty Mannheim, University of Heidelberg, Mannheim, Germany

Fabian J. Theis
Institute of Computational Biology, Helmholtz Zentrum München, Neuherberg, Germany
Department of Mathematics, Technical University of Munich, Garching, Germany

Hermann-Georg Holzhütter
Computational Biochemistry Group, Institute of Biochemistry, Charite—University Medicine Berlin, Berlin, Germany

Nikolaus Berndt
Computational Biochemistry Group, Institute of Biochemistry, Charite—University Medicine Berlin, Berlin, Germany
Institute for Computational and Imaging Science in Cardiovascular Medicine, Charite—University Medicine Berlin, Berlin, Germany

Michael Pimienta
University of California, San Diego School of Medicine, La Jolla, CA, United States
Cedars-Sinai Medical Center, Basic and Translational Pancreas Research, Los Angeles, CA, United States

Mouad Edderkaoui, Ruoxiang Wang and Stephen Pandol
Cedars-Sinai Medical Center, Basic and Translational Pancreas Research, Los Angeles, CA, United States

Changzheng Guo, Daming Sun and Shengyong Mao
Jiangsu Key Laboratory of Gastrointestinal Nutrition and Animal Health, Laboratory of Gastrointestinal Microbiology, National Experimental Teaching Demonstration Center of Animal Science, National Center for International Research on Animal Gut Nutrition, Joint International Research Laboratory of Animal Health and Food Safety, College of Animal Science and Technology, Nanjing Agricultural University, Nanjing, China

Xinfeng Wang
College of Animal Science and Technology, Shihezi University, Shihezi, China

Ni Zhou, Kuifeng Wang, Xiaoyu Zhao, Tingting Huang, Huazhong Chen, Fei Yan, Yongzhi Tang and Jiansheng Zhu
Department of Infectious Diseases, Affiliated Taizhou Hospital of Wenzhou Medical University, Taizhou, China

Shanhua Fang and Hu Zhou
E-Institute of Shanghai Municipal Education Committee, Shanghai University of Traditional Chinese Medicine, Shanghai, China
Department of Analytical Chemistry and CAS Key Laboratory of Receptor Research, Shanghai
Institute of Materia Medica, Chinese Academy of Sciences, Shanghai, China

Julia Rex and Oliver Sawodny
Institute for System Dynamics, University of Stuttgart, Stuttgart, Germany

Anna Lutz
Department of Pharmaceutical Biology and Biotechnology, Albert Ludwigs University Freiburg, Freiburg, Germany

Laura E. Faletti
Institute of Molecular Medicine and Cell Research, Albert Ludwigs University Freiburg, Freiburg, Germany

Ute Albrecht and Johannes G. Bode
Clinic of Gastroenterology, Hepatology and Infection Diseases, Heinrich-Heine-University, Duesseldorf, Germany

Maria Thomas
Dr. Margarete Fischer-Bosch Institute of Clinical Pharmacology, Stuttgart and University of Tuebingen, Tuebingen, Germany

Irmgard Merfort
Department of Pharmaceutical Biology and Biotechnology, Albert Ludwigs University Freiburg, Freiburg, Germany
Spemann Graduate School of Biology and Medicine, Albert Ludwigs University Freiburg, Freiburg, Germany

Christoph Borner
Department of Pharmaceutical Biology and Biotechnology, Albert Ludwigs University Freiburg, Freiburg, Germany
Spemann Graduate School of Biology and Medicine, Albert Ludwigs University Freiburg, Freiburg, Germany
BIOSS Centre for Biological Signaling Studies, Albert Ludwigs University Freiburg, Freiburg, Germany

Juan Tang, Ping Hu, Yansen Li and Chunmei Li
Jiangsu Province Key Laboratory of Gastrointestinal Nutrition and Animal Health, College of Animal Science and Technology, Nanjing Agricultural University, Nanjing, China

Tin-Tin Win-Shwe
Health Effect Assessment Section Center for Health and Environmental Risk Research, National Institute for Environmental Studies, Tsukuba, Japan

Nirupama Benis and Soumya K. Kar
Host Microbe Interactomics, Wageningen University & Research, Wageningen, Netherlands

Maria Suarez-Diez
Systems and Synthetic Biology, Department of Agrotechnology and Food Sciences, Wageningen University & Research, Wageningen, Netherlands

Vitor A. P. Martins dos Santos
Systems and Synthetic Biology, Department of Agrotechnology and Food Sciences, Wageningen University & Research, Wageningen, Netherlands
Lifeglimmer GmbH, Berlin, Germany

Dirkjan Schokker
Wageningen Livestock Research, Wageningen University & Research, Wageningen, Netherlands

Mari A. Smits
Wageningen Livestock Research, Wageningen University & Research, Wageningen, Netherlands
Wageningen Bioveterinary Research, Wageningen University & Research, Wageningen, Netherlands

Tanja Cvitanović Tomaš, Žiga Urlep and Damjana Rozman
Faculty of Medicine, Centre for Functional Genomics and Bio-Chips, Institute of Biochemistry, University of Ljubljana, Ljubljana, Slovenia

Miha Moškon and Miha Mraz
Faculty of Computer and Information Science, University of Ljubljana, Ljubljana, Slovenia

Kalyan C. Vinnakota and Venkat R. Pannala
Henry M. Jackson Foundation for the Advancement of Military Medicine, Inc., Bethesda, MD, United States
Department of Defense Biotechnology High Performance Computing Software Applications Institute, Telemedicine and Advanced Technology Research Center, United States Army Medical Research and Materiel Command, Fort Detrick, MD, United States

Jaques Reifman and Anders Wallqvist
Department of Defense Biotechnology High Performance Computing Software Applications Institute, Telemedicine and Advanced Technology Research Center, United States Army Medical Research and Materiel Command, Fort Detrick, MD, United States

Martha L. Wall, Mohsin Rahim and Irina Trenary
Department of Chemical and Biomolecular Engineering, Vanderbilt University School of Engineering, Nashville, TN, United States

Shanea K. Estes, Tracy P. O'Brien, Richard L. Printz and Masakazu Shiota
Department of Molecular Physiology and Biophysics, Vanderbilt University School of Medicine, Nashville, TN, United States

Lei Mai
Department of Gastroenterology, Fifth Affiliated Hospital, Sun Yat-sen University, Zhuhai, China

Jamey D. Young
Department of Chemical and Biomolecular Engineering, Vanderbilt University School of Engineering, Nashville, TN, United States
Department of Molecular Physiology and Biophysics, Vanderbilt University School of Medicine, Nashville, TN, United States

Dorines Rosario, Rui Benfeitas, Gholamreza Bidkhori, Cheng Zhang and Mathias Uhlen
Science for Life Laboratory, Royal Institute of Technology, Stockholm, Sweden

Saeed Shoaie
Centre for Host-Microbiome Interactions, Dental Institute, King's College London, London, United Kingdom
Centre for Translational Microbiome Research, Department of Microbiology, Tumor and Cell Biology, Karolinska Institute, Stockholm, Sweden

Adil Mardinoglu
Science for Life Laboratory, Royal Institute of Technology, Stockholm, Sweden
Department of Biology and Biological Engineering, Chalmers University of Technology, Gothenburg, Sweden

Jiangnan Ren
Digestive Endoscopy Center, Fifth Affiliated Hospital, Sun Yat-sen University, Zhuhai, China

Wanting Shi, Zhaoshi Liu and Renxu Lai
Department of Gastroenterology, Fifth Affiliated Hospital, Sun Yat-sen University, Zhuhai, China
Digestive Endoscopy Center, Fifth Affiliated Hospital, Sun Yat-sen University, Zhuhai, China

Rongjun Zou
Department of Cardiovascular Surgery, Sun Yat-sen Memorial Hospital, Sun Yat-sen University, Guangzhou, China

Minglei Yang
Department of Genetics, Zhongshan School of Medicine, Sun Yat-sen University, Guangzhou, China

Jialing Wen
Guangdong Institute of Gastroenterology, Guangdong, China
Guangdong Provincial Key Laboratory of Colorectal and Pelvic Floor Diseases, The Sixth Affiliated Hospital, Sun Yat-sen University, Guangzhou, China

Zurah Bibi, Jamil Ahmad, Amnah Siddiqa, Rehan Z. Paracha and Tariq Saeed
Research Centre for Modeling and Simulation, National University of Sciences and Technology, Islamabad, Pakistan

Amjad Ali and Hussnain Ahmed Janjua
Atta-Ur-Rahman School of Applied Biosciences, National University of Sciences and Technology, Islamabad, Pakistan

Shakir Ullah
School of Business, Stratford University, Falls Church, VA, United States

Emna Ben Abdallah and Olivier Roux
IRCCyN UMR Centre National de la Recherche Scientifique 6597, BP 92101, Nantes, France

Sara Zafarnia, Anna Mrugalla, Anne Rix, Dennis Doleschel, Felix Gremse, Fabian Kiessling and Wiltrud Lederle
Institute for Experimental Molecular Imaging, Medical Faculty, RWTH Aachen University, Aachen, Germany

Stephanie D. Wolf, Ute Albrecht and Johannes G. Bode
Department of Gastroenterology, Hepatology and Infectious Diseases, Medical Faculty, Heinrich-Heine-University Düsseldorf, Düsseldorf, Germany

Johannes F. Buyel
Fraunhofer Institute for Molecular Biology and Applied Ecology IME, Aachen, Germany
Institute for Molecular Biotechnology, RWTH Aachen University, Aachen, Germany

Christiane Rennert, Carlo Thiel, Rolf Gebhardt and Madlen Matz-Soja
Rudolf-Schönheimer-Institute of Biochemistry, Faculty of Medicine, Leipzig University, Leipzig, Germany

Sebastian Vlaic
Leibniz Institute for Natural Product Research and Infection Biology, Hans-Knöll-Institute, Jena, Germany

Eugenia Marbach-Breitrück
Rudolf-Schönheimer-Institute of Biochemistry, Faculty of Medicine, Leipzig University, Leipzig, Germany
Institute of Biochemistry, Charité – Universitätsmedizin Berlin, Berlin, Germany
Berlin Institute of Health, Freie Universität Berlin, Humboldt-Universität zu Berlin, Berlin, Germany

Susanne Sales and Andrej Shevchenko
Max Planck Institute of Molecular Cell Biology and Genetics, Dresden, Germany

Bruno Christ
Molecular Hepatology Lab, Clinics of Visceral, Transplantation, Thoracic and Vascular Surgery, University Hospital Leipzig, University of Leipzig, Leipzig, Germany

Uta Dahmen
Experimental Transplantation Surgery, Department of General, Visceral and Vascular Surgery, University Hospital Jena, Jena, Germany

Karl-Heinz Herrmann and Jürgen R. Reichenbach
Medical Physics Group, Institute for Diagnostic and Interventional Radiology, University Hospital Jena, Friedrich Schiller University Jena, Jena, Germany

Matthias König
Department of Biology, Institute for Theoretical Biology, Humboldt University of Berlin, Berlin, Germany

Tim Ricken and Navina Waschinsky
Mechanics, Structural Analysis, and Dynamics, TU Dortmund University, Dortmund, Germany

Jana Schleicher
Experimental Transplantation Surgery, Department of General, Visceral and Vascular Surgery, University Hospital Jena, Jena, Germany
Department of Bioinformatics, Friedrich Schiller University Jena, Jena, Germany

Lars Ole Schwen
Fraunhofer MEVIS, Bremen, Germany

Sebastian Vlaic
Leibniz Institute for Natural Product Research and Infection Biology, Hans Knöll Institute, Jena, Germany

Michaela Bissinger, Peter Schirmacher and Kai Breuhahn
Molecular Hepatopathology, Institute of Pathology, University Hospital Heidelberg, Heidelberg, Germany

Thomas Longerich
Institute of Pathology, RWTH Aachen University Hospital, Aachen, Germany

Index

www.ingramcontent.com/pod-product-compliance
Lightning Source LLC
LaVergne TN
LVHW082129200926
848484LV00008B/2031